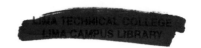

D1359943

MANAGEMENT OF
GENETIC SYNDROMES

MANAGEMENT OF GENETIC SYNDROMES

Edited by

SUZANNE B. CASSIDY
Professor of Genetics and Pediatrics
Case Western Reserve University
University Hospitals of Cleveland

JUDITH E. ALLANSON
Professor of Pediatrics
University of Ottawa
Children's Hospital of Eastern Ontario

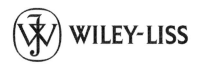

A JOHN WILEY & SONS, INC., PUBLICATION

New York • Chichester • Weinheim • Brisbane • Singapore • Toronto

Published simultaneously in Canada.

For ordering and customer service call 1-800-CALL-WILEY.

Library of Congress Cataloging-in-Publication Data:

Management of genetic syndromes / edited by Suzanne B. Cassidy, Judith E. Allanson.
      p. cm.
   Includes bibliographical references and index.
   ISBN 0-471-31286-X (cloth : alk. paper)
   1. Genetic disorders. I. Cassidy, Suzanne B. II. Allanson, Judith E.
   [DNLM: 1. Hereditary Diseases–diagnosis 2. Hereditary Diseases–therapy 3.
   Abnormalities, Multiple–diagnosis 4. Abnormalities, Multiple–therapy QZ50 M2655 2000]
   RB155.5.M36 2000
   616′.042–dc21   00-038213

Printed in the United States of America.

10 9 8 7 6 5 4 3

We dedicate this book to our families:

Helene and Maurice Bletterman
Joshua Cassidy
Jack and Barbara Robinson

For all they taught us, for their tolerance, and for all their love and encouragement.

CONTENTS

FOREWORD

This is a book whose time has come. Genetic disorders and syndromes are usually thought of as being rare, and yet for affected individuals, their families, and their primary and specialty care physicians, it is essential to have reliable information about the natural history and management of the specific disorders.

The thirty conditions described in this book may seem rare (with incidences between 1 in 600 and 1 in 60,000). However, when you put together all the individual cases of a particular condition in North America, in Europe, and in the world, a very large number of affected individuals will benefit from the information in this book. In the past it has been difficult to bring together information of this type about specific disorders, and that is why this book fills a very important niche. It becomes a model for how to organize information that is needed for the families and primary care providers to manage the many, many other genetic disorders, congenital anomalies, and syndromes that are known to occur. The book is written in understandable language appropriate for families and for primary care and specialty physicians. It is a major contribution.

Over the last two decades, remarkable progress has been made with regard to developing diagnostic tests and unraveling the human genome. Within the next few years all of the human genes will have been defined. The next major goal in genetics will be to understand how genes interact and function, both in the course of development and over a lifetime. In addition to the remarkable progress in basic and clinical genetics, there has been increasing communication and access to information. Through the Internet, the public has access to research reports and data that were usually not readily available in the past. However, it is essential to put that information into a meaningful form and context. That is exactly what this book does. The communication explosion has allowed the networking of researchers and families. The development of parent/lay support groups has led to a cooperation between researchers and families that has helped to define the natural history and the variation that can be seen in a specific disorder.

What every family and physician wants is to provide the best care possible for the affected individual. Nobody wants to miss the opportunity for that individual to reach his or her full potential, to benefit from a useful therapy, or to avoid a complication. Parents need an understanding of what will happen over time so that they can plan. They don't want to waste money and effort going from expert to expert or doing test after test. They need a realistic approach to what they should expect both in childhood and adulthood. They also usually want to know whether there is some risk of recurrence of the condition in their other children, in other family members, and in the affected individual's offspring. They want to know whether prenatal diagnosis is available, and they want to know the spectrum of variation that can occur. The beauty of this new book is that it provides that kind of information for each specific disorder in a logical and understandable form. Most families and physicians will focus in on the chapter relevant to a specific individual. However, they can't help but glance at other chapters and see the remarkable spectrum of complications that are *not* present in the disorder of interest to them. They are likely to benefit from this broader perspective.

Most pediatricians will have heard of all thirty disorders; however, some primary care and specialty physicians may not have heard of a specific disorder until they have the affected individual in their practice. The book should help to alert health care professionals to consider these conditions and should lead to appropriate testing to make a correct diagnosis, reducing the time it takes to make a specific diagnosis. Two-thirds of the conditions in this book have a specific diagnostic test, but the other one-third require "pattern recognition" and an alert, trained health care professional to consider the diagnosis.

It can be expected that additional advances will be made over the next few decades leading to better understanding and better management. So this book is already dated! There is still a lot to be learned! In fact, every family and every affected individual will contribute to that increased knowledge by giving feedback to the authors. Disorder specific-parent/lay support groups will continue to play an important role in improving our understanding. The authors of each chapter have worked together with the support groups and are very aware that it is the process of working together with these groups and the members' willingness to provide information that has led to present-day understanding. We are all very grateful to each of the parents and affected individuals who have taken part in studies that have advanced our knowledge.

To write a book about management, it is necessary to know the natural history of the disorder. The authors of each of these chapters have a wealth of experience and knowledge that has been collected over the last couple of decades. Understanding the natural history not only tells us what to expect at various ages but also how to recognize various complications. It is important to understand the natural history of the condition to determine whether various therapies actually improve the outcome. It is important to understand the natural history to recognize subgroups representing the variability and heterogeneity within the disorder. It is important to understand the natural history to learn the mechanisms that lead to the disorder, e.g., what sort of gene is likely to be involved? Where is the mutation in the gene? How does that mutation relate to severity of complications? How big is the deletion? Does that size relate to severity of complications? How does this gene act against the background of other genes or pathways? Is it possible to recognize a cellular mechanism leading to this disorder? Are there parent-of-origin effects on the expression of the gene or the mutation rate? Are there hot spots that have markedly increased mutation rates? Does the place on the chromosome where the gene lies put it at increased risk for mutation? These are only a few of the questions we hope to answer over the next few decades.

No one is more motivated than the family or the affected individual to learn about these disorders. It is important for them to be as knowledgeable as possible. The families of an affected person usually know more about the condition than most of the physicians they visit. It is important for families to continue to ask questions and to gain as much knowledge as possible to ensure the best outcome for the affected individual. It is important for families and affected individuals to keep their own records about the affected individual, such as a notebook of their visits to health care facilities, copies of the reports, and the results of the tests that have been done. It is also important to keep a photographic record of changes over time.

Once a family or an affected individual becomes involved in collecting information about the disorder, they often develop quite creative ideas that challenge the standard way of thinking about the disorder. Part of the advantage of participating in a support group is that those ideas then can be shared with the medical advisors and researchers and may lead to new knowledge.

Much of our understanding of these disorders is based on the manifestations in childhood, on feeding, on growth and development, and on social skills. However, information on adults is also beginning to accumulate and has been included in this book. In some conditions there is a stable situation, in others there is improvement with aging, and in still others deterioration can be expected. For many of the conditions described in this book, behavioral patterns have been recognized.

How should a family and their primary care physician use the experts? It would be impossible for the authors of these chapters to see every individual with the condition, but it is usually helpful for a family and the affected individual to see a clinical geneticist, to visit a developmental center, or to use the multidisciplinary team that is available in their area. Over the years, specialty clinics to deal with specific conditions have been developed. At some time it is probably appropriate to visit such a clinic at least once to review the affected individual's progress and to consider any special complications or responses. On the other hand, it is very important to have a knowledgeable primary care physician who cares for day-to-day medical needs and is aware of the unique complications of the condition.

The parent/lay support groups form an international network keeping up with new information on the specific disorders, and new information is sure to come. Some new information will come through organized studies of natural history; other data will come through clinical trials of new therapies; and further information will come from basic work on cellular mechanisms and biochemical pathways. For many of these disorders animal models will be developed, such as mice with the specific disorder, so that various therapies can be considered before trials in human beings. We live in a very exciting age and can anticipate major advances over the next few decades for each of the disorders described in this book. The international network of families, affected individuals, and researchers should and will communicate about new ideas, innovative approaches, and better understanding about these conditions.

We have begun to enter an era of evidence-based medicine. Only by having natural history information is it possible to understand the benefits of new interventions and therapies. We will hope that this book is outdated very rapidly because of such new developments, but in the meanwhile this book on management of common genetic syndromes is extremely welcome to families and health care providers alike.

JUDITH G. HALL

Professor and Head, Department of Pediatrics
University of British Columbia and
* British Columbia Children's Hospital*
Professor, Medical Genetics
James and Annabelle McCreary Professor
University of British Columbia

PREFACE

This book is designed to assist primary care physicians, medical specialists, other care providers, and families in assuring optimal care for individuals who have the multiple problems represented by genetic syndromes. It represents the combined experience and knowledge of many experts in medical genetics and related fields, each of whom has spent years participating in the diagnosis and clinical management of a specific genetic syndrome. Most of the chapter authors have conducted major clinical research on "their" disorder.

The syndromes selected for inclusion in this book are those that are sufficiently common as to be regularly encountered in clinics specializing in genetics, development, neurology, or craniofacial disorders. Many of these disorders will not have been seen in the practice of most primary care physicians or non-genetics specialists. When they are encountered, the physician typically has little knowledge of how to confirm the diagnosis, the associated problems and clinical manifestations, and what to do to optimally care for the affected individual. This lack of knowledge is due only partly to infrequent exposure to the disorder. For many

of these conditions, very little has been published concerning management, and a search for such knowledge is extremely time consuming, often provides incomplete information, and is frequently futile. This book was designed to provide that knowledge, based on the cumulative experience of an expert or experts on each condition. As a result, a significant proportion of the information found in this source will be personal experience or observation. In most cases, there is no established "standard of care" based on controlled trials or outcome studies. Other experts may have chosen different approaches in some cases. Nonetheless, the editors have sought to provide the reader with information that is as reliable as possible. Where available, reference to published sources has been included; where unavailable, reference to the author(s) "personal experience" or "personal observation" has been noted, to reflect non-peer-reviewed information.

Deciding upon which disorders to include is no mean task, and there are some disorders for which there is little accumulated experience in management. There are numerous disorders that could have been included with this edition, but were not. In particular, no inborn errors of metabolism were included because other resources are available for such disorders. In addition to 30 genetic (or probably genetic) conditions, one teratogenic disorder, fetal alcohol syndrome, was also included because of its frequency and because genetic factors influence susceptibility.

The editors hope that this proves to be a useful text to primary care physicians, medical geneticists, and other medical specialists, educators, and other providers of care for the individuals and families affected with these common genetic syndromes. Like those with more frequent medical conditions, they deserve the best possible medical, educational, and psychological care.

We are extremely grateful to Florence Stewart for her many long hours of manuscript preparation. We want to thank Stuart Schwartz, Ph.D. for reviewing the cytogenetic and molecular diagnostic nomenclature. We are appreciative to two editors from Wiley-Liss, Collette Bean for giving us the opportunity to compile this book and Luna Han for her assistance in editing. Most importantly, we thank the contributors and the many patients for their willingness to have their photographs published in this book and their participation in the clinical research that provided the information for its content.

SUZANNE B. CASSIDY
JUDITH E. ALLANSON

CONTRIBUTORS

DEBORAH M. ALCORN, M.D., Assistant Professor of Ophthalmology and Pediatrics, Howard Hughes Medical Institute, Departments of Ophthalmology and Genetics, Stanford University School of Medicine, Stanford, California

JUDITH E. ALLANSON, MB ChB, FRCP, DABMG, FCCMG, Professor of Pediatrics, University of Ottawa; Clinical Geneticist, Children's Hospital of Eastern Ontario, Ottawa, ON, Canada

SUSAN J. ASTLEY, Ph.D., Associate Professor of Epidemiology and Pediatrics, University of Washington, School of Public Health and Community Medicine, Research Director, Fetal Alcohol Syndrome Diagnostic and Prevention Network, Division of Genetics and Development, Children's Hospital and Regional Medical Center, Seattle, Washington

BRUCE G. BENDER, Ph.D., Professor of Psychiatry, University of Colorado School of Medicine; Senior Faculty, National Jewish Medical and Research Center, Denver, Colorado

JOHN C. CAREY, M.D., M.P.H., Professor of Pediatrics and Obstetrics & Gynecology, University of Utah Health Science Center, Salt Lake City, Utah

SUZANNE B. CASSIDY, M.D., M.S., Professor of Pediatrics, University of California, Irvine Medical Center, Orange, California

EDITH J. CHERNOFF, M.D., FAAP, Clinical Associate of the Heritable Disorders Branch of the NICHD, National Institutes of Health, Bethesda, Maryland

STERLING K. CLARREN, M.D., ROBERT A. ALDRICH, Professor of Pediatrics, University of Washington School of Medicine, Medical Director, Fetal Alcohol Syndrome Diagnostic and Prevention Network, Seattle, Washington

TREVOR R. P. COLE, MB ChB, FRCP, Consultant Clinical Geneticist and Honorary Senior Lecturer, Department of Clinical Genetics, Birmingham Women's Hospital Healthcare NHS Trust, Birmingham, UK

CHRISTOPHER CUNNIFF, M.D., Associate Professor of Pediatrics and Obstetrics and Gynecology, Chief, Section of Medical and Molecular Genetics, University of Arizona College of Medicine, Tucson, Arizona

DIAN DONNAI, M.B.B.S, FRCP, Consultant Clinical Geneticist and Professor of Medical Genetics, University of Manchester, Department of Medical Genetics, St Mary's Hospital, Manchester, UK

UTA FRANCKE, M.D., Professor of Genetics and Pediatrics, Howard Hughes Medical Institute, Departments of Ophthalmology and Genetics, Stanford University School of Medicine, Stanford, California

CLAIR A. FRANCOMANO, M.D., Medical Genetics Branch, National Human Genome Research Institute, National Institutes of Health, Bethesda, Maryland

ROBERT J. GORLIN, D.D.S., M.S., Regents' Professor Emeritus, Oral Pathology & Genetics, Pediatrics, Laboratory Medicine & Pathology, Otolaryngology, and Dermatology, University of Minnesota, Minneapolis, Minnesota

ANDREA GROPMAN, M.D., Medical Genetics Branch, National Human Genome Research Institute, National Institutes of Health, Bethesda, MD; and Department of Neurology, Children's National Medical Center, Washington, DC

RANDI J. HAGERMAN, M.D., Professor of Pediatrics, University of Colorado Health Sciences Center and The Children's Hospital, Denver, Colorado

BRYAN D. HALL, M.D., Professor of Pediatrics, University of Kentucky, Lexington, Kentucky

LEAH B. HOECHSTETTER, M.S., Genetic Counselor Coordinator, Connective Tissue Clinics, Division of Human Genetics, Children's Hospital Medical Center, Cincinnati, OH

ALASDAIR G. W. HUNTER, M.D., CM, MSc, FCCMG, FRCP, Professor of Pediatrics, University of Ottawa, Head of Genetics Patient Service Unit, Children's Hospital of Eastern Ontario, Ottawa, Canada

MAGGIE IRELAND, M.B.B.S, MSc, MRC, MRCP, Clinician Scientist Fellow, Human Genetics Unit, School of Biochemistry and Genetics, University of Newcastle upon Tyne and Honorary Senior Registrar in Clinical Genetics, Northern Region Genetics Service, Human Genetics Unit, Newcastle upon Tyne, UK

RUTH M. LIBERFARB, M.D., Ph.D., Medical Genetics Branch, National Human Genome Research Institute, National Institutes of Health, Bethesda, MD

MARY G. LINDEN, M.S., Genetic Counselor, National Jewish Medical and Research Center, Denver, Colorado

JOAN C. MARINI, M.D., Ph.D., Chief of the Heritable Disorders Branch, National Institute of Child Health and Development, National Institutes of Health, Bethesda, Maryland

COLLEEN A. MORRIS, M.D., M.S., FACMG, FAAP, Professor of Pediatrics and Pathology and Laboratory Medicine, Chief, Genetics Division, University of Nevada School of Medicine, Las Vegas, Nevada

ROBERT F. MUELLER, M.B.B.S, BSc, FRCP, Professor in Clinical Genetics, Research School of Medicine, University of Leeds, Consultant Clinical Geneticist, St James's Hospital, Leeds, UK

CHRISTINE A. OLEY, M.B.B.S, FRACP, FRCPH., Clinical Geneticist, Queensland Clinical Genetics Service, Senior Lecturer in the Department of Child Health, University of Queensland, Brisbane, Australia

RICHARD M. PAULI, M.D., Ph.D., Professor of Pediatrics and Medical Genetics, Director, Clinical Genetics Center, University of Wisconsin-Madison, Wisconsin

ARTHUR ROBINSON, M.D., Distinguished Professor and Professor Emeritus, Department of Biochemistry and Molecular Genetics, and Department of Pediatrics, University of Colorado School of Medicine, Senior Faculty, National Jewish Medical and Research Center, Denver, Colorado

HOWARD M. SAAL, M.D., Associate Professor of Clinical Pediatrics Head, Clinical Genetics, Division of Human Genetics, Children's Hospital Medical Center, Cinncinati, Ohio

IRIS SCHRIJVER, M.D., Resident Department of Pathology, Stanford University School of Medicine, Stanford, California

ROBERT J. SHPRINTZEN Ph.D., Professor of Otolaryngology, Director, Communication Disorder Unit, Director, Center for the Diagnosis, Treatment, and Study of Velo-Cardio-Facial Syndrome, Director, Center for Genetic Communicative Disorders, State University of New York Health Science Center at Syracuse, New York

CHERYL SHUMAN, M.S., CGC, Assistant Professor, Department of Medical Genetics and Microbiology, Director, Genetic Counselling, Division of Clinical and Metabolic Genetics, The Hospital for Sick Children, University of Toronto, Ontario, Canada

ANN C. M. SMITH, M.D., D.Sc, CGC, Department of Obstetrics and Gynecology, Georgetown University Medical School, Washington, DC; Medical Genetics Branch, National Human Genome Research Institute, National Institutes of Health, Bethesda, Maryland

VIRGINIA P. SYBERT, M.D., Professor of Medicine, Division of Dermatology, University of Washington School of Medicine, Seattle, Washington

DAVID VISKOCHIL, M.D., Ph.D., Associate Professor of Pediatrics, University of Utah, Salt Lake City, Utah

ROSANNA WEKSBERG, M.D., Ph.D., FRCPC, FCCMG, FACMG, Associate Professor of Paediatrics, Head, Division of Clinical and Metabolic Genetics, The Hospital for Sick Children, University of Toronto, Canada

RICHARD J. WENSTRUP, M.D., Associate Professor of Pediatrics, Division of Human Genetics, Cincinnati Children's Hospital Research Foundation, Cincinnati, Ohio

DOUGLAS J. WILKIN, Ph.D., Medical Genetics Branch, National Human Genome Research Institute, National Institutes of Health, Bethesda, Maryland

CHARLES A. WILLIAMS, M.D., Professor of Pediatrics, Chief, Division of Genetics, Department of Pediatrics, University of Florida, Gainesville

CHAPTER 1

INTRODUCTION

SUZANNE B. CASSIDY AND JUDITH E. ALLANSON

THE ORGANIZATION OF THIS BOOK

Each chapter of this book is dedicated to the diagnosis and management of a specific syndrome that is encountered with regularity in specialty programs and occasionally in primary care practice. The authors are acknowledged "experts" who have considerable personal experience in the management of the disorder. Each chapter thus contains unpublished information based on that experience and on the author's personal approach to management in addition to a review of published information. Each chapter format is similar, providing general information on incidence and inheritance, pathogenesis and etiology, diagnostic criteria and testing, and differential diagnosis. The myriad manifestations of each syndrome are presented system by system, with emphasis on the features, evaluation, management, and prognosis. The first two "systems" in each chapter are "Growth and Feeding" and "Development and Behavior." After these, the systems relevant to the specific disorder are discussed, usually in order of importance for that disorder. Each chapter concludes with a listing of family support organizations and some resources available to families and professionals in print and electronic formats. Photographs of physical findings important for diagnosis or management are provided.

Selected references focusing on management issues and citations of good review articles have been included.

This introductory chapter is designed to inform the reader about genetics-related terms used in this book, inheritance patterns, general methods for genetic testing, measurement methods, and the role of the medical geneticist and genetic counselor in the care of genetic disorders. It also provides some important references to additional resources of information about genetic disorders, differential diagnoses, genetic testing, and support organizations.

CATEGORIZATION OF DISORDERS

The descriptive language for patterns of anomalies is somewhat unique to this field and deserves a brief review. The term **sequence** is used to designate a series of anomalies resulting from a cascade of events initiated by a single malformation, deformation, or disruption (Spranger et al., 1982). A well-known example is the Robin sequence, in which thef initiating event is micrognathia. The small mandible then precipitates glossoptosis (posterior and upward displacement of the tongue in the pharynx) with resultant incomplete fusion of the

Management of Genetic Syndromes, Edited by Suzanne B. Cassidy and Judith E. Allanson
ISBN 0-471-31286-X   Copyright © 2001 by Wiley-Liss, Inc.

palatal shelves. The initiating event may be a malformation of the mandible or a deformation caused by in utero constraint and thus inhibiting normal growth of the mandible. The individual components of a sequence may well involve quite disparate parts of the body. For example, lower limb joint contractures and bilateral equinovarus deformity may be found in a child with a meningomyelocele.

An **association** is a nonrandom occurrence in two or more individuals of multiple anomalies not known to represent a sequence or syndrome (Spranger et al., 1982). These anomalies are found together more often than expected by chance alone, demonstrating a statistical relationship but not necessarily a known causal one. For example, the CHARGE association represents a simultaneous occurrence of two or more malformations that include congenital coloboma of the iris, choroid, or optic nerve, heart defects, atresia of choanae, mental and somatic retardation, male genital hypoplasia, and ear anomalies or deafness. An association has limited prognostic significance, and the degree of variability may pose diagnostic problems for the clinician. Most affected children will not have all the anomalies described, which makes establishment of minimal diagnostic criteria difficult. Recognition of an association is useful in that it can guide the clinician, after discovery of two or more component malformations in a newborn, toward a directed search for the additional anomalies. Associations are generally sporadic within a family and have a low empirical recurrence risk. It is most important to remember that associations are diagnoses of exclusion. Any child with multiple anomalies affecting several systems, with or without growth and/or intellectual retardation, should first be assessed to rule out a specific syndrome diagnosis and, lacking such a diagnosis, should have chromosome analysis.

The term **syndrome** is used to describe a broad error of morphogenesis in which the simultaneous presence of more than one malformation is known or assumed to be the result of a single etiology. Its use implies that the group of malformations and/or physical differences has been seen repeatedly in a fairly consistent and unique pattern. The initial definition of any syndrome occurs after the publication of several similar case reports. It becomes refined over time as newly described individuals suggest the inclusion of additional anomalies and the exclusion of others. Thus a syndrome comes to be defined by the coexistence of a small but variable number of "hallmark" anomalies, whereas several other features may be observed at lower frequencies. Even after a particular syndrome is well established, the inherent variability or rarity can make diagnosis difficult. In a specific individual, one or more of the hallmark features of a disorder may be absent and yet the person is affected. It is important to stress that not all syndromes are associated with mental retardation. Generally, no one feature or anomaly is pathognomonic of a syndrome, and even experienced dysmorphologists may disagree about diagnosis. Often, the individual clinician will have had little direct experience of the syndrome. In this environment, the addition of objective methods of evaluation may be useful. Available techniques include direct measurement (anthropometry), standard photographs (photogrammetry), and radiologic assessment (cephalometry). Each method has advantages and disadvantages, and each has its proponents (for details, see Allanson, 1997).

MEASUREMENTS

Selected measurements, with comparison to normal standards, may be helpful in confirming the subjective impression of an abnormality. Common craniofacial dimensions, which provide a great deal of detail about facial shape and size, include head circumference, inner and outer canthal distances, ear length, position, and rotation.

Evaluation of stature should include height (length), upper and lower body segment, arm span, hand length, palm length, and foot length. Normal standards for these and a wide variety of other standardized measurements can be found in the *Handbook of Normal Physical Measurements* (Hall et al., 1989), *Growth References from Conception to Adulthood*, (Saul et al., 1988), and *Smith's Recognizable Patterns of Human Malformation* (Jones, 1997); however, ethnic background, for which norms may vary, should be taken into consideration. Increasingly, standard curves are being developed for particular syndromes. Many syndrome specific standards have been compiled (Saul et al., 1988).

The best way to document dysmorphic features is to photograph them. The prudent clinician will often adopt an attitude of "watchful waiting" if the diagnosis is not apparent at the first assessment (Aase, 1990). As children's facial and body features evolve with time, they may "grow into" a syndrome, and photographs provide serial documentation of these changes. There is great value to reassessment of the dysmorphic individual whose diagnosis is unclear, because there is significant diagnostic yield (Hall et al., 1998). The "art" of dysmorphology is eloquently discussed by Aase (1990). Photographs also facilitate consultations with colleagues and consultants by providing objective evidence of the patient's physical findings. They can be compared with examples of other syndromes in photographic databases such as POSSUM and the London Dysmorphology Database (see below).

COMMON GENETIC TERMINOLOGY

With the recent rapid advances in human genetics has come a proliferation of terms with which many practitioners are unfamiliar. Therefore, a summary of the common terms relating to genes and chromosomes and the major inheritance patterns is in order.

Genes are the individual pieces of coding information that we inherit from our parents,

the blueprint, as it were, for an organism. It is estimated that 80,000 to 100,000 genes are required to develop and "operate" a human being. Individual genes occur in pairs, one inherited from each parent. The balance of the expression of these genes is extremely delicate, with significant abnormality resulting when this balance is disturbed for some genes. Variant forms of the same gene are known as **alleles**, and variation can have no apparent phenotypic effect or major consequences, depending on the specific gene and many other factors. When a variant has minimal phenotypic effect, it is often called a **polymorphism**.

Some syndromes are caused by a permanent structural or sequence change (or **mutation**) in a single gene. Many gene mutations cause their adverse effects through deficient gene expression (and often subsequent protein deficiency), which is called **haploinsufficiency**. This is often the case when a mutation in a gene results in failure to produce the gene product, which can be a so-called **null mutation** or a **protein truncation mutation**. However, other mutations cause their adverse effects by interfering with a process or causing a new adverse effect, and such mutations are called **dominant negative mutations**. The latter is often the result when a structurally abnormal protein is formed. Mutation results in alteration of the sequence and/or length of the bases composing the gene code. Such alterations may result in the substitution of one amino acid for another (a **missense mutation**), in the production of a sequence that does not correspond to the code for an amino acid (a **nonsense mutation**), or in a code that tells the translation machinery to stop prematurely. An unusual form of mutation that is present in a number of neurogenetic disorders, such as fragile X syndrome, myotonic dystrophy, Huntington disease, and the spinocerebellar ataxias, among others, is the so-called **triplet repeat expansion**. Some genes contain within them a string of three bases repeated a number of times. For example,

CGG is repeated up to 50 times in the normal fragile X gene (CGGCGGCGG...). Under certain circumstances, this number becomes amplified, resulting in an increase in the number of such repeated triplets of bases. Thus, in individuals who are affected with fragile X syndrome, there may be hundreds of such repeated triplets. This triplet repeat expansion interferes with the normal function of the gene, causing abnormality (in this case, mental retardation). In fragile X syndrome, the gene actually becomes inactivated if the expansion exceeds a certain number of repeats. Please see Chapter 10 for a more detailed explanation of this type of mutation.

The nomenclature for genes and gene products (proteins) can be quite confusing, despite the best efforts toward a logical approach. The names of genes are often put in italics, and these may represent an abbreviation of the name of the disorder, the name of the protein, or a function of the protein or the gene. For example, the gene causing neurofibromatosis type 1 is called *NF1*, and the protein is named neurofibromin, whereas the gene for Angelman syndrome, *UBE3A*, is named for its protein product, which is one of a family of ubiquitin-protein ligases (enzymes that are part of the protein degradation process). The gene responsible for fragile X syndrome (an X-linked cause of mental retardation) is called *FMR1* (fragile X-linked mental retardation 1), and the protein is called FMRP (fragile X-linked mental retardation protein). Information on the genes is included in the chapters for those who are interested, but aside from genetic testing purposes, it is not critical to know the nomenclature to understand and treat the disorder.

The genes are "packaged" into 46 **chromosomes**, of which 23 chromosomes are transmitted to the offspring in the egg from the mother and 23 in the sperm from the father. One pair of chromosomes, the **sex chromosomes**, differs between males and females. Females have two copies of the X chromosome, whereas males have one copy, the second sex chromosome being the Y chromosome with a largely different set of genes. The remaining 22 pairs, the **autosomes**, do not differ between males and females. The autosomes are numbered in a standard way from largest to smallest. The location of a specific gene on a chromosome is called the **locus** (the plural is **loci**). Some of the syndromes described in this book are caused by the presence of an entire extra chromosome (for example, Down syndrome, Klinefelter syndrome) or duplication of a segment of a chromosome (for example, some cases of Beckwith-Wiedemann syndrome). Others occur because of loss of all (for example, Turner syndrome) or part (for example, some cases of Prader-Willi syndrome) of a chromosome.

PATTERNS OF INHERITANCE

An alteration in a gene can be dominant or recessive. A **dominant** gene mutation only needs to be present in one member of the gene pair to have a clinically evident impact. Any individual with an autosomal dominant gene mutation will have a 1 in 2 chance to pass it on to his or her child, male or female, with each pregnancy. An example is achondroplasia. In achondroplasia, the affected child frequently has two average-stature parents, indicating that the mutation occurred in the egg or sperm that was involved in the conception. This is referred to as a **new mutation** or a **de novo mutation**. Rarely, an apparently normal couple will have more than one child with an apparently new mutation in an autosomal dominant gene. This suggests that the mutation is present in some of the cells of the germ line (gonads) but not in most other cells of the body of one parent. This is known as **germ line (or gonadal) mosaicism**. When a parent has a gonadal cell line with a dominant mutation, the recurrence risk is significantly greater than the risk for a second child with a new mutation but less than the 50% risk expected if the parent had the mutation in all cells of the body and manifested the condition. Several different dominant disorders have been documented to recur in more than one child of an unaffected parent because of germ line mosaicism. Alternately, the autosomal dominant mutation may be carried in a proportion of a parent's somatic cells as well as the germ line. In this situation, the manifestations of the condition may differ, being milder, segmental, or focal. This **somatic mosaicism** may manifest as a streaky alteration in skin pigmentation. Somatic and germ line mosaicism, at the level of the gene or chromosome, occur after conception.

An autosomal **recessive** gene mutation, when present in a single copy in an individual, will be hidden. Such a person is known as a "carrier" and will be normal. If, by chance, a person inherits an abnormal gene for an autosomal recessive disorder from both parents, there is no normal gene partner and the two altered genes will cause symptoms and signs, for example, cystic fibrosis. When each parent carries a recessive mutation for the same disorder, the chance that they both will pass on the mutation to their child, who is then affected, is 25%.

Recessive genes on the X chromosome have different consequences in males and females. A mutated recessive gene on the X will tend to have little impact in a female, because there is a second, normal copy of the gene on the second X chromosome of the pair. In contrast, in the male, a mutation of a **recessive X-linked gene** will have an impact because the genes on the Y chromosome are different from those on the X, and no second gene copy exists. That male must pass the mutated X-linked gene to all his daughters but to none of his sons, because he passes his Y chromosome to his sons. Some disorders are **X-linked dominant**, and females will also be affected. However, males are generally more severely affected in such disorders.

In certain areas of the genetic code, genes behave differently if they have been inherited from the father (**paternally inherited**) rather than from the mother (**maternally inherited**). Only one copy may be active, whereas the other is inactivated, usually by a process of methylation. These genes, whose action differs depending on the parent of origin, are said to be **imprinted**. More can be learned about this phenomenon in the chapters on the imprinted disorders Angelman syndrome (Chapter 3), Beckwith-Wiedeman syndrome (Chapter 4), Prader-Willi syndrome (Chapter 18), and Russell-Silver syndrome (Chapter 20). A more detailed account of patterns of inheritance, imprinting, and mosaicism can be found in any standard text of human or medical genetics, such as those listed under ADDITIONAL RESOURCES, below.

GENETIC TESTING

Several terms used in this book in describing genetic tests are likely unfamiliar to some readers. For some disorders, the appropriate test is a **chromosome analysis** (or **karyotype**, which is an ordered display of an individual's chromosomes). Chromosomes are analyzed by special staining techniques that result in visibility of dark and light bands, which are designated in a very standardized way from the centromere, or major constriction. The short arm of the chromosome is called "p," the long arm is called "q," and bands are numbered up from the centromere on the p arm and down from the centromere on the q arm. Each band is further subdivided according to areas within the bands or between them. Thus the deletion found in velocardiofacial syndrome is in the first band of the q arm of chromosome 22, and is designated del22(q11.2). A standard chromosome analysis has at least 450 bands, which is quite adequate for numerical chromosome anomalies. For some disorders, however, the anomaly cannot be seen reliably on standard chromosome analysis and requires special handling while being processed called **high-resolution banding.** An alternative term, **prometaphase banding**, is used because the cell growth during culturing is adjusted to maximize the number of cells in prometaphase, where the chromosomes are much less condensed and thus longer, rather than in metaphase, where cell growth is stopped in standard chromosome studies. High-resolution banding often has 550 to 800 bands, and allows much more detailed analysis.

A new technique called molecular cytogenetics combines the technique of chromosome analysis with the use of fluorescence-tagged molecular markers (called probes) that are applied after the chromosome preparation is produced. This method is called **fluorescence in situ hybridization**, or **FISH**, and relies on the phenomenon of hybridization (intertwining) of complementary pieces of DNA. Thus, to test whether there is a very small deletion (called a **microdeletion**) that is not visible using chromosome analysis alone, a fluorescence-tagged DNA probe complementary to the deleted material is applied to the chromosome preparation. If the chromosome material is present in the normal amount, a fluorescent signal will be visible at that site under the fluorescence microscope; if the normal chromosome material is absent (deleted), there will be no fluorescence signal. FISH is a very powerful tool not only for diagnosing relatively common microdeletion or **microduplication** disorders but also for identifying the origin of extra chromosome material that cannot be identified by inspection alone and sorting out the origin of the components of a **translocation** (structural rearrangement of chromosomal material).

Other types of genetic testing rely exclusively on molecular diagnostic methodologies. **PCR (polymerase chain reaction)** is a powerful technique for amplifying, thus making many, many copies of a segment of DNA so that it can be analyzed. PCR is used for many genetic disorders with a recurring mutation (such as achondroplasia) or a finite number of common mutations. It can also be used to identify the presence of alterations in the normal methylation pattern in imprinted disorders (see Chapters 3 and 18). **Southern blot** techniques are more time consuming; they involve breaking DNA into small pieces using restriction enzymes and then separating them out using gel electrophoresis and analyzing whether there is a deviation in the distance that a segment of the DNA travels on the gel, indicating that its size is different from usual. Both PCR and Southern blotting usually involve the use of **DNA markers**, or **probes**. These are small segments of DNA complementary to an area of interest. One special type of probe takes advantage of the fact that DNA normally contains many runs of repeated base pairs, such as CACACACACA... , which are usually located between genes and have no phenotypic consequences. These are called **microsatellites**. Such runs occur normally throughout the genome, and the number of repeats is inherited like a genetic trait. There are vast variations in the exact number of repeated doublets, which can be "counted" by molecular techniques and which represent polymorphisms or variants. These so-called **microsatellite markers** form the basis for paternity testing and are also used for diagnostic testing of neighboring genes or the genes within which they occur, although they are not the mutation of the relevant gene that causes disease.

Markers can even be used when the precise gene or mutation is unknown, through a process called **linkage analysis**. This is a gene-hunting technique that uses linked (neighboring) markers to trace patterns of heredity in families in which more than one individual is affected with a disorder in an effort to identify whether a child inherited the chromosome with the relevant marker near a co-inherited disease-causing gene. Although this often does not represent identification of the disease gene itself, it can be very reliable within families with multiple affected and unaffected members, particularly when the disease gene or mutation is unknown. The closer the marker is to the gene of interest, the more accurate the result because proximity reduces the likelihood of crossing over. The disadvantage is that the technique requires DNA from several affected and unaffected family members.

The nomenclature for markers is a bit more uniform than that for genes. Markers are indicated by the letter D (standing for DNA), followed by the number of the chromosome they are on, followed by the letter S (standing for single copy) and the number representing the numerical order in which they were identified. Thus D15S10 was the 10th marker to be identified on chromosome 15. This designation gives no hint as to which gene it is in or near, or where on the chromosome it maps.

THE ROLE OF THE MEDICAL GENETICIST AND GENETIC COUNSELOR

Many syndromes are relatively rare, and any individual physician may have limited personal experience. Medical geneticists, on the other hand, frequently have considerable experience of many cases and have ready access to additional information through the genetics literature. The myriad manifestations of each of the syndromes included in this book often require the care of many diverse specialties. The geneticist can assist in diagnosis, testing, and counseling of affected individuals and their family as a consultant to the non-genetics physician and can orchestrate coordination of care to focus on the whole child or adult. The role of the geneticist extends beyond the individual child to involve the care and well being of the entire family. The primary care physician is encouraged to consult medical geneticists to assist in the management of patients with multiple anomaly syndromes.

An important facet of the care of individuals with syndromes and their families is genetic counseling. This is the provision of nondirective information about the diagnosis and its implications not only for the individual (prognosis) but also for the family (reproductive risks and options). It includes knowledge of the inheritance pattern, likelihood of recurrence in a future pregnancy, and prenatal diagnostic options. Referral to relevant community resources, such as patient support groups, brochures, and web sites and financial, social, and educational services, can also be made during this process. Assisting the patient and/or family to understand the condition and its impact, provide optimal care, and adapt to the existence of a chronic and complex disorder are all part of the process of genetic counseling. Adjustment to a new diagnosis may put considerable strain on a family, and emotional support for the family by care providers is paramount. Genetic counseling is usually provided by medical geneticists or by genetic counselors, who are Masters-prepared professionals who are knowledgeable about genetic disorders and their inheritance, can determine genetic risks, and are trained to assist in the emotional and psychological adjustments necessitated for optimal outcome.

ADDITIONAL RESOURCES

Additional information concerning the included disorders, as well as explanations of inheritance information and diagnostic testing, may be found in standard texts on genetics and genetic disorders. A few particularly useful ones in this context are:

- *Smith's Recognizable Patterns of Human Malformation* (Jones, 1997)
- Syndromes of the Head and Neck (Gorlin et al., 1990)
- Diagnostic Dysmorphology (Aase, 1990)
- Principles and Practice of Genetics (Rimoin, Connor, and Pyeritz, 1996)
- The Metabolic and Molecular Bases of Inherited Disease (Scriver et al.,1995)

In addition, online resources on genetic disorders are readily available, including:

- Online Mendelian Inheritance in Man (OMIM) (*www3.ncbi.nlm.nih.gov/Omim*)
- GeneClinics (*www.geneclinics.org*)

For those with a deeper interest, there are electronic databases that aid in diagnosis and provide photographs and references concerning not only common but also rare genetic disorders. These must be purchased, and include:

- London Dysmorphology Database (*www.hgmp.mrc.ac.uk/lddb*) or (*www. oup.com*)
- POSSUM (Pictures of Standard Syndromes and Undiagnosed Malformations) (*www.possum.net.au*)

A resource of laboratories doing specialized diagnostic testing, both clinically and for research, for genetic disorders and syndromes is:

- GeneTests (*www.genetests.org*)

Further information on individual syndromes for practitioners or families can be obtained from other sources, including:

- National Organization for Rare Diseases (NORD) (*www.rarediseases.org*)
- March of Dimes/Birth Defects Foundation (*www.modimes.org*)

REFERENCES

Aase JM (1990) *Diagnostic Dysmorphology*. New York: Plenum Medical Book.

Allanson JE (1997) Objective techniques for craniofacial assessment: What are the choices? *Am. J. Med. Genet* 70:1–5.

Gorlin RJ, Cohen MM Jr, Hennekam R (2001) *Syndromes of the Head and Neck*, 4th ed. New York; Oxford University Press.

Hall BD, Robl JM, Cadle RG (1998). The importance of diagnostic follow-up of unknown multiple congenital anomaly syndromes. *Am J Hum Genet* 43:A48.

Hall JG, Froster-Iskenius UG, Allanson JE (1989) *Handbook of Normal Physical Measurements*. Oxford: Oxford University Press.

Jones KL (1997) *Smith's Recognizable Patterns of Human Malformation*, 5th ed. Philadelphia; Saunders.

Nussbaum RL, McInnes RR, Willard HF (2001) *Genetics in Medicine*, 6th ed. WB Saunders Co., Philadelphia.

Rimoin DL, Connor JM, Pyeritz RE (1996). *Principles and Practice of Genetics*, 3rd ed. New York; Churchill Livingstone.

Saul RA, Stevenson RE, Rogers RC, Skinner SA, Prouty LA, Flannery DB (1988) *Growth References from Conception to Adulthood*. Proc Greenwood Gen Ctr Suppl 1.

Scriver CR, Beaudet AL, Sly WS, Valle D (1995). *The Metabolic and Molecular Bases of Inherited Disease*, 7th ed. New York; McGraw-Hill.

Spranger J, Benirschke K, Hall JG, Lenz W, Lowry RB, Opitz JM, Pinsky L, Schwarzacher HG, Smith DW (1982): Errors of morphogenesis: Concepts and terms. Recommendations of an International Working Group. *J Pediatr* 100:160–165.

CHAPTER 2

ACHONDROPLASIA

RICHARD M. PAULI

INTRODUCTION

Incidence

The external physical features of achondroplasia have been recognized for millennia and are well represented in art work from diverse cultures in all parts of the world (Enderle et al., 1994). It is the most common, and still most readily recognizable, of the skeletal dysplasias (also known as bone dysplasias, chondrodysplasias, and osteochondrodystrophies), with best estimates of birth prevalence around 1 in 26,000–28,000 (Oberklaid et al., 1979; Orioli et al., 1995). Although achondroplasia is an autosomal dominant, single gene disorder, most cases are sporadic.

Most individuals with achondroplasia can be expected to have a normal life expectancy. Nevertheless, individuals with achondroplasia are at some increased risk for premature death. Hecht et al. (1987) demonstrated that much of that risk arises in infancy and early childhood. Indeed, in their retrospective analysis of 701 persons with this diagnosis, there was a 7.5% risk for death in the first year of life (Hecht et al., 1987). Most of these deaths were sudden and unexpected, probably attributable to acute foraminal compression of the upper cervical cord or lower brain stem (see below) (Pauli et al., 1984). Overall, mean survival was about 10 years less than in the general population. Although it is conceivable that some bias arose from the population studied (e.g., it was derived in part from patients seen at highly specialized referral centers), various corrections did not remove entirely the evident increased risk of premature death.

Diagnostic Criteria

Well-defined clinical and radiologic features allow for virtual certainty of diagnosis in all infants with achondroplasia. External physical characteristics include disproportionately short limbs, particularly the proximal or rhizomelic (upper) segments; short fingers often held in a typical "trident" configuration with fingers deviating distally; moderately enlarged head; depressed nasal bridge; and modestly constricted chest. (Fig. 2.1). In all infants in whom this diagnosis is suspected, radiographic assessment is mandatory. Features that are most helpful in distinguishing achondroplasia from other short-limb disorders include small skull base and foramen magnum; narrowing rather than widening of the interpediculate distance in the lumbar spine and short vertebral bodies; square iliac wings, flat acetabulae narrowing of the

Management of Genetic Syndromes, Edited by Suzanne B. Cassidy and Judith E. Allanson
ISBN 0-471-31286-X Copyright © 2001 by Wiley-Liss, Inc.

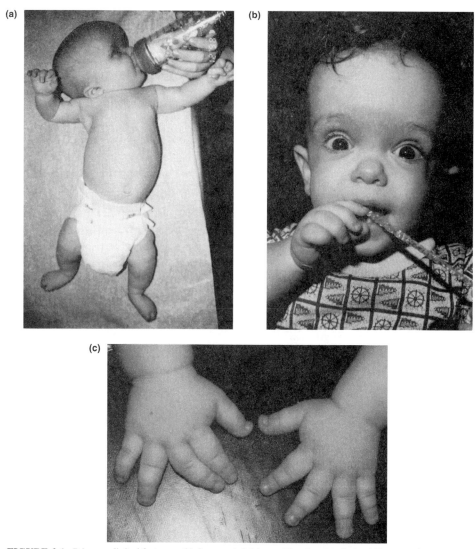

FIGURE 2.1. Primary clinical features of infants and children with achondroplasia. (A): general appearance in a child of about 2 months of age. (B): facial features include a high forehead and depressed nasal bridge. (C): hands show not only shortening of the fingers but also the typical trident configuration (with increased distance particularly between the third and fourth fingers).

sacrosciatic notch and a characteristic radiolucency of the proximal femora (Fig. 2.2); short, thick long bones; flared metaphyses; and short proximal and middle phalanges (Langer et al., 1967). Although both the clinical and the radiologic features evolve with age, in virtually all instances diagnostic uncertainty will only arise in the neonate.

Prenatal diagnosis of achondroplasia using ultrasonographic criteria can be exceedingly difficult (Patel and Filly, 1995; Modaff et al., 1996), particularly because bone foreshortening is often not evident until around 20–24 weeks of gestation (Patel and Filly, 1995).

Etiology, Pathogenesis and Genetics

Most, and perhaps all, of the clinical characteristics and medical complications of

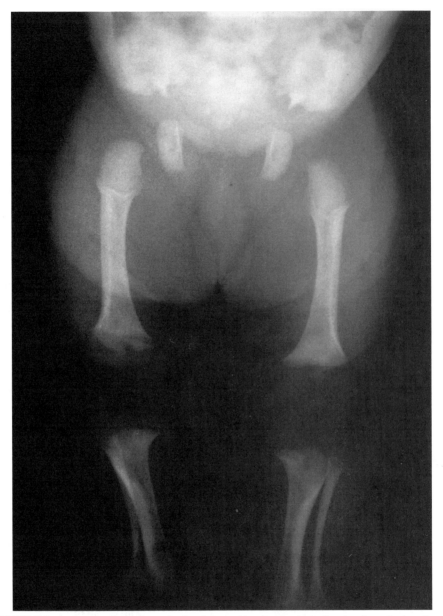

FIGURE 2.2. Anteroposterior radiograph of an infant with achondroplasia showing, in particular, aberrant shape of the ilia and the characteristic radiolucency of the proximal femora.

achondroplasia are explicable on the basis of abnormalities of growth of cartilaginous bone or disproportionate growth of cartilaginous bone when compared with other contiguous tissues.

The molecular origin of this defect in cartilaginous bone development recently has been elucidated (Horton, 1997). All instances of achondroplasia arise from a mutation in one copy of the fibroblast growth factor receptor 3 (*FGFR3*) gene (Shiang et al., 1994; Bellus et al., 1995) and, more remarkably, virtually always from the same nucleotide substitution at the same site in the *FGFR3* gene (Bellus et al., 1995). *FGFR3* is one of four receptors for a large set of growth factors. When *FGFR3* is mutated, as in achondroplasia, its normal inhibitory function is constitutively activated (i.e., turned on whether or not a fibroblast growth factor has bound to it), resulting in increased inhibition of growth of cartilage cells (Webster and Donoghue, 1996).

Because achondroplasia is an autosomal dominant disorder, offspring of affected individuals will have a 50% chance themselves to be affected. However, two additional considerations are important in understanding the transmission genetics of achondroplasia. First, although dominant, most instances of achondroplasia arise from new, spontaneous mutations (Orioli et al., 1995); this means that most individuals with achondroplasia are born to parents both of whom are of average stature. The frequency at which these new mutations arise is correlated with advanced paternal age (Orioli et al., 1995), and, in fact, virtually all of the achondroplasia new mutations arise in the father's germinal cells (Wilkin et al., 1998). Secondly, individuals of small stature may often marry one another. Offspring whose parents both have achondroplasia not only are at a 50% risk to have achondroplasia but have an additional 25% risk to receive two copies of the abnormal allele, resulting in homozygous achondroplasia, a usually lethal condition (Pauli et al., 1983).

Diagnostic Testing

Because virtually all instances of achondroplasia arise from the same base pair substitution (Bellus et al., 1995), molecular testing is straightforward and is currently available commercially. However, the vast majority of affected individuals can be unequivocally diagnosed on the basis of clinical and radiologic features (personal experience). Consultation with a clinician and/or radiologist with expertise in diagnosing skeletal dysplasias would seem to be a more reasonable approach, with *FGFR3* molecular testing reserved for those rare instances in which diagnosis is in doubt (personal observation).

See below, under **Pregnancy**, for a brief discussion of *FGFR3* use for prenatal diagnosis.

Differential Diagnosis

In the broadest sense, achondroplasia may be considered in any individual with disproportionately short stature characterized by greater shortening of the limbs and a relatively normally sized trunk. In practice, only three such diagnoses should cause any confusion: thanatophoric dysplasia, homozygous achondroplasia, and hypochondroplasia.

Thanatophoric dysplasia is nearly always a lethal disorder. It results in profound shortening of the limbs, marked macrocephaly, and marked chest constriction as well as characteristic radiologic features (Maroteaux et al., 1967). Infants with this disorder most often die from respiratory insufficiency either due to a constricted chest or to central apnea related to profound stenosis of the foramen magnum (personal experience). Homozygous achondroplasia closely resembles thanatophoric dysplasia clinically, but has radiologic characteristics that are distinct both from thanatophoric dysplasia and from heterozygous achondroplasia (Pauli et al., 1983). Of course, if an infant has very severe bony changes and is born to parents both of whom have achondroplasia, the differentiation should not be difficult. Another dwarfing disorder due to an *FGFR3* mutation has been described recently (Tavormina et al., 1999). The SADDAN syndrome is characterized by bony changes nearly as severe as those in thanatophoric dysplasia, plus developmental retardation and acanthosis nigricans. In infancy, prior to the onset of acanthosis nigricans and before developmental abnormalities can be identified, distinguishing SADDAN syndrome from achondroplasia and thanatophoric dysplasia may be difficult without molecular evaluation.

Individuals with hypochondroplasia (Hall and Spranger, 1979) have many features resembling achondroplasia, but in most of these individuals the manifestations are uniformly milder. Both clinical and radiologic distinction may be difficult, with a virtual continuum of characteristics ranging from typical achondroplasia to severe hypochondroplasia to mild hypochondroplasia to normal.

It is now recognized that the similarities of these disorders are understandable at a molecular level. Each arises from different mutations of the *FGFR3* gene resulting presumably in different severity of constitutive activation of the receptor (Horton, 1997).

Assessment solely on clinical and radiologic grounds is virtually always sufficient to differentiate achondroplasia from all but hypochondroplasia. Only in this case might molecular testing be needed, looking for the common achondroplasia *FGFR3* mutation. If the mutation is present, diagnosis of achondroplasia is confirmed. If it is absent, then the potentially more difficult task of identifying a molecular basis for a presumptive diagnosis of hypochondroplasia could be pursued.

MANIFESTATIONS AND MANAGEMENT

Unlike many of the disorders discussed in this book, guidelines for care of children with achondroplasia have been previously generated (American Academy of Pediatrics Committee on Genetics, 1995). Although in many ways quite similar, the recommendations made here differ based on materials that have been published since those original guidelines were generated and on the author's personal experience in longitudinally caring for approximately 125 individuals with achondroplasia.

Members of the Medical Advisory Board of Little People of America have special expertise regarding medical assessment and management of individuals with achondroplasia (see below under RESOURCES). Optimal care should include involvement of such an individual as a periodic consultant working in concert with the family physician, pediatrician, or internist who assumes major responsibility for the general care of an individual with this diagnosis.

Growth and Feeding

Moderate to marked short stature is universal in achondroplasia. Ultimate adult heights vary moderately, from about 120 to 145 cm (47 to 57 in.) and a mean of 130 cm (51 in.) in males and from 115 to 137 cm (45 to 54 in.) and a mean of 125 cm (49 in.) in females. Standard growth charts have been generated (Horton et al., 1978) and modified for easier use (Greenwood Genetics Center, 1988; Fig. 2.3A).

In general, individuals with achondroplasia are tall enough to function effectively in most environments with modest adaptive modifications (e.g., appropriately placed stools, seating modification). Reaching may on occasion be problematic, particularly for those with very short arms and concomitant limitation of elbow extension (see below).

Most of those providing care for individuals with achondroplasia concur that obesity is prevalent (Hecht et al., 1988). Indirect methods suggest that between 13% and 43% of adults with achondroplasia are obese (3–8 times the general population rate) (Hecht et al., 1988), although no rigorous studies of body fat content have been completed. Excess weight may contribute to risks related to lumbosacral spinal stenosis (Scott, 1977) and may, in part, account for the modest excess mortality demonstrated in adults (Hecht et al., 1987). Excess weight gain appears to begin in early childhood (Hecht et al., 1988).

Evaluation

- Length or height should be measured at each childhood contact with a health care provider. These measures should

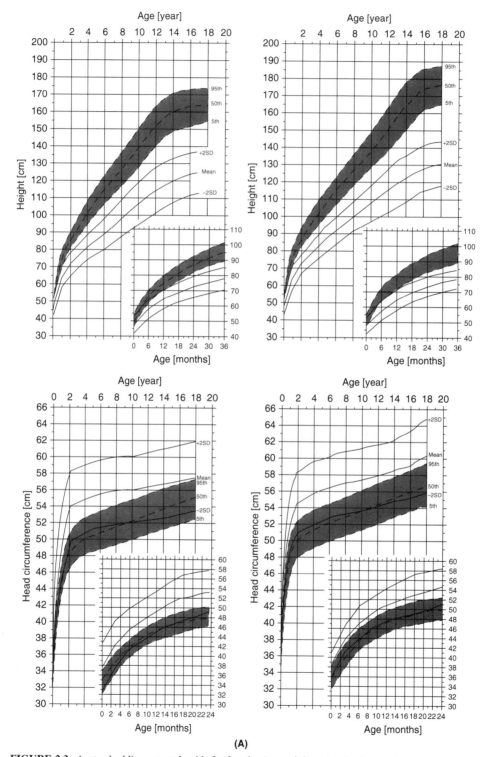

FIGURE 2.3. A: standard linear growth grids for females (*upper left*) and males (*upper right*) and standard head circumference grids for females (*lower left*) and males (*lower right*).

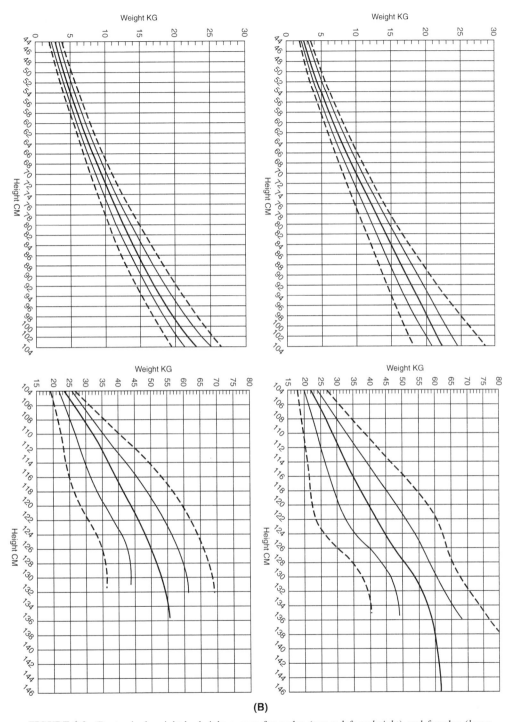

FIGURE 2.3. (B: standard weight-by-height curves for males (*upper left and right*) and females (*lower left and right*).

be plotted on achondroplasia-specific growth charts. Only in this way can growth be used as a nonspecific measure of well-being in children with achondroplasia (as it is used in all average-statured children).

- Standard weight by height curves have been generated (Hunter et al., 1996; see Fig. 2.3B). Note that these are not curves of optimal weight and do not exclude individuals who themselves may be obese. Nevertheless, they are of great value in assessing whether an individual with achondroplasia exceeds the norms for this population. These curves are also of value in identifying failure to thrive that may accompany respiratory compromise in infants and young children with achondroplasia.

Treatment

- There is no effective treatment that will reverse the decremental growth found in achondroplasia.
- Experimental or exceptional interventions may be elected by some families. A series of studies have assessed the effects of growth hormone therapy on children with achondroplasia (Tanaka et al., 1998). Most have shown at least transient increases in growth velocity, with diminishing effect over time. None of the studies has been of sufficient length to demonstrate whether adult stature will be significantly affected.
- Even more controversial is the use of extended limb lengthening (Vilarrubias et al., 1990, Saleh and Burton, 1991). Various techniques have been employed to achieve increases in height of 30 cm (12 in.) or more through osteotomy (cutting through the bone to be lengthened) and distraction (stretching of the bone as the fractured region heals).
- Experience suggests that, at least in North America, most parents embrace the philosophy of modification of the

environment to accommodate the child (see below) rather than attempting to modify the child (personal observation).

- Hunter et al. (1996) suggest that an appropriate aim is to maintain weight in children within +1 SD of the mean and in adults near the mean. Early parental counseling is appropriate — encouraging high-volume, low-calorie food snacks, not using food as reward, involvement in age-appropriate and safe physical activities.
- Nutritional assessment and referral for management is indicated in those developing obesity.

Development and Behavior

Overall, individuals with achondroplasia have normal cognitive development and cognitive function (Hecht et al., 1991). However, when compared with appropriate controls they do have specific differences in development. First, there is clear evidence that children with achondroplasia uniformly have both delayed and unusual motor development (Fowler et al., 1997; Pauli et al., 1997b), principally on the basis of biophysical differences related to stature, disproportion, macrocephaly, joint hypermobility, and hypotonia (Fowler et al., 1997). Secondly, a disproportionate number have language-related problems (Brinkmann et al., 1993); this is most likely caused, at least in part, by an extremely high frequency of middle ear disease and either persistent or fluctuating hearing loss (Brinkmann et al., 1993; personal observations). Finally, a small minority of children with achondroplasia will be more seriously delayed, demonstrate significant learning disabilities, and/or be mentally retarded. The frequency of such problems has not yet been well documented but is almost certainly no greater than 10% (personal experience). A variety of factors could, at least theoretically, contribute to such risk — intrinsic brain abnormalities related to abnormal *FGFR3* expression, hydrocephalus, unrecognized hypoxemia and ischemic damage, or foramen magnum stenosis and cervical myelopathy.

Evaluation

- In infancy, care providers must recognize the anticipated differences in development, particularly motoric development (Hecht et al., 1991; Fowler et al., 1997) and provide reassurance to parents when appropriate.
- Standards have been generated that can be used to compare a child with others with the same diagnosis (Todorov et al., 1981; Fowler et al., 1997; Fig. 2.4). It should be realized, however, that these standards are based either on retrospectively obtained information (Todorov, et al., 1981) or on limited numbers of prospectively generated observations (Fowler, et al., 1997).
- Every child with achondroplasia who diverges significantly from these published standards should be referred for further assessment.

- Marked, persistent hypotonia and gross motor delays, in particular, may be indicative of problems at the craniocervical junction requiring acute multidisciplinary assessment (Pauli et al., 1995).
- Assessment for adaptive needs, particularly at early school age, is crucial.

Treatment

- Various adaptive devices may be needed because of biophysical differences, such as short stature, limited reach, and hypotonia. These include appropriate use of stools, adaptations of school furniture, modifications for toileting, use of a reacher for wiping after toileting, etc. (Pauli et al. 1997c). Adults, too, can benefit from modest adaptations of their work and home environment (Scott, 1977; Crandall et al., 1994). A large body of information is available concerning practical issues of adaptations, much of it through Little People of America (see below under RESOURCES).

Skill	25th-90th %ile for children with achondroplasia	Average age for average statured
Sit without support	9-20.5	5.5
Pull to stand	12-20	7.5
Stand alone	16-29	11.5
Walk	14-27	12
Reach	6-15	3.5
Pass object	8-14	6
Bang two objects	9-14	8.5
Scribble	15-30	13.5

FIGURE 2.4. Developmental observations in young children with achondroplasia (in months).

Neurologic

Hydrocephalus. A large majority of children with achondroplasia are macrocephalic (Horton et al., 1978). Neuroimaging will most often demonstrate both ventriculomegaly and increased extra-axial (subarachnoid) fluid volume, but considerable controversy exists over whether these features represent clinically significant hydrocephalus that should be treated (Steinbok et al., 1989) or are most often a benign process requiring no intervention (Pierre-Kahn et al., 1980). Preponderant opinion appears to favor the latter. Nevertheless, a proportion of children with achondroplasia will develop symptomatic increased intracranial pressure that requires intervention. Using conservative criteria, that proportion appears to be about 5% (personal experience). It seems reasonable to differentiate benign ventriculomegaly and clinically significant hydrocephalus even if, as seems the case, they both arise secondary to increased intracranial venous pressure due to jugular foraminal stenosis (Steinbok et al., 1989).

Evaluation

- At the time of diagnosis, every child with achondroplasia should have assessment of ventricular size and volume of extra-axial fluid by ultrasound, computerized tomography, or magnetic resonance imaging. Because of the need for radiologic neuroimaging for other purposes (see below), ultrasound is the least desirable of these options.
- All children should have serial head circumference measurements plotted on achondroplasia-specific grids (Horton et al., 1978; Fig. 2.3) every 1–2 months in the first years of life and at each well-child visit thereafter.
- The physician should be aware of the signs and symptoms that suggest increased intracranial pressure — accelerating head growth, bulging and tense fontanel, lethargy or irritability, unexplained vomiting, apparent headache, etc. Because of the etiology of the hydrocephalus in achondroplasia (Pierre-Kahn et al., 1980; Steinbok et al., 1989), sudden increase in the prominence of superficial veins over the scalp or eye region (reflecting increased ancillary blood flow bypassing the pressure gradient at the jugular foramina) should be sought. Likewise, parents should be taught the major signs and symptoms of developing hydrocephalus and encouraged to have their child evaluated emergently should such concerns arise.

Treatment

- Should acceleration of head growth arise or should signs and symptoms suggesting increased intracranial pressure develop, then the child should have magnetic resonance imaging of the brain, which can be compared with that obtained at the time of first diagnosis.
- If no acute symptoms persist and if imaging shows preservation of the subarachnoid space and lack of evidence for periventricular parenchymal edema, the physician, in consultation with a neurologist or neurosurgeon, may elect a period of watchful waiting. This compensated hydrocephalus (benign ventriculomegaly) is probably of no consequence, although some have suggested that this may be of greater clinical significance (Steinbok et al., 1989).
- In instances where symptomatic hydrocephalus has unequivocally developed, standard ventriculoperitoneal shunting with an anti-syphon device is appropriate. With appropriate intervention in the minority of affected individuals requiring intervention, prognosis for hydrocephalus should, in general, be favorable. There will be the usual risks and complications related to placement of a ventriculoperitoneal shunt.

Cervicomedullary Junction Constriction. Every infant with achondroplasia has a small foramen magnum due to abnormality of growth of the endochondral cranial base (Hecht et al., 1989). The foramen magnum is not only small but often misshapen, resembling a "keyhole" (Hecht et al., 1989) rather than being round or ovoid. The asynchrony of growth of the foramen magnum compared with its contents (spinal cord and blood vessels) causes risks for either apnea-associated death or high cervical myelopathy and paralysis.

Pauli et al., (1984) and others (for example, Reid et al., 1987) have demonstrated that the diminution of foraminal size may be of considerable consequence in the health and survival of infants with achondroplasia. Without appropriate assessment and intervention some infants will die unexpectedly in the first 1–2 years of life (Pauli et al., 1984; Hecht et al., 1987; Pauli et al., 1995). These apneic deaths likely arise because of vascular compression at the craniocervical junction, resulting in damage to the respiratory control centers in the lower medulla (Pauli et al., 1984; Reid et al., 1987). Such deaths may mimic sudden infant death syndrome but are more likely to be daytime deaths and deaths associated with uncontrolled head movement (Pauli et al., 1984). Without evaluation or management, risk of death is certainly increased over the general population (Pauli et al., 1984) and may approach 10% (Hecht et al., 1987), although experience suggests that a more realistic figure may be in the 2–5% range (personal observation).

Compression of the cervicomedullary cord can also result in high cervical myelopathy, most often in this population presenting with disproportionate and long-persistent hypotonia, weakness, hyperreflexia, asymmetric reflexes, and ankle clonus (Pauli et al., 1995; personal observation). This, too, appears to arise through hypoxic injury or traumatic compression (Hecht et al., 1984).

No accurate estimate of the frequency of these complications seems to be available.

Less frequently, children with achondroplasia and cervicomedullary junction compression may present with chronic, otherwise unexplained respiratory signs and symptoms without demonstrable neurological concomitants (Reid et al., 1987).

Craniocervical junction compression in older children and adults with achondroplasia is much less common (personal experience).

Because complications arise from disproportionate growth of bone compared with the neural tissue it surrounds, efforts at evaluation and management are aimed at minimizing neural damage and, when necessary, decompressing the constraining bone. With appropriate assessment and selective intervention, prognosis is excellent, not only for survival but also for survival without sequelae (Pauli et al., 1995).

Evaluation

A prospective study has been completed that provides support for comprehensive evaluation of every infant with achondroplasia regarding the risk for cervicomedullary junction constriction to identify those who may be at higher than average risk (Pauli et al., 1995). Evaluation that should be completed at the time of initial diagnosis should include the following:

- Complete neurological history
- Careful neurological examination, preferably by a physician with experience, including judging whether severity of hypotonia is outside the expected range for infants with achondroplasia
- Neuroimaging. This could either be computerized tomography with thin cuts and bone windows through the foramen magnum [necessary to obtain measures of the size of the foramen that can be compared with diagnosis specific standards (Hecht et al., 1989)] or magnetic resonance imaging (better visualization of neural structures but

no direct measure of foramen magnum size); note that calvarial ultrasound (American Academy of Pediatrics Committee on Genetics, 1995) cannot assess foraminal structures and should be abandoned as a screening tool in assessing infants with achondroplasia.

- Overnight multichannel polysomnographic evaluation (sleep study) in a sleep center accustomed to assessing infants.

Treatment

- Parents should be counseled regarding careful neck support with handling, using a solid-back stroller and "babysafe," and avoidance of "swing-o-matics," "Johnny-jump-ups," etc., which may precipitate uncontrolled head movement around a constricted foramen magnum. Automatic swings in which an infant is in a sitting or near-sitting position are particularly risky; at least four sudden apneic deaths in infants with achondroplasia have been observed associated with their use (Pauli et al., 1984; personal experience). If initial findings of the comprehensive assessment discussed above are reassuring, no further investigations are needed. However, the infant should continue to have careful periodic monitoring of neurological and respiratory history and clinical and neurological reexaminations about every 6 months.

- In infants with worrisome features [the most highly predictive of which are persisting hypotonia, increased reflexes or clonus in the legs, foramen magnum measurements below the mean for achondroplasia, and central hypopnea (Pauli et al., 1995)], magnetic resonance imaging should be completed (with or without flow studies). If unequivocal evidence for cord compression is present, then surgical decompression should be done immediately (Yamada et al., 1996). With such criteria, around 8% of all children with achondroplasia will undergo suboccipital and cervical decompressive surgery (personal experience).

- All individuals of all ages should be considered to have relative cervical spinal stenosis and, on this basis, to have increased risk related to severe head and neck trauma. Certain physical activities should be strongly discouraged, including full-contact American football, full-contact ice hockey, rugby, downhill skiing, trampoline, dive rolls or other gymnastics in which full-body-weight impact on the head or neck is likely, hanging upside down from knees or feet, and heading in soccer (personal observations).

Respiratory

Infants with achondroplasia have smaller than average thoraces (Stokes et al., 1983) as well as clinical evidence of increased compliance of the rib cage (personal observation). It has been suggested that such features may result in decreased effective lung volumes, decreased respiratory reserve, and increased probability of chronic hypoxemia (Stokes et al., 1983; Reid et al., 1987; Mogayzel et al., 1998). Although this suggestion has been rebutted (Tasker et al., 1998), there remain a few young children with achondroplasia who show chronic hypoxemia often accompanied by failure to thrive (Stokes et al., 1983; personal observation). Living at high altitude predisposes to this complication (personal observation). The frequency of such hypoxemia in isolation is unknown. Appropriate evaluation and treatment should prevent sequelae of chronic hypoxemia. Without treatment, secondary difficulties related to cor pulmonale might be life threatening.

Snoring, when isolated, is a virtually uniform feature in individuals with achondroplasia of all ages and should not be assumed to reflect clinically significant obstruction of the upper airway. Although it is generally conceded that obstructive apnea is common in achondroplasia (at all ages, although more information is available on its occurrence in children), prevalence estimates in the literature vary widely — from about 10% to 75% (Sisk et al., 1999). Most such estimates have suffered from small sample size and/or ascertainment and referral bias. A recent review of experience in one clinic demonstrated that 61% (58/95) had a positive history suggestive of airway obstruction and 36/95 (38%) had confirmation of clinically significant obstructive apnea (Sisk et al., 1999).

A number of factors contribute to the exceedingly high frequency of obstructive apnea. There is hypoplasia of the cranial base and midface resulting in diminution of airway size (Stokes et al., 1983; Waters et al., 1995; Zucconi et al., 1996). Then, with physiologic hypertrophy of the lymphatic ring, obstructive apnea may result, thereby explaining why its onset is so frequently between 2 and 10 years of age (personal observations). In addition, muscular obstruction presumed to be secondary to abnormal innervation may contribute to some instances of serious obstructive apnea in young children with achondroplasia (Tasker et al., 1998); this, in turn, may arise from stenosis of the jugular foramina or hypoglossal canals caused by constriction of the calvarial base (Tasker et al., 1998). Gastroesophageal reflux is also sometimes of considerable importance (Stokes et al., 1983; Tasker et al., 1998). Any of these causes can be compounded by coexisting obesity.

In most children who are adequately assessed and treated, obstructive apnea will resolve without long-term sequelae. In some, and in many adults, long-term use of continuous positive airway pressure at night will be essential both to maintain appropriate oxygen saturations and prevent reemergence of fragmented sleep.

Evaluation

- Nighttime oximetry should be assessed as part of polysomnographic evaluation as discussed above. Many infants less than a year of age with this diagnosis will display transient dips of oxygen saturation into the 85-90% range (personal experience).

- Persistent hypoxemia or desaturations below 85% require further assessment, including pulmonary history and pulmonary evaluation.

- Evaluation of oxygen saturations by spot oximetry during waking hours (e.g., active alert, feeding, crying) is also appropriate.

- Chest circumference measurements compared with achondroplasia-specific standards (Hunter et al., 1995) may be of some utility.

- Parents of affected children should be taught to monitor for signs and symptoms of obstruction during sleep and should be questioned at each visit regarding changes in these signs and symptoms. In adults, the sleep partner or other individual should observe breathing characteristics in sleep for significant features at least yearly. Clinical characteristics in sleep that should be sought include neck hyperextension, loud snoring, glottal stops, observed apneic pauses, deep, compensatory sighs, self-arousals, enuresis, and nighttime emesis (Sisk et al., 1998; personal experience). In addition, daytime symptoms including excessive irritability, hypersomnolence or awake respiratory distress may be of relevance (Sisk et al., 1999).

- Physical assessment, in particular the severity of tonsillar (and, by implication, adenoidal) hypertrophy should be carried out.

- If there is suspicion that clinically significant obstructive apnea is occurring, then overnight polysomnographic studies (preferably with pH probe monitoring) must be completed.

- When significant obstructive apnea is demonstrated, assessment for right ventricular hypertrophy and pulmonary hypertension should be carried out.
- In the presence of obstructive apnea, otolaryngological assessment of the nasopharynx and oropharynx should be completed to help determine whether surgical intervention is likely to be of benefit.
- Simultaneous assessment of neurological status is critical to rule out those less frequent instances when upper airway obstruction is due to central nervous system dysfunction (Reid et al., 1987; Tasker et al., 1998).

Treatment

- In those with small chests, significant hypoxemia, and *no other identified cause* of respiratory problems, transient oxygen supplementation can be effective in blunting the hypoxemic episodes and in allowing resolution of the failure to thrive (Stokes et al., 1983; personal experience).
- Intervention for obstructive apnea, if determined to be present, is a graded series of options that should be pursued in a stepwise fashion depending on response. In children, and some adults, initial management should be tonsillectomy and adenoidectomy [not adenoidectomy alone (Sisk et al., 1999)]. In those who are obese, weight loss efforts should begin as well.
- Should follow-up polysomnography demonstrate persistent clinically significant obstruction then positive airway pressure [continuous positive airway pressure (CPAP), bilevel positive airway pressure (BiPAP), etc.] can be used effectively in both adults and children (Waters et al., 1995).

- Additional surgical intervention may occasionally be required should positive airway pressure be ineffective or not tolerated, including uvulectomy, modified uvulopharyngopalatoplasty, etc. (Sisk et al., 1999).
- Finally, only in a small minority will temporary tracheostomy be needed — around 2% of all individuals with this diagnosis (personal observations).
- Interventions in adults with achondroplasia are similar, although it will be less frequent that adenotonsillar hypertrophy is central and more frequent that obesity is a complicating factor.

Ears and Hearing

Although middle ear dysfunction is generally accepted as a frequent complication in achondroplasia, critical assessments of its frequency and consequences are sparse (see Berkowitz et al., 1991; Shohat et al., 1993). By chart review, Berkowitz et al. (1991) estimated that more than 50% of children with achondroplasia have middle ear dysfunction sufficiently severe to require myringotomy and ventilation tube placement. In one population of approximately 125 children with achondroplasia who have been followed longitudinally, 70% have had chronic or recurrent middle ear abnormalities sufficiently severe to require ventilation tube placement (personal experience). Before surgery most have had either fluctuating or persisting hearing loss of a severity that could interfere with normal language acquisition (personal observation). If not aggressively sought and appropriately treated, hearing loss may be a major contributing factor to language and speech delays.

Outcome depends on aggressiveness of assessment and intervention. Virtually all individuals who are appropriately treated in childhood will have normal hearing in adult life. Hearing loss of sufficient severity to require hearing aids is rare [3/126 in one population (personal observation)].

Evaluation

- Audiometric and tympanometric assessment should be completed first at around 6-10 months of age and then every 6-9 months throughout preschool years.
- A high level of suspicion should be maintained for middle ear problems throughout childhood.

Treatment

- Medical management has, by and large, been ineffective (personal experience), and, therefore, aggressive use of myringotomy and tube placement is encouraged. Experience suggests that in those requiring tube placement once, sufficient autonomous eustachian tube function to allow for normalization of middle ear function usually does not occur until around 6-8 years of age (personal observation). Therefore, in those children maintenance and replacement of ventilating tubes until that age is appropriate.
- During periods of documented or suspected hearing loss, standard interventions *en face* are appropriate (e.g., preferential seating at school, communication).
- Some individuals may show substantial speech and language delay. In those instances, referral for speech and language therapy is essential.

Musculoskeletal

Kyphosis. A transient kyphotic deformity at the thoracolumbar junction of the spine is present in 90–95% of young infants with achondroplasia (Kopits, 1988b; Pauli et al., 1997a). In most it spontaneously resolves after the assumption of orthograde posture. However, around 10% of adults with achondroplasia have a fixed, angular kyphosis that

can result in serious neurological sequelae secondary to tethering of the spinal cord (Kopits, 1988b; Pauli et al., 1997a). Beighton and Bathfield (1981) first suggested that positioning early in life could be determinative in whether the flexible and transient kyphosis of infancy becomes fixed. Other factors contributing to the development of a kyphosis include trunk hypotonia, ligamentous laxity, and macrocephaly, all of which result in an infant with achondroplasia slumping forward if placed in sitting (Pauli et al., 1997a). If long periods are spent in such a position, remodeling in response to anomalous forces results in anterior wedging of vertebrae and fixed kyphosis (Pauli et al., 1997a).

In a sequential series involving 71 infants with achondroplasia, prohibition of unsupported sitting was demonstrated to be effective in decreasing the probability of a fixed kyphosis developing (Pauli et al., 1997a). Furthermore, using a generated algorithm (see Fig. 2.5), the frequency with which a fixed kyphosis of medical significance arises could be reduced to zero (Pauli et al., 1997a). With appropriate care, this is by and large a preventable problem. The use of the protocol summarized below should prevent virtually all clinically significant instances of thoracolumbar kyphosis. In those in whom preventive measures are not taken or in whom they fail, surgical fusion either prophylactically (Kopits, 1988b) or at the first signs of long-track abnormalities can prevent paralysis and/or bowel and bladder incontinence.

Evaluation

- Clinical evaluation of the infant's spine should occur about every 6 months through the first 3 years of life, with particular emphasis on the severity of persisting kyphosis when the child is placed prone.
- If the kyphosis is moderate or marked, then radiographic assessment (sitting lateral and cross-table *prone* lateral X

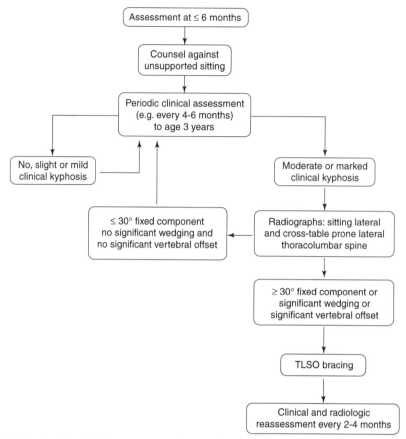

FIGURE 2.5. Algorithm for the assessment and prevention of fixed angular kyphosis (originally published in Pauli et al. 1997a).

rays of the thoracolumbar spine) should be obtained.

- In adolescents or adults who have not been treated in this manner, clinical assessment should include examination of the spine. If a kyphosis is easily palpated, possible consequences should be sought through careful history (e.g., weakness, exercise-induced pain, dysesthesias of the legs, bowel or bladder problems, etc.) and a lateral standing thoracolumbar spine radiograph should be obtained.

Treatment

- Parents of infants should be counseled against allowing unsupported sitting for at least the first 12 months of life

and to avoid devices that cause disadvantageous positioning such as soft infant carriers, umbrella-style strollers, and canvas seats.

- In infants and young children, if the prone radiograph shows that there is an irreversible curve of >30°, the family should be referred for bracing using a thoracolumbosacral orthosis (TLSO) (Kopits, 1988b; Pauli et al., 1997a) (Fig. 2.5).

- In those for whom such anticipatory medical care has not been provided, surgical intervention for kyphosis may be needed (Kopits, 1988b; Lonstein, 1988).

Lumbosacral Spinal Stenosis. Stenosis of the entire spinal canal is uniformly present

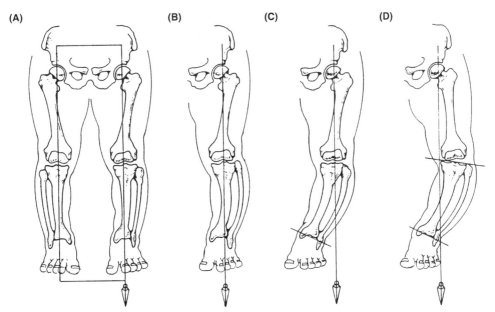

FIGURE 2.6. Diagrammatic representation of increasing severity (B → D; A is normal) of varus deformity. The situation illustrated in D and sometimes that in C will require surgical intervention. (Reprinted with permission from Johns Hopkins University Press).

in individuals with achondroplasia. Although problems related to cervical spinal stenosis are of greater concern in infants and young children, lumbosacral spinal stenosis is more commonly problematic in adults. Exercise-induced spinal claudication (pain, dysesthesias, and motor changes only precipitated by activity and rapidly resolved with rest) is present in most adults with achondroplasia if symptoms are carefully sought (personal experience). However, unless pain is severe and activity markedly compromised, surgical treatment for claudication is elective. In contrast, spinal stenosis that causes either nerve root or cord compression can lead to serious and irreversible sequelae (Pyeritz et al., 1987). Often, signs and symptoms develop in the third or fourth decade of life (Kahanovitz et al., 1982; Pyeritz et al., 1987), and may affect nearly half of young and middle-aged adults (Kahanovitz et al., 1982). Onset of symptoms likely is related to development of additional factors that can exacerbate the intrinsic spinal

stenosis, including intervertebral disc disease, degenerative arthritis, etc. (Kahanovitz et al., 1982; Pyeritz et al., 1987). In addition, those with significant thoracolumbar kyphosis (above) and/or severe hyperlordosis of the lumbar spine are likely at greater risk to develop symptomatic stenosis (Kahanovitz et al., 1982; Pyeritz et al., 1987).

Evaluation

- Every adolescent and young adult should have periodic evaluation searching for signs and symptoms of lumbosacral spinal stenosis. Symptoms to be sought include numbness, dysesthesias, radicular pain, leg weakness, clumsiness, changes in gait, or problems with bladder or bowel continence (Pyeritz et al., 1987). Examination should include complete motor (assessing for weakness or strength asymmetry, abnormal deep tendon reflexes) and sensory evaluation of the legs.
- If abnormalities are discovered, and particularly if there is change in

neurological findings over time, referral for neurological and neurosurgical assessment should be made. At that time, neuroimaging (computerized tomography, magnetic resonance imaging, magnetic resonance myelography) should allow assessment of the severity, level, and associated factors of the stenosis.

Treatment

- Those with severe and/or progressive spinal stenosis require urgent neurosurgical intervention through extended and wide posterior laminectomy (Pyeritz et al., 1987; Lonstein, 1988).
- More complex surgery with both anterior and posterior approaches may be needed in those who also have severe, angulated thoracolumbar kyphosis (Lonstein, 1988).
- Decompression laminectomy usually results in some improvement of symptoms and function (Pyeritz, et al., 1987). Long-term outcomes are less uniformly positive, with only about one-half of patients showing long-term benefit (Pyeritz et al., 1987). Additional surgery is often necessary (Pyeritz et al., 1987).

Knee Instability. Nearly all young children with achondroplasia have unstable knees with both genu recurvatum and moderate lateral instability (personal experience). The recurvatum deformity usually results in hyperextension of between 20° and 70° (Kopits, 1988a; personal observation). It appears to arise primarily from abnormalities of growth of the tibial plateau (Kopits, 1988a). It is usually most severe in the second year of life (Kopits 1988a) and rarely requires intervention but does contribute to the motor delays seen in young children (Fowler et al., 1997). On occasion, however, there may be frank tibiofemoral subluxation [3 of 126 young children in one survey (personal observation)]. Likewise, although

lateral instability may result in local discomfort associated with orthograde activity, probably related more to the need for voluntary muscle stabilization than to the instability *per se* (personal observation), only rarely is this severe enough in itself to require any substantial intervention. In virtually all individuals, these features remit with increasing age (personal observation). Thus instability is usually self-limited or self-resolving.

Evaluation

- Historical and physical determination of the severity of knee hyperextensibility and whether symptoms appear to be arising from it should be sought in young children with achondroplasia.
- A history of activity-precipitated pain over the lateral or posterior knee should be sought.
- When such knee pain is associated with moderate or severe varus deformity, it should precipitate additional referral.

Treatment

- Parents of those with asymptomatic mild or moderate knee instability should be reassured that no intervention is needed.
- In those in whom knee instability causes recurrent pain (most often seen after a day of physical activity), warmth, massage, and nonsteroidal anti-inflammatories can be used.
- *Rarely*, transient bracing for severe knee instability may allow for more normative gross motor development. Transient bracing in 4 of 126 children in one study showed positive benefits (personal experience). Note that bracing is *not* indicated in the treatment of varus deformity and, indeed, may exacerbate that problem (Kopits, 1988a).
- Children with overt knee subluxation appear to benefit markedly from tibial flexion osteotomy surgery (personal experience).

Varus Deformity. A majority of children and adults have bowleg deformity (Kopits, 1988a; personal experience). About 70% of children evaluated in one survey have clinically relevant varus (personal experience). Kopits (1988a) estimated that 93% of adults with achondroplasia have some degree of varus deformity. This arises, at least in part, from overgrowth of the fibula and secondary mechanical stress on the tibia (Kopits, 1988a). In fact, although referred to as tibia varus, the deformity is usually more complex than a simple lateral bow, involving tibia varus, tibia recurvatum, and internal tibial torsion often accompanied by genu recurvatum and lateral instability of the knees and, occasionally, by knee subluxability (Kopits, 1988a; personal experience). With appropriate management, no long-term sequelae should be anticipated. If untreated, worsening pain, increasing disability, and secondary joint damage will arise (Kopits, 1980).

Evaluation

- Examination should include assessment of the child while standing. Serial measurements of loaded distances between the knees, midtibiae, and medial malleoli are helpful in assessing whether deformity is stable, progressing, or accelerating (personal experience).

- Evaluation of whether the three weight-bearing joints remain "in plumb" (Kopits, 1980) (Fig. 2.6) is helpful in deciding if pediatric orthopedic assessment is warranted. If a child is out of plumb when standing, then further evaluation is warranted.

- Evaluation of gait for lateral knee thrust (sudden outward displacement of the knee with weight bearing; Kopits, 1980; personal observation) should be accomplished. This, too, warrants pediatric orthopedic assessment.

Treatment

- For those with varus of sufficient severity to be out of plumb and symptomatic

or in whom a knee thrust has developed, surgery is indicated (Kopits, 1980; personal experience). Surgery in those who are out of plumb but essentially asymptomatic is temporally elective (personal experience), although some investigators have recommended early surgery in this circumstance (Kopits, 1980).

Other Musculoskeletal Complications.
With assumption of standing and walking, most children develop a hyperlordosis (swayback) of moderate or severe degree. This is usually asymptomatic. It may exacerbate risk for lumbosacral spinal stenosis in adulthood (Kahanovitz et al., 1982; Pyeritz et al., 1987). Local pain may develop at the apex of the lordosis in both children and adults (personal experience). In a few children the horizontal sacrum and consequently superficial coccyx may result in chronic coccydynia.

Hypermobility of the shoulders is a virtually constant feature but is only infrequently symptomatic (personal experience). Even in those with inferior subluxability, pain is uncommon (Kopits, 1988a).

The elbows are the one exception to the generalized joint hypermobility seen in individuals with achondroplasia. Although individuals often display marked overpronation and oversupination (personal experience), limitation of extension often develops in early childhood (Kopits, 1988a), frequently of about 20–60 degrees. Less often, there is posterolateral radial head dislocation (Kopits, 1988a) causing more severe limitation of extension as well as limiting pronation and supination. When present this may further limit functionally effective reach (such as for toileting).

Wrists are usually hypermobile. Some individuals have remarkable dorsoventral radiocarpal subluxability (personal observation). The intrinsic joints of the hands are also usually hypermobile and may limit fine motor endurance, particularly in young children (personal observation).

Evaluation

- An assessment of the degree of hyperlordosis should be made, and a history of coccyx pain should be elicited.
- Evaluation for joint hypermobility should be done, and a history of subluxation or pain should be elicited.

Treatment

- When chronic coccydynia is present, it can be treated by padding sewn into the underwear (personal observation).
- Physical therapy for lower abdominal muscle strengthening and teaching of "tucking under" of the buttocks may be warranted in those children with the most marked hyperlordosis (personal experience).
- Surgical intervention for elbow limitation is not indicated. Rather, adaptive devices (such as bottom wipers) should be used as needed.
- Discomfort and fatigue of the wrists when doing fine motor tasks because of hypermobility may be relieved by using a simple stabilizing brace if this proves particularly problematic (personal experience).

Dental

Structural abnormalities of the midface and jaw are exceedingly common in individuals with achondroplasia, including in particular midface hypoplasia and relative mandibular overgrowth. In addition, the palate is often narrow and anteriorly V-shaped (personal observation). The result is a high frequency of malocclusion and crowding of the teeth, including palisading of the upper incisors, anterior open bite, crossbite, and prognathism (personal observation). Outcome depends upon timely assessment and intervention.

Evaluation

- In addition to routine pediatric dental care, children with apparent bite abnormalities should be referred for orthodontic assessment as early as 5–6 years of age.

Treatment

- Options can include palatal expansion, traditional orthodontic manipulations, and, in instances of exceedingly severe midface hypoplasia, consideration of a Le Fort I facial advancement procedure (personal experience).

Anesthetic Risks

Related to many of the problems already discussed, both children and adults with achondroplasia are likely to face one or more operative procedures. Anesthesia presents certain special risks in most dwarfing disorders (Berkowitz et al., 1990). Achondroplasia is no exception. Primary areas of concern include cervical spinal stenosis and consequent risks related to extremes of positioning while sedated or anesthetized; obstructive apnea with or without cor pulmonale and concomitant risks of postsedation obstruction or postextubation pulmonary edema, potentially reduced airway size, and possible restrictive lung disease in young children (Berkowitz et al., 1990). With appropriate care, the complication rate should approach that of the general population.

Evaluation

- Anesthesiologists should be made of aware of the potential risks and of the availability of the excellent review by Berkowitz et al., (1990).

Treatment

- Many pediatric surgeons elect (appropriately) to admit young children with achondroplasia for an overnight stay even for surgery that usually is done as a same-day procedure because of the risk of airway-related complications (personal experience).

Pregnancy

Extraordinarily little information is available on the risks in pregnancy of women with achondroplasia (see Allanson and Hall, 1986). On the basis of a questionnaire administered to a self-selected convenience sample of 87 women with achondroplasia (Allanson and Hall, 1986) the following information appears to be secure. First, women with achondroplasia can continue pregnancies to term, presumably because of relatively normal trunk size. Secondly, complications during pregnancy are relatively infrequent but may include risk for worsening of neurological symptoms related to increasing hyperlordosis and maternal respiratory failure. Antecedently predicting who may develop respiratory compromise seems not to be possible. In two women of similar size and similar baseline pulmonary status, one developed respiratory failure in the early third trimester, whereas the other successfully carried twins to term (personal observation). Except for the small possibility of maternal respiratory failure requiring early delivery, successful pregnancies should be anticipated.

Prenatal testing by *FGFR3* molecular analysis may be elected, principally in two circumstances. First, when both parents have achondroplasia it can be used to distinguish homozygous achondroplasia from other possible outcomes (Shiang et al., 1994). Second, when a sporadic short-limbed dwarfing condition is discovered by ultrasound, presence or absence of achondroplasia as the cause of limb shortening can be determined in this manner (Modaff et al., 1996).

Evaluation

- Women with achondroplasia should be considered at high risk particularly related to the possibility of respiratory compromise later in pregnancy. Baseline pulmonary function studies may provide a basis for monitoring respiratory status as the pregnancy progresses (Allanson and Hall, 1986).

- Careful follow-up for this and other maternal complications is essential.

Treatment

- Women should be counseled to anticipate a scheduled cesarean delivery without a trial of labor.
- There is current controversy and no consensus about appropriate anesthetic management — general, spinal, or epidural — for cesarean delivery in these women.
- Genetic counseling concerning any potential testing of the fetus should precede invasive procedures.

RESOURCES

Little People of America (LPA)

Support group for individuals of marked small stature and for their families; many secondary resources are available through the national LPA and its local district and chapter personnel.
P.O. Box 9897
Washington, D.C. 20016
1-888-LPA-2001
General website:
http://www-bfs.ucsd.edu/dwarfism
Parents' forum website:
http://home1.gte.net/jmayeux/pf1/

LPA Discussion Group On Line

To subscribe: send e-mail to listserv@ucsd.edu; and at message type: subscribe dwarfism
To send messages, send to dwarfism@ucsd.edu

LPA Medical Advisory Board

Charles I. Scott, M.D., Chair
Alfred I. DuPont Institute
1600 Rockland Rd., P.O. Box 289
Wilmington, DE 19899-0269

Thinking Big, Susan Kuklin. New York: Lothrop, Lee and Shepard Books, 1986.

A 48-page picture and textbook appropriate for preschool and young school age children.

Dwarfism. The Family and Professional Guide, Charles Scott, Nancy Mayeux, Richard Crandall, and Joan Weiss. Irvine, CA: Short Stature Foundation, 1994. 195 pages.

Living with Differences. Families with Dwarf Children, Joan Ablon. New York: Praeger (Greenwood), 1988. 194 pages.

A Little of This and a Little of That, available through Rob and Betty Jacobsen, P.O. Box 1747, Longview, WA 98632 (e-mail: rbjake@teleport.com). A compendium of information intended primarily for parents of children with dwarfing disorders.

To Celebrate: Understanding Developmental Differences in Young Children with Achondroplasia. Madison, WI: Midwest Regional Bone Dysplasia Clinic, 1997.

Little People, Big Schools: Preparing the School for Your Young Child with Short Stature. Madison, WI: Midwest Regional Bone Dysplasia Clinic, 1997. (both available from the Midwest Regional Bone Dysplasia Clinic; Clinical Genetics Center; University of Wisconsin-Madison; 1500 Highland Ave., Madison, WI 53705-2280).

REFERENCES

Allanson JE, Hall JG (1986) Obstetric and gynecologic problems in women with chondrodystrophies. *Obstet Gynecol* 67:74–78.

American Academy of Pediatrics Committee on Genetics (1995) Health supervision for children with achondroplasia. *Pediatrics* 95:443–451.

Beighton P, Bathfield CA (1981) Gibbal achondroplasia. *J Bone Joint Surg* 63:328–329.

Bellus GA, Hefferon TW, Ortiz de Luna RI, Hecht JT, Horton WA, Machado M, Kaitila I, McIntosh I, Francomano CA (1995) Achondroplasia is defined by recurrent G380R mutations of *FGFR3. Am J Hum Genet* 56:368–373.

Berkowitz ID, Raja SN, Bender KS, Kopits SE (1990) Dwarfs: Pathophysiology and anesthetic implications. *Anesthesiology* 73:739–759.

Berkowitz RG, Grundfast KM, Scott C, Saal H, Stern H, Rosenbaum K (1991) Middle ear disease in childhood achondroplasia. *Ear Nose Throat J* 70:305–308.

Brinkmann G, Schlitt H, Zorowka P, Spranger J (1993) Cognitive skills in achondroplasia. *Am J Med Genet* 47:800–804.

Crandall R, Crosson T, Scott CI, Mayeux N, Weiss J (1994) *Dwarfism. The Family and Professional Guide*. Irvine, CA: Short Stature Foundation.

Enderle A, Meyerhöfer D, Unverfehrt G (eds) (1994) *Small People—Great Art. Restricted Growth from an Artistic and Medical Viewpoint*. Hamm, Germany: Artcolor.

Fowler ES, Glinski LP, Reiser CA, Horton VK, Pauli RM (1997) Biophysical bases for delayed and aberrant motor development in young children with achondroplasia. *J Dev Behav Pediatr* 18:143–150.

Greenwood Genetics Center (1988) *Growth References from Conception to Adulthood*. Clinton, SC: Jacobs.

Hall BD, Spranger J (1979) Hypochondroplasia: clinical and radiological aspects in 39 cases. *Radiology* 133:95–100.

Hecht JT, Butler IJ, Scott CI (1984) Long-term neurological sequelae in achondroplasia. *Eur J Pediatr* 143:58–60.

Hecht JT, Francomano CA, Horton WA, Annegers JF (1987) Mortality in achondroplasia. *Am J Hum Genet* 41:454–464.

Hecht JT, Hood OJ, Schwartz RJ, Hennessey JC, Bernhardt BA, Horton WA (1988) Obesity in achondroplasia. *Am J Med Genet* 31:597–602.

Hecht JT, Horton WA, Reid CS, Pyeritz RE, Chakraborty R (1989) Growth of the foramen magnum in achondroplasia. *Am J Med Genet* 32:528–535.

Hecht JT, Thompson NM, Weir T, Patchell L, Horton WA (1991) Cognitive and motor skills in achondroplastic infants: Neurologic and respiratory correlates. *Am J Med Genet* 41:208–211.

Horton WA (1997) Fibroblast growth factor receptor 3 and the human chondrodyplasias. *Curr Opin Pediatr* 9:437–442.

Horton WA, Rotter JI, Rimoin DL, Scott CI, Hall JG (1978) Standard growth curves for achondroplasia. *J Pediatr* 93:435–438.

Hunter AGW, Reid CS, Pauli RM, Scott CI (1995) Standard curves of chest circumference in achondroplasia and the relationship of chest circumference to respiratory problems. *Am J Med Genet* 62:91–97.

Hunter AGW, Hecht JT, Scott CI (1996) Standard weight for height curves in achondroplasia. *Am J Med Genet* 62:255–261.

Kahanovitz N, Rimoin DL, Sillence DO (1982) The clinical spectrum of lumbar spine disease in achondroplasia. *Spine* 7:137–140.

Kopits SE (1980) Correction of bowleg deformity in achondroplasia. *Johns Hopkins Med J* 146:206–209.

Kopits SE (1988a) Orthopedic aspects of achondroplasia in children. *Basic Life Sci* 48:189–197.

Kopits SE (1988b) Thoracolumbar kyphosis and lumbosacral hyperlordosis in achondroplastic children. *Basic Life Sci* 48:241–255.

Langer LO, Baumann PA, Gorlin RJ (1967) Achondroplasia. *Am J Roentgenol* 100:12–26.

Lonstein JE (1988) Treatment of kyphosis and lumbar stenosis in achondroplasia. *Basic Life Sci* 48:283–292.

Maroteaux P, Lamy M, Robert JM (1967) Le nanisme thanatophore. *Presse Med* 75:2519–2524.

Modaff P, Horton VK, Pauli RM (1996) Errors in the prenatal diagnosis of children with achondroplasia. *Prenat Diagn* 16:525–530.

Mogayzel PT, Carroll JL, Loughlin GM, Hurko O, Francomano CA, Marcus CL (1998) Sleep-disordered breathing in children with achondroplasia. *J Pediatr* 131:667–671.

Oberklaid F, Danks DM, Jensen F, Stace L, Rosshandler S (1979) Achondroplasia and hypochondroplasia. Comments on frequency, mutation rate, and radiological features in skull and spine. *J Med Genet* 16:140–146.

Orioli IM, Castilla EE, Scarano G, Mastroiacovo P (1995) Effect of paternal age in achondroplasia, thanatophoric dysplasia, and osteogenesis imperfecta. *Am J Med Genet* 59:209–217.

Patel MD, Filly RA (1995) Homozygous achondroplasia: US distinction between homozygous, heterozygous, and unaffected fetuses in the second trimester. *Radiology* 196:541–545.

Pauli RM, Conroy MM, Langer LO, McLone DG, Naidich T, Franciosi R, Ratner IM, Copps SC (1983) Homozygous achondroplasia with survival beyond infancy. *Am J Med Genet* 16:459–473.

Pauli RM, Scott CI, Wassman ER, Gilbert EF, Leavitt LA, Ver Hoeve J, Hall JG, Partington MW, Jones KL, Sommer A, Feldman W, Langer LO, Rimoin DL, Hecht JT, Lebovitz R (1984) Apnea and sudden unexpected death in infants with achondroplasia. *J Pediatr* 104:342–348.

Pauli RM, Horton VK, Glinski LP, Reiser CA (1995) Prospective assessment of risk for cervicomedullary junction compression in infants with achondroplasia. *Am J Hum Genet* 56:732–744.

Pauli RM, Breed A, Horton VK, Glinski LP, Reiser CA (1997a) Prevention of fixed, angular kyphosis in achondroplasia. *J Pediatr Orthop* 17:726–733.

Pauli RM, Modaff P, Fowler E, Reiser CA (1997b) *To Celebrate: Understanding Developmental Differences in Young Children with Achondroplasia.* Madison, WI: Midwest Regional Bone Dysplasia Clinic.

Pauli RM, Modaff P, Reiser CA (1997c) *Little People, Big Schools: Preparing the School for Your Young Child with Short Stature.* Madison, WI: Midwest Regional Bone Dysplasia Clinic.

Pierre-Kahn A, Hirsch JF, Renier D, Metzger J, Maroteaux P (1980) Hydrocephalus and achondroplasia. A study of 25 observations. *Child's Brain* 7:205–219.

Pyeritz RE, Sack GH, Udvarhelyi GB (1987) Thoracolumbar laminectomy in achondroplasia: long-term results in 22 patients. *Am J Med Genet* 28:433–444.

Reid CS, Pyeritz RE, Kopits SE, Maria BL, Wang H, McPherson RW, Hurko O, Phillips JA, Rosenbaum AE (1987) Cervicomedullary compression in young patients with achondroplasia: Value of comprehensive neurologic and respiratory evaluation. *J Pediatr* 110:522–530.

Saleh M, Burton M (1991) Leg lengthening: patient selection and management in achondroplasia. *Orthop Clin North Am* 22:589–599.

Scott CI (1977) Medical and social adaptation in dwarfing conditions. *Birth Defects* 13[2C]:29–43.

Shiang R, Thompson LM, Zhu YZ, Church DM, Fielder TJ, Bocian M, Winokur ST, Wasmuth JJ (1994) Mutations in the transmembrane domain of *FGFR3* cause the most common genetic form of dwarfism, achondroplasia. *Cell* 78:335–342.

Shohat M, Flaum E, Cobb SR, Lachman R, Rubin C, Ash C, Rimoin DL (1993) Hearing loss and temporal bone structure in achondroplasia. *Am J Med Genet* 45:548–551.

Sisk EA, Heatley DG, Borowski BJ, Levenson GE, Pauli RM (1999) Obstructive sleep apnea in children with achondroplasia: surgical and anesthetic considerations. *Otolaryngol Head Neck Surg* 120:248–254.

Steinbok P, Hall J, Flodmark O (1989) Hydrocephalus in achondroplasia: the possible role of intracranial venous hypertension. *J Neurosurg* 71:42–48.

Stokes DC, Phillips JA, Leonard CO, Dorst JP, Kopits SE, Trojak JE, Brown DL (1983) Respiratory complications of achondroplasia. *J Pediatr* 102:534–541.

Tanaka H, Kubo T, Yamate T, Ono T, Kanzaki S, Seino Y (1998) Effect of growth hormone therapy in children with achondroplasia: growth pattern, hypothalamic-pituitary function, and genotype. *Eur J Endocrinol* 138:275–280.

Tasker RC, Dundas I, Laverty A, Fletcher M, Lane R, Stocks J (1998) Distinct patterns of respiratory difficulty in young children with achondroplasia: a clinical, sleep, and lung function study. *Arch Dis Child* 79:99–108.

Tavormina PL, Bellus GA, Webster MK, Bamshad MJ, Fraley AE, McIntosh I, Szabo J, Jiang W, Jabs EW, Wilcox WR, Wasmuth JJ, Donoghue DJ, Thompson LM, Francomano CA (1999) A novel skeletal dysplasia with developmental delay and acanthosis nigricans is caused by a Lys65Met mutation in the fibroblast growth factor receptor 3 gene. *Am J Hum Genet* 64:722–731.

Todorov AB, Scott CI, Warren AE, Leeper JD (1981) Developmental screening tests in achondroplastic children. *Am J Med Genet* 9:19–23.

Vilarrubias JM, Ginebreda I, Jimeno E (1990) Lengthening of the lower limbs and correction of lumbar hyperlordosis in achondroplasia. *Clin Orthop* 250:143–149.

Waters KA, Everett F, Sillence DO, Fagan ER, Sullivan CE (1995) Treatment of obstructive sleep apnea in achondroplasia: Evaluation of sleep, breathing, and somatosensory-evoked potentials. *Am J Med Genet* 59:460–466.

Webster MK, Donoghue DJ (1996) Constitutive activation of fibroblast growth factor receptor 3 by the transmembrane domain point mutation found in achondroplasia. *EMBO J* 15:520–7.

Wilkin DJ, Szabo JK, Cameron R, Henderson S, Bellus GA, Mack ML, Kaitila I, Loughlin J, Munnich A, Sykes B, Bonaventure J, Francomano CA (1998) Mutations in fibroblast growth-factor receptor 3 in sporadic cases of achondroplasia occur exclusively on the paternally derived chromosome. *Am J Hum Genet* 63:711–716.

Yamada Y, Ito H, Otsubo Y, Sekido K (1996) Surgical management of cervicomedullary compression in achondroplasia. *Child's Nerv Syst* 12:737–741.

Zucconi M, Weber G, Castronovo V, Ferini-Strambi L, Russo F, Smirne S (1996) Sleep and upper airway obstruction in children with achondroplasia. *J Pediatr* 129:743–749.

CHAPTER 3

ANGELMAN SYNDROME

CHARLES A. WILLIAMS

INTRODUCTION

Angelman syndrome is a genetic neurobehavioral condition that is characterized by developmental delay, progressive microcephaly, ataxic gait, absence of speech, seizures, and spontaneous bouts of laughter (Angelman, 1965). The first reports from North America appeared in the early 1980s; more recently, many new case reports and several reviews have appeared (Clayton-Smith and Pembrey, 1992; Buntinx et al., 1995; Williams et al., 1995).

Incidence

Angelman syndrome has been reported throughout the world among divergent racial groups. In North America, the great majority of known cases seem to be of Caucasian origin. Although the exact incidence of Angelman syndrome is unknown, an estimate of between 1 in 12,000 to 1 in 20,000 seems reasonable (Clayton-Smith and Pembrey, 1992; Steffenburg et al., 1996; Petersen et al., 1995).

Life span does not appear to be dramatically shortened, and a 62-year-old woman with Angelman syndrome (personal experience) and many individuals in their fourth or fifth decades of life are known.

Diagnostic Criteria

Angelman syndrome is usually not recognized at birth or in infancy because the developmental problems are nonspecific during this time. Parents may first suspect the diagnosis after reading about Angelman syndrome or meeting a child with the condition. The most common age of diagnosis is between three and seven years, when the characteristic behaviors and features become most evident, particularly ambulation. A summary of the developmental and clinical features has been published for the purpose of establishing clinical criteria for the diagnosis (Williams et al., 1995). These are detailed in Tables 3.1 and 3.2. All of the

TABLE 3.1. Developmental History and Laboratory Findings in Angelman Syndrome

Normal prenatal and birth history with normal head circumference; absence of major birth defects; developmental delay evident by 6–12 months of age

Delayed but forward progression of development (no loss of skills)

Normal metabolic, hematologic, and chemical laboratory profiles

Structurally normal brain (MRI or CT may have mild cortical atrophy or dysmyelination)

Management of Genetic Syndromes, Edited by Suzanne B. Cassidy and Judith E. Allanson
ISBN 0-471-31286-X   Copyright © 2001 by Wiley-Liss, Inc.

TABLE 3.2. Clinical Features of Angelman Syndrome

Consistent (100%)

Developmental delay, functionally severe

Speech impairment, none or minimal use of words; receptive and nonverbal communication skills higher than verbal ones

Movement or balance disorder, usually ataxia of gait and/or tremulous movement of limbs

Behavioral uniqueness: any combination of frequent laughter/smiling; apparent happy demeanor; easily excitable personality, often with hand flapping movements; hypermotoric behavior; short attention span

Frequent (>80%)

Delayed, disproportionate growth in head circumference, usually resulting in microcephaly (absolute or relative) by age 2

Seizures, onset usually <3 years of age

Abnormal EEG, characteristic pattern with large-amplitude slow-spike waves

Associated (20–80%)

Strabismus

Hypopigmented skin and eyes

Tongue thrusting; suck/swallowing disorders

Hyperactive tendon reflexes

Feeding problems during infancy

Uplifted, flexed arms during walking

Prominent mandible

Wide mouth, wide-spaced teeth

Frequent drooling, protruding tongue

Sleep disturbance

Flat back of head

Attraction to/fascination with water

Excessive chewing/mouthing behaviors

Increased sensitivity to heat

features do not need to be present for the diagnosis to be made and the diagnosis is often first suspected when the typical behaviors are recognized.

Etiology, Pathogenesis, and Genetics

Angelman syndrome results from absence or nonfunctioning of the normally active maternal allele at 15q11–q13. Angelman syndrome and its counterpart, Prader-Willi syndrome (see Chapter 18), are recognized as classical examples of imprinting; Prader-Willi syndrome usually results from chromosome 15q11–q13 deletions in the paternally derived chromosome, and Angelman syndrome usually results from similar deletions in the maternally derived chromosome (Knoll et al., 1989). Each syndrome thus has associated gene(s) that are active only on one of the parentally derived chromosomes; such genes are considered to exhibit genomic imprinting. There are several distinct genetic events that can perturb the chromosome 15q11–q13 imprinting process and lead to Angelman syndrome. Accordingly, the diagnostic testing and estimation of recurrence risks can be complicated (see below).

There are four types of genetic abnormalities that can cause Angelman syndrome:

- Deletions of region 15q11–q13 of the maternally derived chromosome (70–75% of cases). In addition, there are rare families with unique chromosome 15 translocations and smaller deletions within 15q11–q13. The majority of patients with Angelman syndrome have a relatively large interstitial deletion of 15q11–q13. Molecular analysis has revealed that repeated copies of a large nonfunctional ancestral gene map to both the proximal and distal ends of 15q11–q13, possibly predisposing to unequal recombination resulting in the common large deletions observed in the majority of patients with Angelman syndrome and Prader-Willi syndrome, as well as duplications of this region (Amos-Landgraf et al., 1997). Figure 3.1 illustrates the appearance of individuals with proven large deletions.

- Paternal uniparental disomy (UPD) of chromosome 15 (2–5% of cases). Individuals with Angelman syndrome and paternal uniparental disomy may have a

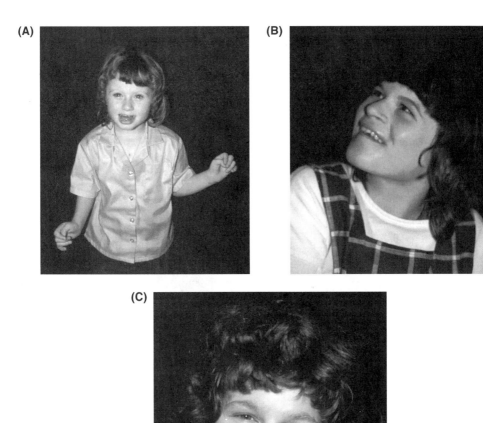

FIGURE 3.1. Individuals with proven large interstitial deletions are pictured. The typical jerky gait with uplifted arms as well as protruding tongue is seen in **A**. Adults with happy demeanor and lack of obvious craniofacial dysmorphia are seen in **B** and **C**.

milder phenotype (i.e., lower incidence of seizures) than that observed in Angelman syndrome caused by other types of genetic mechanisms (Bottani et al., 1994).

- Imprinting defects (2–5% of cases). This subset of patients with Angelman syndrome has mutations or other defects in the mechanism(s) involved in the imprinting process during gametogenesis. Defects in a region termed the imprinting center (IC), located within 15q11–q13, can change the DNA methylation and transcription activity of certain genes that reside within 15q11–q13. Microdeletions in the imprinting center have been found (Ohta et al., 1998).

- *UBE3A* and other presumed single gene mutations (20–25% of cases). The last group has no evidence of the typical large 15q11–q13 deletion, does not have paternal uniparental disomy, and has no imprinting center defect but does show the full Angelman syndrome clinical phenotype. Further study of some of these heretofore genetic test-negative patients found mutations in a new gene, *UBE3A*, encoding the E6AP-3A ubiquitin protein ligase (Kishino et al., 1997; Matsuura et al., 1997). Preliminary mutation analysis of *UBE3A* has revealed a 20% mutation detection rate in this group (Malzac et al., 1998). This group thus comprises those patients with Angelman syndrome caused by *UBE3A* mutations as well as patients with an Angelman syndrome phenotype who have not been found to have *UBE3A* mutations. The latter group is presumed to have a genetic basis for the Angelman syndrome phenotype, perhaps a yet-to-be identified abnormality in *UBE3A* gene function. Alternatively, individuals in this test-negative group could simply have an incorrect clinical diagnosis.

Identification of *UBE3A* has opened doors to the understanding of the biological pathogenesis of Angelman syndrome, although tremendous questions remain to be answered before we can understand how the neurological phenotype emerges. Ubiquitin-related enzymes (ubiquitin molecules are normally attached to proteins to facilitate their degradation) appear to increase during growth factor-induced neural differentiation, and it is possible that *UBE3A* may be involved in the post-translational processing of certain nerve tissue precursor proteins (Smith-Thomas et al., 1994). The demonstration that *UBE3A* is imprinted in certain regions of the brain suggests a stage-specific developmental role in fetal brain development (Rougeulle et al., 1997; Vu and Hoffman, 1997).

The way in which a *UBE3A* mutation leads to the Angelman syndrome phenotype is currently unknown.

When Angelman syndrome is caused by the large deletion, skin and eye hypopigmentation usually result. This occurs because a pigment gene (*P*), located close to the Angelman syndrome gene, is also deleted. *P* appears to code for a tyrosine transporter protein located within the melanosome membrane (Spritz, 1993). In some people with Angelman syndrome, this hypopigmentation can be so severe that a form of albinism is suspected. However, not all of those with deletions of *P* are obviously hypopigmented; they may only have relatively lighter skin color than either parent. In those with uniparental disomy, imprinting defects, or *UBE3A* mutations, *P* is not missing and normal skin and eye pigmentation are seen.

Diagnostic Testing

There are a number of different tests that can detect some causes of Angelman syndrome. None can detect all causes.

- DNA methylation analysis. Imprinted genes within the 15q11–q13 region can be studied by their different degrees of DNA methylation. Certain maternally inherited genes are extensively methylated, and thus inactivated, whereas their paternally inherited contribution (the paternal allele) is unmethylated and active. One gene located within region 15q11–q13 serves as an illustrative example. It is called *SNRPN*, and it produces a small protein (i.e., a small nuclear ribonuclear protein) that helps regulate RNA processing. Normal individuals have a methylated (maternal) and an unmethylated (paternal) *SNRPN* allele, whereas patients with Angelman syndrome caused by uniparental disomy, imprinting center defects, or the typical 15q11–q13 deletion only have unmethylated *SNRPN* allele(s). It is possible to distinguish whether the gene is methylated or unmethylated by molecular techniques. Although DNA methylation testing is the most sensitive single test for diagnosis of Angelman syndrome, it will not detect the presumed single gene mutation class of patients that have *UBE3A* mutations. Also, methylation analysis will not distinguish the molecular class (15q11–q13 deletion, uniparental disomy, or imprinting center defect) to which the patient with Angelman syndrome belongs. It will diagnose approximately 80% of classic Angelman syndrome cases; a negative test does not exclude the diagnosis.

- Fluorescence in situ hybridization (FISH). FISH allows sensitive detection of 15q11–q13 microdeletions using labeled probes that map to 15q11–q13. About 70% of patients with Angelman syndrome will have a positive FISH test; a negative result does not exclude the diagnosis.
- DNA polymorphisms. Analysis of simple sequence repeats (microsatellites) in the parents and affected individual can determine the parental origin of 15q11–q13 and the rest of chromosome 15. It can detect deletions and uniparental disomy. It will not detect the *UBE3A* mutation class of patients. Patients with imprinting center defects will have biparental inheritance of 15q11–q13 but abnormal DNA methylation.
- Mutation detection within *UBE3A* or the imprinting center. This testing is currently available mainly through research labs. Angelman syndrome cases related to mutations in *UBE3A* have normal FISH, methylation, and DNA polymorphism analysis. Angelman syndrome cases related to imprinting defects have abnormal DNA methylation but normal FISH and DNA polymorphism analysis.
- High-resolution chromosome analysis: This analysis can identify the presence of large 15q11–q13 deletions, but false negatives and positives are frequent so this method is no longer solely used to verify deletions. However, all individuals referred with a preliminary clinical diagnosis of Angelman syndrome should have a chromosome analysis because other cytogenetic anomalies can mimic the clinical findings of Angelman syndrome. Also, patients with confirmed Angelman syndrome should have a chromosome study to exclude overt cytogenetic rearrangements (i.e., translocations) involving 15q11–q13.

The choice and sequence of laboratory testing will vary based on the experience of the physician, clinical presentation, availability of laboratory resources, and other factors. Diagnostic testing algorithms have recently been published (American Society of Human Genetics/American College of Medical Genetics Test and Technology Transfer Committee, 1996). In general, the first-line testing is either FISH (which should also include a standard chromosome analysis) or DNA methylation analysis. When FISH detects a deletion, no further diagnostic evaluation typically occurs if the clinical features suggest Angelman syndrome. Additional study may be needed to provide genetic counseling (such as further study of the proband's and mother's chromosome 15 to rule out a cryptic rearrangement or inherited deletion). Cases with an Angelman syndrome-specific methylation pattern require further evaluation such as FISH and/or DNA polymorphism analysis to identify the molecular class of Angelman syndrome (deletion, uniparental disomy, or imprinting center defect) for genetic counseling purposes. Finally, there remains a group of individuals with Angelman syndrome and the classical clinical phenotype who have negative genetic studies, including negative *UBE3A* mutation analyses. Accordingly, the physician must be cautious about excluding the diagnosis when genetic testing is negative.

Genetic Counseling

Most cases of Angelman syndrome result from typical large de novo deletions of 15q11–q13 and are expected to have a low (<1%) risk of recurrence. Angelman syndrome caused by uniparental disomy that has occurred in the absence of a parental translocation is likewise expected to have a <1% risk of recurrence. Parental structurally or functionally unbalanced chromosome complement can lead to 15q11–q13 deletions or to uniparental disomy and will have case-specific recurrence risks. In instances where there is no identifiable large deletion or uniparental disomy, the risk for recurrence may be as high as 50% as the result of either a maternally inherited imprinting center mutation or a *UBE3A* mutation. Individuals with Angelman syndrome who have none of the above abnormalities comprise a significant proportion of cases (currently 10–15%), and some may be at a 50% recurrence risk. Clinical misdiagnoses will also be represented in this group. The causal heterogeneity of Angelman syndrome, as well as the recent detection of maternal germ cell mosaicism (Malzac et al., 1998), can make it difficult to provide recurrence risk estimation. Formal genetic counseling is advised for those families seeking such estimates (Stalker and Williams, 1998).

Differential Diagnosis

Infants with Angelman syndrome commonly present with nonspecific psychomotor delay and/or seizures, and the differential diagnosis is often broad and nonspecific, encompassing such entities as cerebral palsy, pervasive developmental disorder and static encephalopathy. EEG abnormalities may resemble those associated with the Lennox-Gastaut syndrome, a descriptive neurological condition associated with severe seizures and mental retardation. The presence of hypotonia and seizures may raise the possibility of an inborn error of metabolism or a defect in oxidative phosphorylation such as a mitochondrial encephalomyopathy. Subsequent testing for these abnormalities normally includes urine organic acids, serum amino acids, plasma acylcarnitine profiles, and mitochondrial enzyme and DNA mutation screens. Some infants with Angelman syndrome may be suspected of having a myopathic disorder, although the typical presence of brisk deep tendon reflexes suggests that the lower motor neuron and muscle cell units are normal. Subsequent muscle biopsy with routine histology and electron microscopy studies, and EMG, are normal or show mildly abnormal, nonspecific findings (personal experience).

Seizures and severe speech impairment in infants with Angelman syndrome can resemble those seen in the Rett syndrome, but children with Angelman syndrome do not lose purposeful use of their hands. The distinction between these two syndromes is usually resolved by age 3-4 years, when children with Angelman syndrome are progressing developmentally but those with Rett syndrome are clearly at a developmental plateau or have apparent regression. It is unusual for infants with Angelman syndrome to have a dysmorphic facial appearance or to have any congenital anomalies, so chromosomal syndromes are usually not suspected. Infants with Angelman syndrome who do have some degree of apparent facial dysmorphology usually are only manifesting unique parental traits, accentuated by the child's microcephaly and behavioral abnormalities. Rarely, entities such as Williams syndrome (Chapter 30) or Coffin-Lowry syndrome may be initially considered but are quickly ruled out by a complete history and physical examination. Occasionally, an infant will be misdiagnosed as having Prader-Willi syndrome (Chapter 18) when the diagnosis is Angelman syndrome, because of the 15q11–q13 deletion involving the maternally and not the paternally derived chromosome. DNA methylation testing will distinguish between the two.

Older children with nonspecific cerebral palsy are often referred for evaluation for Angelman syndrome because they exhibit gait ataxia, happy affect, and abnormal speech. However, most occurrences of cerebral palsy do not manifest the extent of tremulousness, jerkiness, and the ballismic-like limb movements seen in Angelman syndrome, and some minimal degree of expressive speech is usually present in those with cerebral palsy, whereas speech remains extremely disrupted in Angelman syndrome (only minimal sounds), even in the face of relatively good attention and socialization.

MANIFESTATIONS AND MANAGEMENT

Growth and Feeding

The prenatal and birth periods are usually uncomplicated, and newborns appear to be physically well formed with normal birth weights and head circumferences. In the first 6–12 months, weight gain may be slow because of feeding difficulties and low muscle tone, but the length growth rate is usually preserved. By 12 months of age about 50% show a deceleration of cranial growth that may represent relative or absolute microcephaly (personal experience). Average height is lower than the mean for normal children, but most children with Angelman syndrome will have a head circumference that falls within the normal range. Final adult height has ranged from 144 cm (4.9 in.) to 177 cm (5.10 in.) in a series of 8 adults with Angelman syndrome (personal experience). Familial factors will influence growth so that taller parents have affected children who tend to be taller than the average child with Angelman syndrome (personal experience).

Children with Angelman syndrome are often thin and have low or near normal subcutaneous fat, but by late childhood some increased weight gain can occur and mild to moderate obesity can be seen (Clayton-Smith, 1993). Growth data have been studied in 57 individuals with Angelman syndrome (Whidden et al., 1994). Those with uniparental disomy demonstrated greater height and head circumference growth rates compared to those with deletions or negative genetic tests.

Feeding problems are frequent but not generally severe and usually manifest in infants as difficulty in sucking or swallowing (Fryburg et al., 1991; Zori et al., 1992). Tongue movements may be uncoordinated, with thrusting and generalized oral-motor incoordination. There may be trouble initiating sucking and sustaining breast feeding. The feeding difficulties may first present to the physician as a problem of poor weight gain or as failure to thrive. Frequent spitting up may be interpreted as formula intolerance or gastroesophageal reflux.

During adolescence, puberty may be delayed by 1–3 years, but sexual maturation occurs with development of normal secondary sexual characteristics.

Evaluation

- Evaluate the cause of feeding problems, beginning with an occupational therapy assessment.
- Monitor weight control in adults periodically.

Treatment

- No growth-related treatments are needed.
- Feeding difficulties should prompt feeding therapy, often done by occupational therapists.
- Occasionally, surgery is needed to treat reflux. The surgical technique is the same as that used in the general population.

- Obesity should be treated with individualized diet and exercise.

Development and Behavior

Cognitive Development. In general, cognitive abilities are severely to profoundly impaired in Angelman syndrome. It is known that cognitive abilities in Angelman syndrome are higher than indicated by developmental testing. Most striking is the disparity between receptive and expressive language. Because of their ability to understand language, children with Angelman syndrome often distinguish themselves from those with other causes of severe mental retardation. Attention deficit, hyperactivity, and lack of speech and motor control compromise developmental testing. In such situations, test results are invariably in the severe range of functional impairment. More attentive children can perform in the moderate range, and a minority can perform in the mildly impaired range in some categories such as receptive social skills. Young adults with Angelman syndrome are usually socially adept and respond to most personal cues and interactions. Because of their interest in people, they establish rewarding friendships and communicate a broad repertoire of feelings and sentiments. They participate in group activities, household chores, and the activities and responsibilities of daily living. Like others, they enjoy most recreational activities such as TV and sports.

There is a wide range, however, in developmental outcome, so that not all individuals with Angelman syndrome attain the above-noted skills. A few will be more impaired in terms of their mental retardation and lack of attention, and this seems especially the case in those with difficult-to-control seizures or those with extremely pronounced ataxia and movement problems. Fortunately, most children with Angelman syndrome do not have these severe problems, but even for the less impaired child, inattentiveness and hyperactivity during early childhood often give the impression that profound functional impairment is the only outcome possible. However, with optimal environmental stimulation and consistent behavioral intervention, these children with Angelman syndrome begin to show improved developmental progress. Young adults with Angelman syndrome continue to learn and are not known to have significant deterioration in their mental abilities. Individuals with Angelman syndrome who have severe ataxia and/or scoliosis may lose their ability to walk if ambulation is not encouraged.

Speech and language. The speech disorder in Angelman syndrome has a somewhat typical evolution. Babies and young infants cry less often and have decreased cooing and babbling. A single apparent word, such as "mama," may develop around 10–18 months, but it is used infrequently and indiscriminately without symbolic meaning. By 2–3 years of age, it is clear that speech is delayed but it may not be evident how little the Angelman syndrome child is verbally communicating; crying and other vocal outbursts may also be reduced. By 3 years of age, higher-functioning children with Angelman syndrome are initiating some type of nonverbal language. Some point to body parts and indicate some of their needs by use of simple gestures, but they are much better at following and understanding commands. Others, especially those with severe seizures or extreme hyperactivity, cannot be attentive enough to achieve the first stages of communication, such as establishing sustained eye contact. The nonverbal language skills in those with Angelman syndrome vary greatly, with the most advanced individuals able to learn some sign language and use such aids as picture-based communication boards. Some affected children seem to have enough comprehension to be able to speak, but in even the highest functioning, conversational speech does not develop. Clayton-Smith (1993) reported that a few individuals spoke one to three words, and in a survey of

47 individuals it was reported that 39% spoke up to 4 words, but whether these words were used meaningfully was not noted (Buntinx et al., 1995).

Behavior. The first evidence of this distinctive behavior may be the onset of early or persistent social smiling at the age of 1–3 months. Giggling, chortling, and constant smiling soon develop and appear to represent normal reflexive laughter, but cooing and babbling are delayed or reduced. Later, several types of facial or behavioral expressions characterize the infant's personality. A few have pronounced laughing that is truly paroxysmal or contagious, and "bursts of laughter" occurred in 70% in one study (Buntinx et al., 1995). More often, happy grimacing and a happy disposition are the predominant behaviors. In rare cases, the apparent happy disposition is fleeting, as irritability and hyperactivity are the prevailing personality traits; crying, shrieking, screaming, or short guttural sounds may then be the predominant behaviors. At times apparent aggressive behavior occurs such as pinching, grabbing, biting, slapping, and hitting. These behaviors often represent attention seeking, but if they are not addressed early on they can become persistent. Consistent social disapproval and a structured behavioral modification program will eventually be successful in managing this problem. Physical punishment is usually counterproductive and unsuccessful.

The laughter in Angelman syndrome seems mostly to be an expressive motor event; most reactions to stimuli, physical or mental, are accompanied by laughter or laughterlike facial grimacing. People with Angelman syndrome do, however, experience the entire spectrum of emotionality.

Children with Angelman syndrome are notorious for putting everything in their mouth. In early infancy, hand sucking (and sometimes foot sucking) is frequent. Later, most exploratory play is by oral manipulation and chewing. The tongue appears to be of normal shape and size, but in 30–50% persistent tongue protrusion is a distinctive feature. For the child with Angelman syndrome who has protruding tongue behavior, the problem remains throughout childhood and can persist into adulthood. Drooling is usually associated, and its treatment is problematic, often requiring use of bibs.

Hyperactivity. Essentially all young children with Angelman syndrome have some component of hyperactivity, and males and females appear equally affected. Infants and toddlers may have seemingly ceaseless activity, constantly keeping their hands or toys in their mouth, moving from object to object. Attention span can be so short that social interaction is prevented because the child cannot attend to facial and other social cues; development progress will be difficult unless more attentiveness occurs. In extreme cases, the constant movement can cause accidental bruises and abrasions. Grabbing, pinching, and biting in older children have also been noted and may be heightened by the hypermotoric activity. Hypermotoric activity in Angelman syndrome usually lasts throughout childhood but gradually improves. It is most severe between ages 3 and 10 years.

Sleep Abnormalities. Parents report that decreased need for sleep and abnormal sleep/wake cycles are characteristic of Angelman syndrome (personal experience). Sleep disturbances have been reported in infants with Angelman syndrome, and abnormal sleepwake cycles have been studied in one child with Angelman syndrome who benefited from a behavioral treatment program (Summers et al., 1992). For some individuals with Angelman syndrome, sleep disturbance appears to remain a difficult problem throughout life.

Prognosis is good regarding forward developmental progress (provided such complications as seizures are adequately controlled), but mental retardation is always present.

Evaluation

- Formal evaluation to detect hyperactivity or attention deficit disorder is not necessary. Parental report and observation in the examination room is sufficient.

- Occurrences of marked exacerbation of restlessness and hypermotoric behavior should prompt a careful medical evaluation to detect occult illness such as otitis, urinary tract infection, or dental abscess.

- Clinical psychological evaluation may be helpful, especially in the evaluation of a family's adjustment to a sleep or nighttime behavioral problem. Often, sleep/wake cycles are reversed and family dynamics have accordingly adjusted to this, sometimes without the family's awareness. Also, a behavioral psychology consultation may prove helpful in teaching the family how to implement consistent sleep and daytime schedules.

Treatment

- The severe developmental delay in Angelman syndrome mandates that a full range of early training and enrichment programs be made available.

- Unstable or nonambulatory children may benefit from physical therapy. Special adaptive chairs or positioners may be required at various times, especially for hypotonic or extremely ataxic children.

- Occupational therapy may help improve fine motor and oral-motor control.

- Speech and communication therapy is essential and should focus on nonverbal methods of communication. Augmentative communication aids, such as picture cards or communication boards, should be used at the earliest appropriate time.

- Extremely active and hypermotoric children with Angelman syndrome will require special provisions in the classroom, and teacher's aides or assistants may be needed to integrate the child into the classroom. Children with Angelman syndrome with attention deficits and hyperactivity need room to express themselves and to "grapple" with their hypermotoric activities. The classroom setting should be structured, in its physical design and its curricular program, so that the active child with Angelman syndrome can fit in or adjust to the school environment. Individualization and flexibility are important factors.

- Consistent behavior modification in the school and at home can enable the child with Angelman syndrome to be toilet trained (schedule trained) and to perform most self-help skills related to eating, dressing, and performing general activities in the home.

- Use of medications such as scopolamine patches or glycopyrrolate to dry secretions may be beneficial for drooling, but often these medications do not provide an adequate long-term effect (personal experience).

- Tongue protrusion is not so extensive that tongue reduction surgery is performed, although that is an option in severe cases. Likewise, surgical reimplantation of salivary gland ducts could be an option in cases of severe drooling, but this has yet to be reported in Angelman syndrome.

- Most affected people do not receive drug therapy for hyperactivity, and the hypermotoric behavior is tolerated, for better or worse, by the parents and the school (personal experience). Some parents report that changes in diet can affect activity levels, but no consistent dietary associations seem apparent. Some may benefit from use of stimulant medications such as methylphenidate, dexedrine, and Adderal, whereas others are given antihistamines such as diphenhydramine and hydroxyzine. Clonidine has also been used. Use of the phenothiazines as a sedating or calming drug is not recommended because of side effects.

- A structured environment, consistent behavioral modification, and often one-on-one personal interaction may be required in the school or home to deal with the hyperactivity and provide viable developmental training.
- Many families construct safe but confining bedrooms to accommodate disruptive nighttime wakefulness.
- Use of sedatives such a chloral hydrate or diphenhydramine (Benadryl) may be helpful if wakefulness excessively disrupts home life. Recently, administration of purified melatonin (0.3 mg) one hour before bedtime has been shown to be of help in some, but this should not be given in the middle of the night if the child wakes (Wagstaff, 1997). Customary dosing of routinely available melatonin uses higher dosing amounts, given at 3–5 mg per night (personal experience). Nevertheless, most infants and children with Angelman syndrome do not receive sleep medications, and those who do usually do not require long-term use.

Neurologic

Microcephaly. The prevalence of absolute microcephaly in deletion-positive individuals varies from 88% (Zori et al., 1992) to 34% (Saitoh et al., 1994) and may be as low as 25% when non-deletion cases are also included (Clayton-Smith and Pembrey, 1992). A significant proportion of affected individuals, however, will not develop microcephaly. Most individuals with Angelman syndrome have head circumference less than the 25th percentile by age 3 years, often accompanied by a flattened occiput. The brain in Angelman syndrome is structurally normal, although occasional abnormalities have been reported, including cerebellar hypoplasia, unilateral temporal lobe hypoplasia, and vermian cyst.

The most common MRI or CT changes, when any are present, are mild cortical atrophy, mild generalized ventriculomegaly, thin corpus callosum, and mildly decreased myelination (Zori et al., 1992; Buntinx et al., 1995). Several detailed microscopic and chemical studies of the brain in Angelman syndrome have been reported, but the findings generally have been nonspecific. Leonard et al. (1993) used MRI to study convolutional and gyral patterns in Angelman syndrome and Prader-Willi syndrome and found that people with Angelman syndrome had longer sylvian fissures and more anomalous gyral convolutions when compared to Prader-Willi syndrome. The significance of this remains to be further delineated and confirmed.

Severe microcephaly is very unusual; most have normal cranial growth rates in later childhood but maintain low percentiles or mild absolute microcephaly on the growth points.

Seizures. The seizure prevalence in Angelman syndrome has been reported to be as high as 90%, but this is probably an overestimation. Fewer than 25% develop seizures before 12 months of age; most have onset before 3 years, but initial occurrence in older children or in teenagers is not exceptional (Zori et al., 1992). Those with the large 15q11–q13 deletion may have intractable epilepsy, the most frequent being atypical absence or myoclonia type. Less frequently, generalized extensor tonic seizures or flexor spasms occur (Minassian et al., 1998). The seizures can be of any type and occur in all genotypic classes of Angelman syndrome. Most seizures are effectively controlled with anticonvulsants. At times, seizures may be difficult to recognize or distinguish from the child's usual tremulousness, hyperkinetic limb movements, or attention deficits.

Gait and movement disorders. In early childhood, the mildly impaired child can have almost normal walking. There may be only mild toe-walking or an apparent prancing gait. This may be accompanied by a tendency to lean or lurch forward. The tendency to lean forward is accentuated during running, and, in addition, the arms are held uplifted. For these children, balance and coordination does not appear to be a major problem. More severely affected children can be very stiff and robotlike or extremely shaky and jerky when walking. Voluntary movements are often irregular, varying from slight jerkiness to uncoordinated coarse movements that prevent walking, feeding, and reaching for objects. Although they can crawl fairly effectively, affected individuals may become rigid or appear anxious when placed in the standing position. The legs are kept wide based, and the feet are flat and turned outward. This, accompanied by uplifted arms, flexed elbows, and downward turned hands, produces the characteristic gait of Angelman syndrome. Most of those with Angelman syndrome are so ataxic and jerky that walking is often delayed until age 3 or 4 years (Zori et al., 1992; Buntinx et al.,1995), when they are better able to compensate motorically for the jerkiness; about 10% may fail to achieve walking (Clayton-Smith, 1993). Although many children with Angelman syndrome require a lengthy period of training and assistance, the prognosis for independent ambulation is good.

Evaluation

- Microcephaly in Angelman syndrome seems to be a reflection of generalized decrease in brain growth, so MRI and/or CT imaging does not appear warranted unless other factors (e.g., focal neurological findings or unexplained psychomotor regression) are present.

- An EEG is recommended during the early phase of diagnosis and treatment. EEGs do vary at different times, and apparently normal tracings, especially in young infants, are not infrequent. The typical EEG is often more abnormal than expected, and it may suggest seizures when in fact there appear to be none clinically. It usually has symmetrical high-voltage slow wave activity (4–6 cycles per second) persisting for most of the record and unrelated to drowsiness and very-large-amplitude slow activity at 2–3 cycles per second occurring in runs and more prominent anteriorly. In addition, spikes or sharp waves, mixed with large-amplitude 3–4 cycles per second components, are seen posteriorly and usually provoked by passive eye closure (Boyd et al., 1988; Sugimoto et al., 1992; Minassian et al., 1998).

- Orthopedic and physical and occupational therapy evaluations may be needed.

Treatment

- Educational strategies should be targeted to amelioration of effects of the developmental delay.

- There is no agreement as to the optimal seizure medication, but there are patterns of use that are more frequent. Anticonvulsant medications used for minor motor seizures (e.g., valproic acid, clonazepam, lamotrigine) are more commonly prescribed than those for major motor seizures (e.g., diphenylhydantoin, phenobarbital). Almost all people with Angelman syndrome have breakthrough seizures and seizure exacerbations. However, most are controlled with a single anticonvulsant medication, and the prognosis for adequate seizure control is good. Perhaps 10% will have clinically severe seizures that require multiple medications and periodic hospitalizations (personal experience). Many adults have infrequent seizures and can be tapered off medications, but, after a long period of abatement, seizures may recur. For many, seizure medications can be discontinued in the early adolescent or adult years.

- Some children with uncontrollable seizures have been placed on a ketogenic diet, and this has proved helpful in some but not all cases of intractable seizures (personal experience).

- Tremulous movements may be severe enough in themselves to require treatment and may improve with benzodiazepines; a recent report suggests a benefit with piracetam as adjunct treatment, but that medication is currently not available in the U.S. (Guerrini et al., 1996).
- Children with Angelman syndrome are at risk for medication overtreatment because their movement abnormalities or attention deficits can be mistaken for seizures and because EEG abnormalities can persist even when seizures are controlled.
- For some children with Angelman syndrome who have a cerebral palsy-like presentation there may be significant heel cord tightening, and tendon lengthening surgery can be helpful.
- Some have marked out-toeing and pes planus and thus have a valgus gait, often with subluxing ankles; ankle bracing is helpful, and some require surgical stabilization.
- Walkers are helpful for many until independent walking begins.
- Ongoing physical and occupational therapies are often needed throughout childhood. Physical therapy is usually helpful in improving ambulation. Scoliosis can develop in adolescence, is especially a problem in those who are nonambulatory and can be treated with early bracing to prevent progression; surgical correction or stabilization may be necessary for severe cases. Sometimes bracing or surgical intervention may be needed to properly align the legs.

Ophthalmologic

Surveys of patients with Angelman syndrome demonstrate a 30–60% incidence of strabismus. Strabismus appears to be more common in a number of genetic disorders that cause ocular hypopigmentation, because pigment in the retina is crucial to normal development of the optic nerve pathways. Long-term retinal function, anterior chamber function, and other measures of ocular health appear to be normal.

Evaluation

- Referral to an ophthalmologist is indicated for all affected individuals, regardless of genetic origin for the Angelman syndrome.

Treatment

- Management of strabismus in Angelman syndrome is similar to that in other children: evaluation by an ophthalmologist, correction of any visual deficit, and, where appropriate, patching and surgical adjustment of the extraocular muscles. The hypermotoric activities of some children with Angelman syndrome will make wearing of patches or glasses difficult. Surgical outcome for strabismus repair is probably equivalent to that in other conditions involving developmental delay; most cases are successful.

RESOURCES

Angelman Syndrome Foundation, USA National Office

414 Plaza Drive, Suite 209, Westmont, IL 60559
www-angelman.org
Tel: 1-800-432-6435
Fax: 212-779-7728

Internet Resources

Angelman Syndrome Link sites:
http://www.chem.ucsd.edu/asf
http://shell.idt.net/
Angelman Syndrome:
http://people.zeelandnet.nl/

Angelman Syndrome

http://www.castlegate.net/

Angelman syndrome information for families and professionals:

http://asclepius.com/angel/

Angels Among Us: Angelman Syndrome Information and Resources:

http://shell.idt.net/~julhyman/angel.htm

Dutch information (also English) and the "Angelman Photo Album":

http://people.zeelandnet.nl/fhof/angel-man.htm

lls sont aux anges! (French information—extensive):

http://www.mygale.org/02/angelman/

Organizzazione Sindrome di Angelman (Italian Angelman syndrome society):

http://www.netgroup.it/medico/orsa/

Norwegian Angelman syndrome page:

http://home.sol.no/hevo/angel.htm

ACKNOWLEDGMENTS

This document was developed in part with grant funding from the Raymond C. Philips Research and Education Contract, Children's Medical Services, Department of Health, State of Florida.

REFERENCES

American Society of Human Genetics/American College of Medical Genetics Test and Technology Transfer Committee. Diagnostic testing for Prader-Willi and Angelman syndromes (1996): Report of the ASHG/ACMG Test and Technology Transfer Committee. *Am J Hum Genet* 58:1085-1088.

Amos-Landgraf JM, Ji Y, Wandstrat AE, Driscoll DJ, Schwartz S, and Nicholls RD (1997) Recombination between large, transcriptionally active repeated elements at the proximal and distal breakpoints in Prader-Willi and Angelman syndromes. *Am J Hum Genet Supplement* 61S; (4):A3.

Bottani A, Robinson WP, DeLozier-Blanchet CD, Engel E, Morris MA, Schmitt B, Thun-Hohenstein L, Schinzel A (1994) Angelman syndrome due to paternal uniparental disomy of chromosome 15: A milder phenotype? *Am J Med Genet* 51:35–40.

Boyd SG, Harden A, Patton MA (1998) The EEG in early diagnosis of the Angelman (happy puppet) syndrome. *Eur J Pediatr* 147: 508–13.

Buntinx IM, Hennekam RCM, Brouwer OF, Stroink H, Beuten J, Mangelschots K, Fryns JP (1995) Clinical profile of Angelman syndrome at different ages. *Am J Med Genet* 56:176–183.

Clayton-Smith J, Pembrey ME (1992) Angelman syndrome. *J. Med Genet* 29:412–415.

Clayton-Smith J (1993) Clinical research on Angelman syndrome in the United Kingdom: Observations on 82 affected individuals. *Am J Med Genet* 46(1):12–15.

Fryburg JS, Breg WR, Lindgren V (1991) Diagnosis of Angelman syndrome in infants. *Am J Med Genet* 38:58-64.

Glenn CC, Saitoh S, Jong MTC, Filbrandt MM, Surti U, Driscoll DJ and Nicholls RD (1996) Expression, DNA methylation, and gene structure of the human *SNRPN* gene. *Am J Hum Genet* 58:335–346.

Guerrini R, De Lorey TM, Bonanni P, Moncla A, Dravet C, Suisse G, Livet MO, Bureau M, Malzac P, Genton P, Thomas P, Sartucci F, Simi P, Serratosa JM (1996) Cortical myoclonus in Angelman syndrome. *Ann Neurol* 40:39-48

Kishino T, Lalande M, Wagstaff J (1997) *UBE-3A/E6-AP* mutations cause Angelman syndrome. *Nat Genet* 15:70–73.

Knoll JHM, Nicholls RD, Magenis RE, Graham JM, Lalande M, Latt SA(1989) Angelman and Prader-Willi syndromes share a common chromosome 15 deletion but differ in parental origin of the deletion. *Am J Med Genet* 32:285–290.

Kubota T, Das S, Christian SL, Baylin SB, Herman JG, and Ledbetter DH (1997) Methylation-specific PCR simplifies imprinting analysis. *Nat Genet* 16:16–17.

Ledbetter D, Niikawa N (1994) Molecular and clinical study of 61 Angelman syndrome patients. *Am J Med Genet* 52:158–163.

Leonard CM, Williams CA, Nicholls RD, Agee OF, Voeller KK, Honeyman JC, Staab EV (1993) Angelman and Prader-Willi syndrome: A magnetic resonance imaging study of differences in cerebral structure. *Am J Med Genet* 46(1):26–33.

Malzac P, Webber H, Moncla A, Graham Jr JM, Kukolich M, Williams C, Pagon R, Ramsdell L, Kishino T, Wagstaff J (1998) Mutation analysis of *UBE3A* in Angelman syndrome patients. *Am J Hum Genet* 62: 1353–1360.

Matsuura T, Sutcliffe JS, Fang P, Galjaard RJ, Jiang YH, Benton CS, Rommens JM, Beaudet AL (1997) De novo truncating mutations in E6-AP ubiquitin-protein ligase gene (*UBE3A*) in Angelman syndrome. *Nat Genet* 15:74-77.

Minassian BA, DeLorey TM, Olsen RW, Philippart M, Bronstein Y, Zhang Q, Guerrini R, Van Ness P, Livet MO, Delgado-Escueta AV (1998) Angelman syndrome: Correlation between epilepsy phenotypes and genotypes. *Ann Neurol* 43:485–493.

Ohta T, Buiting K, Kokkonen H, McCandless S, Heeger S, Driscoll DJ, Cassidy SB, Horsthemke B, Nicholls RD (1999) Molecular mechanism of Angelman syndrome in two large families involves an imprinting mutation. *Am J Hum Genet* 64:385–386.

Petersen MB, Brondum-Nielsen K, Hansen LK, Wulff K (1995) Clinical, cytogenetic, and molecular diagnosis of Angelman syndrome: Estimated prevalence rate in a Danish county. *Am J Med Genet* 60:261–262.

Rougeulle C, Glatt H, Lalande M (1997) The Angelman syndrome candidate gene, *UBE3A/E6-AP*, is imprinted in brain. *Nat Genet* 17:14–15.

Saitoh S, Harada N, Jinno Y, Hashioto K, Imaizumi K, Kuroki Y, Fukushima Y, Sugimoto T, Renedo M, Wagstaff J, Lalande M, Mutirangura A, Kuwano A (1994) Molecular and clinical study of 61 Angelman syndrome patients. *Am J Med Genet* 52:158–63.

Smith-Thomas LC, Kent C, Mayer RJ, Scotting PJ (1994) Protein ubiquitination and neuronal differentiation in chick embryos. *Brain Res Dev Brain Res* 81:171–177.

Spritz, R. (1993) Molecular genetics of oculocutaneous albinism *Seminars Dermatol* 12(3): 167–172.

Stalker HJ, Williams CA (1998) Genetic counseling in Angelman syndrome: The challenges of multiple causes. *Am J Med Genet* 77:54–59.

Steffenburg S, Gillberg CL, Steffenburg U, Kyllerman M (1996) Autism in Angelman syndrome: A population-based study. *Ped Neurol* 14:131–135.

Sugimoto T, Yashuhara A, Ohta T, Nishida N, Saitoh S, Hamabe J, Niikawa N (1992) Angelman syndrome in three siblings: Characteristic epileptic seizures and EEG abnormalities, Epilepsia 33:1078–82.

Summers JA, Lynch PS, Harris JC, Burke JC, Allison DB, Sandler L (1992) A combined behavioral/pharmacological treatment of sleep-wake schedule disorder in Angelman syndrome. *Dev Behav Pediatr* 13(4):284–287.

Vu TH, Hoffman AR. (1997) Imprinting of the Angelman syndrome gene, *UBE3A*, is restricted to brain *Nat Genet* 17:12–13.

Wagstaff J (1997) Genetic and Clinical Studies of Angelman Syndrome. Angelman Syndrome Foundation Medical and Scientific Symposium. July 3, Seattle, Washington.

Whidden EM, Kubilis P, Marum T, Driscoll DJ, Zori R, Williams CA (1994) Growth in individuals with Angelman syndrome. *Am J Hum Genet* 55:3, A96.

Williams CA, Angelman H, Clayton-Smith J, Driscoll DJ, Hendrickson JE, Knoll JHM, Magenis RE, Schinzel A, Wagstaff J, Whidden EM, Zori RT (1995a) Angelman syndrome: Consensus for diagnostic criteria. *Am J Med Genet* 56:237–238.

Williams CA, Zori RT, Hendrickson JE, Stalker H, Marum T, Whidden EM, Driscoll DJ (1995b) Angelman syndrome. *Current Problems in Pediatrics* 25(7):216–231.

Zeeschnigk M, Lich C, Buiting K, Doerfler W, Horsthemke B (1997) A single-tube PCR test for the diagnosis of Angelman and Prader-Willi syndromes based on allelic methylation differences at the *SNRPN* locus. *Eur J Hum Genet* 5(2):94–98.

Zori RT, Hendrickson J, Woolven S, Whidden EM, Gray B, Williams CA (1992) Angelman syndrome: Clinical profile. *J Child Neurol* 7(3):279–280.

CHAPTER 4

BECKWITH-WIEDEMANN SYNDROME

ROSANNA WEKSBERG AND CHERYL SHUMAN

INTRODUCTION

Beckwith (1998a) has collated a comprehensive and entertaining history of overgrowth and related syndromes. In this review, he provides a translation of a case report from 1861 of a patient with features suggestive of Beckwith-Wiedemann syndrome and shows a ceramic figure from west Mexico dating back to 200 BC–200 AD with macroglossia and a possible umbilical defect. Although there were numerous early reports of individuals with features of Beckwith-Wiedemann syndrome, a syndromic designation awaited Beckwith's (1963) report of three unrelated children with exomphalos, hyperplasia of the kidneys and pancreas, and adrenal cytomegaly. The following year, Wiedemann (1964) published a report of siblings with exomphalos, macroglossia, and macrosomia. The triad of exomphalos, macroglossia, and gigantism was considered characteristic of this newly described syndrome, hence the designation EMG syndrome, now commonly referred to as Beckwith-Wiedemann syndrome or Wiedemann-Beckwith syndrome.

In 1822, Meckel first documented hemihypertrophy in the medical literature, whereas the first clinical case report by Wagner appeared in 1839 (cf. Ringrose et al., 1965). Hemihypertrophy, referring to increased cell size, was widely used until recently to describe "unilateral overgrowth of the body, including the structures of the head, trunk and limbs" (Viljoen et al., 1984). The term hemihyperplasia has replaced hemihypertrophy and refers to an abnormality of cell proliferation restricted to one or more regions of the body leading to asymmetric overgrowth (Cohen, 1989). Isolated hemihyperplasia is a diagnosis of exclusion, because hemihyperplasia can be associated with numerous genetic conditions (Hoyme et al., 1998) (see **Differential Diagnosis** below).

Incidence

The population incidence of Beckwith-Wiedemann syndrome is estimated to be 1 in 13,700, with equal incidence in males and females (Thornburn et al., 1970; Pettenati et al., 1986). This is likely an underestimate, as cases with milder phenotypes may not be diagnosed. For hemihyperplasia, incidence is estimated to be 1 in 86,000 (Parker and Skalko, 1969), with some authors reporting greater frequency in females (Ringrose et al., 1965; Hoyme et al., 1998).

Management of Genetic Syndromes, Edited by Suzanne B. Cassidy and Judith E. Allanson
ISBN 0-471-31286-X Copyright © 2001 by Wiley-Liss, Inc.

It appears that some cases of isolated hemihyperplasia may, in fact, represent cases of Beckwith-Wiedemann syndrome with reduced expressivity. Evidence for this view comes from several common associations with isolated hemihyperplasia: 1) increased birth weight (mean 3.8 kg) (Leisenring et al., 1994); 2) renal findings (medullary sponge kidney, abnormal collecting system) (Parker and Skalko, 1969; Tomooka et al., 1988); and 3) a well-documented increase in risk for embryonal tumor, especially Wilms tumor (Ringrose et al., 1965; Hoyme et al., 1998). In addition, preliminary data from molecular testing appear to support this theory in a portion of cases (see below).

Diagnostic Criteria

Consensus criteria are yet to be established for Beckwith-Wiedemann syndrome, but the presence of three or more of the findings detailed below is generally regarded as necessary to establish a firm diagnosis. Where there are fewer findings, such as macroglossia with umbilical hernia or isolated hemihyperplasia, the differential diagnosis should include possible Beckwith-Wiedemann syndrome and consideration should be given to offering screening for embryonal tumors, the more so because a fraction of Beckwith-Wiedemann syndrome cases demonstrate somatic mosaicism (see below).

Beckwith-Wiedemann syndrome is defined clinically by the presence of macrosomia (prenatal and/or postnatal gigantism), hemihyperplasia, macroglossia (typically present at birth but also reported to develop postnatally) (Chitayat et al., 1990b), abdominal wall defect (omphalocele, umbilical hernia, diastasis recti), embryonal tumors, adrenocortical cytomegaly, ear anomalies (anterior linear lobe creases, posterior helical pits), visceromegaly, renal abnormalities, and neonatal hypoglycemia (Pettenati et al., 1986; Weng et al., 1995a). Additional supportive findings may include polyhydramnios and prematurity, enlarged placenta, cardiomegaly and occasional structural cardiac anomalies, nevus flammeus or other hemangiomata, cleft palate, advanced bone age, and characteristic facies with midfacial hypoplasia and infraorbital creases (Fig. 4.1A). This characteristic facial appearance tends to regress over time, especially if macroglossia and the attendant prognathism is mild or treated (Fig. 4.1B). Most individuals with Beckwith-Wiedemann syndrome have a good prognosis for long-term physical health and development, but there remains a subgroup with serious and life-threatening findings. About 20% will die in the perinatal period of complications of prematurity, macroglossia, or, rarely, cardiomyopathy (Pettenati et al., 1986; Weng et al., 1995a).

When dealing with apparently isolated hemihyperplasia, one must distinguish hemiatrophy, in which the smaller body part is not normal but hypoplastic. Hemihyperplasia can involve a single organ or region of the body or several regions. When several regions are involved, these may be on one side of the body (ipsilateral) or opposite sides (contralateral). The degree of asymmetry is variable and may be rather mild in appearance. When asymmetry is limited to one limb, a measurable difference of greater than 1 cm in length should exist and/or a significant measurable difference in girth. Since hemihyperplasia can be very mild, there exists a clinical "gray zone" within which it is difficult to define the significance of asymmetry in some individuals because some degree of asymmetry exists in the normal population. Once asymmetric overgrowth is established, other additional findings may lead to a diagnosis of Beckwith-Wiedemann syndrome or to numerous other diagnoses (see **Differential Diagnosis**).

Etiology, Pathogenesis, and Genetics

Beckwith-Wiedemann syndrome is believed to be a complex, multigenic disorder caused by alterations in growth regulatory genes

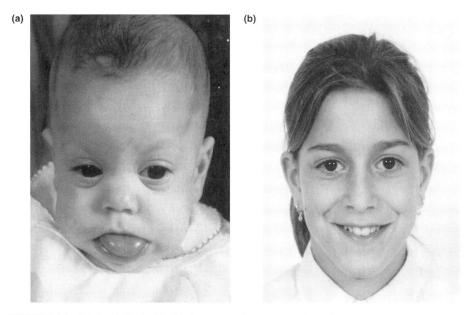

FIGURE 4.1. Child with Beckwith-Wiedemann syndrome at age 6 months (a) and at age 10 years (b).

on chromosome 11p15 (Fig. 4.2) (Li et al., 1997, 1998). The phenotypic variability in Beckwith-Wiedemann syndrome reflects its genetic heterogeneity. As a result, perhaps the most straightforward approach to understanding etiology involves grouping individuals with Beckwith-Wiedemann syndrome according to family history, karyotype, and molecular data. Each group highlights specific features of Beckwith-Wiedemann syndrome.

At present, Beckwith-Wiedemann syndrome can be categorized into eight distinct genetic groups (Table 4.1). A large proportion of Beckwith-Wiedemann syndrome cases, about 85%, are sporadic and karyotypically normal (groups A–D). Very few families are reported with chromosome abnormalities of 11p15 (groups E and F), yet 10–15% have autosomal dominant pedigrees (groups G and H) with demonstrated linkage, at least in some families, to chromosome 11p15. Therefore, a detailed family history is an important part of the initial evaluation. Because the phenotype may be variable even within a family, pedigree review

should survey parental birth weights, history of abdominal wall defect, increased tongue size or tongue surgery, and other features of Beckwith-Wiedemann syndrome. In adults, the most helpful physical features include hemihyperplasia, prominence of jaw, enlarged tongue, and ear creases and pits. Abdominal ultrasound may help to evaluate abnormalities of kidneys and other abdominal organs. Adult heights are usually normal, and other features may be quite subtle or even surgically altered; hence, early childhood photographs are very useful adjuncts to family assessment and estimation of recurrence risk.

Approximately 10–20% of patients with Beckwith-Wiedemann syndrome have paternal uniparental disomy (UPD), with two paternally derived copies of chromosome 11p15 and no maternal contribution for that region (group A). All patients with uniparental disomy exhibit somatic mosaicism. This implies that uniparental disomy arises postzygotically and may be found only in some tissues, e.g., in fibroblasts or renal tissue but not in lymphocytes. Because most somatic tissues are not available for testing,

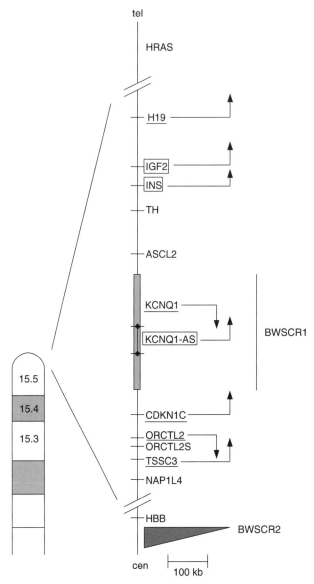

FIGURE 4.2. Map of 11p15. The arrows indicate transcriptional orientation. Underlined genes are preferentially expressed from the maternal allele; boxed elements are preferentially expressed from the paternal allele. Locations and sizes are approximate.

the quoted frequency of uniparental disomy in Beckwith-Wiedemann syndrome most certainly is an underestimate of the actual frequency.

In some groups of patients with Beckwith-Wiedemann syndrome there are effects on multiple genes (Fig. 4.3A). Both maternally expressed growth suppressor genes and paternally expressed growth promoter genes would be affected. Thus, in paternal uniparental disomy of 11p15, the Beckwith-Wiedemann syndrome clinical phenotype and tumor predisposition could be caused by the combination of increased expression of paternally expressed growth promoter genes (such as *IGF2*) and loss of maternally

TABLE 4.1. Beckwith-Wiedemann Syndrome: Genetic and Molecular Groups

Group Designation	Group Name	Frequency of BWS Cases in This Group (%)	Inherited/ Sporadic	Recurrence Risk to Parents of a Child with BWS
A	Paternal UPD	10–20	Sporadic	Low
B	MZ twins	<1	Sporadic	Low
C	*IGF2* loss of imprint	50–60	Unknown	Unknown
D	*KCNQ1-AS*	~50	Unknown	Unknown
E	11p15 chromosome translocation/ inversion	<1	Inherited or sporadic	May be as high as 50% if maternal translocation[1]
F	11p15 chromosome duplication	<1	Inherited or sporadic	Increased[1]
G	AD pedigrees[2] Normal karyotype	10–15	Inherited	May be as high as 50% with preferential maternal transmission[1]
H	*CDKN1C* mutations[2]	5–10	Usually inherited	May be as high as 50% with preferential maternal transmission[1]

Overall, 85% of Beckwith-Wiedemann syndrome (BWS) cases are sporadic and 15% are associated with vertical transmission; the subgroups listed in this table do not include all patients with BWS and are not mutually exclusive. [1]Specific figure not known. [2]These subgroups overlap. UPD, uniparental disomy; MZ, monozygous; AD, autosomal dominant.

expressed growth suppressor genes (such as *H19*). Figure 4.3B illustrates this model, depicting the gene dosages of paternally expressed growth promoter genes and maternally expressed growth suppressor genes.

Chromosomal rearrangements involving 11p15 are observed in which the inheritance pattern of the Beckwith-Wiedemann syndrome phenotype is influenced by the parent of origin. Translocations and inversions typically show inheritance from the maternal side (group E), whereas duplications are typically paternally inherited (group F).

Patients with 11p15 translocations or inversions exhibit typical features of Beckwith-Wiedemann syndrome. In contrast, patients with 11p15 duplications have more atypical clinical features as well as a significant risk of developmental delay (Waziri et al., 1983; Slavotinek et al., 1997). For this patient group, as well as for the uniparental disomy group, the model of an imbalance of growth promoter and growth suppressor genes could be applied (Fig. 4.3C).

The observations of uniparental disomy, preferential maternal transmission of Beckwith-Wiedemann syndrome in autosomal

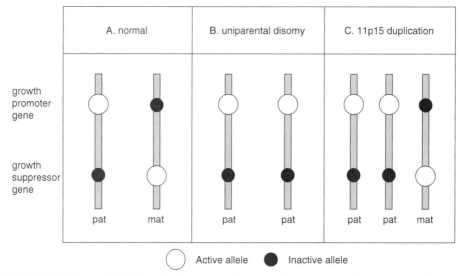

growth promoter gene

growth suppressor gene

○ Active allele ● Inactive allele

FIGURE 4.3. Effect of 11p15 duplication and uniparental disomy on growth promoter and growth suppressor gene expression.

dominant pedigrees, and parent-of-origin effects in chromosome abnormalities associated with Beckwith-Wiedemann syndrome, together provide convincing evidence that Beckwith-Wiedemann syndrome arises from alterations in imprinted genes on 11p15. Genomic imprinting is an epigenetic phenomenon whereby the two alleles of a gene are differentially modified such that only one parental allele, parent-specific for a given gene, is normally expressed (see page 5). During gametogenesis, imprinting marks from the previous generation are erased and imprinting is reset according to the sex of the current transmitting parent (Barlow, 1994). Imprinted genes cluster in distinct regions on chromosomes, and an imprinting center is believed to control resetting of a cluster of closely linked imprinted genes during transmission through the opposite sex (Nicholls, 1994).

The 11p15 region associated with Beckwith-Wiedemann syndrome spans 1000 kb containing several imprinted genes implicated in Beckwith-Wiedemann syndrome (Fig. 4.2). Our current understanding of the role of some of these imprinted genes in Beckwith-Wiedemann syndrome is outlined below (where possible, we have used gene names preferred by the Human Genome Organisation Nomenclature Committee).

IGF2. *IGF2* is a paternally expressed (maternally imprinted) embryonic growth factor. Disruption of *IGF2* imprinting (biallelic expression) (group C) has been observed in some patients with Beckwith-Wiedemann syndrome (Weksberg et al., 1993) as well as in multiple tumors, including Wilms (Ogawa et al., 1993; Rainier et al., 1993). Group C, in fact, represents a large proportion of Beckwith-Wiedemann syndrome cases. However, the significance of this finding is unknown. In theory, those patients with loss of imprinting of *IGF2* could have an imbalance of growth promoter with or without altered growth suppressor gene expression resulting in dysregulated growth (Li et al., 1998).

H19. *H19* is a maternally expressed gene encoding a biologically active nontranslated mRNA that may function as a tumor suppressor (Hao et al., 1993). Even when *IGF2* is biallelically expressed, expression of *H19* from the normal maternal allele is usually maintained in cases of Beckwith-Wiedemann syndrome (Weksberg et al., 1995). This may be due to hypermethylation with loss of expression (Joyce et al., 1997) at this locus.

CDKN1C. The *CDKN1C* gene (also known as *p57^{KIP2}*) is a member of the cyclin-dependent kinase inhibitor family acting to negatively regulate cell proliferation. It is both a tumor suppressor gene and a potential negative regulator of fetal growth. Both these functions and the imprinted expression of this gene suggested it as a candidate for a maternally expressed growth inhibitory gene in Beckwith-Wiedemann syndrome. Mutations in this gene have been reported in 5–10% of Beckwith-Wiedemann syndrome cases (group H) and appear to be associated with the clinical finding of omphalocele (Lam et al., 1999) and cleft palate (personal observation). Such mutations are found more frequently in cases with a positive family history (Hatada et al., 1996; O'Keefe et al., 1997). However, *CDKN1C* mutations have not been found for all cases of Beckwith-Wiedemann syndrome with dominant transmission (group G).

KCNQ1. The *KCNQ1* (also known as *KvLQT1*) gene product forms part of a potassium channel and has been implicated in at least two cardiac arrhythmia syndromes. *KCNQ1* is maternally expressed in most tissues, with the notable exception of the heart. It had been proposed that *KCNQ1* might serve as an imprinting center for the 11p15 region. Disruption of such an imprinting center could affect transcription and DNA replication through an effect on chromatin structure.

KCNQ1-AS. *KCNQ1-AS* is an imprinted transcript that is antisense to *KCNQ1* and may represent an additional imprinting control element in human 11p15.5 (Smilinich et al., 1999; Lee et al., 1999).

Other Imprinted Genes. *TSSC3* (also known as *IPL, BWRIC*) and *ORCTL2* (also known as *TSSC5, BWRIA, IMPT1*) are two

recently identified imprinted genes in the 11p15 region (Qian et al., 1997; Dao et al., 1998). Both genes show preferential maternal expression in the fetus and are located centromeric to *CDKN1C*. Although neither gene has been directly implicated in Beckwith-Wiedemann syndrome, both are hypothesized to have negative growth regulatory functions.

In some patient groups, the molecular etiology for Beckwith-Wiedemann syndrome remains unidentified. The underlying mutation may be in regions of known genes not currently screened by mutation analysis (Algar et al., 1999), or there may be mutations in other, independent genes.

An enigmatic clinical group among patients with Beckwith-Wiedemann syndrome (group B) consists of monozygotic ("identical") twin pairs, raising the possibility of a postzygotic mutation or recombination event. There have been approximately 20 such twin pairs reported, most commonly female and discordant for Beckwith-Wiedemann syndrome. However, a small number of male monozygotic twins discordant for Beckwith-Wiedemann syndrome, and both male and female monozygotic twin pairs concordant for Beckwith-Wiedemann syndrome, have been reported (Leonard et al., 1996). The excess number of female discordant monozygotic twins in Beckwith-Wiedemann syndrome may reflect temporally related developmental processes involving imprinting, X inactivation, and twinning (Lubinsky and Hall, 1991).

For apparently isolated hemihyperplasia, somatic mosaicism for paternal uniparental disomy may be the underlying molecular lesion. This hypothesis is supported by several observations including the risk of embryonal tumor development, the known spectrum of tumors, and certain clinical features (birth weight and renal findings) suggesting that at least a portion of patients with hemihyperplasia represent "mild" Beckwith-Wiedemann syndrome. Although chromosomal abnormalities have been associated with

TABLE 4.2. Diagnostic Testing

Karyotype	All children presenting with features of BWS should have a karyotype in a cytogenetic service laboratory, as there are prognostic implications if 11p15 duplication is present (see **Development**).
UPD of 11p15	Many molecular service laboratories now offer this; however, a negative result is not conclusive (see below).
CDKN1C (*p57^{KIP2}*)	This testing is currently available only on a research basis.

hemihyperplasia, molecular lesions have not been reported to date.

Elucidation of the molecular etiology of each Beckwith-Wiedemann syndrome clinical group is critical for the definition of recurrence risks for these families. The risk of recurrence for Beckwith-Wiedemann syndrome is believed to be low in the absence of clinical findings in either parent or of a positive family history. This risk clearly would be adjusted for those families presenting with autosomal dominant transmission, as well as for some individuals for whom a molecular etiology has been characterized. The risk for this latter group may be increased or decreased depending on the molecular finding (see **Diagnostic Testing**). More specific recurrence risks (Table 4.1) for individuals or families in certain of the Beckwith-Wiedemann syndrome clinical groups are discussed in **MANIFESTATIONS AND MANAGEMENT**. It is imperative, however, to ensure that the clinical features are not consistent with another overgrowth syndrome (such as Simpson-Golabi-Behmel syndrome), where the recurrence risk may be significantly higher.

The recurrence risk for isolated hemihyperplasia appears to be very low but would be dependent on the underlying etiology. Once again, caution must be used to rule out other associated genetic syndromes for families presenting with apparently isolated hemihyperplasia.

Diagnostic Testing

At this time, diagnostic testing is useful for confirming the diagnosis and for defining recurrence risks rather than for phenotype/genotype correlations and medical management issues (Table 4.2). One exception to this would involve the finding of a chromosome abnormality such as a duplication of 11p15, because this has a significant association with developmental delay (Slavotinek et al., 1997). Therefore, chromosomal analysis including high-resolution banding for chromosome 11p should be undertaken on all children with Beckwith-Wiedemann syndrome.

Uniparental disomy can be assessed by restriction fragment length polymorphism (RFLP) analysis of multiple 11p15 loci or by methylation studies of multiple imprinted genes on 11p15. Because all cases of uniparental disomy associated with Beckwith-Wiedemann syndrome reported to date involve somatic mosaicism, failure to detect uniparental disomy in one tissue (usually lymphocytes) is not conclusive. One should consider obtaining another tissue (such as skin), especially in the event of surgery. 11p15 uniparental disomy may be found in many tissues of patients with Beckwith-Wiedemann syndrome or may be limited to normal kidney tissue surrounding a Wilms tumor in a phenotypically normal child. The presence of mosaicism for 11p15 uniparental disomy would confer a low recurrence risk, as this results from a postzygotic event.

CDKN1C testing is currently available only through research laboratories. If a mutation in *CDKN1C* is found in a child with Beckwith-Wiedemann syndrome, the parents should be offered testing because this mutation carries a 50% risk of transmission. Although mutations in *CDKN1C* are usually maternally transmitted, both parents should be tested because there have been two cases of paternal transmission of a *CDKN1C* mutation associated with Beckwith-Wiedemann syndrome in the child (Lee et al., 1997b; personal data). If no mutation were found in either parent, prenatal testing for recurrence of a *CDKN1C* mutation remains an option in view of the theoretical possibility of gonadal mosaicism. There are no published data for such a situation in Beckwith-Wiedemann syndrome.

Currently, *IGF2* expression studies and *H19* methylation studies remain research tools and should not be considered part of the diagnostic work-up. *IGF2* expression studies can be undertaken only on tissues expressing *IGF2*, which include skin fibroblast samples, and only on those individuals informative (i.e., heterozygous) for transcribed *IGF2* polymorphisms.

With respect to *KCNQ1-AS*, testing is restricted to research laboratories and there are no data as yet regarding the significance of these findings or the associated recurrence risks.

Differential Diagnosis

There are a number of overgrowth syndromes that should be considered in the differential diagnosis of children presenting with macrosomia or other features of Beckwith-Wiedemann syndrome. The possibility of maternal diabetes mellitus during pregnancy should be considered and investigated. In addition, other features not commonly associated with Beckwith-Wiedemann syndrome might suggest other diagnoses. Some children with hypotonia appear to have enlarged tongues. Especially when developmental delay is present, other diagnoses should be seriously considered. Several syndromes with phenotypes overlapping that of Beckwith-Wiedemann syndrome are discussed below. Some cases involving overgrowth do not fit into any of these defined

syndromes; clearly, other new overgrowth syndromes remain to be defined.

Simpson-Golabi-Behmel syndrome shares the following features with Beckwith-Wiedemann syndrome: macrosomia, visceromegaly, macroglossia, and renal cysts. Findings unique to Simpson-Golabi-Behmel syndrome that do not occur in Beckwith-Wiedemann syndrome include coarse features, cleft lip, high frequency of cardiac defects (Lin et al., 1999), supernumerary nipples, polydactyly, and other skeletal anomalies. Simpson-Golabi-Behmel syndrome, like Beckwith-Wiedemann syndrome, has an increased risk of neonatal mortality, and an increased risk for developing embryonal tumors, including Wilms tumor. The actual risk figure for tumor development has not been quantified. Simpson-Golabi-Behmel syndrome is caused by mutations in an X-linked gene, *GPC3*, encoding an extracellular proteoglycan (glypican-3) believed to function in growth control regulation during development (Weksberg et al., 1996; Neri, 1998).

Perlman syndrome is defined by macrosomia, increased risk of neonatal mortality, mental retardation, nephroblastomatosis, and a high incidence of bilateral Wilms tumor, occurring usually in the first year of life. There is a characteristic facial appearance: round face, upsweep of anterior scalp hair, depressed nasal bridge, and micrognathia. At present, the molecular basis of Perlman syndrome is unknown, but it likely represents a distinct genetic entity in light of its autosomal recessive inheritance (Greenberg et al., 1986; Grundy et al., 1992).

Costello syndrome overlaps clinically with Beckwith-Wiedemann syndrome only in the neonatal period, with patients presenting with overgrowth, cardiac defects, and edema. These patients can easily be distinguished from Beckwith-Wiedemann syndrome patients over time by their distinctive facial coarsening and failure to thrive (Johnson et al., 1998; van Eeghen et al., 1999).

Hemihyperplasia may be a feature of a number of syndromes other than Beckwith-Wiedemann syndrome, including neurofibromatosis type I (see Chapter 14), Klippel-Trenaunay-Weber syndrome, Proteus syndrome, McCune-Albright syndrome, epidermal nevus syndrome, triploid/diploid mixoploidy, Maffucci syndrome, and osteochondromatosis or Ollier disease (Hoyme et al., 1998).

MANIFESTATIONS AND MANAGEMENT

In many cases, absolute frequencies for the clinical features associated with Beckwith-Wiedemann syndrome are not well documented. The figures vary widely in published reports; some of the variability may be due to overlap with Simpson-Golabi-Behmel syndrome and some to ascertainment bias. Therefore, the features listed below will in many instances be presented as approximate frequencies.

Growth and Feeding

A large percentage (87%) of individuals with Beckwith-Wiedemann syndrome have birth weights and lengths around the 97th centile for gestational age (Weng et al., 1995a). However, onset of rapid growth can occur from the prenatal period to as late as one year of age in some cases (personal experience). Overgrowth is not an absolute requisite for clinical diagnosis. Head circumference varies in that there may be a large head in keeping with other growth parameters, or relative microcephaly. As long as the head circumference remains in the normal range, relative microcephaly does not correlate with poor developmental outcome.

The increased rate of somatic growth typically continues through the first few years of life. Growth generally parallels the normal growth curve (Pettenati et al., 1986), with bone age often at the upper limits of normal. In some studies, growth rate decreases somewhat beyond midchildhood (Weng et al., 1995a). Adult heights cluster between the 50th and 97th centiles (Pettenati et al., 1986; Weng et al., 1995a).

Hemihyperplasia occurs in about 25% of Beckwith-Wiedemann syndrome cases; it may not be evident at birth and may become more marked in the first few years of life (Elliott et al., 1994a). Hemihyperplasia of the face, either as part of Beckwith-Wiedemann syndrome or isolated, should be carefully distinguished from plagiocephaly (asymmetric cranial shape). If plagiocephaly is labeled hemihyperplasia, then an increased risk for tumor development would be inappropriately applied.

Macroglossia can occasionally lead to serious difficulties with respect to feeding.

Evaluation

- Height, weight, and head circumference should be measured annually. Familial heights, especially parental, should be obtained and considered in determining whether macrosomia is truly present. A bone age may assist in predicting adult height.
- If hemihyperplasia is observed, measurements of affected regions such as limbs should be taken regularly, including both length and girth. If the leg length discrepancy is greater than 1 cm, referral to orthopedics is indicated.
- It is important to follow these children over several years to evaluate relative growth potential of the two limbs so that surgical treatment, if necessary, can be carried out at the optimal time.
- If the hemihyperplasia involves the limbs or trunk, examination for possible scoliosis should be undertaken.

Treatment

- There is no specific treatment recommended for macrosomia.
- For children with leg length discrepancy, annual follow-up through orthopedics

during childhood is important to determine whether surgical intervention is indicated during puberty.

- Epiphysiodesis of the hyperplastic leg may be considered when that leg attains the final length predicted for the other.
- Significant facial hemihyperplasia may require referral to a craniofacial surgeon.
- Feeding difficulties encountered because of macroglossia may be ameliorated by use of a longer nipple such as those used for babies with cleft palate; rarely, nasogastric tube feedings are indicated for a period of time.

Development and Behavior

Contrary to early reports, development is usually normal for individuals with Beckwith-Wiedemann syndrome unless there are serious complications associated with prematurity, a period of uncontrolled or undetected hypoglycemia, or chromosomal duplication involving 11p15. Individuals with molecular findings of uniparental disomy for 11p15 or *CDKN1C* mutations do not generally exhibit developmental delay. Some parents have commented that their children with Beckwith-Wiedemann syndrome are behaviorally different from their other children; however, this was not confirmed in a small sample (personal observation). For isolated hemihyperplasia, which is clearly etiologically heterogeneous, an increased incidence of developmental delay (15–20%) has been reported (Viljoen et al., 1984; Ringrose et al., 1965). There may be some ascertainment bias in this figure, as hemihyperplasia is more likely to be identified if there are other associated findings such as developmental delay. The association of hemihyperplasia and developmental delay may be due to an underlying genetic syndrome or to somatic mosaicism for a chromosome abnormality.

Evaluation

- Developmental screening evaluation should be part of every routine visit for children with Beckwith-Wiedemann syndrome.
- Individuals with developmental delay associated with Beckwith-Wiedemann syndrome or hemihyperplasia should be carefully evaluated for related syndromes or for chromosome abnormalities (for the latter group, this may include chromosome studies of the skin).
- Those with developmental delay should have a careful, complete developmental assessment.

Treatment

- Any individual with developmental delay associated with Beckwith-Wiedemann syndrome and/or hemihyperplasia should be offered standard interventions such as infant stimulation programs, occupational and physical therapy, and individualized education programs.

Cardiovascular

Much of the information regarding cardiovascular problems in Beckwith-Wiedemann syndrome is anecdotal. The reported incidence of structural cardiac malformations ranges from 9% to 34%, with about one-half involving cardiomegaly (Pettenati et al., 1986; Elliott et al., 1994a). Cardiomyopathy has been rarely reported.

Cardiomegaly of early infancy in Beckwith-Wiedemann syndrome usually resolves spontaneously. Cardiomyopathies in these children can be severe and lethal despite current interventions. The prognosis for other structural cardiac anomalies depends on the specific defect identified and current treatment options.

Evaluation

- In cases of Beckwith-Wiedemann syndrome, there should be a high index of suspicion for cardiac problems and standard cardiac evaluation should precede any surgical or dental procedure.

- If a cardiac abnormality is suspected on clinical evaluation, a comprehensive and systematic cardiac evaluation would be recommended, including ECG and echocardiogram.
- If a conduction defect is found, the possibility that the diagnosis is Costello syndrome or Simpson-Golabi-Behmel syndrome should be considered.

Treatment

- Treatment of cardiac abnormalities is the same as in the general population for the specific cardiac abnormality detected.

Pregnancy and Perinatal Period

Pregnancies with affected fetuses are associated with a high incidence (~50%) of premature births (Weng et al., 1995a), polyhydramnios (~50%) and fetal macrosomia (~90%) (Elliott et al., 1994b). Other notable features of many births of babies with Beckwith-Wiedemann syndrome are enlarged placentae, with many averaging almost twice the normal weight for gestational age (Weng et al., 1995a), and long umbilical cords.

Prognosis depends on the severity of the presenting perinatal problems. An increased perinatal mortality rate (~20%) is associated with Beckwith-Wiedemann syndrome (Pettenati et al., 1986; Weng et al., 1995a).

Evaluation

- Fetal evaluations in pregnancies with suspected fetal Beckwith-Wiedemann syndrome should include serial ultrasounds and biophysical profiles.
- Because of the increased risk of fetal macrosomia and maternal preeclampsia and eclampsia, women suspected to be carrying a fetus with Beckwith-Wiedemann syndrome should be closely monitored and perinatal management should be undertaken in a high-risk unit.

- Level II ultrasound at 19–20 weeks and again at 32 weeks gestation as well as serum α-fetoprotein (at 16 weeks gestation) could be offered to parents of a child with Beckwith-Wiedemann syndrome in subsequent pregnancies or for pregnancies undertaken by an individual with Beckwith-Wiedemann syndrome. Ultrasound screening, in conjunction with α-fetoprotein screening, should be used to look for an abdominal wall defect. Ultrasound can also be used to assess growth parameters advanced for gestational age (likely not detectable until late in the second trimester) and to detect organomegaly, renal anomalies, cleft palate, cardiac abnormality, and macroglossia. In addition, there has been one report of an early ultrasound, between 10 and 14 weeks gestation, revealing increased nuchal translucency thickness and exomphalos in a fetus later found to have Beckwith-Wiedemann syndrome (Souka et al., 1998).
- If a molecular lesion has been identified (e.g., *CDKN1C* mutation), the possibility of prenatal diagnosis by chorionic villus sampling (CVS) or amniocentesis may be considered. Some families may wish to undertake such testing for pregnancy and delivery management and others possibly to decide whether or not to continue with the pregnancy. Even in the absence of obvious clinical findings on prenatal investigation, the newborn should be considered at risk and monitored for hypoglycemia as outlined above.

Treatment

- When Beckwith-Wiedemann syndrome is suspected in pregnancy, delivery planning should anticipate the possible perinatal complications such as polyhydramnios, prematurity, macrocephaly, large birth weight, omphalocele, macroglossia, and hypoglycemia.

BECKWITH-WIEDEMANN SYNDROME

Less frequent complications may include hypocalcemia or polycythemia.

- Management may need to include the delivery of an infant with an omphalocele. Thus it is preferable to plan the delivery in a center equipped to handle these issues.

Endocrine

Hypoglycemia is reported to occur in approximately 30–50% of babies with Beckwith-Wiedemann syndrome (Pettenati et al., 1986; Engstrom et al., 1988). The underlying cause of the hypoglycemia appears to be hyperinsulinemia and islet cell hyperplasia. This may be related to 11p15 uniparental disomy and/or other mechanisms involved in dysregulation of genes on 11p15. Mosaicism for 11p15 uniparental disomy is in fact the underlying pathogenetic mechanism in focal nesidioblastosis of the pancreas (de Lonlay et al., 1997).

No data are available concerning long-term outcome of hypoglycemia associated with Beckwith-Wiedemann syndrome. In general, children without Beckwith-Wiedemann syndrome who have hypoglycemia have significantly smaller head circumferences and more neurological deficits, including lower IQ scores at 5–7 years of age than their unaffected counterparts. Neonates with seizures due to hypoglycemia tend to have the worst overall neurological prognosis (Halamek and Stevenson, 1998). Newborns with asymptomatic hypoglycemia, although not completely without risk for sequelae, have the best prognosis. None of these studies adequately assesses the risks faced by neonates who do not experience seizure activity (Halamek and Stevenson, 1998).

Other abnormal laboratory findings noted in patients with Beckwith-Wiedemann syndrome include polycythemia (19.5%), hypocalcemia (4.6%), hypercholesterolemia, or hyperlipidemia (2.3%) (Engstrom et al., 1988). Hypothyroidism has been reported in several cases of Beckwith-Wiedemann syndrome (Martinez y Martinez et al., 1985).

Evaluation

- Any neonate suspected of having Beckwith-Wiedemann syndrome should be screened for hypoglycemia for the first few days of life. Serial blood glucose measurements to detect asymptomatic hypoglycemia as well as frequent examination for clinical signs of symptomatic hypoglycemia are recommended for neonates with Beckwith-Wiedemann syndrome. For term infants, plasma glucose concentrations <30 mg/dL in the first 24 hours of life and <45 mg/dL thereafter are abnormal. Although it has been suggested that preterm infants may require less glucose than term infants, it is recommended that the same plasma glucose concentrations be maintained in preterm neonates (Halamek and Stevenson, 1998).

- If early discharge is planned, parents should be advised about the typical clinical manifestations of hypoglycemia and health care professionals should ensure that rapid access to medical care is available.

- If hypoglycemia persists beyond the first few days, evaluation by a pediatric endocrinologist is suggested.

- A high index of suspicion should be maintained for hypocalcemia and hypothyroidism.

Treatment

- Either oral or IV glucose should be administered while awaiting laboratory confirmation of hypoglycemia if clinical manifestations of hypoglycemia are present.

- Any patient treated for hypoglycemia should be carefully followed with serial glucose determinations at 15- to

30-min intervals until the level rises to 60–100 mg/dL.

- If hypoglycemia persists, referral to a pediatric endocrinologist is advised because hypoglycemia in a small number of cases can be very refractory to baseline treatment.

- A number of drugs, such as diazoxide or somatostatin, can be used for refractory cases (Halamek and Stevenson, 1998).

- Early intervention for hypocalcemia or hypothyroidism is indicated. Treatment for these issues is not known to be different from treatment in patients without Beckwith-Wiedemann syndrome.

Craniofacial

Distinctive facial features of Beckwith-Wiedemann syndrome include macroglossia, anterior ear lobe creases and posterior helical pits, facial nevus flammeus, and prominent eyes with infraorbital creases. Macroglossia can occasionally lead to serious difficulties with respect to feeding and respiratory complications. Macroglossia may also lead to difficulties with speech articulation. Later childhood problems may include malocclusion, as mandibular (or lower jaw) growth accelerates in response to tongue size. In addition, hemihyperplasia may affect one side of the face and/or tongue, which may lead to an asymmetric appearance.

Evaluation

- Issues related to facial appearance are optimally assessed by a multidisciplinary team including plastic surgeons, speech pathologists, and orthodontists. It is recommended that these health care providers have experience with the natural history of children with Beckwith-Wiedemann syndrome to anticipate growth patterns and potential long-term impact of macroglossia and/or hemihyperplasia so that medical, dental, and surgical interventions can be optimally planned.

- Concerns about speech difficulties due to macroglossia should be assessed by a speech pathologist familiar with the macroglossia associated with Beckwith-Wiedemann syndrome and its natural history.

Treatment

- Children with only mild to moderate macroglossia tend to be able to accommodate their tongues as their facial bone structures grow, so that they can keep their tongues fully in their mouths.

- Partial tongue resection is generally considered for children encountering orthodontic and/or cosmetic concerns that have not resolved by preschool ages. Children anticipated to require such intervention should be followed longitudinally by a craniofacial team as noted above. Rarely, tongue resection may be required at an earlier age because of severe airway obstruction (Weng et al., 1995b).

- Many procedures have been described for tongue reduction. The most common involve excision of either the central portion of the tongue or excision of the anterior portion. Excision of the central portion is indicated when the goal is primarily to reduce the central thickness of the tongue. On the other hand, excision of the anterior portion is indicated when tongue protrusion, with its associated problems related to aesthetics, speech, and mandibular deformities, is the primary problem. Neither approach is perfect, but both can be of assistance aesthetically and functionally. Early complications include bleeding and dehiscence, as well as respiratory obstruction with postoperative swelling. Late complications range from an ankylosed, misshapen tongue to an organ that remains thick and, with the resultant scarring, has less mobility than required. Fortunately, these complications are unusual, although they are of significance when they occur (Zuker, personal communication).

- Orthodontic treatment as well as plastic surgery may be considered to alter a prognathic appearance.
- Implementation of therapeutic exercises for the tongue has not been successful (personal experience).

Gastrointestinal and Other Abdominal

Abdominal wall defects are a very common finding in children with Beckwith-Wiedemann syndrome. These defects include omphalocele, umbilical hernia, and diastasis recti. Other less common findings are inguinal hernia, prune belly sequence, and gastrointestinal malformations including atresia, stenosis, and malrotation.

Visceromegaly is a common finding and may involve any or all of the following: liver, spleen, pancreas, kidneys, and adrenals. Adrenocortical cytomegaly is a cardinal feature of Beckwith-Wiedemann syndrome. Renal findings are further discussed in a separate section below. Functional problems associated with enlarged liver and spleen are generally not reported. However, hyperplastic changes in the pancreas are associated with the hypoglycemia seen in this condition.

Diaphragmatic eventration, which is uncommon, may be detected during ultrasound screening for embryonal tumors.

The outcome for omphalocele surgery for children with Beckwith-Wiedemann syndrome depends on the size of the defect and whether or not the liver is involved. In addition, the prognosis may be affected by the presence of associated medical and surgical complications. Early detection and surgical intervention of gastrointestinal malformations are important for a good outcome.

Evaluation

- Evaluation for abdominal wall defects and visceromegaly includes standard physical examination as well as ultrasound. This should be undertaken at the time of diagnosis.
- There should be a high index of suspicion for gastrointestinal malformations, which may require imaging of the tract for diagnosis of stenosis, atresia, or malrotation.

Treatment

- Usually, abdominal wall defects and gastrointestinal malformations are amenable to early closure with a good prognosis. Standard surgical intervention is indicated.
- Surgical risks may result from hypoglycemia or intubation difficulties related to macroglossia, as well as to any findings detected on prior assessment, such as cardiac abnormalities.

Genitourinary

Patients with Beckwith-Wiedemann syndrome frequently have renal anomalies, including nephromegaly, which may be unilateral or bilateral. Reports also note the following findings: renal medullary dysplasia, duplicated collecting system, nephrocalcinosis, medullary sponge kidney, cystic changes, hydronephrosis, nephrolithiasis, and diverticulae (Choyke et al., 1998; Borer et al., 1999).

Prognosis for renal function is generally good. However, it is important to identify those individuals at high risk for loss of renal function from congenital malformation, nephrocalcinosis, medullary sponge kidney, or medullary dysplasia. Active surveillance and appropriate treatment are required to maximize long-term renal function.

Enlargement of the bladder, uterus, phallus, clitoris, ovaries, and testes has been reported. The natural history of other genitourinary organomegalies is not well documented but has not been reported as problematic. Given the natural history of other types of somatic overgrowth in Beckwith-Wiedemann syndrome, surveillance without active intervention should be the first course of action.

Evaluation

- Serial ultrasound in patients with Beckwith-Wiedemann syndrome is valuable not only for tumor surveillance but also to assess the integrity of the renal tract.
- If congenital malformations are identified, further imaging studies may be indicated.
- Referral to a pediatric nephrologist and/or urologist is appropriate if such malformations are identified.
- If there is evidence of calcium deposition on ultrasound screening, evaluation of urinary calcium excretion (calcium-to-creatinine ratio) is indicated.
- Prospective studies are underway to evaluate whether patients with Beckwith-Wiedemann syndrome over 8 years of age should continue to have annual clinical assessments along with renal ultrasounds. The primary reason for this is to define the risk of developing renal changes that require medical intervention, such as nephrocalcinosis or medullary sponge kidney. The risk for such renal complications is believed to be low.

Treatment

- Surgical intervention may be indicated for congenital malformations of the renal tract, as for the general population.
- If abnormalities of urinary calcium-to-creatinine ratio are found, referral to a pediatric nephrologist is recommended.
- Treatment consists first of increased fluid intake with possible addition of diuretics.

Neoplasia

Children with Beckwith-Wiedemann syndrome and/or hemihyperplasia are predisposed to certain malignancies (Sotelo-Avila et al., 1980; Wiedemann, 1983; Pettenati et al., 1986). The overall risk for tumor development in individuals with Beckwith-Wiedemann syndrome is estimated to be 7.5% (Wiedemann, 1983). For the two most common tumors, Wilms tumor and hepatoblastoma, the general population risks are 1 in 10,000 and 1 in 100,000, respectively. Most of the increased tumor risk for both Beckwith-Wiedemann syndrome and isolated hemihyperplasia is in the first 5–8 years of life.

The tumors reported in Beckwith-Wiedemann syndrome consist primarily of embryonal tumors such as Wilms tumor, hepatoblastoma, rhabdomyosarcoma, adrenocortical carcinoma, and neuroblastoma. Also seen are a wide variety of other tumors, both malignant and benign (Sotelo-Avila et al., 1980; Wiedemann, 1983). Several factors appear to be associated with tumor development in Beckwith-Wiedemann syndrome. These include the presence of hemihyperplasia (Wiedemann, 1983), nephromegaly (DeBaun et al., 1998), and nephrogenic rests or nephroblastomatosis (Coppes et al., 1999). Beckwith proposed the terms "nephrogenic rest" for a focus of abnormally persistent nephrogenic cells that can be induced to form a Wilms tumor and "nephroblastomatosis" for the diffuse or multifocal presence of nephrogenic rests (Beckwith et al., 1990).

For children with isolated hemihyperplasia, the risk for tumors is reported to be approximately 5.9% (Hoyme et al., 1998). The anatomic site of the tumor does not always correlate with the laterality of the hemihyperplasia (Hoyme et al., 1998). For hemihyperplasia, the reported range of tumor types overlaps significantly with that of Beckwith-Wiedemann syndrome (Hoyme et al., 1998). This suggests that some individuals with hemihyperplasia may represent a *forme fruste* of Beckwith-Wiedemann syndrome and that the majority of tumors arise from genetic events that overlap the underlying mechanisms responsible for Beckwith-Wiedemann syndrome. However some tumors, such as leiomyosarcoma, are more likely to be related to disorders other than Beckwith-Wiedemann syndrome.

Although the oldest patient with Beckwith-Wiedemann syndrome who had a Wilms tumor detected was 10 years 2 months, 96% of all Wilms tumors in a series of 121 Beckwith-Wiedemann syndrome cases presented by 8 years (Beckwith, 1998b). In one study, the outcome in children with Beckwith-Wiedemann syndrome was not improved through regular abdominal ultrasound screening (Craft et al., 1995). More recently, however, another report found that a regular screening protocol reduced the percentage of stage III and IV Wilms tumors (Choyke et al., 1999). As imaging studies improve, the need for invasive follow-up investigation resulting from such screening (Choyke et al., 1999) should be considerably reduced.

No specific data are available for long-term survival of children with Beckwith-Wiedemann syndrome and tumors. In general, it is appropriate to counsel patients with Beckwith-Wiedemann syndrome and Wilms tumor, hepatoblastoma, or other tumors that the prognosis is not known to be different in children with Beckwith-Wiedemann syndrome than in those without Beckwith-Wiedemann syndrome. Although one study reported a better prognosis for 10 children with Beckwith-Wiedemann syndrome and Wilms tumor than for Wilms tumor alone (Vaughan et al., 1995), in another small cohort there was no difference in prognosis for these two groups (personal experience). Prognosis is generally very good (>80%) for long-term survival; the best prognostic indicators are smaller tumor size (Breslow et al., 1991), absence of anaplasia, and absence of metastatic spread.

Evaluation

- It is recommended that children with suspected or diagnosed Beckwith-Wiedemann syndrome or isolated hemihyperplasia be followed on a 3-month basis with abdominal ultrasound until the age of 8 years (Beckwith 1998b).
- Common ultrasound findings include hepatomegaly, nephromegaly, and splenomegaly. As ultrasound technology continues to improve, findings such as "bulky" pancreas and/or mesenteric nodes may be detected. Generally, the above findings are not associated with neoplasm but should be carefully followed for several intervals of ultrasound screening.
- Masses detected in the liver or kidney must be distinguished from malformations such as hemangioma. Depending on the type of lesion, appropriate imaging studies such as CT or MRI can be used for better definition.
- In this context, a baseline CT or MRI has been recommended for patients entering a tumor surveillance program (Clericuzio et al., 1992; Beckwith 1998b).
- Consultation with an oncologist and/or relevant subspecialist may be useful to evaluate specific imaging findings.
- If nephrogenic rests are detected or suspected, careful follow-up should be undertaken. In future, better MRI technology should facilitate visualization of macroscopic nephrogenic rests (Gylys-Morin et al., 1993), possibly identifying the subgroup of patients with Beckwith-Wiedemann syndrome at increased risk for Wilms tumor.
- In some centers, parents are advised to perform abdominal palpation for tumor surveillance. Some concern has been raised that this might place undue pressure on the parent-child relationship and lead to added feelings of guilt in the event that a mass were not detected via palpation. However, some parents may in fact feel empowered by becoming involved in this manner in their child's medical management.

- Screening for neuroblastoma with urinary homovanillic acid (HVA) and vanillylmandelic acid (VMA) (Chitayat et al., 1990a) as well as chest X ray has been suggested, but these are generally not incorporated into baseline tumor screening protocols because of the relatively low risk for this tumor.

- α-Fetoprotein (AFP) can be used as an additional marker in the first few years of life for early detection of hepatoblastoma. α-Fetoprotein levels tend to be somewhat higher in children with Beckwith-Wiedemann syndrome in the first year of life (Everman, in press), but the most important indicator for management is to determine whether the α-fetoprotein is falling or rising. If α-fetoprotein is elevated, a high index of suspicion must be maintained. The authors suggest early follow-up at a one-month interval with repeat α-fetoprotein (to determine whether it is falling), liver function studies, and repeat imaging including chest X ray. In any case of a rising α-fetoprotein, an exhaustive search for an underlying tumor, including germ cell tumors, is indicated. Consultation with an oncologist may also be useful.

Treatment

- For all tumors detected, treatment follows standard oncology protocols with the added caveat that these children are at risk for second primaries.

- Children with Beckwith-Wiedemann syndrome do not appear to show increased sensitivity to chemotherapeutic agents, and the nephrogenic rests in the kidneys of these children show a marked reduction in size in response to chemotherapy (Regalado et al., 1997).

- Treatment should be aimed at preserving as much functional renal tissue as possible.

RESOURCES

Beckwith-Wiedemann Support Network

2711 Colony Road, Ann Arbor, MI 48104
Tel: 734-973-0263
Fax: 734-973-9721
Parents toll-free 1-800-837-2976

REFERENCES

Algar EM, Deeble GJ, Smith, PJ (1999) *CDKN1C* expression in Beckwith-Wiedemann syndrome patients with allele imbalance. *J Med Genet* 36:524–531.

Barlow DP (1994) Imprinting: a gamete's point of view. *Trends Genet* 10:194–199.

Beckwith JB (1963) Extreme cytomegaly of the adrenal fetal cortex, omphalocele, hyperplasia of kidneys and pancreas, and Leydig-cell hyperplasia: Another syndrome? Abstract, Western Society for Pediatric Research, Los Angeles, November 11, 1963.

Beckwith JB, Kiviat NB, Bonadio JF (1990) Nephrogenic rests, nephroblastomatosis, and the pathogenesis of Wilms' tumor. *Pediatr Pathol* 10:1–36.

Beckwith JB (1998a) Vignettes from the history of overgrowth and related syndromes. *Am J Med Genet* 79:238–248.

Beckwith JB (1998b) Nephrogenic rests and the pathogenesis of Wilms tumor: Developmental and clinical considerations. *Am J Med Genet* 79:268–273.

Borer JG, Kaefer M, Barnewolt CE, Elias ER, Hobbs N (1999) Renal findings on radiological followup of patients with Beckwith-Wiedemann syndrome. *J Urol* 161:235–239.

Breslow N, Sharples K, Beckwith JB, Takashima J, Kelalis PP, Green DM, D'Angio GJ (1991) Prognostic factors in nonmetastatic, favorable histology Wilms' tumor. Results of the Third National Wilms' Tumor Study. *Cancer* 68:2345–2353.

Chitayat D, Friedman JM, Dimmick JE (1990a) Neuroblastoma in a child with Wiedemann-Beckwith syndrome. *Am J Med Genet* 35:433–436.

Chitayat D, Rothchild A, Ling E, Friedman JM, Couch RM, Yong SL, Baldwin VJ, Hall JG

(1990b) Apparent postnatal onset of some manifestations of the Wiedemann-Beckwith syndrome. *Am J Med Genet* 36:434–439.

Choyke PL, Siegel MJ, Craft, AW, Green, DM, DeBaun MR (1999) Screening for Wilms tumor in children with Beckwith-Wiedemann syndrome or idiopathic hemihypertrophy. *Med Pediatr Oncol* 32:196–200.

Choyke PL, Siegel MJ, Oz O, Sotelo-Avila C, DeBaun MR (1998) Nonmalignant renal disease in pediatric patients with Beckwith-Wiedemann syndrome. *Am J Roentgenol* 171:733–737.

Cohen MM Jr. (1989) In Harris H and Hirschhorn K, eds. *Advances in Human Genetics*, New York: Plenum, 18:181–303; Addendum, 373–376.

Coppes MJ, Arnold M, Beckwith JB, Ritchey ML, D'Angio GJ, Green DM, Breslow NE (1999) Factors affecting the risk of contralateral Wilms tumor development: A report from the National Wilms Tumor Study Group. *Cancer* 85:1616–1625.

Clericuzio CL, D'Angio GJ, Duncan M, Green DM, Knudson AG Jr. (1992) Summary and Recommendations of the Workshop Held at the First International Conference on Molecular and Clinical Genetics of Childhood Renal Tumors, Albuquerque, New Mexico, May 14–16.

Craft AW, Parker L, Stiller C, Cole M (1995) Screening for Wilms' tumour in patients with aniridia, Beckwith syndrome, or hemihypertrophy. *Med Pediatr Oncol* 24:231–234.

Dao D, Frank D, Qian N, O'Keefe D, Vosatka RJ, Walsh CP, Tycko B (1998) *IMPT1*, an imprinted gene similar to polyspecific transporter and multi-drug resistance genes. *Hum Mol Genet* 7:597–608.

DeBaun MR, Siegel MJ, Choyke PL (1998) Nephromegaly in infancy and early childhood: A risk factor for Wilms tumor in Beckwith-Wiedemann syndrome. *J Pediatr* 132:401–404.

de Lonlay P, Fournet JC, Rahier J, Gross-Morand MS, Poggi-Travert F, Foussier V, Bonnefont JP, Brusset MC, Brunelle F, Robert JJ, Nihoul-Fekete C, Saudubray JM, Junien C (1997) Somatic deletion of the imprinted 11p15 region in sporadic persistent hyperinsulinemic hypoglycemia of infancy is specific of focal adenomatous hyperplasia and endorses partial pancreatectomy. *J Clin Invest* 100:802–807.

Elliott M, Maher ER (1994a) Beckwith-Wiedemann syndrome. *J Med Genet* 31:560–564.

Elliott M, Bayly R, Cole T, Temple IK, Maher ER (1994b) Clinical features and natural history of Beckwith-Wiedemann syndrome: Presentation of 74 new cases. *Clin Genet* 46:168–174.

Engstrom W, Lindham S, Schofield P (1988) Wiedemann-Beckwith syndrome. *Eur J Pediatr* 147:450–457.

Everman DB, Shuman C, Dzolganovski B, O'Riordan MA, Weksberg R, Robin NH (2000) Serum alpha-fetoprotein levels in Beckwith-Wiedemann syndrome. *J Pediatr* 137:123–127.

Greenberg F, Stein F, Gresik MV, Finegold MJ, Carpenter RJ, Riccardi VM, Beaudet AL (1986) The Perlman familial nephroblastomatosis syndrome. *Am J Med Genet* 24:101–110.

Grundy RG, Pritchard J, Baraitser M, Risdon A, Robards M (1992) Perlman and Wiedemann-Beckwith syndromes: Two distinct conditions associated with Wilms' tumor. *Eur J Pediatr* 151:895–898.

Gylys-Morin V, Hoffer FA, Kozakewich H, Shamberger RC (1993) Wilms tumor and nephroblastomatosis: Imaging characteristics at gadolinium-enhanced MR imaging. *Radiology* 188:517–521.

Halamek LP, Stevenson DK (1998) Neonatal hypoglycemia, part II: Pathophysiology and therapy. *Clin Pediatr (Phila)* 37:11–16.

Hao Y, Crenshaw T, Moulton T, Newcomb E, Tycko B (1993) Tumour-suppressor activity of *H19* RNA. *Nature* 365:764–767.

Hatada I, Ohashi H, Fukushima Y, Kaneko Y, Inoue M, Komoto Y, Okada A, Ohishi S, Nabetani A, Morisaki H, Nakayama M, Niikawa N, Mukai T (1996) An imprinted gene *p57KIP2* is mutated in Beckwith-Wiedemann syndrome. *Nat Genet* 14:171–173.

Hoyme HE, Seaver LH, Jones KL, Procopio F, Crooks W, Feingold M (1998) Isolated hemihyperplasia (hemihypertrophy): Report of a prospective multicenter study of the incidence of neoplasia and review. *Am J Med Genet* 79:274–278.

Johnson JP, Golabi M, Norton ME, Rosenblatt RM, Feldman GM, Yang SP, Hall BD, Fries MH (1998) Costello syndrome: Phenotype, natural history, differential diagnosis, and possible cause. *J Pediatr* 133:441–448.

Joyce JM, Lam WK, Catchpoole DJ, Jenks P, Reik W, Maher ER, Schofield PN (1997) Imprinting of *IGF2* and *H19*: Lack of reciprocity in sporadic Beckwith-Wiedemann syndrome. *Hum Mol Genet* 6:1543–1548.

Lam WW, Hatada I, Ohishi S, Mukai T, Joyce JA, Cole TR, Donnai D, Reik W, Schofield PN, Maher ER (1999) Analysis of germline *CDKN1C* (*p57KIP2*) mutations in familial and sporadic Beckwith-Wiedemann syndrome (BWS) provides a novel genotype-phenotype correlation. *J Med Genet* 36:518–523.

Lee MP, DeBaun MR, Mitsuya K, Galonek HL, Brandenburg S, Oshimura M, Feinberg AP (1999) Loss of imprinting of a paternally expressed transcript, with antisense orientation to *KVLQT1*, occurs frequently in Beckwith-Wiedemann syndrome and is independent of insulin-like growth factor II imprinting. *Proc Natl Acad Sci USA* 96:5203–5208.

Lee MP, DeBaun M, Randhawa G, Reichard BA, Elledge EJ, Feinberg AP (1997b) Low frequency of *p57KIP2* mutation in Beckwith-Wiedemann syndrome. *Am J Hum Genet* 61:304–309.

Lee MP, Hu RJ, Johnson LA, Feinberg AP (1997a) Human *KVLQT1* gene shows tissue-specific imprinting and encompasses Beckwith-Wiedemann syndrome chromosomal rearrangements. *Nat Genet* 15:181–185.

Leisenring WM, Breslow NE, Evans IE, Beckwith JB, Coppes MJ, Grundy P (1994) Increased birth weights of National Wilms' Tumor Study patients suggest a growth factor excess. *Cancer Res* 54:4680–4683.

Leonard NJ, Bernier FP, Rudd N, Machin GA, Bamforth F, Bamforth S, Grundy P, Johnson C (1996) Two pairs of male monozygotic twins discordant for Wiedemann-Beckwith syndrome. *Am J Med Genet* 61:253–257.

Li M, Squire JA, Weksberg R (1997) Molecular genetics of Beckwith-Wiedemann syndrome. *Curr Opin Pediatr* 9:623–629.

Li M, Squire JA, Weksberg R (1998) Molecular genetics of Wiedemann-Beckwith syndrome. *Am J Med Genet* 79:253–259.

Lin AE, Neri G, Hughes-Benzie R, Weksberg R (1999) Cardiac anomalies in the Simpson-Golabi-Behmel syndrome. *Am J Med Genet* 83:378–381.

Lubinsky MS, Hall JG (1991) Genomic imprinting, monozygous twinning, and X inactivation. *Lancet* 337:1288.

Martinez y Martinez R, Ocampo-Campos R, Perez-Arroyo R, Corona-Rivera E, Cantu JM (1985) The Wiedemann-Beckwith syndrome in four sibs including one with associated congenital hypothyroidism. *Eur J Pediatr* 143:233–235.

Neri G, Gurrieri F, Zanni G, Lin A (1998) Clinical and molecular aspects of the Simpson-Golabi-Behmel syndrome. *Am J Med Genet* 79:279–283.

Nicholls RD (1994) New insights reveal complex mechanisms involved in genomic imprinting. *Am J Hum Genet* 54:733–740.

Ogawa O, Eccles MR, Szeto J, McNoe LA, Yun K, Maw MA, Smith PJ, Reeve AE (1993) Relaxation of insulin-like growth factor II gene imprinting implicated in Wilms' tumour. *Nature* 362:749–751.

O'Keefe D, Dao D, Zhao L, Sanderson R, Warburton D, Weiss L, Anyane-Yeboa K, Tycko B (1997) Coding mutations in *p57KIP2* are present in some cases of Beckwith-Wiedemann syndrome but are rare or absent in Wilms tumors. *Am J Hum Genet* 61:295–303.

Parker DA, Skalko RJ (1969) Congenital asymmetry: Report of 10 cases with associated developmental abnormalities. *Pediatrics* 44:584–589.

Pettenati MJ, Haines JL, Higgins RR, Wappner RS, Palmer CG, Weaver DD (1986) Wiedemann-Beckwith syndrome: Presentation of clinical and cytogenetic data on 22 new cases and review of the literature. *Hum Genet* 74:143–154.

Qian N, Frank D, O'Keefe D, Dao D, Zhao L, Yuan L, Wang Q, Keating M, Walsh C, Tycko B (1997) The *IPL* gene on chromosome 11p15.5 is imprinted in humans and mice and is similar to *TDAG51*, implicated in Fas expression and apoptosis. *Hum Mol Genet* 6:2021–2029.

Rainier S, Johnson LA, Dobry CJ, Ping AJ, Grundy PE, Feinberg AP (1993) Relaxation of imprinted genes in human cancer. *Nature* 362:747–749.

Regalado JJ, Rodriguez MM, Toledano S (1997) Bilaterally multicentric synchronous Wilms' tumor: Successful conservative treatment despite persistence of nephrogenic rests. *Med Pediatr Oncol* 28:420–423.

Ringrose RE, Jabbour JT, Keele DK (1965) Hemihypertrophy. *Pediatrics* 36:434–448.

Slavotinek A, Gaunt L, Donnai D (1997) Paternally inherited duplications of 11p15.5 and Beckwith-Wiedemann syndrome. *J Med Genet* 34:819–826.

Smilinch NJ, Day CD, Fitzpatric GV, Caldwell GM, Lossie AC, Cooper PR, Smallwood AC, Joyce JA, Schofield PN, Reik W, Nicholls RD, Weksberg R, Driscoll DJ, Maher ER, Shows TB, Higgins MJ (1999) A maternally methylated CpG island in *KvLQT1* is associated with an antisense paternal transcript and loss of imprinting in Beckwith-Wiedemann syndrome. *Proc Natl Acad Sci USA* 96:8064–8069.

Sotelo-Avila C, Gonzalez-Crussi F, Fowler JW (1980) Complete and incomplete forms of Beckwith-Wiedemann syndrome: Their oncogenic potential. *J Pediatr* 96:47–50.

Souka AP, Snijders RJ, Novakov A, Soares W, Nicolaides KH (1998) Defects and syndromes in chromosomally normal fetuses with increased nuchal translucency thickness at 10–14 weeks of gestation. *Ultrasound Obstet Gynecol* 11:391–400.

Thorburn MJ, Wright ES, Miller CG, Smith-Read EH (1970) Exomphalos-macroglossia-gigantism syndrome in Jamaican infants. *Am J Dis Child* 119:316–321.

Tomooka Y, Onitsuka H, Goya T, Hayashida Y, Kuroiwa T, Kudo S, Miyazaki S, Torisu M (1988) Congenital hemihypertrophy with adrenal adenoma and medullary sponge kidney. *Br J Radiol* 61:851–853.

Van Eeghen AM, Van Gelderen I, Hennekam RC (1999) Costello syndrome: Report and review. *Am J Med Genet* 82:187–193.

Vaughan WG, Sanders DW, Grosfeld JL, Plumley DA, Rescoria FJ, Scherer 3rd LR, West KW, Breitfeld PP (1995) Favorable outcome in children with Beckwith-Wiedemann syndrome and intraabdominal malignant tumors. *J Pediatr Surg* 30:1042–1044.

Viljoen D, Pearn J, Beighton P (1984) Manifestations and natural history of idiopathic hemihypertrophy: A review of eleven cases. *Clin Genet* 26:81–86.

Waziri M, Patil SR, Hanson JW, Bartley JA (1983) Abnormality of chromosome 11 in patients with features of Beckwith-Wiedemann syndrome. *J Pediatr* 102:873–876.

Weksberg R, Shen DR, Fei YL, Song QL, Squire J (1993) Disruption of insulin-like growth factor 2 imprinting in Beckwith-Wiedemann syndrome. *Nat Genet* 5:143–150.

Weksberg R, Squire J (1995) In *Genomic Imprinting: Causes and Consequences*, Ohlsson R, Hall K, Ritzen M, eds. Cambridge, UK: Cambridge University Press, p. 237–251.

Weksberg R, Squire JA, Templeton DM (1996) Glypicans: A growing trend. *Nat Genet* 12:225–227.

Weng EY, Moeschler JB, Graham, Jr. JM (1995a) Longitudinal observations on 15 children with Wiedemann-Beckwith syndrome. *Am J Med Genet* 56:366–373.

Weng EY, Mortier GR, Graham, Jr. JM (1995b) Beckwith-Wiedemann syndrome. An update and review for the primary pediatrician. *Clin Pediatr (Phila)* 34:317–326.

Wiedemann H-R (1964) Complexe malformatif familial avec hernie ombilicale et macroglossie, un "syndrome nouveau." *J Genet Hum* 13:223–232.

Wiedemann H-R (1983) Tumours and hemihypertrophy associated with Wiedemann-Beckwith syndrome. *Eur J Pediatr* 141:129.

Zuker RM (1999) Personal communication.

CHAPTER 5

CHARGE ASSOCIATION

CHRISTINE A. OLEY

INTRODUCTION

Incidence

The various abnormalities that together comprise the CHARGE association were first described by Hall in 1979, although there had been several reports in the 1950s and 1960s of children with choanal atresia and congenital heart disease, coloboma and congenital heart disease, and coloboma and choanal atresia. Pagon et al. in 1981 reported a further 21 cases and coined the acronym "CHARGE association" to describe this pattern of anomalies (Table 5.1).

More than 200 cases have now been reported, and CHARGE association is probably one of the most common multiple-anomaly conditions encountered by clinicians. Good reviews are available (Pagon et al., 1981; Davenport et al., 1986; Oley et al., 1988; Blake et al., 1990; Tellier et al.,

TABLE 5.1. Most Common Anomalies Seen in CHARGE Association

C = Coloboma
H = Heart defects
A = Atresia choanae
R = Retardation of growth and/or development
G = Genital defects
E = Ear anomalies and/or deafness

1998). The frequency is probably the same in males and females. However, a preponderance of males has been reported, probably because the diagnosis is made more readily in males because of hypogonadism, rather than there being a true male preponderance. It is evident that although the most consistent features are still those represented by the letters in the acronym CHARGE, there are additional abnormalities that occur frequently. These include facial palsy, renal abnormalities, orofacial clefts, and tracheoesophageal fistula. Often, the presence of these additional anomalies can be useful as confirmatory evidence of the diagnosis. However, the total clinical spectrum and the criteria for the diagnosis of the CHARGE association need to be refined. Only when this happens will the true incidence be known.

Most recent reports of children with CHARGE association suggest that in some infants who survive the newborn period, the prognosis may be better than expected.

Diagnostic Criteria

CHARGE is usually known as an association, as distinct from a syndrome, although not everyone is in agreement with this designation (Davenport et al., 1986; Lubinsky, 1994). A **syndrome** is a pattern of anomalies

Management of Genetic Syndromes, Edited by Suzanne B. Cassidy and Judith E. Allanson
ISBN 0-471-31286-X   Copyright © 2001 by Wiley-Liss, Inc.

with a specific cause, such as Down syndrome related to trisomy 21, or single gene disorders such as Marfan syndrome. An **association** is usually a heterogeneous group of anomalies that occur together more often than would be expected by chance. All the included anomalies are not necessarily present in an affected individual, and for CHARGE association, the number of anomalies that must be present for a confident diagnosis has not been determined.

It has been proposed that at least four of the major features included in the acronym must be present to make a confident diagnosis of the CHARGE association and that these should include either coloboma or choanal atresia (Pagon et al., 1981). The reported frequency of the major anomalies in patients with the CHARGE association varies and is dependent on how these patients have been ascertained, for example, through ophthalmology, cardiology, or developmental clinics.

Several reviews document the frequency of the major features (Pagon et al., 1981; Oley et al., 1988; Harvey et al., 1991; Tellier et al., 1998). Colobomas involving iris, retina, or optic disc can be bilateral or unilateral. They are found in 80–90% of patients. Vision loss varies according to the size and location of the coloboma. Congenital heart defects occur in 60–85%. No specific heart lesion predominates, and many are complex defects. Choanal atresia or stenosis is found in 55–85% and is frequently bilateral. Growth retardation is documented in 70–85%, with retardation of development ranging from 60–100%. Genital abnormalities have mainly been reported in males, with reports varying from 53–100%. Ear anomalies and/or deafness occur in 85–100%. The ears are quite distinctive, described as short and wide, low-set, protruding, lop or cup-shaped, and simple (Figs. 5.1–5.3). The antihelix is unusual and distinctive.

Other relatively common findings include facial asymmetry, unilateral facial palsy, cleft lip and/or palate, swallowing dysfunction, gastroesophageal reflux, esophageal atresia and/or tracheoesophageal fistula, and renal anomalies (including vesicoureteric reflux, hydronephrosis, rotated kidneys, and small kidneys) (Davenport et al., 1986; Oley et al., 1988).

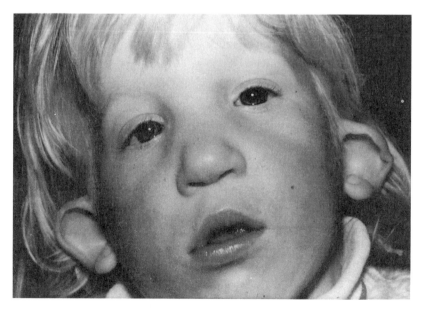

FIGURE 5.1. Note asymmetry of ears with protruding simple right ear and low-set, cup-shaped left ear.

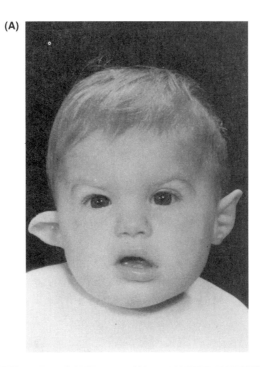

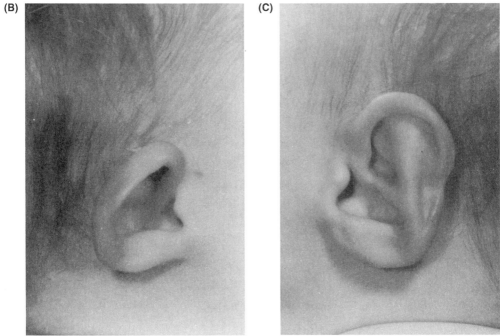

FIGURE 5.2. A: Note asymmetry of ears with low-set, protruding, lop right ear, slightly prominent left ear, and right facial palsy. **B:** Lateral view of right ear showing overfolded helix. **C:** Lateral view of left ear showing a triangular concha, deep triangular fossa, and prominent antihelix.

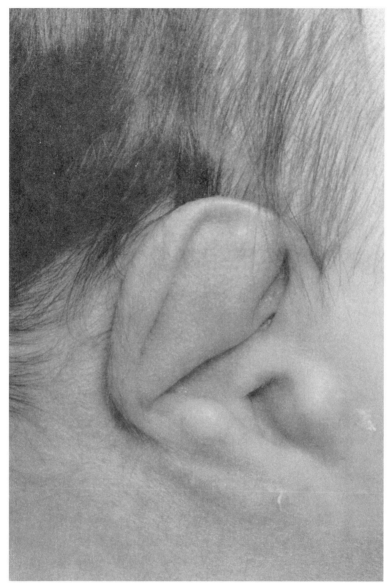

FIGURE 5.3. Square-shaped ear with triangular concha, discontinuity between antihelix and antitragus, and absent lobe.

Etiology, Pathogenesis, and Genetics

There is increasing evidence that the various defects seen in the CHARGE association may result from abnormal neural crest cell growth, migration, differentiation, or survival (Siebert et al., 1985). At present, the cause of the CHARGE association remains unknown. Most cases reported are sporadic. However, many aspects favor the view that a genetic abnormality is involved. The strongest of such evidence includes *1*) the concordance of phenotype in monozygotic twins and discordance in dizygotic twins, *2*) absence of definite identified environmental factors, *3*) a significantly higher paternal age at conception than in the general population, *4*) the existence of chromosomal anomalies in some cases, and, finally, *5*) rare familial forms (Levin et al., 1973; Oley et al., 1988; Tellier et al., 1998). Although concordance in monozygotic twins does not prove a genetic cause, it does indicate an increased likelihood of a genetic contribution to the occurrence of the defects in some cases. Several chromosomal abnormalities have been reported in patients with the constellation of anomalies seen in CHARGE association, including two cases with a microdeletion of 22q11.2 (Clementi et al., 1991; Emmanuel et al., 1992). Both of these had features compatible with both CHARGE association and DiGeorge syndrome. The majority of reported cases of CHARGE association have had normal chromosomes.

Although some of the features seen in the CHARGE association are also seen in thalidomide embryopathy and diabetic embryopathy, there have been no reports of these being implicated as the cause of CHARGE association in other cases. Nor have other teratogens been definitely implicated in the etiology of the CHARGE association, with the exception of two reports. One patient had a history of in utero exposure to hydantoin and presented with the clinical manifestations of CHARGE association (Bartoshesky et al., 1982), and one was exposed to carbon monoxide during the 7th month of pregnancy (Courtens et al., 1996). All these factors suggest the possible role of a *de novo* dominant mutation or a hitherto undetectable chromosomal abnormality in CHARGE association.

Diagnostic Testing

There is no specific diagnostic testing possible for CHARGE association. It should be kept in mind that this is a diagnosis of exclusion and should only be concluded when chromosome analysis and FISH for 22q11.2 deletion are negative. When it is suspected,

evaluation for the other anomalies and functional problems should occur. Diagnosis is based on the diagnostic criteria.

Differential Diagnosis

Between 40% and 50% of children with choanal atresia have other abnormalities (Harris et al., 1997), and in some of these cases there is an obvious chromosomal anomaly, such as trisomy 13, 18, or 21, or a single gene disorder, such as Treacher Collins syndrome. Oculo-auriculo-vertebral spectrum (see Chapter 16) shares some features with CHARGE association (Van Meter and Weaver, 1996). However, Oculo-auriculo-vertebral spectrum is frequently associated with eyelid coloboma, which is rarely seen in CHARGE association. Because of the overlap between CHARGE association and DiGeorge syndrome (see Chapter 29), a 22q11.2 deletion needs to be excluded in any child with CHARGE association. Ocular features may help to separate the different phenotypes of DiGeorge syndrome, VATER association (see Chapter 28), cat-eye syndrome, and Oculo-auriculo-vertebral spectrum, which have systemic characteristics in common with CHARGE association.

MANIFESTATIONS AND MANAGEMENT

For optimal management, the patient with CHARGE association should ideally be referred to a center that can undertake all areas of specialist treatment and management. This helps in long-term follow-up and benefits the parents, and, most importantly, it offers an integrated, multidisciplinary approach. In this way, surgical management can be combined with investigations that also require a general anesthetic. This requires active coordination and cooperation between the appropriate specialities.

Growth and Feeding

Although the majority of patients with CHARGE association have appropriate birth weight and length, over 70% experience postnatal growth retardation, with weight and length falling below the third centile. Feeding difficulties are a major feature in patients who fail to thrive in infancy. Pharyngeal incoordination and laryngeal and pharyngeal abnormalities are common findings in many of those with CHARGE association (Blake et al., 1990). This, in addition to the occurrence of gastroesophageal reflux, may account for the difficulties children have initially with feeding and in introduction of solid food to their diet. Early feeding problems are likely to improve, however, and catch-up growth to the low normal range can occur. Those children who maintain their weight in the early months are often the ones who have nutritional intervention (usually in the form of gastrostomy tube feeding). In the others, catch-up growth by 3 years of age and normal height velocity are reported to be achieved (Harvey et al., 1991). Many children with severe cardiac problems show poor early growth. In most individuals ultimate height is at or below the third centile. Growth hormone deficiency and gonadotropin deficiency have been reported in a few patients (Tellier et al., 1998). There is no correlation between the degree of growth retardation and the abnormalities present in patients with CHARGE association.

Evaluation

- Because gastroesophageal reflux and swallowing difficulties occur commonly, early assessment of feeding should be instituted by a multidisciplinary team, including gastroenterologists, speech and language pathologists, occupational therapists, and dietitians.
- Esophageal pH studies for reflux, barium swallow, and endoscopy must be considered.

- If growth remains poor in early childhood, then growth hormone secretion should be assessed.

Treatment

- Feeding problems in infants with CHARGE association continue to be one of the most difficult management issues. Medical management with antispasmodics may benefit a few. Controversy reigns over whether early insertion of gastrostomy feeding tubes gives better long-term results. This mode of treatment is more common in the United States than in the United Kingdom, where the trend is for a Nissen fundoplication if management with oral feeding fails. Interestingly, the U.S. children appear to have more long-term problems with oral intake (Blake et al., 1998).
- In the children with ongoing growth deficiency but normal growth hormone levels, there is insufficient information as yet to know whether treatment with growth hormone is beneficial.

Development and Behavior

It is difficult to determine the frequency and degree of developmental retardation in patients with CHARGE association from the literature because of differences in ascertainment and definition and frequent lack of formal psychometric testing. When assessed, learning difficulties have been reported in between 60% and 100% of patients. However, some of the reports suggesting that most children had learning problems did not involve long-term follow-up. Early motor delay is seen in the majority of patients with severe visual problems; deafness and the effects of chronic illness contribute greatly to the delay. However, early gross motor delay does not necessarily indicate a worse prognosis.

To achieve as normal a level of functioning as possible it is essential that all of the patients' deficits be identified and treated as early as possible, particularly the hearing, visual, motor, and language deficits. This may be overlooked by surgical teams intent on achieving survival from a major cardiac, choanal, or tracheoesophageal repair.

The diagnosis of mental retardation should be made with caution in anyone with impaired hearing and vision, as they are inherently understimulated. Deafness, if not recognized early, may present with delay in language; poor vision may cause delay in fine motor skills. Children with both defective hearing and vision may present at an earlier date with delay in gross motor skills and problems with balance. In some cases they may also appear autistic. Mental retardation may be present but should only be diagnosed when the extent of the sensory deficit is known and when the child is in an adequate educational program. Severe mental retardation/learning disability appears to be uncommon, although there are few long-term studies. In one study of 7 children, only one had severe mental retardation (Harvey et al., 1991). Major strides in development are often made by patients with CHARGE association once parents realize that mental retardation is not inevitable and their child's potential is explained fully.

Because it is now clear that mental retardation is uncommon, it should not be used as one of the features of the CHARGE association. Instead, the term "developmental delay" may be more appropriate (Blake et al., 1990). Because the majority of children with the CHARGE association will have some early motor delay, it may appear that a child is going to have significant problems since early intellectual assessments look particularly at gross and fine motor development as well as speech development. Thus there can be a discrepancy between the results of these early assessments and later cognitive abilities once motor performance and language skills have improved.

There is some evidence that significant learning problems may be more common in patients with bilateral choanal atresia, particularly in those who experience consequent hypoxia (Lin et al., 1990). The presence of central nervous system malformation is strongly associated with choanal atresia. There is a predominance of forebrain anomalies, particularly arrhinencephaly and holoprosencephaly.

Although concurrence of cyanotic congenital heart disease and choanal atresia has been associated with a worse prognosis for survival, no clinical features in infancy seem to be predictive of developmental outcome (Harvey et al., 1991).

Developmental outcome in many of these children will be influenced greatly by factors such as the presence of structural brain abnormalities, the presence and severity of visual and hearing deficits, early management of these sensory deficits, adequate feeding and nutrition, adverse perinatal factors, coexistent medical and surgical problems, and implementation of early intervention strategies and family supports. Physicians need to be particularly alert to the problems of visual and hearing deficits, which may be difficult to detect in infancy or may develop during later childhood.

Evaluation

- Assessment of vision and hearing as well as early referral for appropriate developmental and educational services are essential within the first few months of life.

- If there are multiple sensory deficits then evaluation should be done by specially trained therapists.

Treatment

- Early evaluation and therapy is vital and should be accomplished by a team of specialists including developmental pediatricians, speech and language therapists, occupational therapists and physiotherapists, as well as therapists dealing with deaf-blind children.

- Hearing aids and intensive speech/language therapy should be initiated for children with hearing loss as soon as it is identified.
- If visual correction is needed, it should be accomplished expeditiously. If this is not possible, then an intensive program for the visually handicapped should be instituted.

Ophthalmologic

The major ocular feature of the CHARGE association is coloboma. Colobomas are frequent abnormalities, occurring in 80–90% of patients. They are frequently bilateral and can involve iris, retina, or optic disc. They rarely involve the iris alone. Lid colobomas occur infrequently (Davenport et al., 1986). Vision loss varies according to the size and location of the coloboma, with a range from no impairment to severe visual loss with lack of light perception (Russell-Eggitt et al., 1990). However, over 50% of children with the CHARGE association have some visual impairment (Kaplan, 1989).

Other ocular abnormalities are common. These include microphthalmia, which has been described in about 30% (Kaplan, 1989); nystagmus, which may be related to macular or optic nerve involvement or may be central in origin and can be horizontal, vertical, or rotatory (Russell-Eggitt et al., 1990); and strabismus. Refractive errors are also common.

Rarer abnormalities reported include atresia of lacrimal canaliculi, blocked nasolacrimal duct, and congenital glaucoma. True ptosis is uncommon, and more often pseudoptosis is associated with microphthalmia or orbital asymmetry (Russell-Eggitt et al., 1990). Delayed visual maturation has been reported occasionally, particularly in infants who are severely ill from various causes (Davenport et al., 1986).

Not all patients are sick infants, and some are diagnosed later in life. The coloboma seen in the CHARGE association is not specific to it, but additional findings such as facial nerve palsy may point to this diagnosis in a child with multiple abnormalities.

There is no correlation between the severity of the ocular defect and the other abnormalities seen in CHARGE association, including learning problems.

Evaluation

- It is important for the clinician to be aware of the ophthalmic features of the CHARGE association, because some, such as chorioretinal coloboma, may be undetected until complicated by retinal detachment. Chorioretinal coloboma often occurs without an iris defect and may not be easily detected.
- Early review by an ophthalmologist is important to determine whether chorioretinal colobomas or other eye anomalies are present.
- Assessment of visual function is important to maximize potential for education.

Treatment

- Corrective lenses or low-vision aids may improve visual performance.
- If strabismus is present, then appropriate treatment by occlusion or surgery may be necessary.
- Surgery should be done for retinal detachment and cataracts.

Cardiovascular

Between 60% and 85% of patients with the CHARGE association have congenital heart defects. The severity and spectrum of congenital heart defects varies, with no specific heart defect predominating, although there is a preponderance of right-sided heart lesions and conotruncal defects. Tetralogy of Fallot and atrio-ventricular septal defects are the most common cyanotic cardiac defects. Patent ductus arteriosus is a common finding either alone or associated with more severe lesions.

Conotruncal anomalies (tetralogy of Fallot, double-outlet right ventricle, truncus arteriosus) are found in approximately 40% of those with congenital heart disease (Cyran et al., 1987; Lin et al., 1987; Wyse et al., 1993). Aortic arch anomalies (vascular ring, aberrant subclavian artery, interrupted aortic arch) have been reported to occur in 36% in one study (Lin et al., 1987), but this has not been validated in other studies.

About 75% of congenital heart defects require surgical management, with the remaining 25% being comparatively mild heart defects, small atrial septal defect, ventricular septal defect, pulmonary stenosis, patent ductus arteriosus, or a combination of these (Wyse et al., 1993).

If a complex congenital heart defect is present, the mortality rate can be significant (30–40%), but in few is death directly related to the underlying congenital heart disease (Wyse et al., 1993). Outlook for survival appears to be poor if more than one of the following three features are present: cyanotic cardiac lesion, bilateral posterior choanal atresia, or tracheoesophageal fistula. Mortality seems largely not to be caused by the structural heart or choanal abnormalities but instead reflects the underlying pharyngeal and laryngeal incoordination that results in aspiration of secretions.

Evaluation

- If a neonate presents with cyanosis, it could be due to congenital heart disease, choanal atresia or a combination of both. If the child remains cyanotic despite an oral airway being established, the cause is likely to be congenital heart disease. The child should then be stabilized and transported to a tertiary referral center.
- All patients with CHARGE association should undergo a full cardiac examination even if the heart appears to be normal at birth.
- Careful imaging is essential before surgery, as complex and multiple cardiovascular abnormalities can be present that may not be easily detectable.
- Patients with CHARGE association may require an early shunt procedure before a later definitive repair. It may be possible to send patients directly for cardiac surgery on the basis of echocardiographic findings alone. However, cardiac catheterization may be necessary to identify anomalous subclavian vessels and/or to rule out peripheral pulmonary stenosis.

Treatment

- Cardiac surgery is no different in patients with CHARGE association than in patients with the same cardiac lesion in the general population.
- Caution must be exercised if prostaglandin administration is indicated to maintain ductal patency before surgery, as there may be a high mortality in neonates with CHARGE association who receive prostaglandins (Blake et al., 1990). These should only be administered once a neonate is adequately ventilated and has good venous access and cardiac anatomy has been well defined.
- Outcome is likely to be improved if collaboration between specialist surgical teams allows necessary procedures to be performed using the minimum of anesthetics.

Respiratory

Choanal atresia is caused either by failure to develop patency between the nasal cavity and nasopharynx, which normally occurs between the 25th and 45th day of embryonic life, or to an abnormality in the migration of cephalic neural crest after neural tube closure (Kaplan, 1989). It can involve both bone and soft tissue and results in either partial or total obstruction of the posterior nasal airway. Between 55% and 85% of patients with CHARGE association have choanal atresia or stenosis. It is usually bilateral and can be bony or membranous. A female predominance has been reported (Hengerer and Strome, 1982; Tellier et al., 1998). The typical presentation of bilateral choanal atresia is respiratory distress in the neonatal period, usually very soon after birth. There may be a history of polyhydramnios in the pregnancy. Because newborns are obligate nose breathers, unilateral choanal atresia may also present as respiratory distress, but this often occurs later and is less severe. The usual presentation of unilateral choanal atresia is noisy breathing, persistent nasal discharge, or feeding difficulty. In unilateral cases the condition may not be detected until after the early neonatal period.

Apart from choanal atresia, other upper airway abnormalities are common and include laryngomalacia, subglottic stenosis, and laryngeal clefts or webs (Stack and Wyse, 1991). Tracheoesophageal fistula occurs infrequently. Laryngomalacia may result in such significant airway problems that tracheostomy is needed. If micrognathia is present, intubation may be difficult because of the combination of small jaw and anterior larynx. Intubation may continue to be a problem with increasing age. With subglottic stenosis, either congenital or acquired, the airway will usually increase in size with age (Stack and Wyse, 1991).

Evaluation

- Typically, the nasal alae are patent, and direct visualization of the posterior nasal space may not reveal evidence of deeper obstruction. In the delivery room, inability to pass a standard nasogastric or suction catheter beyond the nares should alert the physician to the possibility of choanal atresia. The diagnosis of atresia may be inferred by simple clinical tests of airway patency such as passing a soft rubber catheter, observing misting on a metal spatula, auscultation of the nares, or using a wisp of cotton wool.

- CT scanning is the investigation of choice to diagnose choanal atresia or stenosis (Morgan and Bailey, 1990). There have been reports of misleading CT scans caused by accumulation of mucus in the nasal cavities, so careful preparation using vasoconstrictor drops and nasal suction is essential if high-quality images are to be obtained.

Treatment

- Initial management is establishment of the airway using an oral airway or, failing that, by endotracheal intubation.

- A tracheostomy is only indicated if there is an associated anomaly preventing oral intubation.

- Three surgical approaches have been advocated in the treatment of choanal atresia, transpalatal, transnasal, and transseptal. Although the transpalatal route allows good access, it is associated with longer operating time, greater blood loss, longer convalescence, and stunted palatal growth in some patients (Morgan and Bailey, 1990). Some studies found no difference in the success rate compared with the transnasal route (Black et al., 1983), but used the transpalatal approach only in older patients who had a failed transnasal repair. The advantages of the transnasal repair are preservation of the developing hard palate, shorter operating time, and minimal blood loss. After transnasal correction using a diamond burr, polyethylene tube stents are normally left in situ for 6 weeks, followed by dilation where necessary. The overall eventual success rate has been up to 94% (Morgan et al., 1993). The transnasal approach is now considered by most to be the technique of choice. CT scan evidence suggests that the choanal atresia in the CHARGE association may lead to a narrower posterior choanal region with a more contracted nasopharynx than in patients who have isolated choanal atresia. The reoperation rate is much higher in the CHARGE association (Stack and Wyse, 1991) than in isolated choanal atresia.

Ears and Hearing

Distinctive ear anomalies and/or deafness are reported in 85–100% of patients. Many clinicians believe that the external ear anomalies in the CHARGE association are sufficiently distinctive that a tentative diagnosis can be made on those features alone and a search for the other associated anomalies instituted. Although the ear abnormality is frequently bilateral, asymmetry is common. The most typical ear findings are low-set ears (64%), asymmetry (34%), small or absent lobes (32%), posterior angulation (25%), and "square" shape (Tellier et al., 1998). The patterns of more severe ear anomalies appear distinct, with Kaplan (1989) describing most ears in the CHARGE association as "cupped, trumpet, lop, or pixie-like" (Figs. 5.1–5.3).

When present, hearing loss may be variable, although the most common finding is moderate to severe progressive mixed loss. The conductive component can be attributed to ossicular anomalies and/or middle ear effusion. The ossicular defects may affect hearing primarily in the low frequencies, but deficits in the mid- to high-frequency range have also been reported. The conductive loss secondary to middle ear effusion may persist beyond childhood. The sensorineural component can be mild to severe and tends to be greatest in the high frequencies. The resultant audiogram yields a "wedge-shaped" pattern, with a low-frequency conductive loss and concomitant high-frequency sensorineural loss. The bone conduction threshold curve may slope downward from low to high frequencies, whereas the air conduction threshold curve is flat (Brown and Israel, 1991). It is thought that in most cases the conductive and sensorineural loss are progressive, although the rate of progression

tends to be slow and may arrest (Davenport et al., 1986).

Histologic evaluation of the temporal bones has revealed multiple malformations throughout the middle and inner ears. These include ossicular anomalies, absence of the stapedius muscle, absence of the oval window, aberrations of the facial nerve, Mondini-type malformation of the cochlea, and numerous malformations of the vestibular apparatus (Wright et al., 1986).

Evaluation

- Initial assessment consists of examination of the tympanic membranes to exclude a middle ear effusion.
- Brain stem-evoked audiometry may subsequently be used to help assess the level of hearing.
- Computed tomography of temporal bone is used to exclude ossicular or inner ear abnormalities.
- Assessment of hearing is often difficult in children who have multisensory deprivation, and this must be undertaken by a team of specialists.

Treatment

- Chronic serous otitis media is very common in CHARGE association and may require early and repeated myringotomies with insertion of ventilation tubes. These tubes may make an enormous difference to the quality of life, and tube insertion needs to be undertaken early, because the first 2 years of life are vitally important in the development of speech.
- Involvement of a teacher of the deaf at an early age will allow counseling for parents and offer better provision for educational needs.
- Most patients with CHARGE association and hearing loss are candidates for hearing aids. However, there are several factors that reduce the success rate. Malformations and softness of the

pinnae as well as small ear canals make fitting of hearing aids difficult. Many patients have sufficiently large cochlear losses that bone conduction aids will not provide adequate amplification as an alternative. The children are often supplied with hearing aids too late, and this can result in poor compliance, especially if they have acquired the habit of disregarding sounds.

- Cochlear implants may be useful in some patients.

Genitourinary

The presence of micropenis and undescended testes makes the early diagnosis of CHARGE association easier in boys. Hypospadias is uncommon, and penile agenesis and microtestis are rare. Most studies have not described obvious external genital defects in females, but labial hypoplasia has been noted in two women over the age of 15 years (Davenport et al., 1986). Pubertal development in both sexes may be delayed or absent and may be correlated with pituitary or hypothalamic deficiency. Only a small number of patients with recognized CHARGE association have entered puberty, and there is no information available about their fertility.

Evaluation

- If micropenis and cryptorchidism are present, then assessment of pituitary function is indicated. Basal follicle stimulating hormone (FSH), luteinizing hormone (LH), and testosterone levels should be measured. A three- to five day intramuscular stimulation test with human chorionic gonadotropin (hCG) to evaluate testicular function for testosterone production, as well as an intravenous stimulation test with luteinizing hormone-releasing hormone (LH-RH) to evaluate the integrity of

the hypothalamic-pituitary axis should be considered. Evaluation of other hormones such as growth hormone, adrenocorticotropic hormone (ACTH), cortisol, and thyroid-stimulating hormone is recommended to rule out hypopituitarism.

- If the initial physical changes of puberty are not present by age 13 years in girls or age 14 years in boys, evaluation of the hypothalamic-pituitary-gonadal axis should be considered. This would include bone age and gonadotropin levels, both before and after gonadotropin-releasing hormone (GnRH) stimulation. However, a moderate delay in the onset of puberty is common in CHARGE association, even when pituitary function appears normal. This "normal" delay should be taken into consideration when contemplating investigation in these teenagers.

Treatment

- In a patient with micropenis and a normal response to an hCG stimulation test, a short course of either testosterone or hCG should be considered in early infancy. Adequate penile growth with this form of therapy may avoid some of the psychological problems these boys face as they are growing up with a very small penis.

- Treatment of cryptorchidism can be medical, surgical, or a combination of both. Therapy with intramuscular hCG for 4–6 weeks has been helpful in treating some patients. If testicular descent does not occur with this treatment, then orchiopexy before age 2 years should be carried out. However, atrophic testes have been found in some boys even after surgical correction (Blake et al., 1998).

- Patients with CHARGE association may require hormone therapy to achieve puberty. This would involve intramuscular testosterone in males, and in females low-dosage estrogen therapy initially and then cyclic estrogen-progesterone therapy.

RESOURCES

USA Support Group

CHARGE Syndrome Foundation, Inc.
2004 Parkade Boulevard, Columbia,
MO 65202-3121
Phone: (573) 499-4694
E-mail: mnorbury@mall.coin.missouri.edu

UK Support Group

Contact Sheila Draper, 115 Boundary Road, Colliers Wood, London
SWI9 2DE, UK
Phone: (020) 8540 2142

Australia/New Zealand Support Group

C/o P.O. Box 91, Glenfield, NSW,
Australia 2167
Phone: (02) 9605 8475

ACKNOWLEDGMENTS

I am grateful to Dr Judith Allanson, Ottawa, Canada, for providing Figure 3 and to the editors of the *Journal of Medical Genetics* for allowing me to reproduce Figures 1, 2A, and 2B.

REFERENCES

Bartoshesky LE, Bhan L, Nagpaul K, Pushayan H (1982) Severe cardiac and ophthalmologic malformations in an infant exposed to diphenylhydantoin in utero. *Pediatrics* 69:202–203.

Black RJ, Pracy R, Evans JNG (1983) Congenital posterior choanal atresia. *Clin Otolaryngol* 8:251–255.

Blake KD, Russell-Eggitt IM, Morgan DW, Ratcliffe JM, Wyse RYH (1990) Who's in CHARGE? Multidisciplinary management of patients with CHARGE association. *Arch Dis Child* 65:217–223.

Blake KD, Davenport SLH, Hall B, Hefner MA, Pagon RA, Williams MS, Lin AE, Graham JM (1998) CHARGE association: An update and review for the primary pediatrician. *Clin Pediat* 37:159–173.

Brown DP, Israel SM (1991) Audiologic findings in a set of fraternal twins with CHARGE association. *J Am Acad Audiol* 2:183–188.

Clementi M, Tenconi R, Turolla L, Silvan C, Bortotto L, Artifoni L (1991) Apparent CHARGE association and chromosome anomaly: Chance or contiguous gene syndrome. *Am J Med Genet* 41:246–250.

Courtens W, Hennequin Y, Blum D, Vamos E (1996) CHARGE association in a neonate exposed *in utero* to carbon monoxide. *Birth Defects Orig Artic Ser* 30:407–412.

Cyran SE, Martinez R, Daniels S, Dignan PSJ, Kaplan S (1987) Spectrum of congenital heart disease in CHARGE association. *J Pediatr* 110:576–578.

Davenport SLH, Hefner MA, Mitchell JA (1986) The spectrum of clinical features in CHARGE syndrome. *Clin Genet* 29:298–310.

Emmanuel BS, Budarf ML, Sellinger B, Goldmuntz E, Driscoll DA (1992) Detection of microdeletions of 22q11.2 with fluorescence in situ hybridization (FISH): Diagnosis of DiGeorge syndrome (DGS), velo-cardio-facial (VCF) syndrome, CHARGE association and conotruncal cardiac malformations. *Am J Hum Genet* 51(suppl):A3.

Hall BD (1979) Choanal atresia and associated multiple anomalies. *J Pediatr* 95:395–398.

Harris J, Robert E, Källén B (1997) Epidemiology of choanal atresia with special reference to the CHARGE association. *Pediatrics* 99:363–367.

Harvey AS, Leaper PM, Bankier A (1991) CHARGE association: Clinical manifestations and developmental outcome. *Am J Med Genet* 39:48–55.

Hengerer AS, Strome M (1982) Choanal atresia: A new embryologic theory and its influence on surgical management. *Laryngoscope* 92:913–921.

Kaplan LC (1989) The CHARGE association: Choanal atresia and multiple congenital anomalies. *Otolaryngol Clin North Amer* 22:661–672.

Levin DL, Muster AJ, Newfeld EA, Paul MH (1973) Concordant aortic arch anomalies in monozygotic twins. *J Pediatr* 83:459–461.

Lin AE, Chin AJ, Devine W, Park SC, Zackai E (1987) The pattern of cardiovascular malformation in the CHARGE association. *Am J Dis Child* 141:1010–1013.

Lin AE, Siebert JR, Graham JM (1990) Central nervous system malformations in the CHARGE association. *Am J Med Genet* 37:304–310.

Lubinsky MS (1994) Properties of associations: Identity, nature, and clinical criteria, with a commentary on why CHARGE and Goldenhar are not associations. *Am J Med Genet* 49:21–25.

Morgan DW, Bailey CM (1990) Current management of choanal atresia. *Int J Pediatr Otorhinolaryngol* 19:1–13.

Morgan D, Bailey M, Phelps P, Bellman S, Grace A, Wyse R (1993) Ear-nose-throat abnormalities in the CHARGE association. *Arch Otolaryngol Head Neck Surg* 119:49–54.

Oley CA, Baraitser M, Grant DB (1988) A reappraisal of the CHARGE association. *J Med Genet* 25:147–156.

Pagon RA, Graham JM, Zonana J, Yong SL (1981) Coloboma, congenital heart disease, and choanal atresia with multiple anomalies: CHARGE association. *J Pediatr* 99:223–227.

Russell-Eggitt IM, Blake KD, Taylor DSI, Wyse RKH (1990) The eye in the CHARGE association. *Br J Ophthalmol* 74:421–426.

Siebert JR, Graham JM, MacDonald C (1985) Pathologic features of the CHARGE association: Support for involvement of the neural crest. *Teratology* 31:331–336.

Stack CG, Wyse RKE (1991) Incidence and management of airway problems in the CHARGE association. *Anaesthesia* 46:582–585.

Tellier AL, Connier-Daire V, Abadle V, Amiel J, Sigaudy S, Bonnet D, de Lonlay-Debeney P, Morrisseau-Durand MP, Hubert P, Michel JL, Jan D, Dollfus H, Baumann C, Labrune P, Lacombe D, Philip N, LeMerrer M, Briard ML, Munnich A, Lyonnet S (1998): CHARGE syndrome: Report of 47 cases and review. *Am J Med Genet* 76:402–409.

Van Meter TD, Weaver DD (1996) Oculo-auriculo-vertebral spectrum and the CHARGE association: Clinical evidence for a common pathogenetic mechanism. *Clin Dysmorphol* 5:187–196.

Wright CG, Brown OE, Meyerhoff WL, Rutledge JC (1986) Auditory and temporal bone abnormalities in CHARGE association. *Ann Otol Rhinol Laryngol* 95:480–486.

Wyse RKE, Al-Mahdawl S, Bum J, Blake K (1993) Congenital heart disease in CHARGE association. *Pediatr Cardiol* 14:75–81.

CHAPTER 6

CORNELIA DE LANGE SYNDROME

MAGGIE IRELAND

INTRODUCTION

Cornelia de Lange syndrome is a rare developmental malformation syndrome characterized by mental retardation, short stature, limb abnormalities, and distinctive craniofacial features (Ireland, 1996). Because there are no diagnostic biochemical, cytogenetic, or molecular abnormalities, diagnosis depends on recognition of the characteristic pattern of malformations and, in particular, the distinctive craniofacial features (Allanson et al., 1997). As a consequence, misdiagnosis of the syndrome is common and has complicated the assessment of cases of Cornelia de Lange syndrome in the literature, including those with biochemical or cytogenetic abnormalities or unusual inheritance patterns that might provide clues to the underlying gene defect.

The syndrome is named after Cornelia de Lange, who described 2 children whom she felt had a new and distinct pattern of malformations not previously described in the medical literature (de Lange, 1933). She later described an additional case of the syndrome and the detailed post-mortem results of one of her original cases who had subsequently died (de Lange, 1938). The syndrome is also sometimes called Brachmann-de Lange

syndrome in recognition of a German doctor who described an earlier case (Brachmann, 1916). Recently, a case earlier than Brachmann's has come to light, that described by Vrolik, a Dutch anatomist working in Amsterdam in the late nineteenth century (Oostra et al., 1994). The first cases to appear in the English literature were described by Ptacek and colleagues in 1963, and there are now several hundred cases in the literature (Ptacek et al., 1963).

Within the phenotypic pattern there is a wide range of severity. The most severely affected infants are usually born with diaphragmatic hernia, which is occasionally bilateral, and severe limb reduction defects with missing fingers, hands, or forearms (Cunniff et al., 1993). Most of the early reported cases of the syndrome were severely mentally retarded with little or no speech. However, over the last decade there have been increasing numbers of reports of more mildly affected individuals (Ireland and Burn, 1993; Ireland et al., 1993; Saal et al., 1993; Clericuzio, 1993; Van Allen et al., 1993). It is now generally accepted that there is a milder form of the syndrome. At the mild end of the spectrum are adults who are able to live independently and reproduce (de Die-Smulders et al., 1992). To discriminate

Management of Genetic Syndromes, Edited by Suzanne B. Cassidy and Judith E. Allanson
ISBN 0-471-31286-X   Copyright © 2001 by Wiley-Liss, Inc.

between the two forms, the term "classical" is used for those individuals who are severely growth retarded and the term "mild" is reserved for those who have less severe growth retardation and developmental delay.

Incidence

The published estimates of incidence for Cornelia de Lange syndrome vary from 1 in 10,000 to 1 in 100,000 live births (Pearce et al., 1967; Opitz, 1985). The most accurate study of incidence was carried out by Beck and Fenger and was based on the complete ascertainment of all cases of Cornelia de Lange syndrome in Denmark over a 5-year period. They calculated an incidence of 1 in 50,000 (Beck and Fenger, 1985). An unpublished study based on cases of the syndrome in the north of England found an incidence of 1 in 48,000 for classical Cornelia de Lange syndrome and 1 in 37,000 if individuals with the mild form of the syndrome were also included (M. Ireland, personal data).

Diagnostic Criteria

The phenotype in Cornelia de Lange syndrome is characterized by the presence of mental retardation, short stature, limb abnormalities, and distinctive craniofacial features. The limb abnormalities range from short forearms with small hands and tapering fingers to severe limb reduction defects with missing fingers, hands, and forearms. Developmental abnormalities and short stature are common to a large number of malformation syndromes so that the diagnosis of Cornelia de Lange syndrome is usually clinched by the recognition of the distinctive craniofacial features (Fig. 6.1).

The facial features are so striking that they usually override the features that are commonly associated with the genetic and ethnic background of the individual (Ptacek et al., 1963; Huang et al., 1967). Affected individuals have microbrachycephaly with a short neck and a low posterior hairline. The anterior hairline often extends down onto the forehead. The eyebrows are usually neat and

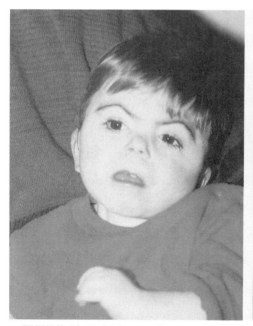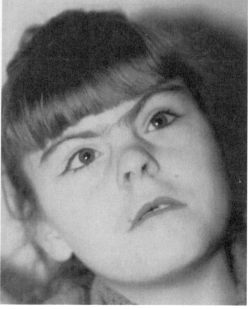

FIGURE 6.1. Facial features of two individuals with the classical Cornelia de Lange syndrome phenotype. Note the neat, arched eyebrows that have a "pencilled" quality to them, the depressed nasal bridge, anteverted nares, long smooth philtrum, and thin lips.

arched and give the impression that they have been "pencilled on" (Ireland et al., 1993; Smithells, 1965). Bushy eyebrows are not characteristic (Ireland et al., 1993; Van Allen et al., 1993). The eyes are usually normally set but occasionally can be down-slanting (Smithells, 1965; Levin et al., 1990). The eyelashes are often long and curled, giving the impression that they have been enhanced by mascara (Ireland et al., 1993; Van Allen et al., 1993). Ptosis of the upper eyelids is common and is responsible for the compensatory upward tilt of the head that is so characteristic of affected children. At birth the nasal bridge is usually depressed and the nares anteverted. With increasing age the nasal bridge becomes more prominent and the nares less anteverted. The philtrum is usually long and smooth and protrudes forward so much that it can often be detected antenatally (Bay et al., 1993; Saal et al., 1993; Van Allen et al., 1993). The lips are usually thin with a central cupid's bow on the upper lip. The mouth is often crescent shaped with the outer corners turned down. The mandible is usually smaller than expected for the size of the face and some cases can have severe micrognathia. Although rarely commented on, the supraorbital ridges and zygomatic arches are poorly developed (Ireland et al., 1993; Krajewska-Walasek et al., 1995). The ears may be normally set or posteriorly rotated and low set. The morphology of the ears is often simple, and, occasionally, they can appear large in relation to the face.

Figures 6.1 and 6.2 show individuals with the classical and mild forms of the syndrome, respectively.

In a detailed review of 31 cases previously diagnosed as having Cornelia de Lange syndrome, Ireland and colleagues felt that only 20 of the individuals had the syndrome (Ireland et al., 1993). A detailed comparison between the craniofacial features of the two groups identified those features that were most specific to the syndrome. These were

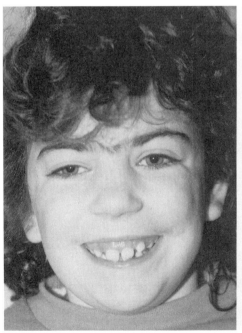 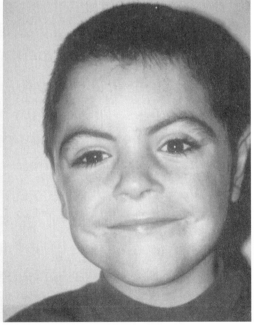

FIGURE 6.2. Facial features of two individuals with the mild Cornelia de Lange syndrome phenotype. Note the increased facial expression and the presence of the neat, arched eyebrows, depressed nasal bridge, smooth philtrum, and thin lips.

the combination of the characteristic eyebrows, the long, smooth philtrum, thin lips, and crescent-shaped mouth. Those features that were felt to be nonspecific were hypertrichosis, synophrys, and bushy eyebrows.

Halal and Preus devised a scoring system for the diagnosis of Cornelia de Lange syndrome based on measurements of the metacarpophalangeal profile originally described by Poznanski (Halal and Preus, 1979). Their system was based on scoring those metacarpophalangeal measurements that allowed the greatest discrimination between a group that was very typical for Cornelia de Lange syndrome and a group that was referred as possible Cornelia de Lange syndrome but for whom the diagnosis was rejected. In their study, they found that the first metacarpal was shorter than the second, third, fourth, and fifth, whereas the second and fifth were usually shorter than the third and fourth. They found that all the measurements in the Cornelia de Lange syndrome group showed greater deviation from the mean.

On reviewing detailed radiological studies of 20 patients with Cornelia de Lange syndrome, Peeters found no radiological abnormality that was diagnostic but suggested that a short first metacarpal with relatively long third and fourth metacarpals in the presence of rounding and subluxation of the radial head is highly suggestive of the diagnosis (Peeters, 1975).

Preus and Rex sought to improve diagnostic accuracy by constructing a scoring system based on numerical taxonomy (Preus and Rex, 1983). They used 30 characteristics to construct a diagnostic index, which allowed them to separate 99% of cases into those who were very typical of the syndrome and those who were not. They were able to confirm the diagnosis in those who had Cornelia de Lange syndrome in 84% of cases using measurements from the metacarpophalangeal index. In practice, both the numerical taxonomy scoring system and the analysis of metacarpophalangeal measurements are time consuming to perform and add little to diagnostic acumen.

Etiology, Pathogenesis, and Genetics

The pathogenesis of Cornelia de Lange syndrome is currently unknown. Most cases of the syndrome are sporadic and thought to result from a new autosomal dominant mutation (Ireland, 1996). There are several reports in the literature of familial cases that have included affected siblings and transmission from parent to child. There are also cases of discordant dizygotic and concordant monozygotic twins. The transmission from affected mother or father to child confirms that the condition is dominantly inherited, and this is further strengthened by the occurrence of affected and unaffected offspring (Mosher et al., 1985; de Die-Smulders et al., 1992; Chodirker and Chudley, 1994). The cases of recurrence in a sibship with normal parents are too few to be explained by autosomal recessive inheritance and are most likely caused by germline mosaicism in one or the other parent (Ireland, 1996). To take into account the possible risk of germ line mosaicism, a recurrence risk of 1% is normally quoted.

Because there are no diagnostic tests for the syndrome, management of pregnancies subsequent to the birth of an affected child usually centers on detailed ultrasonography looking for structural abnormalities such as a cystic hygroma, limb reduction defect, diaphragmatic hernia, heart abnormality, or the characteristic facial profile. The facial profile consists of severe micrognathia with a long, bulging philtrum and small nose and is well illustrated in a publication that shows scan pictures of the fetal face at 33 weeks of gestation (Manouvrier et al., 1996). Intrauterine growth retardation, although present in most cases at birth, is rarely present before the third trimester.

There has been no consistently identified chromosome abnormality associated with Cornelia de Lange syndrome. Only two significant abnormalities have been reported since chromosome banding techniques became available (Wilson et al., 1983; Ireland et al., 1991); both were *de novo* translocations. In one case, the long arm of chromosome 21 was translocated onto chromosome 14 [t(14;21)(q32;q11)] (Wilson et al., 1983). This individual had classical Cornelia de Lange syndrome but no reduction deformity of the limbs. The other translocation involved band 3q26.3 and 17q23.1(Ireland et al., 1991). This patient was more severely affected, having bilateral absence of both hands and forearms. The involvement of band 3q26.3 is of particular interest given the initial confusion between the Cornelia de Lange syndrome and the 3q duplication phenotype (see **Differential Diagnosis** below) in which 3q26 is the 3q duplication critical region. A review reveals a lack of deletions involving band 3q26.3, suggesting that this may be the site of an important developmental gene, which is vital for early embryonic development. Infants with deletions involving band 17q23.1 do not resemble infants with Cornelia de Lange syndrome. Given the severity of the phenotype in the patient with the *de novo* 3q;17q translocation and the involvement of band 3q26.3, it has been hypothesized that the gene for Cornelia de Lange syndrome may be located at 3q26.3 and that the translocation break point has disrupted either the gene or its regulatory sequences (Ireland et al., 1991).

Diagnostic Testing

No diagnostic biochemical, cytogenetic, or molecular tests are available. The diagnosis rests entirely on the recognition of the characteristic pattern of delayed growth and development with associated abnormalities of limb development and, in particular, the characteristic craniofacial features. In cases where there are atypical features or there is any doubt about the diagnosis, it is probably advisable to seek a second opinion from a physician with experience with the syndrome.

In 1983 Westergaard and colleagues reported the total absence of pregnancy associated plasma protein-A (PAPP-A) in serial serum samples from a pregnant women who later gave birth to a child with Cornelia de Lange syndrome (Westergaard et al., 1983). A recent study by this author found PAPP-A to be present in 19 second-trimester maternal serum samples analyzed but found the levels to be significantly reduced (Aitken et al., 1999). On the basis of this data we have produced a table of likelihood ratios. Although not a diagnostic test, PAPP-A may prove to be a valuable additional marker for those at risk of recurrence or in pregnancies in which abnormalities consistent with a diagnosis of Cornelia de Lange syndrome are detected.

Differential Diagnosis

In 1979 Fryns described a new pattern of malformations characterized by a coarse face, diaphragmatic hernia (85%), cleft palate (30%), and distal limb hypoplasia (75%) (Fryns, 1979), which is referred to as Fryns syndrome. Recurrence within sibships suggested an autosomal recessive pattern of inheritance. Unlike Cornelia de Lange syndrome, in pregnancies affected by Fryns syndrome polyhydramnios and premature labor are common and birth weight, length, and head circumference are usually normal for gestation. There is considerable overlap in facial dysmorphism with Cornelia de Lange syndrome, including hypertrichosis, narrow palpebral fissures, flat nasal bridge, upturned nose, and micrognathia. Fryns syndrome can be discriminated from Cornelia de Lange syndrome facially by the presence of a short upper lip and macrostomia. Cardiac, renal, and genital abnormalities are common and overlap with those seen in Cornelia de Lange syndrome (Bishun and Morton, 1965; Lubinsky et al., 1983; Bamforth, et al., 1989).

Individuals exposed to large quantities of alcohol often are small at birth, fail to thrive, and have mild to severe developmental abnormalities (see Chapter 9). Craniofacial features overlap with those seen in Cornelia de Lange syndrome. The features common to both conditions include microcephaly, short palpebral fissures, a short, upturned nose, a smooth underdeveloped philtrum, and a thin upper lip (Clarren and Smith, 1978; Clarren, 1981; Frias et al., 1982). Small distal phalanges are common. Cardiac defects similar to those seen in Cornelia de Lange syndrome are also well recognized. Children with fetal alcohol syndrome are more likely to be confused with mild rather than classical Cornelia de Lange syndrome.

Partial duplication of the long arm of chromosome 3 can present as a *de novo* event or, more commonly, as an unbalanced product of a familial balanced translocation or inversion. In the case of translocations or inversions, the duplication for 3q is commonly associated with a deletion of other variable regions of the genome (Wilson et al., 1978; Sciorra et al., 1979). Infants with duplication 3q are mentally retarded and fail to thrive, although they are usually of normal birth weight and length (Tranebjaerg et al., 1987). Facially they resemble Cornelia de Lange syndrome in that their hair extends down over the forehead (Fineman et al., 1978; Anneren and Gustavson, 1984). The eyelashes may be prominent, the nasal bridge depressed, and the nares anteverted. The philtrum is usually long and prominent, although it continues to show a central philtral groove, which infants with Cornelia de Lange syndrome do not have. Micrognathia is also common, but it is unusual for the lips to be thin or the mouth crescent shaped. The facial features of 3q duplication that differentiate it from Cornelia de Lange syndrome are a sloping forehead, bushy eyebrows, hypertelorism, upward slanting palpebral fissures, epicanthal folds, a rather broad nose, maxillary prognathism, and relatively normal lips. Eye abnormalities including congenital cataract and glaucoma are common in duplication 3q and are almost never seen in Cornelia de Lange syndrome (Fear

and Briggs, 1979; Mulcahy et al., 1979). Malformations common in duplication 3q include central nervous system, cardiac, and renal abnormalities, cleft palate, and genital hypoplasia (Mulcahy et al., 1979; Rosenfeld et al., 1981). Craniosynostosis, camptodactyly, and talipes are the most commonly associated skeletal abnormalities. Occasionally, polydactyly of the hands or syndactyly of the toes is seen. Rhizomelic shortening of the limbs has been described in a number of cases (Kawashima and Maruyama, 1979; Chen et al., 1996). Chromosome analysis of the affected child and parents will confirm the diagnosis.

Scott et al. described three brothers with a new malformation syndrome that was characterized by growth deficiency, mental retardation, and brachycephaly (Scott, et al., 1971), now known as Scott craniodigital syndrome. A further affected male has also been described (Lorenz et al., 1990), making linkage to the X chromosome a strong possibility. The affected males have a number of facial features that overlap with Cornelia de Lange syndrome, including prominent eyebrows, long, dark eyelashes that give the face a startled expression, small nose, and micrognathia. Additional features in the syndrome include syndactyly of the fingers and toes.

A family history, details of the pregnancy, and birth weight will aid in making the diagnosis. Chromosome analysis, ophthalmologic assessment, and assessment of facial anomalies by a physician experienced in dysmorphology will allow the discrimination of these entities from Cornelia de Lange syndrome.

MANIFESTATIONS AND MANAGEMENT

Growth and Feeding

Affected individuals are usually small at birth as a result of intrauterine growth retardation, which can often be detected by ultrasound during the third trimester

(Froster and Gortner, 1993; Kliewer et al., 1993). There are, however, many reports of infants affected with Cornelia de Lange syndrome who have normal birth weights (Bay et al., 1993; Kousseff et al., 1993; Kline et al., 1993; Krajewska-Walasek et al., 1995). Height, weight, and head circumference during childhood are all usually less than third centile (Ireland et al., 1993). Individuals with the mild form of Cornelia de Lange syndrome commonly have less severe growth retardation (Bay et al., 1993).

The most comprehensive study of growth in Cornelia de Lange syndrome was undertaken by Kline and colleagues (Kline et al., 1993). They used serial measurements of height, weight, and head circumference taken from 180 individuals aged birth to 29 years and constructed centile charts for Cornelia de Lange syndrome that were superimposed on charts for unaffected individuals. The mean birth weight in their study was 2.27 kg, and 68% of individuals had a birth weight less than the fifth centile. There was, however, a wide range of birth weight, with some weights on the 90th centile. There was also a large variation in birth lengths, with some as high as the 95th centile. By 2 years of age all heights were below the fifth centile, but subsequent height velocity for all individuals in the study was normal. The pubertal growth spurt occurred at the normal time (mean of 15 years for males and 13 years for females), but the magnitude of the pubertal growth spurt was less than that seen in the general population. The mean adult height was 155.78 cm for males and 131.13 cm for females. The 5th and 95th centiles for adult heights were 141 and 170 cm for males and 106 and 156 cm for females. In contrast to height velocity, in affected individuals between 2 years and puberty, weight velocity was less than that seen in unaffected individuals, and weights for the group as a whole were under the fifth centile. However, in males after the age of twelve there was a significant increase in weight, with some individuals having weights at the 50th centile.

Kousseff and colleagues studied growth in 30 individuals with Cornelia de Lange syndrome, although they did comment that the diagnosis was questionable in a number of the patients and no clinical photographs were included. They found that 90% of the studied individuals had poor growth and 40% had birth weight less than 2.7 kg. Of particular interest was the finding of endocrine abnormalities in 6 individuals. Four were found to have growth hormone deficiency, one was found to have end-organ resistance to growth hormone, and one was found to have the empty sella syndrome.

Feeding is usually poor from birth, and it is not uncommon for affected infants to require nasogastric tube feeding. In a few cases it is necessary to insert a gastrostomy tube. Interestingly, those who have gastrostomy tubes usually thrive and have height and weight in the normal range (personal data). Gastroesophageal reflux is common, and it contributes to feeding problems and failure to thrive. Lack of coordination of oral musculature and difficulty in chewing may also play a part.

Prognosis for normal growth rate is good if underlying gastroesophageal reflux is diagnosed and treated early.

Evaluation

- Head circumference, length, and weight should be measured at birth and every 6–12 months thereafter throughout childhood.
- Growth velocity should be calculated, and if it is less than normal underlying pathology such as gastroesophageal reflux should be sought (see below).

Treatment

- Adequate caloric intake should be ensured through nasogastric feeding if the child is unable to bottle feed.
- In cases with severe gastroesophageal reflux and feeding difficulties it may be necessary to place a gastrostomy tube at the time of fundoplication.

Development and Behavior

A number of studies and case reports have documented IQ in affected individuals, and the results have ranged from 30 to 60 for classically affected individuals and up to 102 for those who are more mildly affected (Barr et al., 1971; Cameron and Kelly, 1988; Ireland et al., 1993; Bay et al., 1993; Van Allen et al., 1993; Jackson et al., 1993; Kline et al., 1993). In a study of psychosocial development of 36 individuals with Cornelia de Lange syndrome at ages ranging from 5 to 47 years, specific deficits in verbal communication were identified but relatively good self-help skills were found (Beck, 1987).

Berney et al. (1999) carried out a detailed study of behavior in 49 individuals with the classical and mild phenotypes. The ages of those in the study ranged from early childhood to adulthood. They found a wide variety of symptoms, including hyperactivity (40%), self-injury (44%), daily aggression (49%), and sleep disturbance (55%). The behavioral difficulties correlated closely with the presence of an autistic-like syndrome and the degree of mental retardation. They also found that the behavioral difficulties continued into adulthood.

Kline and colleagues obtained developmental assessments on 122 individuals with Cornelia de Lange syndrome using a variety of methods and were able to construct developmental milestone charts with 25th, 50th, 75th, and 95th centiles covering gross motor, fine motor, social skills, and speech development (Kline et al., 1993). The 25th, 50th, 75th, and 95th centiles for walking independently were 18 months, 2 years, 3-1/2 years, and 10 years. The same centiles for the first word were 13 months, 18 months, 2 years, and 5 years. There was no regression in skills for any of the individuals, and strengths were found in visual spatial memory and perceptual organization skills including fine motor skills. Of particular interest was a finding of higher IQs in the younger age group. It was not possible to determine whether this was a

consequence of earlier educational intervention or of the improved diagnosis of individuals with mild Cornelia de Lange syndrome, because they did not comment on the numbers in their study with classical and mild forms of the syndrome. In a smaller study, we have found that classically affected individuals walked between the ages of 2 and 6 years whereas those with the mild form walked between 1 and 2-1/2 years (Ireland et al., 1993). Those with the classical form had only single words or no speech, whereas those with the mild form could often construct sentences.

There are many reports in the literature of speech being absent in individuals with Cornelia de Lange syndrome. At the other end of the spectrum, one female with mild Cornelia de Lange syndrome was reported to be able to talk in sentences at 14 years (Ireland et al., 1993; Bay et al., 1993; Krajewska-Walasek et al., 1995).

In a study of the prognostic indicators for the development of speech, birth weight less than 2.27 kg, moderate to severe hearing impairment, upper limb malformations, poor social interactions, and severe motor delay indicated a poor prognosis (Goodban, 1993). The 116 patients in the study ranged in age from 2 months to 29 years, although more than 70% were less than 6 years old, thus limiting the power of the study in assessing speech in later childhood and adolescence. Of those over the age of 4, 53% could construct sentences of 2 or more words whereas 33% had up to two words. Four percent of individuals were thought to have language skills in the normal or low-normal range. Overall, the study found that expressive language was inferior to comprehension and that individuals with highly developed vocabularies often had poor syntactic skills. Individuals were usually quiet and rarely talked even if they had well-developed vocabularies. The overall results suggested that speech and language skills were better than previous reports in the literature, but it was not possible to ascertain whether this was because few individuals in the study were institutionalized, the parents of the children in the study had higher expectations, the parents were more likely to have had their child's hearing impairment diagnosed and treated, or the children had more intensive educational input.

Harland and Bowden (1998) focused their study of speech and language on 9 individuals with the mild form of the syndrome. The individuals ranged in age from 5 to 30 years with a mean of 15 years. All 9 could communicate verbally, and both receptive and expressive language was delayed. In contrast to the study by Goodban, Harland and Bowden (1993) found no discrepancy between comprehension and expression. Syntactic skills were found to be restricted and utterances telegraphic. They found no word finding or naming problems. With respect to pragmatic skills they found poor eye contact, restricted facial expression, and limited attempts at initiation of speech. Four of the individuals in the study had a dysphonic voice, and 5 had hypernasality with nasal escape, which was confirmed on videofluoroscopy. Examination of the palate revealed one individual with a submucous cleft, and the other 8 had an unusual midline ridge of the soft palate that occasionally also involved the hard palate.

Several reports in the literature have commented on the low-pitched growling cry that is so characteristic of the syndrome in infancy (Ptacek et al., 1963; Barr et al., 1971; Saal et al., 1993; Van Allen et al., 1993; Jackson et al., 1993). Fraser and Campbell (1978) comment on the dysphonic nature of the speech in older individuals in their study, although spectrographic analysis did not reveal abnormally low fundamental frequencies. They suggest that a connection may exist between the glottal "fry" (a nonperiodical phonation of the vocal folds in frequencies below the normal pitch register) observed in the cries of the younger non-speaking individuals and the hoarseness in the speech of the older subjects.

It has not been possible to assess the effect of the combined neural and conductive deafness seen in the syndrome (see below) on impaired speech because none of the studies of speech in Cornelia de Lange syndrome has included an assessment of hearing. Because individuals with Cornelia de Lange syndrome are now treated with hearing aids and the insertion of ventilation tubes, the development of speech may appear to improve in years to come.

Almost all children with the syndrome will eventually learn to walk. Those with the mild phenotype will be sitting by one year and walking by two years, whereas most of those with the classical syndrome will be over two years old before they are sitting and over 3 years old before they are walking (personal experience). A minority of those with the classical form of the syndrome will produce a few words, whereas the majority of those with the mild form will ultimately be able to talk in sentences.

Behavioral disturbance is common in Cornelia de Lange syndrome and is more frequent in those with severe mental retardation (Shear et al., 1971; Johnson et al., 1976; Sarimski, 1997). Difficulties in communication often exacerbate the situation and highlight the need to use a method of sign language from an early age to improve communication and reduce frustration. It is important to rule out a medical cause such as gastroesophageal reflux when there is deterioration in behavior. Dramatic improvements in behavior are not uncommon after treatment of the reflux. Reported abnormal behaviors that have been described in the syndrome include autistic features such as lack of social relatedness and impassivity, rejection of physical contact, rigidity, and inflexibility to change. Pleasure in vestibular stimulation is common. Restlessness, hyperactivity, distractibility, irritability, and self-injurious behavior have all been described.

The prognosis for management of behavior problems is good if an underlying medical problem is identified and treated or if a communication difficulty was the underlying problem and the difficulties are circumvented with the addition of sign language. In the absence of such underlying problems, however, behavior remains a difficult management issue for families and care providers.

Evaluation

- Early referral should be made to an intervention program or child development center for identification of special intervention and education needs.
- Assessment of hearing should be accomplished by otoacoustic emission and auditory brain stem responses at diagnosis.
- Hearing should be checked every 6 months during childhood to detect conductive deafness related to middle ear disease.
- Any deterioration in behavior should be investigated promptly, and a medical cause such as gastroesophageal reflux should be considered.
- Communication skills should be evaluated.

Treatment

- Speech therapy should be instituted for those with the mild form of Cornelia de Lange syndrome.
- Enrollment in an early intervention program and subsequently in a special education program should take place as early as possible.
- Sign language or other techniques should be introduced to aid communication.
- Middle ear disease should be treated with antibiotics and, if needed, ventilation tubes.
- Any medical problem such as gastroesophageal reflux underlying behavioral deterioration should be treated.
- Long-standing behavior problems are difficult to change but may be improved

with behavioral modification. Guidance in techniques of behavior modification may be sought from a behavioral psychologist or developmental pediatrician.
- There are no studies indicating good responses from medication, such as methylphenidate (Ritalin), in this condition.

Ears and Hearing

Some degree of hearing impairment is present in over 90% of individuals with Cornelia de Lange syndrome. This has now been shown to be sensorineural in origin and usually bilateral (Sataloff et al., 1990; Ichiyama et al., 1994; Kaga et al., 1995). Superimposed otitis media and chronic middle ear disease ("glue ear") are common and can be difficult to diagnose because the external auditory canals tend to be very narrow in this disorder. Middle ear disease is less of a problem later in childhood and in adulthood.

Hearing aids tend to be better tolerated when fitted early. Early diagnosis and treatment of hearing impairment is imperative if the development of language in those with the mild form of the syndrome is not to be impaired.

Evaluation

- Otoacoustic emission and auditory evoked brain stem response testing should be conducted.
- Hearing should be checked every 6 months to detect conductive loss secondary to "glue ear".

Treatment

- Antibiotic treatment should be used for otitis media.
- Hearing aids should be fitted early.
- Insertion of ventilatory tubes should be accomplished to treat chronic middle ear disease.

Limb Abnormalities

A spectrum of limb abnormalities is seen in Cornelia de Lange syndrome that ranges from small hands with tapering fingers to bilateral reduction deformities with missing hands and forearms (Geudeke et al., 1963; France et al., 1969; Berg et al., 1970; Barr et al., 1971; Stratton et al., 1988; Cunniff et al., 1993; Ireland and Burn, 1993; Van Allen et al., 1993; Froster and Gortner, 1993; Krajewska-Walasek et al., 1995; Ireland, 1996). More minor hand abnormalities include proximally placed thumbs, single palmar creases, and clinodactyly of the fifth finger (Barr et al., 1971). The characteristic shape of the hands is well illustrated by Barr (Barr et al., 1971). More rarely, fusion of two fingers or polydactyly may be seen, and there is one report of a finger with two nails (Beck and Fenger, 1985).

Dermatoglyphic analysis of the hands has revealed relatively underdeveloped dermal ridges throughout childhood (Berg et al., 1970; Barr et al., 1971; Filippi, 1989). Overall, there is an increased frequency of radial loops and arches and a decrease in the number of whorls. The total finger ridge count is low, and interdigital triradii are also common (Abraham and Russel, 1968; Berg et al., 1970; Barr et al., 1971; Filippi, 1989). Jackson and colleagues (1993) found that 27% of individuals in their study had severe limb reduction defects, whereas others have suggested that 14% of classically affected individuals have severe limb reduction defects (Ireland, 1996). In the upper limbs the humerus, ulna, and radius are reduced in length, and occasionally the radius or ulna is aplastic (Geudeke et al., 1963; Froster and Gortner, 1993). Shortening of the metacarpals and in particular of the first metacarpal is common (Peeters, 1975). The second and fifth metacarpals are usually shorter than the third and fourth, and measurements of all the metacarpophalangeal bones are several standard deviations below the mean (Peeters, 1975; Halal and Preus, 1979). Flexion contractures of the elbows are common and are secondary to deformation of the proximal metaphysis of the radius, which is usually subluxed (Peeters, 1975; Filippi, 1989; Van Allen et al., 1993). The severe limb reduction defects may be unilateral or bilateral and when unilateral show no predilection to a particular side (Berg et al., 1970). Even those individuals with severe limb reduction defects have good fine motor skills.

Although more than 100 cases of severe upper limb reduction defects have been reported in the literature, there are only a handful of cases with major lower limb reduction defects. The reported lower limb abnormalities have included partial syndactyly of the second and third toes, absent toes with clefting of the foot, talipes equinovarus, absence of the tibia, bowed fibula, and bifid femur (Filippi, 1989; Pfeiffer and Correll, 1993; Van Allen et al., 1993).

Evaluation

- Measurement of the metacarpophalangeal index and X rays of the elbow may aid diagnosis.

Treatment

- There are no published reports of benefit from surgical approaches to limb anomalies, and even those with severe mental retardation often have remarkably good fine motor control.

Gastrointestinal

Gastroesophageal reflux is by far the most common gastrointestinal problem in Cornelia de Lange syndrome and affects those with both the classical and mild forms of the syndrome (Jackson et al., 1993; Leroy et al., 1993; Bull et al., 1993; Ireland, 1996).

Untreated, the reflux can lead to significant morbidity and mortality. The development of Barrett's esophagus and esophageal stenosis is common and the development of adenocarcinoma of the esophagus can occur. The condition can present in affected individuals with failure to thrive, reduced growth velocity, anemia, recurrent pneumonia, apnea, or behavioral disturbance. Because the association between reflux and Cornelia de Lange syndrome has only relatively recently come to light, damage to the esophagus has often been severe at the time of diagnosis.

Malformations of the gastrointestinal tract presenting shortly after birth include pyloric stenosis in approximately 1% of affected individuals or, very rarely, an annular pancreas presenting as duodenal obstruction (Berg et al., 1970; Froster and Gortner, 1993; Bay et al., 1993). Uncommonly, abnormalities of mesenteric insertion and failure of normal rotation of the bowel during embryonic development can lead to malrotation and in some cases have resulted in life-threatening volvulus with ischemia and infarction of the bowel (Jackson et al., 1993).

In practice, very few individuals respond to conservative management of gastroesophageal reflux, and most need surgery (personal experience). Postoperative problems such as bloating and the inability to belch are common and can be avoided by the use of a "floppy" fundoplication. Stories of the dramatic improvement in behavior and development postoperatively are common. Children with the syndrome who have a gastrostomy are often considerably larger than those who do not. Although prognosis is good if reflux is diagnosed and treated early, it is poor if there is a delay in diagnosis and there is already evidence of a Barrett's esophagus. Death from adenocarcinoma of the esophagus has occurred (DuVall and Walden, 1996).

Evaluation

- It is important to have a high index of suspicion and to consider the diagnosis of gastroesophageal reflux when anemia, deterioration in behavior, or a decrease in growth velocity occurs. Symptoms occurring when the child lies down at night and the appearance of dystonic posturing are good clues.

- Barium studies are of little help in making the diagnosis, and few affected individuals will tolerate 24-hour monitoring with a pH probe.
- It is not uncommon to resort to endoscopic examination under anesthesia. The benefits to the patient can be increased if hearing, eye, and dental examinations can be organized while the child is anesthetized.

Treatment

- Initial treatment should consist of advice on small, thickened feeds and keeping the individual as upright as possible.
- Pharmacotherapy with antacids, H_2-receptor blockers, and proton pump inhibitors should be tried.
- Fundoplication, occasionally with the insertion of a gastrostomy tube, is usually necessary.

Cardiovascular

Congenital heart defects are present in 20–25% of people with the classical form of Cornelia de Lange syndrome but are rare in mild Cornelia de Lange syndrome (Ireland, 1996; Mehta and Ambalavanan, 1997; Tsukahara et al., 1998). The most common abnormality is stenosis of the pulmonary valve either alone or in combination with a ventricular septal defect. A wide range of other cardiac defects has also been reported in the syndrome, including tetralogy of Fallot, coarctation of the aorta, atrial septal defect, hypoplastic left heart, single ventricle, and atrioventricular canal defect. Mild pulmonary branch stenosis is seen in 2% of children with the mild form of the syndrome but rarely requires treatment (Ireland, 1996). The most severe cardiac defects are often seen in infants with diaphragmatic hernia and severe limb reduction defects.

Children with the more complex congenital heart defects usually fail to thrive and die before or during corrective surgery. Those with the more straightforward defects do well.

Evaluation

- All babies with Cornelia de Lange syndrome should have a cardiac assessment shortly after birth, usually including echocardiography and ECG.

Treatment

- As in all cases of congenital heart disease, antibiotic prophylaxis is indicated before and during any procedure that induces a transient bacteremia, such as dental work, to prevent infective endocarditis.
- Referral should be made to a pediatric cardiology unit for management.
- The indications for and method of cardiac surgery are the same as in the general population.

Craniofacial

A high, arched palate is a common finding in individuals with Cornelia de Lange syndrome. The reported incidence of cleft palate varies between 18 and 59% (Jackson et al., 1993). In contrast to many of the other abnormalities, it also occurs in individuals with the mild form of the syndrome. Submucous clefts are also occasionally seen. The cleft palate is never associated with a cleft lip. The prognosis is usually good, but those with mild Cornelia de Lange syndrome and a cleft are less likely to develop speech than those without a cleft.

Evaluation

- Examination of the palate should occur at diagnosis.

Treatment

- If symptoms or signs suggest a submucous cleft, referral for a specialist assessment is indicated.

- Repair of the cleft palate is ideally accomplished in a unit experienced in this area. The methods are no different from those in the general population.
- Speech therapy is indicated postoperatively to maximize the development of speech in those with mild Cornelia de Lange syndrome.

Ophthalmologic

Ptosis of the upper eyelid is a common finding, especially in classical Cornelia de Lange syndrome (45%), in which it can range from a mild cosmetic problem to obstruction of the visual axis (Levin et al., 1990). It frequently results in the upward tilt of the head that is so characteristic of the syndrome. Myopia is also very common and has been reported in 60% of those with classical Cornelia de Lange syndrome. Symptoms suggestive of nasolacrimal duct obstruction such as watery eyes and recurrent conjunctivitis are very common. However, the symptoms usually resolve spontaneously with time and are rare after the age of six. It is common for these children to be referred for probing of the tear ducts, but in practice this has little effect on resolving the symptoms (personal experience).

Evaluation

- Referral for ophthalmologic assessment should be made in the first six months of life.

Treatment

- Correction of refractory errors should begin early because glasses are poorly tolerated if not fitted early.
- Surgery to correct ptosis is indicated if there is obstruction to the visual axis.
- Prompt treatment of conjunctivitis should occur.
- Because probing of the nasolacrimal duct has little effect on the symptoms, it should be avoided.

Genitourinary

The most common abnormality of the renal tract seen in Cornelia de Lange syndrome is a horseshoe kidney (Wick et al., 1982; Van Allen et al., 1993). Cryptorchidism is an extremely common finding in males with Cornelia de Lange syndrome and may occur in association with hypospadias and a hypoplastic scrotum (Leroy et al., 1993; Froster and Gortner, 1993; Krajewska-Walasek et al., 1995). The most common genital abnormality in females is a bicornuate uterus (Van Allen et al., 1993).

During early childhood the umbilicus and nipples are characteristically hypoplastic. Puberty occurs in both sexes at the usual time, and secondary sexual development is normal. Individuals with the mild form of the syndrome have reproduced, and offspring with and without the syndrome have been reported. This is in keeping with the presumed autosomal dominant nature of the condition.

Evaluation

- Ultrasound evaluation of the kidneys should be accomplished at diagnosis.
- Pubertal development should be followed to identify the time at which reproduction is possible.

Treatment

- Orchiopexy should be undertaken before 2 years of age, ideally between 6 months and 18 months, with the repair of any concomitant hypospadias being organized at the same time.
- If recurrent urinary tract infections result from kidney malformations, they should be treated with antibiotics and/or surgery as in the general population. However, the structural abnormalities of the kidneys that have been reported rarely require surgical intervention.

Neurological

A large number of CNS abnormalities have been reported, but most have been single case reports and no consistent abnormality has emerged. The reported incidence of seizures varies from 11 to 23%. Seizures are usually infrequent and can be well controlled with medication.

Evaluation

- Elucidation of the type and frequency of seizures is accomplished by clinical history and EEG, as in the general population.

Treatment

- Anticonvulsant medication should be used as for seizures in the general population. No studies have been undertaken to compare the use of different anticonvulsants.

RESOURCES

Cornelia de Lange Syndrome Foundation

302 West Main Street, #100, Avon, CT 06001, USA. Tel: 1 800 223 8355, Fax: 860 676 8337.

Alan and Jane Peaford, Cornelia de Lange Syndrome Foundation UK

"Tall Trees", 106 Lodge Lane, Grays, Essex, RM16 2UL, England. Tel +44 01375 376439.

Brochures

Facts About Cornelia de Lange Syndrome
Fact sheet that can be obtained from the Cornelia de Lange Syndrome Foundation, UK or US
Cornelia de Lange Syndrome
A booklet produced by the Cornelia de Lange syndrome Foundation UK summarizing the main features of the syndrome

Cornelia de Lange Syndrome Foundation Family Album

Photographs and details of over 100 individuals with Cornelia de Lange syndrome whose parents are members of the Cornelia de Lange Syndrome Foundation US

On-Line Resources

Cornelia de Lange Syndrome Foundation:
www.cdls.co.uk
www.cdlsoutreach.org

National Organization for Rare Disorders (NORD)

http://www.nord-rdb.com/~orphan

REFERENCES

Abraham JM, Russel A (1968) De Lange syndrome: A study of nine examples. *Acta Paediatr Scand* 57:339–353.

Aitken DA, Ireland M, Berry E, Crossley JA, Macri JN, Burn J, Connor JM (1999) Second trimester pregnancy associated plasma protein-A levels are reduced in Cornelia de Lange syndrome pregnancies. *Prenat Diag* 19:706–710.

Allanson JE, Hennekam RCM, Ireland M (1997) de Lange syndrome: Subjective and objective comparison of the classical and mild phenotypes. *J Med Genet* 34:645–650.

Anneren G, Gustavson KH (1984) Partial trisomy 3q (3q25—qter) syndrome in two siblings. *Acta Paediat Scand* 73:281–284.

Bamforth JS, Leonard CO, Chodirker BN, Chitayat D, Gritter HL, Evans JA, Keena B, Pantzar T, Friedman JM, Hall JG (1989) Congenital diaphragmatic hernia, coarse facies, and acral hypoplasia: Fryns syndrome. *Am J Med Genet* 32:93–99.

Barr AN, Grabow JD, Matthews CG, Grosse FR, Motl ML, Opitz JM (1971) Neurologic and psychometric findings in the Brachmann-de Lange syndrome. *Neuropaediatrie* 3:46–66.

Bay C, Mauk J, Radcliffe J, Kaplan P (1993) Mild Brachmann-de Lange syndrome. Delineation of the clinical phenotype, and characteristic behaviors in a six-year-old boy. *Am J Med Genet* 47:965–968.

Beck B (1987) Psycho-social assessment of 36 de Lange patients. *J Ment Defic Res* 31:251–257.

Beck B, Fenger K (1985) Mortality, pathological findings and causes of death in the de Lange syndrome. *Acta Paediat Scand* 74:765–769.

Berg JM, McCreary BD, Ridler MAC, Smith GF (1970) *The de Lange Syndrome.* Pergamon Press, Oxford.

Berney TP, Ireland M, Burn J (1999). Behavioural phenotype of Cornelia de Lange syndrome. *Arch Dis Child* 81:333–336.

Bishun NP, Morton WRM (1965) Brachmann/De Lange syndrome. *Lancet* 1:439.

Brachmann W (1916) Ein Fall von symmetrischer Monodaktylie durch Ulnadefedkt, mit symmetrischer Flughautbildung in den Ellenbeugen, sowie anderen Abnormalitaten. Jahr Kinderheilkunde 84:225–235.

Bull MJ, Fitzgerald JF, Heifetz SA, Brei TJ (1993) Gastrointestinal abnormalities: A significant cause of feeding difficulties and failure to thrive in Brachmann-de Lange syndrome. *Am J Med Genet* 47:1029–1034.

Cameron TH, Kelly DP (1988) Normal language skills and normal intelligence in a child with de Lange syndrome. *J Speech Hear Disord* 53:219–222.

Chen C, Liu F, Jan S, Lan C (1996) Partial duplication of 3q and distal deletion of 11q in a stillbirth with an omphalocele containing the liver, short limbs, and intrauterine growth retardation. *J Med Genet* 33:615–617.

Chodirker BN, Chudley AE (1994) Male-to-male transmission of mild Brachmann-de Lange syndrome. *Am J Med Genet* 52:331–333.

Clarren SK (1981) Recognition of fetal alcohol syndrome. *JAMA* 254:2436–2439.

Clarren SK, Smith DW (1978) The fetal alcohol syndrome. *N Engl J Med* 298:1063–1067.

Clericuzio CL (1993) Mild mental retardation with classic somatic phenotype in the Brachmann-de Lange syndrome. *Am J Med Genet* 47:992–994.

Cunniff C, Curry CJ, Carey JC, Graham JM, Jr., Williams CA, Stengel-Rutkowski S, Luttgen S, Meinecke P (1993) Congenital diaphragmatic hernia in the Brachmann-de Lange syndrome. *Am J Med Genet* 47:1018–1021.

de Die-Smulders C, Theunissen P, Schrander-Stumpel C, Fryns JP (1992) On the variable expression of the Brachmann-de Lange syndrome. *Clin Genet* 41:42–45.

de Lange C (1933) Sur un type nouveau de dégénération (typus amstelodamensis). *Arch Med Enfants* 36:713–719.

de Lange C (1938) Nouvelle observation du "Typus Amstelodamensis" et examen anatomo-pathologique de ce type. *Arch Med Enfants* 41:193–203.

DuVall GA, Walden DT (1996) Adenocarcinoma of the esophagus complicating Cornelia de Lange syndrome. *J Clin Gastroenterol* 22:131–133.

Fear C, Briggs A (1979) Familial partial trisomy of the long arm of chromosome 3 (3q). *Arch Dis Child* 54:135–138.

Filippi G (1989) The de Lange syndrome. Report of 15 cases. *Clin Genet* 35:343–363.

Fineman RM, Hecht F, Ablow RC, Howard RO, Breg WR (1978) Chromosome 3 duplication q/deletion p syndrome. *Pediatr* 61:611–618.

France NE, Crome L, Abraham JM (1969) Pathological features in the de Lange syndrome. *Acta Paediatr Scand* 58:470–480.

Fraser WI, Campbell BM (1978). A study of six cases of de Lange Amsterdam dwarf syndrome, with special attention to voice, speech, and language characteristics. *Develop Med Child Neurol* 20:189–198.

Frias JL, Wilson AL, King GJ (1982) A cephalometric study of fetal alcohol syndrome. *J Pediatr* 101:870–873.

Froster UG, Gortner L (1993) Thrombocytopenia in the Brachmann-de Lange syndrome [letter]. *Am J Med Genet* 46:730–731.

Fryns JP (1979) A new lethal syndrome with cloudy cornea, diaphragmatic defects, and distal limb deformities. *Hum Genet* 50:65–70.

Fryns JP, Dereymaeker AM, Hoefnagels M, D'Hondt F, Mertens G, van den Berghe H (1987) The Brachmann-de Lange syndrome in two siblings of normal parents. *Clin Genet* 31:413–415.

Geudeke M, Bijlsma JB, Bruijne JI (1963) Chromosomen-onderzoek bij typus degenerativus amstelodamensis. *Maandschr Kindergeneesk* 31:248–258.

Goodban MT (1993) Survey of speech and language skills with prognostic indicators in 116 patients with Cornelia de Lange syndrome. *Am J Med Genet* 47:1059–1063.

Halal F, Preus M (1979) The hand profile on de Lange syndrome: diagnostic criteria. *Am J Med Genet* 3:317–323.

Harland K, Bowden M (1998) Speech and language evaluation in mild Cornelia de Lange syndrome. *R Coll Speech Lang Therapists Bull* 555: 12–13.

Huang C, Emanuel I, Huang SW, Chen TY (1967) Two cases of the de Lange syndrome in Chinese infants. *J Pediatr* 71:251.

Ichiyama T, Hayashi T, Tanaka H, Nishikawa M, Furukawa S (1994) Hearing impairment in two boys with Cornelia de Lange syndrome. *Brain Dev* 16:485–487.

Ireland M (1996) Cornelia de Lange syndrome: Clinical features, common complications and long-term prognosis. *Curr Paediatr* 6:69–73.

Ireland M, Burn J (1993) Cornelia de Lange syndrome — photo essay. *Clin Dysmorphol* 2:151–160.

Ireland M, Donnai D, Burn J (1993) Brachmann-de Lange syndrome. Delineation of the clinical phenotype. *Am J Med Genet* 47:959–964.

Ireland M, English C, Cross I, Houlsby WT, Burn J (1991) A de novo translocation t(3;17)(q26.3;q23.1) in a child with Cornelia de Lange syndrome. *J Med Genet* 28:639–640.

Jackson L, Kline AD, Barr MA, Koch S (1993) De Lange syndrome: a clinical review of 310 individuals. *Am J Med Genet* 47:940–946.

Johnson HG, Ekman P, Friesen W (1976) A behavioral phenotype in the de Lange syndrome. *Pediatr Res* 10:843–850.

Kaga K, Tamai F, Kitazumi E, Kodama K (1995) Auditory brainstem responses in children with Cornelia de Lange syndrome. *Int J Pediat Otorhinolaryngol* 31:137–146.

Kawashima H, Maruyama S (1979) A case of chromosome 3 duplication q deletion p syndrome born to the mother with a pericentric inversion, inv(3)(p25q21). *Jpn J Hum Genet* 24:9–12.

Kliewer MA, Kahler SG, Hertzberg BS, Bowie JD (1993) Fetal biometry in the Brachmann-de Lange syndrome. *Am J Med Genet* 47:1035–1041.

Kline AD, Barr M, Jackson LG (1993) Growth manifestations in the Brachmann-de Lange syndrome. *Am J Med Genet* 47:1042–1049.

Kline AD, Stanley C, Belevich J, Brodsky K, Barr M, Jackson LG (1993) Developmental data on individuals with the Brachmann-de Lange syndrome. *Am J Med Genet* 47:1053–1058.

Kousseff BG, Thomson-Meares J, Newkirk P, Root AW (1993) Physical growth in Brachmann-de Lange syndrome. *Am J Med Genet* 47:1050–1052.

Krajewska-Walasek M, Chrzanowska K, Tylki-Szymanska A, Bialecka M (1995) A further report of Brachmann-de Lange syndrome in two sibs with normal parents [review]. *Clin Genet* 47:324–327.

Leroy JG, Persijn J, Van de Weghe V, Van Hecke R, Oostra A, De Bie S, Craen M (1993) On the variability of the Brachmann-de Lange syndrome in seven patients. *Am J Med Genet* 47:983–991.

Levin AV, Seidman DJ, Nelson LB, Jackson LG (1990) Ophthalmologic findings in the Cornelia de Lange syndrome. *J Pediat Ophthalmol Strabismus* 27:94–102.

Lorenz P, Hinkel GK, Hoffmann C, Rupprecht E (1990) Scott's craniodigital syndrome — report of a second family. *Am J Med Genet* 37:224–226.

Lubinsky M, Severn C, Rapoport JM (1983) Fryns syndrome: A new variable multiple congenital anomalies (MCA) syndrome. *Am J Med Genet* 14:461–466.

Manouvrier S, Espinasse M, Vaast P, Boute O, Farre I, Dupont F, Puech F, Gosselin B, Farriaux JP (1996) Brachmann-de Lange syndrome: Pre- and postnatal findings. *Am J Med Genet* 62:268–273.

Mehta AV, Ambalavanan SK (1997) Occurrence of congenital heart disease in children with Brachmann-de Lange syndrome. *Am J Med Genet* 71:434–435.

Mosher GA, Schulte RL, Kaplan PA, Buehler BA, Sanger WG (1985) Pregnancy in a woman with the Brachmann-de Lange syndrome. *Am J Med Genet* 22:103–107.

Mulcahy MT, Pemberton PJ, Sprague P (1979) Trisomy 3q: Two clinically similar but cytogenetically different cases. *Ann Genet* 22:217–220.

Oostra RJ, Baljet B, Hennekam RC (1994) Brachmann-de Lange syndrome "avant la lettre" [letter]. *Am J Med Genet* 52:267–8:35.

Opitz JM (1985) The Brachmann-de Lange syndrome [review]. *Am J Med Genet* 22:89–102.

Pashayan H, Whelan D, Guttman S, Fraser FC (1969) Variability of the de Lange syndrome: Report of 3 cases and genetic analysis of 54 families. *J Pediatr* 75:853–858.

Pearce PM, Pitt DB, Roboz P (1967) Six cases of de Lange's syndrome; parental consanguinity in two. *Med J Aust* 1:502–506.

Peeters KLM (1975) Radiological manifestations of the Cornelia de Lange syndrome. *Pediatr Radiol* 3:41–46.

Pfeiffer RA, Correll J (1993) Hemimelia in Brachmann-de Lange syndrome (bdls): a patient with severe deficiency of the upper and lower limbs. *Am J Med Genet* 47:1014–1017.

Preus M, Rex AP (1983) Definition and diagnosis of the Brachmann-de Lange syndrome. *Am J Med Genet* 16:301–312.

Ptacek LJ, Opitz JM, Smith DW, Gerritsen T, Waisman HA (1963) The Cornelia de Lange syndrome. *J Pediatr* 63:1000–1021.

Rosenfeld W, Verma RS, Jhaveri RC, Estrada R, Evans H, Dosik H (1981) Duplication 3q: Severe manifestations in an infant with duplication of a short segment of 3q. *Am J Med Genet* 10:187–192.

Saal HM, Samango-Sprouse CA, Rodnan LA, Rosenbaum KN, Custer DA (1993) Brachmann-de Lange syndrome with normal IQ [review]. *Am J Med Genet* 47:995–998.

Sarimski K (1997) Communication, social-emotional development and parenting stress in Cornelia-de-Lange syndrome. *J Intellect Disabil Res* 41:70–75.

Sataloff RT, Spiegel JR, Hawkshaw M, Epstein JM, Jackson L (1990) Cornelia de Lange syndrome. Otolaryngologic manifestations. *Arch Otolaryngol Head Neck Surg* 116:1044–1046.

Sciorra LJ, Bahng K, Lee ML (1979) Trisomy in the distal end of the long arm of chromosome 3. A condition clinically similar to the Cornelia de Lange syndrome. *Am J Dis Child* 133:727–730.

Scott CR, Bryant JL, Graham CB (1971) A new craniodigital syndrome with mental retardation. *J Pediatr* 78:658–663.

Shear CS, Nyhan WL, Kirman B, Stern J (1971) Self-mutilative behaviour as a feature of the de Lange syndrome. *J Pediatr* 78:506–509.

Smithells RW (1965) De Lange's Amsterdam dwarfs syndrome: Introductory review with two case reports. *Dev Med Child Neurol* 7:27–30.

Stratton RF, Koehler N, Morrow WR (1988) An unusual cardiomelic syndrome. *Am J Med Genet* 29:333–341.

Tranebjaerg L, Baekmark UB, Dyhr-Nielsen M, Kreiborg S (1987) Partial trisomy 3q syndrome inherited from familial t(3;9)(q26.1; p23). *Clin Genet* 32:137–143.

Tsukahara M, Okamoto N, Ohashi H, Kuwajima K, Kondo I, Sugie H, Nagai T, Naritomi K, Hasegawa T, Fukushima Y, Masuno M, Kuroki Y (1998) Brachmann-de Lange syndrome and congenital heart disease. *Am J Med Genet* 75:441–442.

Van Allen MI, Filippi G, Siegel-Bartelt J, Yong SL, McGillivray B, Zuker RM, Smith CR, Magee JF, Ritchie S, Toi A, Reynolds JF (1993) Clinical variability within Brachmann-de Lange syndrome: A proposed classification system. *Am J Med Genet* 47:947–958.

Westergaard JG, Chemnitz J, Teisner B, Poulsen HK, Ipsen L, Beck B, Grudzinskas JG (1983) Pregnancy-associated plasma protein A: A possible marker in the classification and prenatal diagnosis of Cornelia de Lange syndrome. *Prenat Diagn* 3:225–232.

Wick MR, Simmons PS, Ludwig J, Kleinberg F (1982) Duodenal obstruction, annular pancreas, and horseshoe kidney in an infant with Cornelia de Lange syndrome. *Minn Med* 65:539–41: 35.

Wilson GN, Hieber VC, Schmickel RD (1978) The association of chromosome 3 duplication and the Cornelia de Lange syndrome. *J Pediatr* 93:783–788.

Wilson WG, Kennaugh JM, Kugler JP, Wyandt HE (1983) Reciprocal translocation 14q;21q in a patient with the Brachmann-de Lange syndrome. *J Med Genet* 20:469–471.

CHAPTER 7

DOWN SYNDROME

ALASDAIR G. W. HUNTER

INTRODUCTION

Incidence

The prevalence of Down syndrome is highly dependent on maternal age and the gestational timing at ascertainment. Trisomy 21 accounts for about 1 in 150 first-trimester spontaneous abortions, and 35% of cases diagnosed between 15 and 28 weeks of gestation are lost naturally, the actual loss rate varying inversely with gestation at ascertainment (Hook et al., 1995). Estimates of birth prevalence must allow for underascertainment, which is more common to older studies based on birth certificate and registry data. In more recent studies, allowance must be made for case loss due to prenatal diagnosis and termination of pregnancy.

Bray et al. (1998) undertook a meta-analysis of 9 published data sets of birth prevalence and have provided maternal age-specific rates from age 16–50 years. Those rates rise from 0.69 in 1000 (1/1445) live births at age 20 years to 38.89 in 1000 (1/25) at the age of 45, with an overall prevalence of 1.42 in 1000 (1/704). All 9 populations were of largely European extraction, but there are few data to suggest that age-specific rates differ significantly by race, although they

may be somewhat higher in Mexican Americans and Jews of African/Asian origin (Hook et al., 1995).

Life expectancy tables are estimated on the basis of cross-sectional survival rates to specific ages. If the birth prevalence of Down syndrome is constant, one can compare the rate of Down syndrome at age 50 years with that at birth in different decades and calculate and compare survival rates to age 50. However, such comparisons of survival for Down syndrome over time are complicated by a changing birth prevalence and other factors such as improved neonatal ascertainment and uneven improvement in survival across different age groups. Down syndrome is highly maternal age dependent, and if more mothers over 35 begin having children, and thus increase the birth prevalence, more children are available to survive, thus causing an 'apparent' increased survival to age 50. Increased use of maternal serum screening and prenatal diagnosis would have the opposite effect. An improvement in early survival will again present more cases surviving at later ages, without necessarily signaling improved longevity for older patients.

Notwithstanding these caveats, several geographically disparate studies have concluded that survival for patients with Down syndrome has shown marked improvement,

Management of Genetic Syndromes, Edited by Suzanne B. Cassidy and Judith E. Allanson
ISBN 0-471-31286-X   Copyright © 2001 by Wiley-Liss, Inc.

particularly over the past 25–30 years. Most of the improvement has resulted from the treatment of congenital heart disease and respiratory infections during the first decade, but reduced institutionalization with increased mobility and integration into society have probably also played a role. In a study of 2412 cases born between 1976 and 1980, Dupont et al. (1986) estimated a survival of 58 years for a child who was then age 5. Baird and Sadovnick (1988) used the British Columbia registry data on 1610 live births with Down syndrome born from 1908 to 1981 to predict a 44% and 13.6% survival to ages 60 and 68 years, respectively. This compared with 86.4% and 78.4% in the general population. The survival curves for Down syndrome do not parallel those of the general population. Mortality during the first 5 years continues to be high because of factors such as congenital heart disease, possibly a higher rate of sudden infant death syndrome, pneumonia, infections, and leukemia. From 5 to 39 years the curves parallel but somewhat exceed the general population. There then follows an increase in mortality rate that is more rapid than that of both the general population and other retarded individuals. Higher age-specific rates of stroke and senility appear as major factors responsible for this reduced survival.

Diagnostic Criteria

The diagnosis of Down syndrome is usually straightforward and is based on the characteristic appearance (gestalt) and behavior of affected individuals. This may be more challenging in premature infants, in some older adults, in an unfamiliar racial/ethnic group, or in patients whose signs are modified by significant mosaicism or a structural chromosome change that results in only partial duplication of 21q22. As with any syndrome, the signs and symptoms are variable from patient to patient.

The neonate with Down syndrome is characteristically hypotonic and hyperextensible and has poor behavioral reflexes. The skull is mildly microcephalic and brachycephalic with a flat occiput. The fontanels tend to be large, a third may be palpable, and they close late. The posterior hair whorl is more likely to be midline, and the hair is fine. The face is round in the neonate and infant (Fig. 7.1) and becomes more oval with age (Figs. 7.2 and 7.3). Underdevelopment of the midface gives a flat appearance, and the upper facial depth and length of the maxillary arch are disproportionately reduced. Epicanthal folds and upslanting palpebral fissures are typical, and the palpebrae 'purse' on laughing or crying. Brushfield spots of the iris are common and are more peripherally placed than those seen in the general population. Ophthalmologic evaluation often reveals fine opacities of the lens, but true cataracts are uncommon until adulthood. The optic disc is rosy colored and has an increased number of retinal vessels. The nose is short with a low nasal bridge and, usually, small nares. The mouth is downturned, and a small oral cavity contributes to a tendency to protrude the tongue and to mouth breathe, which results ultimately in cracked lips and possibly the fissured appearance of the tongue. Dental anomalies are common in older children and adults. Growth of the mandible tends to outpace that of the palate, leading to prognathism. The ears are small and may be cupped or show a folded-over upper helix. The neonate often has redundant nuchal skin, and with age the neck may appear wide when viewed from behind, perhaps partly because of the relative microbrachycephaly. The chest may reveal signs of congenital heart disease that affects about 40–50% of patients.

The hands are short with a high frequency of single palmar creases (which are in no way pathognomonic or significant in and of themselves). The middle phalanx of the fifth finger is short and/or triangular, resulting in a single flexion crease or clinodactyly, respectively. Dermatoglyphic analysis is not performed as often today, but characteristic

(A) 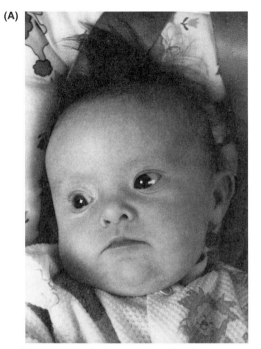   (B)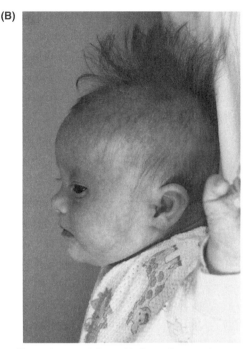

FIGURE 7.1. **A** Six-week-old girl with Down syndrome illustrating round face with flat malar area, low nasal bridge, epicanthal folds, and upslanting palpebral fissures. Even at rest there is some pursing around the eyes. Her nose is short and her mouth downturned. **B** A lateral view of the same child shows mottling of the skin, malar flatness, and a small nose. The ear is slightly small with mild overfolding of the helix.

findings include a higher frequency of arches and ulnar loops on the thumb, ulnar loops on the index and middle fingers and radial loops on the fourth and fifth fingers, a distal palmar triradius, and interdigital loops at I1 and I3. Dermatoglyphics have provided the backbone for a number of diagnostic indices for Down syndrome (Preus, 1977). The space between the first and second toes is increased and accompanied by a vertical plantar crease with an origin at the space. Cutis marmorata is common. The diagnosis may be aided by radiologic evidence of an additional manubrial ossification center, a flat acetabular angle, and hypoplastic iliac wings that flare outward.

The relative frequency and discriminant value of specific signs may vary between racial/ethnic groups. For example, the flat occiput, face, and nasal bridge and epicanthal folds have been shown to be more common in the general population of South African Blacks than in Caucasians, whereas a protruding tongue, excess nuchal skin, and Brushfield spots are less common in Black children with Down syndrome (Christianson et al., 1995). Although several authors have developed clinical diagnostic indices that have good discriminant power for Down syndrome (Preus, 1977), the gold standard for the diagnosis is karyotypic demonstration of trisomy 21.

Both Down syndrome and congenital malformations are common, and so the chance occurrence of a wide variety of birth defects in children with Down syndrome is to be expected. Comparison of the rates of specific malformations between children with and those without Down syndrome is required to determine which malformations are causally related to Down syndrome. Torfs and Christianson (1998) have provided a

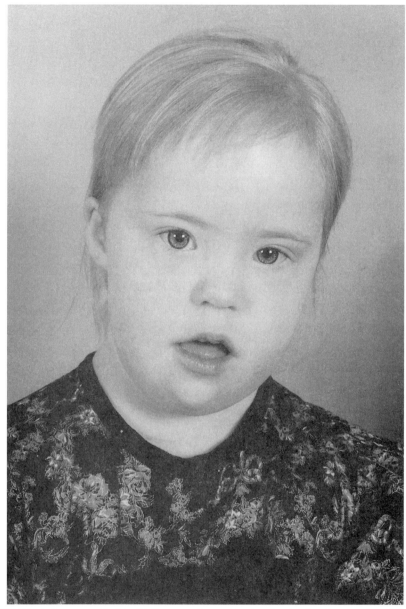

FIGURE 7.2. A four-year-old girl with Down syndrome showing that the face has lengthened from that of the newborn but maintains the characteristic low nasal bridge, epicanthal folds, and upslanting palpebral fissures. Brushfield spots can be seen close to the iris margin. There is malar underdevelopment and a tendency to mouth breathe. The ear is small with a slight overfolding and crimping of the upper helix.

review of the literature and a comparison of the rates of 61 anomalies between 2,894 patients with Down syndrome and a control population of 2.5 million from the same newborn surveillance registry. Forty-five of the malformations occurred significantly more frequently in Down syndrome, and every major system was represented. Risk ratios varied from nonsignificant to 1009 (atrioventricular canal defect). Risk ratios of over 100

(A)

(B)

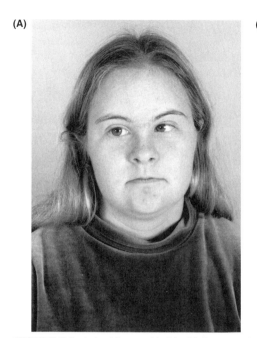
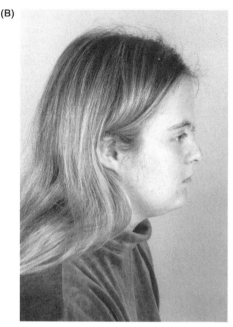

FIGURE 7.3. **A** An 18-year-old girl with Down syndrome demonstrating mild upslanting of the palpebral fissures, epicanthus, strabismus and Brushfield spots. Although there has been growth of the nose, it remains small and short with a relatively low bridge. There continues to be a downturn to the mouth, and the lower jaw is small. **B** The lateral view demonstrates brachycephaly, a small ear with a slightly overfolded helix, and a small nose and jaw.

were obtained for patent ductus arteriosus (152), overriding aorta (200), stenosis of the small intestine (142), duodenal atresia (265), Hirschsprung disease (102), annular pancreas (430), and hernia of Morgagni (246). Of equal interest are malformations that did not show an increased rate, including other types of diaphragmatic hernia, cleft lip with or without cleft palate, renal agenesis, neural tube defects, omphalocele, pyloric stenosis, and most cardiac malformations classified as conotruncal or looping defects. Blasto-genic and midline field defects are under-represented, with the exception of holo-prosencephaly, tetralogy of Fallot, tracheoe-sophageal fistula, and anal atresia. Almost all anal atresia in Down syndrome is low and without a fistula and has a good prognosis.

The association of Down syndrome with maternal age was the major impetus for the development of prenatal cytogenetic programs in many countries. However,

amniocentesis and chorionic villus sampling are costly, risk causing miscarriage, and have a relatively low yield, especially if applied to younger women. This has driven the search for a population-based screen-ing method. Most of such screening has focused on second-trimester maternal serum screening with one or more of the follow-ing: elevated α-fetoprotein, high β-human chorionic gonadotropin (β-hCG or free β-hCG), and low estriol. Now a variety of first-trimester biochemical markers, notably preg-nancy associated plasma protein-A (PAPP-A) and free β-hCG, are increasingly being uti-lized. Maternal serum screening can ascer-tain about 70% of cases for a false-positive rate of about 5%. Urine markers have also been explored. These screening tests only modify the prior age-specific risk figure, and positive screens require follow-up assess-ment, which may include invasive testing for karyotype analysis. In regions where there is extensive utilization of maternal serum screening, about 2 fetuses are detected by screening for each case diagnosed neonatally. The rate of amniocenteses per case detected with maternal serum screening is about 70 as compared to 200 when maternal age over 35 is used as the indication for amniocentesis.

With increased use of middle-trimester ultrasound it has become apparent that, in addition to the obvious major malformations associated with Down syndrome, there are a number of biophysical signs seen more commonly in the fetus with Down syndrome than in normal fetuses. Careful comparison of the rates of such markers in Down syndrome and in the general population allows calculation of a likelihood ratio for Down syndrome when such a sign is found. These can then be used alone, or in combination when they are shown to be independent, with the maternal age-specific risk to estimate a modified odds for Down syndrome and to make recommendations about further invasive diagnostic testing. Likewise, the absence of such markers will decrease the age-specific risk of Down syndrome.

Presently the definition of each ultrasonographic sign and the estimation of likelihood ratios vary between publications, and it is beyond the scope of this chapter to establish a consensus. Of the markers, typical cardiac malformations, duodenal atresia, echogenic bowel, and nuchal thickening have likelihood ratios of over 5, short humerus/femur, intracardiac echogenic foci, fifth finger clinodactyly, and pleural effusion are in the range of 2 to 2.5, and pyelectasis and brachycephaly are closer to 1.5. Recent estimates are that a combination of fetal ultrasound at 11–14 weeks of gestation and maternal age may detect up to 80% of fetuses with Down syndrome for a false-positive rate of 5%, and algorithms for combining ultrasound with maternal serum screening are being developed and evaluated. Some of these include graduated risk ratios dependent on the degree to which a specific sign or measurement is abnormal. However, ultrasonographic skills are highly variable, and their use in prenatal screening for Down syndrome requires a high level of training and a standardized approach.

Questions of personal ethics and choice are intrinsic to prenatal diagnosis. All couples should receive education appropriate to their level of understanding that includes a discussion of Down syndrome and an explanation of screening and where it may lead, as well as counseling that provides an explicit discussion of the ethical issues and the choices that may be required. This is as true for ultrasound screening and maternal serum screening as it is for amniocentesis.

Etiology, Pathogenesis and Genetics

Down syndrome is caused by trisomy for chromosome 21, specifically, duplication (trisomy) of 21q22. About 95% of cases result from nondisjunction and resultant standard trisomy 21. The remaining 5% are relatively evenly split between patients with Robertsonian translocations, of which the 14;21 translocation is the most common and about half are familial, and mosaic Down syndrome. Mosaicism may arise by postzygotic (mitotic) nondisjunction of a normal zygote or the postzygotic loss of a chromosome 21 from a trisomic zygote. The lack of any maternal age association with mosaicism suggests that the former is the more important. A small minority of patients have other types of chromosome rearrangements, some of which result in partial duplications (trisomy) of chromosome 21.

Maternal age is the single most important determinant of nondisjunction trisomy 21, and molecular techniques have shown that 85–90% of cases result from maternal and 5–10% from paternal meiotic errors, whereas up to 5% of cases may represent postzygotic mitotic nondisjunction. About 75% of maternal and 50% of paternal nondisjunction occurs in meiosis I, with the remainder occurring in meiosis II. The observation that the odds ratio increases for both maternal meiosis I and II errors with age suggests that there is an age-sensitive risk factor acting at the time of conception (Yoon et al., 1996).

It has been suggested that maternal smoking may reduce the birth rate of Down syndrome, perhaps through greater fetal wastage, and that maternal thyroid disease may increase the risk, but these factors are of insignificant importance at the level of the individual woman. The potential of a paternal age effect on incidence has been the subject of debate (Stene et al.,1987), but it must be considered of minor, if any, importance given our current knowledge of the origin of the trisomy. Verger (1997) reviewed evidence concerning natural, medical, and accidental radiation exposure and the risk of trisomy and concluded that the data are contradictory and unconvincing but that there is need for further properly designed studies.

The pathogenesis of the characteristic appearance and specific associated malformations of Down syndrome are presumed to relate to dosage effects of genes on 21q22. That only certain malformations occur more frequently supports the view that specific genes, rather than a generalized embryological disturbance, are at play. Efforts are underway using patients with partial 21q duplications, animal models of Down syndrome, and modern molecular mapping and cloning techniques to isolate key Down syndrome genes (Hubert et al., 1997).

The recurrence risks for parents of children with trisomy 21 Down syndrome vary with the age of the mother at the time of the birth of the child. Mothers who have had a child with Down syndrome and who were of late maternal age maintain their current age-related risk, whereas those who were young (<30 years) are at increased risk (up to 6-fold) compared with their age peers. The basis for this increased risk remains unknown but could relate to a decreased likelihood of spontaneous abortion of trisomic fetuses or to an age-independent increased propensity to nondisjunction. There has been some evidence of increased prior fetal loss in young mothers of children with Down syndrome (Lippman and Aymé, 1984). Properly designed studies have shown that second- and third-degree relatives of patients with trisomy 21 are not themselves at increased risk (Berr et al., 1990). A common question is that of the risk to a couple in which one member has a relative with Down syndrome of unknown karyotype. The known age-specific rates of trisomy versus translocation Down syndrome and the likelihood of male and female transmission of a translocation can be used to calculate the risks for specific relatives of the affected person. The highest risk is about 1 in 640, and it applies to the children of the sister of the affected person. This is not greatly different from the population prevalence, and the risks decline rapidly with the degree of relationship and are lower when the connection is through a male.

Parents of children with *de novo* translocations are not at significantly increased risk for recurrence, whereas a man with a balanced Robertsonian translocation is at a 3–5% risk and a woman at a 10–15% risk for recurrent Down syndrome. Note must be taken of the special circumstance of a parental 21;21 translocation, where the risk is 100%.

Diagnostic Testing

Chromosome studies are indicated in all cases to eliminate even the remote possibility of diagnostic error and to uncover instances of chromosome translocation that result in complete or partial duplication (trisomy) of chromosome 21. Discovery of a translocation requires testing of the parents, and ultimately possibly other family members, to determine future reproductive risks. The diagnosis of Down syndrome can be made on interphase nuclei using fluorescence *in situ* hybridization (FISH), but a standard karyotype is more usual and provides information about translocations. For patients suspected of having Down syndrome and in whom a normal chromosome result is reported, it may be appropriate to refer to a specialist in dysmorphology, who may assess whether to look for mosaicism through the study of more cells or another tissue.

Differential Diagnosis

Down syndrome is common and distinctive and should not often be confused with other syndromes. In our referral experience, the most common confusion is with a normal neonate who has one or more of the common signs or minor anomalies that physicians associate with Down syndrome (e.g., hypotonia, 'large' tongue, single palmar creases). Absence of the other common signs and the facial gestalt of Down syndrome should avoid this error. Likewise, hypothyroidism and Beckwith-Wiedemann syndrome (see Chapter 4) can be distinguished by their own typical signs and the lack of other characteristics of Down syndrome.

A number of young children with Smith-Magenis syndrome (see Chapter 22) have been diagnosed fortuitously when the diagnostic deletion of 17p11.2 was detected on a karyotype requested for suspected Down syndrome. The overlapping features include brachycephaly, round face, upslanting palpebral fissures, midface hypoplasia, a small, wide nose, and Wölfflin-Krückmann iris spots that may be confused with Brushfield spots. Other signs of Down syndrome are absent, however, and with time the more typical appearance and behavior of Smith-Magenis syndrome become apparent.

Zellweger syndrome, a peroxisomal disorder, shares a number of findings with Down syndrome including hypotonia, large fontanels, flat occiput and face, anteverted nares, epicanthal folds, Brushfield spots, cataracts, abnormal helices, single palmar crease, and cardiac septal defects. Distinguishing signs include severe early developmental delay, seizures, a high forehead, shallow orbits, hepatomegaly, joint contractures, stippled epiphyses, and brain migrational anomalies. The diagnosis can be confirmed by finding elevated plasma very-long-chain fatty acids.

MANIFESTATIONS AND MANAGEMENT

Health care providers are a vital link in helping parents adapt to the initial shock and disappointment of learning that their child has Down syndrome. Studies have demonstrated that parents prefer to be told as a couple, as soon as possible, and by an informed professional who is known to them. In many cases, the primary physician may accompany, or quickly introduce, a specialist as required. Where there is delay in informing, the parents often come to suspect a problem through cues from others, and this delay leaves them with the task of 'reinforming' their family and friends that the baby is not 'OK'. Some studies have shown that parents perceive physicians to have been overly pessimistic in their initial communications. Written information, referral to other parents, support groups, experts, and community services, as well as ongoing follow-up are perceived as important.

It is perhaps surprising that, at least in France, there may have been a recent increase in the proportion of children with Down syndrome being given up for adoption (Dumaret et al., 1998). This study showed that lack of associated malformations, birth rank greater than 2, maternal age of 15–24 years, residence in a large urban area, and birth outside France were factors associated with a lower likelihood of abandonment. Although these are largely sociocultural determinants, the authors believed that professionals can have a major impact in the way that options are presented to parents.

Growth and Feeding

Any of the known associated gastrointestinal malformations such as duodenal atresia, annular pancreas, Hirschsprung disease, or anal atresia/stenosis may complicate early feeding. A high index of suspicion and prompt intervention will reduce morbidity and mortality.

The relative placidity and hypotonia, particularly of the tongue, together with a small oral cavity and narrow nares may cause some initial difficulty with attachment to the breast and sucking. The same oral and motor difficulties may cause a delay in the introduction of solid foods, and the primary care physician has an important role in ensuring that a balanced diet is being maintained throughout infancy.

Patients with Down syndrome show a decreased growth rate and length (height) from birth throughout the growth period, with the most marked failure in infancy and adolescence. There is evidence that those raised in the community are taller than those raised in institutions. Females tend to fall 1.5–2.5 SD below the population mean until age 12 years and then fall to more than 3 SD below. The comparable figures for males are 2–3 SD below the mean to age 13 years and then 2–4 SD below to adulthood (Pueschel, 1990).

From late infancy, children with Down syndrome show a relative increase in mean weight for height and in weight/height^2, and excessive weight is a significant problem in adulthood. Prasher (1995) used the body mass index (BMI) in a sample of 201 adults with Down syndrome to show that only 13% of males and 10% of females were within their desirable weight range, whereas 31% of men and 22% of women were overweight and a further 48% of men and 47% of women were obese. In about one-third of subjects, the obesity was considered a significant health concern, and women were overrepresented in this group. The highest body mass indexes were seen in patients living at home, followed by those in group homes and then those in institutions.

The majority of children who remain in good general health should reach their genetic height potential. Management of weight gain may prove to be a challenge, but early anticipatory guidance, close monitoring and management, together with a multifaceted intervention will hopefully be successful, while at the same time making patients more participatory and improving their self-image and self-esteem.

Evaluation

- Length, weight and head circumference curves for Down syndrome are available in print and from the Internet and should be used to best monitor patients for other potential causes of growth failure and for problems with weight (Cronk et al., 1988; Pueschel, 1990)(see Resources).
- There should be a high index of suspicion for gastrointestinal malformations, which should be evaluated as in the general population.

Treatment

- For infants with difficulty sucking, assuring that the child is well awake and properly supported with the chin steadied, that the mouth and nose are clear of mucus (a syringe with a small amount of normal saline may help clear the nose), and that the child is burped regularly will usually overcome these minor, self-limited problems. In breast feeding, it may be helpful to facilitate attachment to the breast by first expressing a small amount of milk and by feeding more often (every 2–3 hours) to stimulate milk production. In a minority of cases the difficulties may be more marked and persistent and require referral to an expert in feeding.
- Gastrointestinal malformations should be treated as for the general population.
- Treatment of identifiable causes of a falloff from the appropriate growth curves, such as hypothyroidism or chronic bowel disease, should allow

resumption of the normal Down syndrome growth pattern.

- People with Down syndrome are short and do have a specific reduction in insulin-like growth factor-1 (IGF-1), which can be increased by therapeutic growth hormone with a concomitantly increased growth rate. However, there are no long-term studies of growth hormone treatment. Use of growth hormone in this context is not recommended outside properly approved scientific study where long-term follow-up is intended.

- There is every reason to believe that the solution to the problem of excess weight begins with careful childhood monitoring of weight and with special emphasis on aspects of diet and exercise. Prasher (1995) did find evidence of a fall in age-specific weight, more marked in men and over the age of 60 years.

Development and Behavior

The newborn with Down syndrome is hypotonic and, although tone will improve, developmental delay is the rule. Many aspects of development in Down syndrome have been reviewed by Hartley (1986). Eye contact with the mother is delayed, and once it is established it is maintained longer, which may inhibit development of other spheres of eye contact. The early temperament is very similar to that of the average child, but reactions tend to be muted. At an early stage, language is acquired in a pattern similar to mental-age-equivalent average children. By school age, children with Down syndrome lack the normal correlation between the production and comprehension of language, and the relative level of vocalization and grammatical usage falls in those over the age of 10 years. Children with Down syndrome show greater asynchrony in their sensorimotor development and less permanence to the acquisition of new abilities. The types of errors differ from those of normal children and they show more restricted play, as well as stereotypic and repetitive behavior, which is less goal oriented and organized. Children with Down syndrome who enter the normal school system require the intervention of qualified individuals and specialized programs to help them cope with those cognitive difficulties that prevent them from demonstrating adequate comprehension, problem solving, and communication (Hartley, 1986).

Although studies have shown there is some truth to the stereotype of children with Down syndrome as good, happy, affectionate, and outgoing, the picture is more complex and there are many exceptions. Children with Down syndrome show an age-related increase in anxiety, depression, and withdrawal, and although they show no overall increase in abnormal scores on the Child Behavior Checklist compared to others with mental retardation, they do show comparatively greater disobedience, stubbornness, speech problems, and preference for being alone, and less impulsiveness and hyperactivity (Dykens and Kasari, 1997).

In general, rates of neuroses, conduct disorders, and psychoses are lower in Down syndrome than in others who are learning disabled. On the other hand, depression, with a mean age of onset of 29 years, has been reported in up to 10% of adults in one study, and another study has shown that rates of psychopathology rise from less than 20% under age 20 to over 30% by the age of 28 years (Carr, 1994).

More normal tone and the absence of major malformations have been shown to correlate with higher Vineland scores, as well as better parental action on professional guidance. The former has predictive value for future developmental success. Although some IQ data based on patients not integrated into society and the general school system may be overly pessimistic, most studies show the mean IQ in Down syndrome to be less than 50 and include a trend to a decline with age. Social development may significantly outstrip mental age. Some (Carr, 1994) have suggested that the decline may be reversed during the third and fourth decades. The mean IQ in children and young adults ranges from 45 to 48, with a wide range and an upper limit of about 70. The mental age equivalent of the range is from 1 to 9 years, with a mean of 5.5 years. The IQ of children with Down syndrome does correlate approximately as expected with mean parental IQ. Mean IQs as low as 25 are recorded from adult samples; however, the confounding impacts of institutionalization, depression, and Alzheimer disease need to be assessed in a sample of individuals with Down syndrome who have shared some of the advantages denied to earlier cohorts. It is axiomatic that overall IQ is a poor measure of the spectrum of abilities that may be highly variable and that specific assessment of the individual components of development is required.

Today, many children with Down syndrome receive input from a number of sources such as child development, physiotherapy, and occupational therapy. Although there is some evidence of early benefit from such interventions, the ultimate value as compared to a stimulating home environment is yet to be adequately demonstrated. Although some parents are responsive to such interventions, others may feel overwhelmed, and it is important that parents be reassured that they can select a comfortable level of outside intervention without fear that they may be depriving their child of an essential need.

To a large extent, prospects for independent living and employment must be considered to be in flux. There has yet to be a generation of people with Down syndrome who have grown up with every effort made to integrate them fully into the school system and society. Several studies have shown that a significant proportion of individuals remain dependent in one or more of the daily skills of feeding, washing, dressing, and toileting, and that fewer than one-half of young adults are independent in all four. Other authors

report competencies of 80% to over 90% in these domains (Carr, 1994). It is not clear whether these differences between studies are methodological or represent true differences in the populations due to successful intervention. Although a significant proportion of adults with Down syndrome may be left alone for a few hours or more and can get out and around familiar territory and prepare simple meals, some level of day-to-day supervision remains a requirement for virtually all.

In the past, those not at home were cared for in institutions or hospitals. This led to a pattern of increasing rates of institutionalization with age. Although many individuals with Down syndrome continue to spend a longer period with their parents than the average child, there is a trend to increasing residence within the community with different levels of supervision depending on the degree of independence. Current goals are therefore to maximize self-help skills and foster independence.

A major challenge now and in the future will be to find meaningful employment for individuals with Down syndrome. Appearance, mental disability, slowness, poor acquisition of new skills, and, in some cases, overdependence fostered by overprotective parents probably all contribute to the currently small proportion of individuals who are employed. Only about 10% of persons with Down syndrome are in work placements, and less than 5% are in paying jobs. This appears equally true for recent school graduates (Carr, 1994). Again, there is the need to foster skills and independence and, some have even argued, to alter appearance.

A decline in mental faculties in Down syndrome during the third and fourth decades of life was noted as early as 1876 and was seen to be associated with the neuropathologic changes of Alzheimer disease in the 1930s and 1940s. As greater numbers of patients began to survive to middle age, the clinical significance of these early observations became apparent, and it is now well established that virtually 100% of individuals with Down syndrome show the neuropathologic changes of Alzheimer disease by the age of 35–40 years. The pathology shows the same pattern of susceptible neurons as in the general population for both neurofibrillary tangles and senile plaques. The plaques of the amyloidogenic Aβ peptide are deposited at the same rate as in typical Alzheimer disease, but the process begins as early as the second decade, as opposed to the fifth decade in the general population (Holtzman, 1997). Atrophic changes on MRI also mirror those of standard Alzheimer disease, but age-matched patients with Down syndrome show more atrophic lesions in the white matter and T2 weighted hypodensity in the basal ganglia. Although there are remarkable similarities between the Alzheimer-like changes in Down syndrome and those in the general population, the pathological processes have not been proven identical.

Onset of clinical dementia lags significantly behind the appearance of the neuropathologic changes, but current evidence suggests that it is highly penetrant, with the average age of onset at 51–54 years and an average survival from diagnosis of about 5 years. Tests of cognitive function to detect early dementia have shown declining scores in Down syndrome across the age categories 25–34, 35–44, 45–54 and 55–64 years, a pattern not seen in control retarded individuals (Thase et al., 1982). The presence of an apolipoprotein Eε4 allele has the same effect in reducing the age of onset of Alzheimer disease as in the general population (Schupf et al., 1998). In a young cohort of individuals with Down syndrome, Del Bo et al. (1997) found that an inverse correlation between age and IQ in Down syndrome was limited to those cases with at least one Eε4 allele. Alzheimer disease in Down syndrome does differ from that in the general population in showing an earlier onset in males as well as an excess of affected males (Schupf et al., 1998) and a higher frequency of associated

seizures (15% to 20%). However, associated parkinsonian signs may be less common. Alzheimer disease is an important contributing cause to death in adults with Down syndrome.

Evaluation

- Evaluation of the developmental needs of the child with Down syndrome includes assessment of the acceptance by, and comfort of, the family with the diagnosis and of their support network.

- Physical health and sensory systems may also have a significant impact upon development, and these should be carefully assessed (see below).

- The approach to development should be multidisciplinary and may include, among others, a primary care physician, a physical and occupational therapist, a developmental specialist, a teacher with specialized expertise, and a speech therapist.

- Early signs of Alzheimer disease in high-functioning individuals include a decline in memory and verbal capability, whereas others may show a decrease in social interaction and attention and increasing apathy. It is important to rule out hypothyroidism and depression in such cases.

Treatment

- Intervention can be expected to involve all those listed above and may also require social support, various medical specialists, and those with skills in behavioral management.

- Those working with the child and family must have a realistic but also positive and optimistic approach. Today, children in countries with well-developed educational and health care systems will be enrolled in early organized infant and then childhood educational programs. The best are likely to be those that recognize that children with Down syndrome are not simply delayed but may have specific deficits that require imaginative approaches to teaching that which the average child would simply acquire. Innovative methods may be particularly important in the area of communication.

- Early behavioral intervention may be an important preventive measure for some children.

- There is a long history of claims of therapeutic value for drugs, hormones, vitamins, and related therapies to improve the motor and cognitive function of individuals with Down syndrome. Included have been growth and thyroid hormone, vitamins, 5-OH-tryptophan, glutamic acid, injection of fetal cells, and various "cocktail" mixtures. It can be stated that those with Down syndrome are not deficient in any of these substances, that properly controlled trials have failed to show benefit, that studies claiming benefit are anecdotal or uncontrolled, and that in general the benefit can be ascribed to a placebo effect resulting from increased intervention and attention.

- Currently there is no curative treatment for Alzheimer disease, and although some therapies show promise in slowing the process or alleviating the symptoms, it cannot be assumed that their effect will be comparable in Down syndrome. Institution of any such treatments should be as part of properly designed scientific studies.

Neurologic

Stereotypic movements are common in those with mental handicap and may be even more prevalent in those with Down syndrome. In a study of 145 patients with a mean age of 40 years, Haw et al. (1996) found that at least 90% had dyskinesias, almost all with orofacial and about 20% with limb or trunk signs. Tongue thrust (68%), an impassive face

(57%), and decreased arm swing occurred in 50% or more of cases. Bradykinesias (33%) and global parkinsonism (4%) were only seen in those with dementia, and this has been confirmed in other studies. Brief random movements, grimacing, abnormal facial movements, and postural and gait abnormalities were very commonly observed. About 40% of patients showed stereotypic movements including trunk rocking, rubbing a hand on the chest, or waving the hands in front of the eyes. There appears to be a positive correlation between the occurrence of dyskinesia and the severity of mental disability and lack of academic and practical skills.

Seizures occur in about 5–7% of children with Down syndrome compared with a range of 20–50% in those with other forms of mental retardation. In one series of 47 cases with seizures, the cause was known in 29 cases and included cardiac hypoxia (8), cerebral artery occlusion (3), perinatal complications (7), infections (5), febrile (2), trauma (2), and chemotherapy (2) (Stafstrom et al., 1991). There was no significant difference in the rate of tonic-clonic (61–69%), myoclonic, and infantile spasms between those of known and unknown cause, and the 4 cases of atonic seizures were in the unknown and the 6 cases of focal seizures in the known causation group.

In contrast to the relatively low rate of seizures in children, adults with Down syndrome and Alzheimer disease appear to have a higher frequency of seizures than those with Alzheimer disease in the general population.

Evaluation

- Abnormal movements do not usually require treatment, although medication or other toxicity should be ruled out.

- Evaluation of seizures does not differ from that in the general population. EEG should be performed if there is a suspicious history.

Treatment

- Treatment of seizures does not differ from that in the general population.

Endocrine

Hypothyroidism. Thyroid disease, particularly hypothyroidism, is significantly more common in Down syndrome than in the general population. This includes congenital hypothyroidism as detected by newborn screening programs. The sex ratio is even. Prevalence varies with the definition, and there is an age-related inverse correlation between detection of a number of different antithyroid antibodies and levels of free and bound T_3 and T_4, and of thyroid-binding globulin (Pueschel, 1990). The prevalence of antithyroid antibodies and of patients with elevated TSH but normal T_4 far exceeds the number of patients with low T_4, and it is unclear which of such cases will become hypothyroid. An inverse correlation between elevated TSH and growth parameters has been reported in young patients, raising the question of possible resistance to thyroid hormone. Hypothyroidism is reported in between 20% and 40% of those with Down syndrome, whereas hyperthyroidism is found in about 2.5% and may be a phase in the course of thyroid disease. Several studies have found an increased rate of thyroid disease in parents, particularly mothers, of children with Down syndrome.

Pueschel (1990) noted a lower IQ in patients with Down syndrome and a low T_4 than in those with normal or elevated TSH but normal T_4 and questioned whether hypothyroidism might account for some of the age-associated decline in IQ seen in Down syndrome. With continued early ascertainment through screening, treated hypothyroidism should have no significant negative impact.

Sexual maturation. Much of the literature regarding sexual development and function in Down syndrome is based on older reports of institutionalized patients, and there are relatively few detailed hormonal data available. Such studies suggested that men with Down syndrome had relatively small genitalia and that there was a high incidence of testicular failure with elevated FSH and LH, decreased Leydig cell function, and germinal cell hypoplasia. In contrast, Pueschel (1990) reported that 45 males raised at home had normal onset and chronology of puberty, with normal penile and testicular size and hormonal levels equivalent to normative data. It remains unclear as to whether the differences are environmental or age related.

Female development also appears to be normal (see Pueschel, 1990 for review). The mean age at menarche of 12.6 years does not differ from that of normal sibs, and there does not appear to be any excess of menstrual problems or irregularities. FSH and LH rise normally with maturation, and levels of FSH, LH, and estradiol are equivalent to controls. Although earlier studies have reported high rates of ovarian abnormalities and anovulatory cycles, a 1992 study of 10 27-year-old females by Scola and Pueschel found that 88% of cycles had a biphasic temperature curve indicative of ovulation. Again, differences from earlier reports may be age or environmentally related.

Despite evidence of normal sexual development, there remain fewer than 50 cases of documented fertility in women, and apparently only one in a non-mosaic man with Down syndrome. Whether the paucity of examples of offspring born to parents with Down syndrome represents reduced opportunity for sexual activity and/or biologically reduced fertility remains unclear. Studies of some earlier populations have found that a significant minority of young adolescents showed age-appropriate interest in the opposite sex and that this proportion increased with maturity. Interest in marriage was more frequent among women (>40%), and interest in children was virtually confined to them (~20%). However, caregivers generally considered sex education inappropriate and fewer than one-third had received any such instruction (Carr, 1994).

Evaluation

- Screening for neonatal hypothyroidism is important for children with Down syndrome. This is done through mandatory newborn screening in most jurisdictions.
- There is compelling evidence that clinical examination is inadequate to detect thyroid disease in Down syndrome, at least in part because of the overlap of signs. Growth velocity may decline or other symptoms may develop at least a year before the clinical recognition of hypothyroidism in children, and it may masquerade as depression or even Alzheimer disease in adults. Therefore, annual screening with TSH and T$_4$ throughout life is currently recommended.
- Any variation from normal physiological sexual maturation is unexpected and requires a standard evaluation for cause.
- The testes should be examined periodically because of the higher rate of testicular tumors, and women require standard gynecological care. The latter may be facilitated if carried out by a familiar health care provider and by taking special care to preeducate the woman about any examinations or procedures.

Treatment

- Treatment of hypothyroidism is standard replacement with L-thyroxine and continued monitoring of blood levels.
- Some centers treat with low-dose thyroxine in the face of markedly elevated TSH and normal T$_4$ levels.
- With integration of individuals with Down syndrome into society, adolescents and young adults with Down syndrome need properly tailored education, advice, and counsel concerning interpersonal relationships, appropriate social behavior, sexual activity, risks of pregnancy, sexually transmitted disease, and situations that may place them at increased risk for sexual abuse. Success will generally require the understanding and participation of parents.
- Women with adequate intellectual ability can be taught menstrual hygiene, whereas hysterectomy may be appropriate for those who cannot manage. Today, a formal approval mechanism is generally required for the latter.
- Long-term contraceptive methods may be most appropriate for those who are sexually active and potentially fertile.
- Vigilance is important because of the increased risk of sexual abuse of retarded persons.

Ophthalmologic

The periocular dysmorphic signs have been described above. Hypoplastic peripheral irides and Brushfield spots are common. Down syndrome accounts for about 4% of congenital cataracts. Careful examination in childhood may reveal early opacities but, although cataracts develop in over half of patients, most are on the lens periphery and cause visual impairment in a minority of adult cases. Findings may include heterotopic or accessory lacrimal glands, strabismus (30–40%), nystagmus, optic nerve hypoplasia, keratoconus (15%), ectropion and/or upper lid eversion, and blepharoconjunctivitis. About 60–70% of patients with Down syndrome have a significant refractive error, of which astigmatism is the most common, followed by hyperopia and myopia; the latter may be severe.

Ahmad and Pruett (1976) reported attenuated retinal pigment, peripapillary and patchy peripheral pigment epithelial atrophy, and choroidal vascular sclerosis in 63 eyes from 32 patients. Eleven eyes from 6 other patients had retinal detachment, and trauma was considered an important contributing factor.

With good care, the prognosis for vision in childhood and young adulthood is good. The optic nerve hypoplasia does not appear to be of clinical significance. There does appear to be some concern for vision later in life because infranasal limbus and degenerative retinal changes may be seen in adults. Keratoconus occurs at a younger age than in the general population and is more subject to development of acute hydrops with its accompanying severe visual impairment.

Evaluation

- Early eye assessment for refractory extraocular muscle imbalance (most often esotropia) with appropriate therapy and follow-up is important to prevent loss of binocular vision and/or amblyopia and to maximize visual acuity. Strabismus must be distinguished from pseudostrabismus caused by epicanthal folds.
- Periodic reevaluation, with the precise interval influenced by age and prior findings, is important to reduce the likelihood of secondary complications and to anticipate new problems such as cataract.
- Causes of eye irritation or behavior that may increase the risk of self-induced ocular trauma should be sought and treated.

Treatment

- Refractive errors are the most common and important visual problems and require early refraction studies and prescription for glasses.
- Strabismus may respond to eye patching or may require surgery.
- Blepharitis usually will respond to lid cleansing and topical antibiotics.
- Cataract may require removal of the lens and a prosthetic implant, and significant keratoconus may be treated with penetrating keratoplasty and a corneal transplant.

Ears and Hearing

Over 90% of ear lengths in Down syndrome fall below the third percentile for the general population; the helix is often angulated and over-folded and the lobes small to absent. The osteocartilaginous junction is narrow to stenotic and may compromise visualization of the tympanic membrane and increase the susceptibility to obstruction by wax.

Eustachian tube dysfunction, in part anatomic and probably also due to muscular hypotonia, including the tensor veli palatini, likely explains the high rate of asymptomatic middle ear effusion, which has a prevalence of about 60% from infancy to adulthood (Schwartz and Schwartz, 1978). Thus persons with Down syndrome are at high risk for conductive hearing loss, although mixed and pure sensorineural hearing loss may also occur. A small minority have been found to have congenitally malformed stapes, and other ossicular anomalies may be acquired. Malformations of the inner ear may also be seen. Some degree of hearing loss occurs in over 60% of those with Down syndrome.

Recurrent ear infections and middle ear effusions are to be anticipated, but with a team approach to hearing care most children with Down syndrome can obtain adequate hearing to prevent interference with speech and educational efforts.

Evaluation

- Management of the structural and functional ear anomalies requires early and complete assessment of hearing, which may include electrophysiological studies.
- Ongoing monitoring for middle ear infections and effusions with tympanometry and/or pneumootoscopy is important. Evaluation should begin before 6 months of age and should be repeated frequently in infancy with the intervals decreasing with age, keeping in mind that adults will be found to have a significant rate of middle ear effusion.

Treatment

- Treatment of acute and chronic complications, which may compromise hearing and thereby interfere with speech and education, should be aggressive.
- A significant proportion of individuals may benefit from some means of amplification.

Cardiovascular

Congenital heart disease occurs in 40–50% of individuals with Down syndrome and is an important determinant of survival. The actual rate and relative frequency of specific anomalies vary with ascertainment. An apparent increase in the incidence of congenital heart disease in Down syndrome from 1970 to the 1980s was the result of better detection, primarily of patent ductus arteriosus and atrial septal defect (Khoury and Erickson, 1992). The cardiac malformations in Down syndrome are typically embryologically simple, with perimembranous ventricular septal defect the most common, followed by endocardial cushion defect, then patent ductus arteriosus and atrial septal defect, endocardial cushion defect (ostium primum type), tetralogy of Fallot and, finally, others accounting for less than 1%. Endocardial cushion defect is more common in Black than in White children with Down syndrome, and muscular ventricular septal defect is relatively underrepresented in both.

Hijii et al. (1997) reported 87.8% survival to age 24 years for their patients with Down syndrome and congenital heart disease who were treated surgically. This compared with 92.2% for those without heart anomalies and 41.4% for those with cardiac lesions who were not operated upon. They also showed that those patients who either had no heart malformation or underwent surgical repair had better functional adaptation than the non-surgically treated group.

Pulmonary hypertension occurs more often and earlier in children with congenital heart disease and Down syndrome, especially in the presence of large right to left shunts.

Evaluation

- Echocardiography is the current standard for evaluation, and in comparison the sensitivity of clinical assessment is 0.53, radiology 0.44, electrocardiogram 0.41, and all three combined 0.73 (Tubman et al., 1991).
- Patients with Down syndrome should be followed with echocardiography into adulthood because of the potential to develop aortic regurgitation.

Treatment

- Although there has been controversy regarding the merits of medical versus surgical management of significant congenital heart malformations in Down syndrome, and over the timing of surgery, there now appears to be a consensus favoring early surgical intervention.
- Medical treatment of endocardial cushion defect has less than a 5% 5-year survival as compared to almost 70% for surgically treated patients, which compares favorably with children without Down syndrome who have the equivalent lesion. Tubman et al. (1991) found that surgical mortality was twice as high in patients with endocardial cushion defect treated after 1 year of age.

Musculoskeletal

Recognized in the 1960s, the association of atlantoaxial instability with Down syndrome gained notoriety in the early 1980s when there were several reports of patients with significant signs of cervical cord damage. About 15% of individuals with Down syndrome have an atlanto-odontoid distance of 5 mm or greater, which is not seen in the general population. The instability is primarily anterior and is due to laxity. Atlanto-occipital instability is also relatively common in Down syndrome. Being male and over the age of 10 is associated with radiologic instability. An alert was issued by a consensus group (Cooke, 1984) that recommended a temporary restriction of children with Down syndrome from all sports that might cause neck flexion, a permanent restriction for those found to have atlantoaxial instability, and a return to activities for those with normal cervical spine radiographs. Although the majority of organizations and authorities supported these recommendations, a few argued against the use of radiographic screening because of very poor sensitivity and specificity and the real risk that many children would be unnecessarily restricted from sports. They pointed out that by 1984 over 500,000 individuals with Down syndrome had participated in the Special Olympics without a single known occurrence of serious neck injury and that although up to 17% may have radiologic instability, there were only 37 reports in the literature of neurological damage. The majority of those cases had forewarning and recovered, and there was no evidence that radiographs could predict those who would become symptomatic.

Arguing against acute trauma as the cause of the majority of symptomatic cases is the fact that in many cases there is no such history, and, furthermore, a significant majority of case reports have been of females, whereas trauma is more common in males. With time some patients will develop an os odontoideum, which is considered an avulsion fracture of the odontoid and is therefore evidence of chronic instability and secondary bony changes.

A small minority of those with Down syndrome will develop neurologic complications of atlantoaxial instability, and an even smaller number will suffer a catastrophic event in the absence of some earlier neurological signs. These events can be minimized through encouraging lower-risk sports and neurological monitoring. Intervention in the presence of neurological signs

attributable to the cervical spine should not be delayed, as chronic changes are unlikely to be reversible and complications appear higher in late-treated cases.

Evaluation

- After a decade of support for routine periodic radiographic screening of children with Down syndrome, the American Academy of Pediatrics Committee on Sports concluded that such evaluation may not be valuable in identifying those at risk (American Academy of Pediatrics, 1995). It stated that it was more important to attempt to clinically evaluate those with complaints or physical findings that might be compatible with spinal cord injury. One of the most sensitive signs for impending damage is a problem with gait. A change in bladder or bowel function may also be important.

- Appropriate management of the active child or young adult with Down syndrome requires a regular and careful neurologic history and physical examination.

- It seems reasonable to carry out flexion-extension neck radiographs on those who plan to participate in high-risk activities such as tumbling or diving.

Treatment

- Participation in high-risk activities should be discouraged if there is evidence of chronic instability, such as an os odontoideum or 7 mm or more of instability.

- A small minority of children with Down syndrome will require stabilizing surgery with a C1–C2 and/or atlanto-occipital fusion. A Gallie C1–C2 fusion appears to be a satisfactory approach for symptomatic anterior atlantoaxial subluxation, and some authors suggest a period of prior traction as well as a postoperative halo to assure stability and fusion.

- A number of authorities have argued that, because an increased atlanto-dens interval is common and complications are rare and usually forewarned, neurologically asymptomatic patients with Down syndrome should not have surgery (Goldberg, 1993). Others stress the necessity to distinguish a simple stable increased atlanto-dens space from an unstable increased space with atlantoaxial movement noted on flexion-extension films. Pueschel et al (1981) noted that all their patients with over 7 mm of instability developed neurologic signs. In favor of early intervention is the fact that late surgery is associated with a high morbidity and mortality.

- Decisions regarding surgery require the involvement of experienced and expert surgeons, a careful weighing of the evidence of present or impending neurological damage, and consideration of the benefits and risks of the surgical approach.

Gastrointestinal

A number of the gastrointestinal malformations that occur with increased frequency in Down syndrome may not lead to symptoms until several months after birth. These include Hirschsprung disease, duplication cysts, and duodenal or anal stenosis. In addition, there is evidence to suggest that gastrointestinal reflux and celiac disease are more common in Down syndrome.

Hypotonia and relative inactivity may account for a higher rate of constipation in the euthyroid and otherwise healthy child with Down syndrome.

Evaluation

- Digestive difficulties should be evaluated aggressively, given the high rate of gastrointestinal malformations.

- Rectal biopsy should be carried out before ascribing severe chronic constipation to hypotonic bowel.

Treatment

- Malformations and functional gastrointestinal problems should be treated as in the general population.

- Adequate response to chronic constipation is generally obtained with a standard pediatric approach when not due to a malformation or Hirschsprung disease.

Immunologic

The introduction of antibiotics and the deinstitutionalization of patients has greatly reduced the impact of the well-known diminished functioning of the immune syndrome in Down syndrome. The relative mortality rate from pneumonia has fallen from 124 times the general population in 1949–1959 to 62-fold for 1960–1971. The comparable figures for other infections declined from 52- to 12-fold, and they are undoubtedly lower today. However, these data, together with the known increased incidence of certain malignancies (see below) and a greater risk of becoming a chronic hepatitis B carrier, emphasize the presence of a significant immunological deficiency.

Abnormalities have been reported in virtually all aspects of the immune system, including immunoglobulin levels, titers of specific antibodies, phagocytic and chemotactic responses, T, B, and natural killer (NK) cells, and the production of cytokines (Ugazio et al., 1990). Not all findings have been consistent, and their individual contributions to the functional immune defects remain unclear. Some changes may be acquired, perhaps secondary to the primary abnormalities. However, many of the defects appear to be intrinsic, and fetuses with Down syndrome at 17–24 weeks gestation have been found to have low T, B, and NK cells relative to normal controls (Thilaganathan et al., 1993).

The fetal thymus appears normal with normal cell populations but shows changes in function including abnormalities of specific antigen responses and receptor formation. There may be a small reduction in cellular response to phytohemagglutinin stimulation. Although the percentage of T cells is maintained, the total number of circulating lymphocytes and of T cells is reduced, with alterations in specific subsets of cells and an impaired T cell-mediated response. A change is seen with age wherein the absolute number of cells with low NK activity increases while those with high NK activity decrease in number. This may explain reduced function in the face of normal total numbers. The percent and absolute number of B cells are diminished. $CD4^+$ helper lymphocytes are significantly reduced, whereas the absolute number of $CD8^+$ cells is normal, resulting in an inverted CD4-to-CD8 ratio. Findings with respect to immunoglobulin levels have been variable but are generally reported as low. Poor responses to specific antigens have also been reported and may, to some extent, be age related.

Both monocytes and neutrophils have been shown to have a depressed chemotactic and phagocytic response. The latter display poor intracellular killing that may relate to diminished superoxide, secondary to the dosage effect on superoxide dismutase, which is located on chromosome 21. This fits with an increased susceptibility to catalase-positive but not to catalase-negative bacteria seen in Down syndrome. A gene-dosage effect for other immune system genes on chromosome 21, including interferon receptor and CD18, may play specific roles in the immunological disturbances of Down syndrome.

Despite advances in the treatment of infectious disease, children and adults with Down syndrome continue to show an increased morbidity and mortality from infectious disease. However, survival has greatly improved over the past decades, and it is to be hoped that increasing normalization within society, greater awareness of risks, and the prudent and appropriate use of antibiotics may lead to further gains.

Evaluation

- Although children with Down syndrome show a greater susceptibility to infectious disease, and several anomalies of immune responsiveness may be found, there does not appear to be justification for routine immunologic evaluation of patients. Such studies should be reserved for those patients with unusually severe problems and/or evidence of frank immunodeficiency.

Treatment

- Although response to vaccination may not be as effective in people with Down syndrome, it is recommended that they follow a normal vaccination schedule, including hepatitis B, for which they are at significant risk to become chronic carriers.

- The possible role of vitamin A and zinc in normalizing some aspects of the immunodeficiency in Down syndrome remains controversial. It is the opinion of this author that any such intervention should only occur as part of a large, multicenter, scientifically valid double-blind controlled trial that includes accurate measurement of these compounds before and during treatment as well as providing laboratory and clinical assessment of immunological function.

Neoplasia

The incidence of leukemia in Down syndrome is about 20 times that in the general population and includes both acute lymphocytic leukemia and acute nonlymphocytic leukemia. Acute lymphocytic leukemia occurs in 1.7–2.1% of patients, which is about 14 times the expected rate. About half the cases of acute nonlymphocytic leukemia are acute megakaryoblastic (M7), a rate about 40 times higher than in the general population. After the age of 3 years the ratio of acute lymphocytic leukemia to acute nonlymphocytic leukemia parallels the usual distribution.

Neonates with Down syndrome may show a transient leukemoid reaction, also referred to in the literature as transient leukemia or transient megaloblastic leukemia. This condition appears to be virtually limited to patients with a trisomy 21 cell line and has been reported in only one normal individual who had 200 normal cells karyotyped. There is some evidence that transient leukemoid reaction may be more common in those with a mosaic karyotype. Several cases have been diagnosed on fetal blood samples obtained during prenatal diagnostic procedures. The leukemoid reaction generally disappears by 1–2 months, but about 25% of cases go on to develop leukemia within a mean interval of 16 months. Transient leukemoid reaction most commonly precedes acute nonlymphocytic leukemia, in which it occurs in 18% of reported cases according to Iselius et al. (1990). In the review by those authors of 215 cases of leukemia and transient leukemoid reaction, they found 72 cases of transient leukemoid reaction, 86 of acute nonlymphocytic leukemia, 19 of acute lymphocytic leukemia, 25 of acute leukemia of unknown type, 9 of acute undifferentiated leukemia, and 4 of myelofibrosis. Additional acquired chromosomal abnormalities appeared more common in patients with Down syndrome and acute nonlymphocytic leukemia, of which about half were M7. These included higher rates of trisomy 8, 19, and an additional 21, as well as a lower rate of hypodiploidy than in the general population. None of the 19 cases of M7 had a normal karyotype.

It is of note that chromosome 21 is the most common acquired aneuploidy in acute lymphocytic leukemia and is frequently involved in acquired translocations [most common being t(12;21)(p13;q22)], and unequal amplification of certain areas of 21 is related to some cell markers of acute lymphocytic leukemia (Berger, 1997).

In addition to leukemia, a number of other tumors appear to be more frequent in Down syndrome. These include testicular and possibly central nervous system germ cell tumors, retinoblastoma, syringomata, and pancreatic and bone tumors (Satgé et al., 1998), whereas neuroblastoma, nephroblastoma, gastrointestinal, uterine, breast, and other central nervous system malignancies may be underrepresented.

It appears that children with Down syndrome and acute myeloid leukemia have a better event-free survival and overall survival (65–70%) than does the average child. The outcome for children who present at less than 2 years of age is significantly better than for those who present later. Fungal and bacterial infections are more common and post-chemotherapy recovery time is longer in children with Down syndrome treated with arabinosyl cytosine (Ravindranath et al., 1993). Although Down syndrome has been shown to be a negative prognostic factor in acute lymphocytic leukemia treated by conventional therapy, event-free survival and overall survival are equivalent to the general population when both are treated with an intensive regime.

Evaluation

- The signs and symptoms of the patient with Down syndrome and leukemia do not differ significantly from those in the general population. Specifically in acute lymphocytic leukemia, there is no difference in presenting signs, race, sex ratio, organomegaly, percentage of blasts, or rates of the different immunophenotypes (Ragab et al., 1991). Patients with Down syndrome are slightly older and have slightly higher initial hemoglobin values.

- No routine screening is indicated.

Treatment

- Treatment should be carried out in experienced tertiary care centers that participate in standard and research protocols and where there is experience in treating children with Down syndrome.
- The current consensus is that the results of treatment of acute myeloid leukemia with chemotherapy, which includes high-dose arabinosyl cytosine, are comparable to those obtained with bone marrow replacement in the general population. This makes bone marrow transplant inappropriate as initial therapy for patients with Down syndrome (Ravindranath et al., 1993). The differences may in part reflect varying metabolism of some chemotherapeutic agents.
- Patients with Down syndrome appear more sensitive to toxicity from chemotherapy, particularly from methotrexate, because of slower clearance, but this increased morbidity is not reflected in higher mortality from treatment.
- Survival in acute lymphocytic leukemia is comparable to that in the general population when treatment is with an intensive regime that includes a consolidation phase (Ragab et al., 1991).

Sleep

The relative underdevelopment of the midface, sometimes associated with a narrow nasopharynx, and the high rate of hypotonia appear to place children with Down syndrome at increased risk for obstructive sleep apnea, even in the face of fairly normal-sized tonsils and adenoids.

The majority of children will respond to fairly simple intervention. It is important to note that obstructive sleep apnea may increase the risk for pulmonary hypertension in susceptible individuals.

Evaluation

- Suspicion should be raised if parents or care providers note an unusual sleeping position, such as with the head hyperextended or on the stomach with the knees drawn up, significant snoring, or restless, disturbed sleep with awakenings. Poor sleep may be associated with daytime drowsiness or a decline in behavior.
- A polysomnogram may be helpful in clarifying concerns about sleep apnea.
- A careful assessment of the cause of sleep apnea should be sought before treatment, especially surgery, is suggested.

Treatment

- Most symptomatic cases will respond to tonsillectomy and adenoidectomy.
- Continuous positive airway pressure may be the appropriate intervention for some.
- Very occasionally, more involved surgery, such as enlargement of the midface, may be required.

Craniofacial

The subject of the oral cavity and dentition was recently reviewed by Desai (1997). The hypoplastic midface is associated with a reduced height, length, and depth, but not width, of the palate and is likely an important factor in the tendency to protrude the tongue and to mouth breathe. The tongue is hypotonic with a midline diastasis and increased concavity of the anterior two-thirds. Tongue scalloping and fissuring is possibly developmental and may potentiate halitosis. Hypotonia of the facial muscles causes passive elevation of the upper lip and eversion of the lower, which may be exacerbated by tongue protrusion. The result is chronic drooling, chapping and cheilitis, and it may play a role in the increased rate of upper respiratory infections and peridontitis, which may begin as early as 6–15 years.

Facial plastic surgery to alter the appearance of one who is developmentally delayed is highly controversial both because of the issues of informed consent and the argument that society should accept persons as they are rather than have them change to an arbitrary norm. Pueschel et al. (1986) surveyed parental and physician attitudes toward facial cosmetic surgery for Down syndrome, including that for epicanthal folds, upslanting fissures, lower lip and tongue reduction, and nasal augmentation. They found that over 80% of parents but only 10% of physicians held a positive view toward the acceptance of a child with Down syndrome by society and that significantly more physicians than parents thought that appearance was a significant detriment to socialization, progress in language, and self-help skills. A significant proportion of both groups thought that surgery would decrease preconceived prejudices and increase employability, but both groups were also concerned about the surgical risks, the reaction of the child, and the possible development of unrealistic teacher and societal expectations from a more 'normal'-appearing child. Of parents, 61% would not want such surgery, 26% were undecided, and 13% were in favor.

Evaluation

- Medical history and physical examination should be obtained to identify any ill effects of a large tongue.

Treatment

- There may be an argument for reduction of the tongue when there continues to be a significant orolingual disproportion that interferes with pronunciation and chewing or causes drooling. Selected cases may benefit from improved speech and eating, and the closed mouth may improve appearance and self-confidence, reduce oral inflammation and cheilosis, and perhaps reduce dental problems.

Dental

Dental anomalies are common in Down syndrome and include delayed and asynchronous primary dentition (completed by 4–5 years) and secondary dentition. Microdontia affects between 35% and 55% of primary and secondary dentition. Primary teeth may be retained and there is a greater rate of supernumerary teeth, taurodontism (0.5–5%), tooth hypoplasia, hypocalcification, and crown variants, especially on the labial surfaces. Crowns are more likely to be conical, small, and short. The roots are complete but short, and this may contribute to instability and susceptibility to tooth loss associated with periodontal disease, which is more common than in the general retarded population. Partial anodontia affects about half the patients with Down syndrome as compared to 2% of the general population. Tooth agenesis occurs in a pattern different from that seen in the general population and most often affects the mandibular central incisors. Occlusal problems, most often of the central and lateral incisors and canines, are common and result from mouth breathing, impaired chewing, bruxism, tooth agenesis, shortness and asymmetry of the maxillary arch, and temporomandibular problems.

Hypotonia of the facial muscles may play a role in the increased rate of upper respiratory infections and peridontitis, which may begin as early as 6–15 years. There is some evidence that at least part of the increased susceptibility is caused by the response of the gums to plaque, which forms at a normal rate. Decreased salivary flow and an increase in pH and bicarbonate buffer may result in mucosal thinning and xerostomia while offering some protection against dental caries.

Evaluation

- Early referral for regular semiannual dental care is important both for repeated instruction in dental hygiene for the prevention of gum disease and the longer-term planning of possible orthodontics.

Treatment

- Instruction in dental hygiene and one-on-one help and instruction with brushing and flossing must begin at an early age in all children with Down syndrome, and dental hygiene must become a lifelong habit.
- Specific dental anomalies will vary widely from individual to individual and will require a tailored approach.
- In the absence of a successful program of gum care, early tooth loss can be anticipated. Dental caries are much more likely to be a problem.
- Antibiotic prophylaxis is required at the time of dental care for many affected people with congenital heart disease.
- Significant malocclusion can be treated in a standard fashion, although braces may complicate gum care.

Dermatologic

The skin in infancy is generally soft, and cutis marmorata is common. Seborrheic dermatitis may occur in up to 30% of patients, with red cheeks being common, and with time the skin has a tendency to become dry and rough and may show local thick and scaly hyperkeratotic patches on the limbs. A wide variety of skin disorders are reported in Down syndrome, and many are age related (Ercis et al., 1996). The most common include palmoplantar keratosis seen in about 75% of those over the age of 5 years, and a chronic, erythematous follicular papular dermatosis that is most common between 20 and 40 years. The latter is uncommon in teens and over the age of 45 years and is

most obvious over the sternum and between the scapulae. Adolescents commonly suffer from pustular follicular lesions in the perigenital, thigh, and buttock areas.

Five to fifteen percent of patients may show one or more of alopecia totalis, geographic tongue, cheilitis, or xerosis. Lentigines, blepharitis, syringomata, and sun-induced atrophy appear more commonly than in the general population.

Evaluation

- A careful skin examination should be part of routine anticipatory care.

Treatment

- These problems should be treated as in the general population.

RESOURCES

There is a wealth of written, visual, electronic, and direct contact resources available for parents and health care providers. Only a sampling are listed, as many web sites provide suggested reading and other information services. Many countries have national associations, often with local chapters, and many hospitals serving children have special Down syndrome clinics and an organized network of services.

Books

Stray-Gunderson K., editor (1995) *Babies with Down Syndrome: A New Parents Guide*, 2nd ed. Rockville, MD: Woodbine House. ISBN:0933149646 (tel 301-468-8800,1-800-843-7323)

Rogers PT, Coleman M, editors (1992) *Medical Care in Down Syndrome: A Preventative Medicine Approach*, Volume 8, Pediatric Habilitation, New York:Marcel Decker. ISBN: 0-8247-8684-X

Edwards JP, Elkins TE (1998) *Just Between Us: A Social Sexual Training Guide for Parents and Professionals Who Have*

Concerns for Persons with Retardation. Portland, OR: Ednick Communications.

Web sites

US National Down Syndrome Society: *www.ndss.org*

Canadian Down Syndrome Society: *http//home.ican.net/~cdss/index/html*

National Down Syndrome Congress (US): *http://members.carol.net/~ndsc*

World-wide organizations: *www.nas.com/downsyn/org.html*

Down Syndrome Quarterly: *www.denison.edu/dsq* (health, vitamin, growth hormone policy statements)

Checklist for Health Care: *http://members.carol.net/~ndsc /hw_table.html*

Growth Charts: Height and Weight (metric and imperial) *www.growthcharts.com/ charts/ds/charts.html*

Head circumference: *www.growthcharts.com /charts/ds/hccharts.html*

Dr Len Leshin's Health Page: *www.davlin. net/users/leshin/*

Telephone contacts

US National Down Syndrome Society, 666 Broadway, New York, NY, 10012-2317, email *info@ndss.org*, 1-800-221-4602 (US), 212-460-9330

Canadian Down Syndrome Society, 811-14th St NW, Calgary, AB T2N 2A4, tel 403-270-8500, fax 403-270-8291

REFERENCES

Ahmad A, Pruett RC (1976) The fundus in Mongolism. *Arch Ophthal* 94:772–776.

American Academy of Pediatrics (1995) Atlantoaxial instability in Down syndrome: Subject review. *Pediatr* 96:151–154.

Baird PA, Sadovnick AD (1988) Alzheimer disease: Life expectancy in Down syndrome adults. *Lancet II*:1354–1356.

Berger R (1997) Acute lymphoblastic leukemia and chromosome 21. *Cancer Genet Cyto Genet* 94:8–12.

Berr C, Borghi E, Rethoré M-O, Lejeune J, Alperovitch A (1990) Risk of Down syndrome in relatives of trisomy 21 children. A case-control study. *Ann Génét* 33:137–140.

Bray I, Wright DE, Davies C, Hook EB (1998) Joint estimation of Down syndrome risk and ascertainment rates: A meta-analysis of nine published data sets. *Prenatal Diag* 18:9–20.

Carr J (1994) Annotation: Long term outcome for people with Down's syndrome. *J Child Psychol Psychiat* 35:425–439.

Christianson AL, Kromberg JGR, Viljeon E (1995) Clinical features of black African neonates with Down's syndrome. *East African Med J* 72:306–310.

Cooke RE (1984) Atlantoaxial instability in individuals with Down's syndrome. *Adapted Physical Activity Quarterly* 1:194–196.

Cronk C, Crocker AC, Pueschel NSM, Shea AM, Zackai E, Pickens G, Reed RB (1988) Growth charts for children with Down syndrome: 1 month to 18 years. *Pediatr* 81:102–109.

Del Bo R, Comi GP, Bresolin N, Castelli E, Conti E, Degiuli A, Ausenda CD, Scarlato G (1997) The apolipoprotein Eε4 allele causes a faster decline of cognitive performances in Down's syndrome. *J Neurol Sci* 145:87–91.

Desai SS (1997) Down syndrome. A review of the literature. *Oral Surg Oral Med Oral Pathol Oral Radiol Endodont* 84:279–285.

Dumaret CA, de Vigan C, Julian-Reynier C, Goujard J, Rosset D, Aymé S (1998) Adoption and fostering of babies with Down syndrome: A cohort of 593 cases. *Prenat Diagn* 18:437–445.

Dupont A, Vaeth M, Videbeck P (1986) Mortality and life expectancy in Down's syndrome in Denmark. *J Ment Defic Res* 30:111–120.

Dykens EM, Kasari C (1997) Maladaptive behavior in children with Prader-Willi syndrome, Down syndrome, and nonspecific mental retardation. *Am J Ment Retard* 102:228–237.

Ercis M, Balci S, Ataken N (1996) Dermatological manifestations of 71 Down syndrome patients admitted to a clinical genetics unit. *Clin Genet* 50:317–320.

Goldberg MJ (1993). Spine instability and the Special Olympics. *Clinics in Sports Med* 12(3):507–515.

Hijii T, Fukushige J, Igarashi H, Takahashi N, Ueda K (1997) Life expectancy and social adaptation in individuals with Down syndrome and without surgery for congenital heart disease. *Clin Pediatr June* 97:327–332.

Hartley XY (1986) A summary of recent research into the development of children with Down's syndrome. *J Ment Defic Res* 30:1–14.

Haw CM, Barnes TRE, Clark K, Crichton P, Kohen D (1996) Movement disorders in Down's syndrome: A possible marker of the severity of the mental handicap. *Movement Disorders* 11:395–403.

Holtzman DM (1997) Alzheimer disease and Down syndrome. *Cytogenet Cell Genet* 77: (Suppl. 1),17.

Hook EB, Mutton DE, Ide R, Alberman E, Bobrow M (1995) The natural history of Down syndrome conceptuses diagnosed prenatally that are not electively terminated. *Am J Hum Genet* 57:875–881.

Hubert RS, Mitchell S, Chen X-N, Ekmekji K, Gadomski C, Sun Z, Noya D, Kim U-J, Chen C, Shizuya H, Simon M, De Jong PJ, Korenberg JR (1997) BAC and PAC contigs covering 3.5 Mb of the Down syndrome congenital heart disease region between D21S55 and MX1 on chromosome 21. *Genomics* 41:218–226.

Iselius L, Jacobs P, Morton N (1990) Leukemia and transient leukemia in Down syndrome. *Hum Genet* 85:477–485.

Khoury MJ, Erickson JD (1992) Improved ascertainment of cardiovascular malformations in infants with Down's syndrome, Atlanta, 1968 through 1989. *Am J Epidemiol* 136:1457–1464.

Lippman A, Aymé S (1984) Fetal death rates in mothers of children with trisomy 21 (Down syndrome). *Ann Hum Genet* 48:303–312.

Prasher VP (1995) Overweight and obesity amongst Down's syndrome adults. *J Int Disability Res* 39:437–441.

Preus M (1977) A diagnostic index for Down syndrome. *Clin Genet* 12:47–55.

Pueschel SM, Scola FH, Perry CD, Pezzullo JC (1981) Atlanto-axial instability in children with Down syndrome. *Pediatr Radiol* 10:129–132.

Pueschel SM, Montiero LA, Erickson M (1986) Parents' and physicians' perceptions of facial plastic surgery in children with Down syndrome. *J Ment Defic Res* 30:71–79.

Pueschel SM (1990) Growth, thyroid function, and sexual maturation in Down syndrome. *Growth, Genetics and Hormones* 6(1):1–5.

Ragab AH, Abdel-Mageed A, Shuster JJ, Frankel LS, Pullen J, van Eys J, Sullivan MP, Boyett J, Borowitz M, Crist WM (1991) Clinical characteristics and treatment outcome of children with acute lymphocytic leukemia and Down's syndrome. *Cancer* 67:1057–1063.

Ravindranath Y, Abella E, Krischer J, Weinstein H (Pediatric Oncology Group) (1993) Acute myeloid leukemia (AML) in Down syndrome (DS) Response and toxicity with high dose arabinosyl cytosine (ARA-C). *Proc ASCO* 12:323.

Satgé D, Sommelet D, Geneix A, Nishi M, Malet P, Vekemans MJ (1998) A tumor profile in Down syndrome. *Am J Med Genet* 78:207–216.

Schupf N, Kapell D, Nightingale B, Rodriguez A, Tycko B, Mayeux R (1998) Earlier onset of Alzheimer's disease in men with Down syndrome. *Neurology* 50:991–995.

Schwartz DM, Schwartz RH (1978) Acoustic impedance and otoscopic findings in young children with Down's syndrome. *Arch Otolaryngol* 104:652–656.

Scola PS, Pueschel SM(1992) Menstrual cycles and basal body temperature curves in women with Down syndrome. *Obstet Gynecol* 79:91–94.

Stafstrom CE, Patxot OF, Gilmore HE, Wisniewski KE (1991) Seizures in children with Down syndrome: Etiology, characteristics and outcome. *Dev Med Child Neurol* 33:191–200.

Stene E, Stene J, Stengel-Rutkowski S (1987) A reanalysis of the New York State prenatal diagnosis data on Down's syndrome and paternal age effects. *Hum Genet* 77:299–302.

Thase ME, Smeltzer LL, Maloon J (1982) Clinical evaluation of dementia in Down's syndrome: A preliminary report. *J Ment Defic Res* 26:239–244.

Thilaganathan B, Tsakonas D, Nicolaides K (1993) Abnormal fetal immunological development in Down's syndrome. *Fetal Neonatal Med* 100:60–62.

Torfs CP, Christianson RE (1998) Anomalies in Down syndrome individuals in a large population based registry. *Am J Med Genet* 77:431–438.

Tubman TRJ, Shields MD, Craig BG, Mulholland HC, Nevin NC (1991). Congenital heart disease in Down's syndrome: Two year prospective early screening study. *Br Med J* 302:1425–1427.

Ugazio AG, Maccario R, Notorangelo LD, Burgio GR (1990) Immunology of Down syndrome: A review. *Am J Med Genet Supp* 7:204–212.

Verger P (1997) Down syndrome and ionizing radiation. *Health Physics* 73:882–893.

Yoon PW, Freeman SB, Sherman SL, Taft LF, Gu Y, Pettay D, Flanders WD, Khoury MJ, Hassold TJ (1996) Advanced maternal age and the risk of Down syndrome characterized by the meiotic stage of the chromosome errors. *Am J Hum Genet* 58: 628–633.

CHAPTER 8

THE EHLERS-DANLOS SYNDROMES

RICHARD J. WENSTRUP AND LEAH B. HOECHSTETTER

INTRODUCTION

Incidence

The Ehlers-Danlos syndromes are a genetically, biochemically, and clinically diverse group of heritable connective tissue disorders having joint laxity and dermal features in common (Beighton et al., 1988; Beighton, 1992; Steinmann et al., 1993). Prior classifications of Ehlers-Danlos syndrome have included up to 11 disorders. Recently, a simplified classification has been proposed that takes into account increasing clinical experience and recent advances in our understanding of the molecular pathogenesis of these disorders. Table 8.1 provides the new classification and its relationship to the most recent prior classification in 1988 (Beighton et al., 1988, 1998). There are no well-founded figures for the prevalence of Ehlers-Danlos syndrome. Beighton's figure of 1:156,000 in southern England seems extremely low to clinicians who see patients with Ehlers-Danlos syndrome (Beighton et al., 1989). For all forms of Ehlers-Danlos syndrome, combined prevalence estimates of 1 in 5,000 have been made (Barabas, 1967).

Diagnosis

For clarity, the diagnostic criteria, pathogenesis and genetics, and testing of each type of Ehlers-Danlos syndrome will be discussed separately. Generalized joint hypermobility can be a feature of all forms of Ehlers-Danlos syndromes. Determination of hypermobility in adults and adolescents can be assessed using the scale derived by Beighton and Wolf (Beighton et al., 1989). A score of 5/9 or greater defines hypermobility:

- Passive dorsiflexion of the little fingers beyond 90 degrees (Fig. 8.1). One point for each hand.
- Passive apposition of the thumbs to the flexor aspect of the forearm. One point for each hand.
- Hyperextension of the elbows beyond 10 degrees. One point for each elbow.
- Hyperextension of the knees beyond 10 degrees. One point for each elbow.
- Forward flexion of the trunk with knees fully extended so the palms of the hand rests flat on the floor. One point.

THE CLASSICAL TYPE

Diagnostic Criteria

Because Ehlers-Danlos syndrome types I and II were shown to be allelic disorders with overlapping clinical features, it has been

Management of Genetic Syndromes, Edited by Suzanne B. Cassidy and Judith E. Allanson
ISBN 0-471-31286-X   Copyright © 2001 by Wiley-Liss, Inc.

TABLE 8.1. Clinical Features, Inheritance Patterns, and Biochemical Defects of the Ehlers-Danlos Syndromes

Villefranche Classification (1997)	Berlin Classification (1988)	Clinical Features	Inheritance	Biochemical Defects
Classical Type	I Gravis II Mitis	Soft, hyperextensible skin; easy bruising; thin, atrophic scars: hypermobile joints; varicose veins; prematurity of affected newborns.	AD	Mutations in proα1(V) or proα2(V) chains of type V collagen (*COL5A1, COL5A2*) in some families.
Hypermobility Type	III	Soft skin; large and small joint hypermobility	AD	Not known
Vascular Type	IV Arterial-ecchemotic	Thin, translucent skin with visible veins; easy bruising; absence of skin and joint extensibility; arterial, bowel, and uterine rupture	AD	Mutations in *COL3A1*: abnormal type III collagen synthesis, secretion, or structure
Kyphoscoliosis Type	VI	Soft skin; muscle hypotonia; scoliosis: joint laxity; hyperextensible skin	AR	Lysyl hydroxylase deficiency; mutations in *PLOD1* gene
Arthrochalasia Type	VIIA, VIIB Arthro-chalasia multiplex	Congenital hip dislocation, severe joint hypermobility; soft skin with or without abnormal scarring	AD	Deletion of exons from type I collagen genes that encode the amino-terminal propeptide cleavage site of *COL1A1* (type A) or *COL1A2* (type B).
Dermatospor-axis Type	VIIC	Severe skin fragility; sagging, redundant skin	AR	Recessive mutations in type I collagen N-peptidase
Other Variants	VIII Periodontal	Generalized periodontitis; soft, hyperextensible skin; chronic purple-hued scarring over shins	AD	Not known
	V X-linked	Similar to mild classical type	XLR	Not known
	X	Joint laxity; clotting disorder	AR	Not known; proposed defect in fibronectin

AD, autosomal dominant; AR, autosomal recessive; XLR, X-linked recessive.

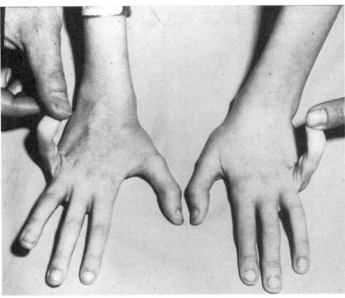

FIGURE 8.1. Clinical test for hypermobility: passive dorsiflexion of the fifth digits beyond 90° from the horizontal plane.

proposed that they be combined into a single entity. The classical form of Ehlers-Danlos syndrome is characterized by joint laxity, hyperextensibility of skin, and poor wound healing. The skin is soft and velvety and can be stretched easily. The dermis is fragile and is easily bruised. Scars after trauma or surgical procedures are thin and atrophic and may stretch considerably after healing (Fig. 8.2). More severely affected individuals have scars with a characteristic "cigarette paper" appearance. Molluscoid pseudotumors are present at the extensor surfaces of joints, in the foot, and on the shins. About one-half of affected individuals with Ehlers-Danlos syndrome I are delivered up to 1 month prematurely as infants because of premature rupture of fetal membranes. A significant number of individuals with Ehlers-Danlos syndrome have cardiac abnormalities. Mitral valve prolapse is particularly common in the vascular form of Ehlers-Danlos syndrome (type IV) (Jaffe et al., 1981) but can be seen in all types (personal observation). Aortic root dilatation with occasional rupture has been reported

in the classical and hypermobile types of Ehlers-Danlos syndrome (types I–III) (Tiller et al., 1998). Musculoskeletal features seen in Ehlers-Danlos syndrome type I include joint hyperextensibility in all patients and a fairly high frequency of scoliosis and pes planus. The joint hypermobility can lead to the onset of osteoarthritis in the third or fourth decade.

Skin hyperextensibility, widened atrophic scars, and joint hypermobility are the major diagnostic criteria.

Etiology, Pathogenesis, and Genetics

The classical form of the Ehlers-Danlos syndrome is an autosomal dominant single-gene disorder. Ultrastructural findings show thickened collagen fibrils in skin; so-called "cauliflower" deformities of collagen fibrils have been reported as well. Mutations in type V collagen are a major cause of the classical type of Ehlers-Danlos syndrome. Abnormalities in the proα1(V) and proα2(V) chains were identified in several families described as the classical form of Ehlers-Danlos syndrome, Ehlers-Danlos syndrome type I, or

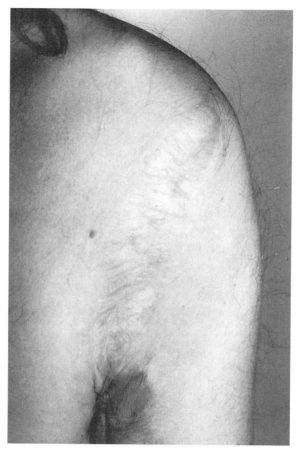

FIGURE 8.2. Widened "cigarette" paper scar in a 25-year-old man with classical Ehlers-Danlos syndrome 6 months after a surgically repaired injury from a motor vehicle accident.

Ehlers-Danlos syndrome type II (Chessler et al., 1993; Toriello et al., 1996; Wenstrup et al., 1996; Nicholls et al., 1996; Burrows et al., 1996; De Paepe et al., 1997; Michalickova et al., 1998; Lichonds et al., 1998; Schwarze et al., 2000; Wenstrap et al., 2000). At least three loci are involved, since several families are discordant for linkage to both *COL5A1* and *COL5A2* (Greenspan et al., 1995; Wenstrup et al., 1996).

Diagnostic Testing

At the time of writing, neither biochemical nor DNA-based methods have been developed that provide reliable results in this form of Ehlers-Danlos syndrome.

THE HYPERMOBILITY TYPE

Diagnostic Criteria

This form is Ehlers-Danlos syndrome type III, unchanged from earlier classifications. It is characterized primarily by hyperextensibility of large and small joints and soft, velvety skin. Individuals with Ehlers-Danlos syndrome type III have normal scarring but may have stretchy skin. Molluscoid pseudotumors are absent. As discussed in the section on the classical form, a significant number of individuals with both the classical form and the hypermobile form have dilatation and/or rupture of the ascending aorta. Musculoskeletal features seen in the classical form of Ehlers-Danlos syndrome, such as scoliosis and pes planus, are also common. The joint hypermobility can be associated with the onset of osteoarthritis in the third or fourth decade.

Skin involvement (hyperextensibility and/or smooth, velvety skin) and joint hypermobility are the major diagnostic criteria.

Etiology, Pathogenesis, and Genetics

This form of Ehlers-Danlos syndrome is an autosomal dominant single-gene disorder. At the time of writing, the genetic basis of this form of Ehlers-Danlos syndrome is unknown.

Diagnostic Testing

Diagnostic testing is based on fulfillment of clinical criteria.

THE VASCULAR TYPE

Diagnostic Criteria

This form represents a refined definition of Ehlers-Danlos syndrome type IV in that it is limited to those patients with dominant mutations in the gene for the proα1(III) chain of type III collagen Pepin et al. (2000). Patients

with this condition often have a characteristic face (Fig. 8.3) and thin, translucent skin with easy bruisability; scar formation is usually normal (Byers et al., 1980; De Paepe, 1994). In fair-skinned individuals, subcutaneous vasculature is easily visible beneath the skin (Fig. 8.4). Affected individuals are at high risk for life-threatening rupture of the intestine, uterus, or medium-sized arteries. The most common sites of arterial rupture are the mesenchymal arteries in the abdomen, the splenic artery, the renal arteries, and the descending aorta. There may also be an increased incidence of stroke. Another life-threatening complication is uterine rupture in the peripartum period.

Characteristic facial appearance, thin, translucent skin, arterial/intestinal/uterine fragility or rupture, and extensive bruising are the major diagnostic criteria.

Etiology, Pathogenesis, and Genetics

The vascular form of Ehlers-Danlos syndrome was initially thought to be autosomal recessive in inheritance, but most individuals have family histories compatible with autosomal dominant single-gene inheritance, and linkage analysis has documented dominant inheritance in several families. The vascular form of Ehlers-Danlos syndrome is caused

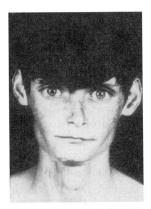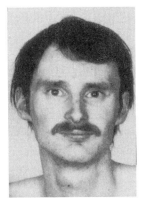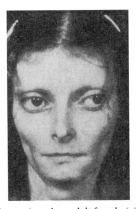

FIGURE 8.3. Typical face in a 14-year-old male (*left*), an adult male (*center*), and an adult female (*right*) with the vascular form of Ehlers-Danlos syndrome. The nose is thin, delicate appearing, and somewhat "pinched". The lips are thin, and the cheeks appear hollow. Some individuals have a staring appearance because of decreased adipose tissue below the eyes.

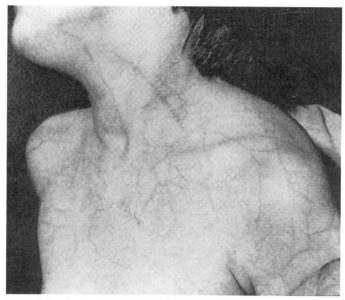

FIGURE 8.4. Thinned dermis, with visible superficial vasculature, in an individual with the vascular form of Ehlers-Danlos syndrome.

by abnormal synthesis, structure, or secretion of type III collagen (Byers, 1995; Byers et al., 1980; Beighton et al., 1988; Steinmann et al., 1993; De Paepe, 1994). Collagen fibers are small and irregular in skin and blood vessels. Several mutations have been described in the triple helical region of the type III collagen molecule. These include multiexon deletions, single point mutations, and splicing defects. In contrast to mutations of type I collagen that result in osteogenesis imperfecta, mutations that result in Ehlers-Danlos syndrome type IV are equally likely to be single-exon splicing defects as substitutions for glycine residues in the triple helical domain. Surprisingly, splicing defects and multiexon deletions do not result in more severe disease phenotypes than glycine substitutions, as they often do in osteogenesis imperfecta. All mutations associated with Ehlers-Danlos syndrome IV appear to deleteriously affect type III collagen structure. A small number of cases are due to null mutations resulting in loss of expression of one *COL3A1* allele (Pepin et al., 2000).

Diagnostic Testing

Testing for this form of Ehlers-Danlos syndrome can be reliably accomplished by analysis of type III procollagen and collagen chains harvested from cultured dermal fibroblasts.

THE KYPHOSCOLIOSIS TYPE

Diagnostic Criteria

The cardinal features of the kyphoscoliosis type of Ehlers-Danlos syndrome, also called Ehlers-Danlos syndrome type VI, are neonatal onset of joint laxity, kyphoscoliosis, and hypotonia (Wenstrup et al., 1989). These features are found in virtually all patients. Ocular fragility, which was observed in the original reports, is found in only a minority of patients. Skin fragility, easy bruisability, and dermal hyperextensibility occur to some extent in most patients, although they are much less prominent than in patients with classical Ehlers-Danlos syndrome. Individuals with the kyphoscoliosis form of Ehlers-Danlos syndrome, like those with the vascular form, are at risk of having a potentially catastrophic arterial rupture (Wenstrup et al., 1989). Most patients have radiologically detectable osteopenia, but pathological fractures are rare (personal experience).

Generalized joint laxity, severe muscle hypotonia at birth, progressive scoliosis at birth or within the first year of life, and scleral fragility and rupture of the ocular globe are the diagnostic criteria.

Etiology, Pathogenesis, and Genetics

In patients with this form of Ehlers-Danlos syndrome, collagen is hydroxylysine-deficient because of a deficiency of lysyl hydroxylase (procollagen lysyl 2-oxoglutarate 5 dioxygenase; *PLOD1*) (Heikkinen et al., 1994). Many of the cross-links that normally occur between adjacent collagen monomers within a fibril begin as chemical modifications of hydroxylysyl residues. Therefore, although hydroxylysine-deficient collagen is efficiently secreted from cells, it is not capable of normal cross-linking. All patients with Ehlers-Danlos syndrome type VI have decreased hydroxylysine content in dermal tissues (Pinnell et al., 1972). Hydroxylysine content in dermal collagen is typically less than 10% of normal, or <0.5 per 1,000 residues in all patients with Ehlers-Danlos syndrome type VI. The deficiency is highly tissue- and collagen type specific, apparently affecting only type I and III collagens (Eyre and Glimcher, 1972; Ihme et al., 1984). Several patients have been reported who have defects at both *PLOD* alleles. Hautala et al. (1993) reported homozygosity for an intragenic duplication of exons 9–15 in two patients. The duplication appears to be the only common mutant allele, with an allele frequency of 19.1% in 35 families with Ehlers-Danlos syndrome type VI (Heikkinen et al., 1997). There appears to be a rare subtype that is clinically indistinguishable but has normal lysyl hydroxylase activity and normal hydroxylysyl content in skin (Steinmann et al., 1993).

Diagnostic Testing

The laboratory is a key element in the diagnosis of this form of Ehlers-Danlos syndrome. Patients will often show a reduction of lysyl hydroxylase activity in cultured dermal fibroblasts in assays that use [14C] lysine-labeled underhydroxylated collagen; prolyl 4-hydroxylase activity is used as a positive control (Wenstrup et al., 1989). Unfortunately, values for enzyme activity differ considerably from assay to assay, and from laboratory to laboratory, so maximum activity values consistent with the disease phenotype cannot be uniformly stated. More recently, measurement of the ratio of urinary excretion of pyridinium cross-links has become widely used as a screen for this disorder. Affected individuals demonstrate a narrow range of deoxypyridinoline-to-pyridinoline ratios that is at least one order of magnitude greater than age-matched controls (Pasquali et al., 1994; Steinmann et al., 1995). This method shows great promise in providing a rapid, inexpensive diagnostic test for Ehlers-Danlos syndrome type VI.

THE ARTHROCHALASIA TYPE

Diagnostic Criteria

This form of Ehlers-Danlos syndrome, which corresponds to Ehlers-Danlos syndrome types VIIA and VIIB in previous classifications, is characterized by extreme joint laxity, multiple joint dislocations, and congenital hip dislocations that are difficult to repair surgically. Dermal features include tissue fragility and widened scars; these dermal findings are less prominent than in the classical form of Ehlers-Danlos syndrome (types I and II).

Severe generalized joint hypermobility with recurrent subluxations and congenital bilateral hip dislocation are the major diagnostic criteria. Minor diagnostic criteria include tissue fragility, including atrophic scars, kyphoscoliosis, and skin hyperextensibility.

Etiology, Pathogenesis, and Genetics

The biochemical defect that results in this form of Ehlers-Danlos syndrome is the failure to accomplish normal cleavage of the amino-terminal propeptide of type I collagen in all tissues. Electron micrographs of collagen fibrils from skin of a patient with this disorder show abnormal collagen fibrils that are irregular in outline and vary widely in diameter. Patients have autosomal dominant mutations that remove the exon containing the N-peptidase recognition sequence in proα 1(I) (type A) or proα 2(I) (type B) chains. This recognition sequence is contained in exon 6 of both *COL1A1* and *COL1A2*, which are highly homologous and have well-conserved intron-exon boundaries. The molecular mechanism for Ehlers-Danlos syndrome types VIIA and VIIB is almost always mutations that disrupt the splice acceptor or splice donor sequences 5' or 3' to exon 6, causing removal of that exon during processing of mRNA (Barabas, 1967; Beighton, 1992; Steinmann et al., 1993; Byers, 1995).

Diagnostic Testing

Confirmation of the diagnosis is accomplished by electrophoretic demonstration of pNα1(I) or pNα2(I) chains extracted from dermal collagen or harvested from cultured skin fibroblasts. Direct demonstration of exon 6 skipping in cDNAs of *COL1A1* or *COL1A2* can be performed, followed by mutation analysis.

THE DERMATOSPORAXIS TYPE

Diagnostic Criteria

This very rare form of Ehlers-Danlos syndrome, which corresponds to Ehlers-Danlos syndrome type VIIC in previous classifications, is characterized by striking dermal fragility. The skin is lax but not stretchy, and joint dislocation is usually not a feature of this disorder. Infants have been reported with premature rupture of membranes, and umbilical/inguinal hernias occur as well.

Diagnostic criteria include severe skin fragility and sagging, redundant skin.

Etiology, Pathogenesis, and Genetics

The biochemical defect that results in this form of Ehlers-Danlos syndrome is the failure to cleave off the amino-terminal propeptide of type I collagen due to deficiency of the procollagen I N-peptidase gene (Colige et al., 1999). In skin, procollagen metabolites that contain the N-propeptides are present, and cultured dermal fibroblasts secrete procollagens in which the N-propeptide but not the C-propeptide is retained. Procollagen molecules from mutant cell strains are normally cleaved when placed into control cultures, indicating that the defective processing is not caused by abnormalities in the procollagen substrate, as it is in the arthrochalasia type of Ehlers-Danlos syndrome.

Diagnostic Testing

This is performed by electrophoretic demonstration of pNα1(I) or pNα2(I) chains extracted from dermal collagen or harvested from cultured skin fibroblasts.

OTHER EHLERS-DANLOS SYNDROME VARIANTS

Ehlers-Danlos syndrome type VIII is a rare autosomal dominant condition characterized by soft, hyperextensible skin, abnormal scarring, easy bruising, hyperextensible joints, and generalized periodontitis. It resembles Ehlers-Danlos syndrome type I, but in the few available clinical reports it is distinguished from the latter disorder by periodontitis with early loss of teeth and by the characteristic purplish discoloration of scars on the shins. The molecular basis of Ehlers-Danlos syndrome type VIII is unknown. It is unclear whether this entity is truly distinct from the classical form of Ehlers-Danlos syndrome (types I and II).

Arneson and co-workers reported a single family in which two siblings of unaffected parents had joint hyperextensibility, mitral valve prolapse, easy bruisibility, and poor wound healing (Arneson et al., 1980). Clotting studies performed to evaluate excessive bleeding at incision sites were normal except for a striking defect in the platelet adhesion that is normally observed in response to exposure of platelets to collagen. Addition of purified fibronectin to the patients' plasma improved platelet adhesiveness. The authors suggested that this disorder, referred to in subsequent classifications of Ehlers-Danlos syndrome as type X, may be caused by a defect in fibronectin.

MANIFESTATIONS AND MANAGEMENT

Because Ehlers-Danlos syndrome in all its forms is a generalized connective tissue disorder, there are pleiotropic effects. A wide variety of medical complications of Ehlers-Danlos syndrome has been reported, but two major caveats must be made. First, many clinical reports, particularly those written before the mid-1980s, do not distinguish between the different Ehlers-Danlos syndrome subtypes. Lack of this distinction will substantially limit the usefulness of published case reports except in those rare instances when the subtype can be clearly surmised from the clinical report. This is particularly true with regard to management of pregnancy and delivery and for vascular complications, because the vascular form of Ehlers-Danlos syndrome (type IV) and the classical form (types I and II) have substantially different underlying pathology, complications, and management recommendations. The second caveat is that most clinical reports are of single cases or a small series of patients. There are very few large or population-based series that might provide information about the full range of therapeutic outcomes or accurate estimates of the prevalence of certain complications of Ehlers-Danlos syndrome.

Pregnancy

Because of the multiple complications that can occur during pregnancy in a patient with Ehlers-Danlos syndrome, it is recommended that all cases should be referred to a high-risk obstetric practice, where one is available. In addition to problems directly related to carriage and delivery of the fetoplacental unit, pregnancy is a period of increased risk of vascular rupture for those with susceptible Ehlers-Danlos syndrome subtypes, particularly the vascular form (Ehlers-Danlos syndrome IV), the kyphoscoliotic form (Ehlers-Danlos syndrome VI), and the classical form (Ehlers-Danlos syndrome I and II).

Prematurity is a complication primarily of the classical form of Ehlers-Danlos syndrome (types I and II). There are two potential causes for premature rupture of membranes in an Ehlers-Danlos syndrome pregnancy. The first is abnormal membranes of an affected fetus, whether or not the mother is affected. Rupture of membranes typically occurs 3 or 4 weeks early but rarely occurs earlier than 35 weeks of gestation. Thus delivery of an affected infant typically does not increase the risk for respiratory distress syndrome because lung development is complete by 36–37 weeks, when delivery most often occurs.

There may also be cervical incompetence in a woman with Ehlers-Danlos syndrome, whether or not the fetus is affected. Pregnant women with all forms of Ehlers-Danlos syndrome, except the hypermobility form (Ehlers-Danlos syndrome III), are apparently at risk. Painless cervical dilatation has been reported as early as the second trimester of pregnancy and has been associated with spontaneous abortion or precipitous delivery.

Although a mild to moderate increase in peripartum bleeding is common in all forms of Ehlers-Danlos syndrome, the risk of severe uterine hemorrhage and/or rupture is a hallmark of the vascular form of Ehlers-Danlos syndrome. Although earlier reports of 25% mortality in each pregnancy due to these complications now appear to be an overestimate, the risk of severe hemorrhagic complications from labor and vaginal delivery, including death or shock, remain unacceptably high, in the range of 10% per pregnancy (Pepin et al., 2000).

Evaluation

- Pregnant women with the vascular form of Ehlers-Danlos syndrome must undergo extremely careful monitoring of blood pressure during gestation.
- Cervical incompetence should be investigated.
- Before delivery, clotting studies including bleeding time should be performed.
- No published standards of care exist for delivery in affected women; however, pregnant individuals with the vascular form of Ehlers-Danlos syndrome should be delivered by cesarean section and not allowed to enter into labor. For other Ehlers-Danlos syndrome subtypes, vaginal delivery is possible.

Treatment

- Active consultation between a high-risk obstetrics practice and a clinician familiar with the clinical and genetic heterogeneity of the Ehlers-Danlos syndrome is strongly recommended.
- If the bleeding time is prolonged, one should consider giving fresh frozen plasma concentrate or DDAVP to improve bleeding times (Rochelson et al., 1991).
- Cervical incompetence is conservatively treated with bed rest and the Trendelenburg position. If dilatation progresses, cervical incompetence is

typically treated with cerclage. However, in patients with evidence of tissue fragility, the likelihood of suture displacement and local infection may contraindicate this procedure. An alternative procedure is placement of a Smith-Hodge pessary, which may avoid the above complications (Leduc and Wasserstrum, 1992).

Growth and Feeding

Growth or feeding problems in the Ehlers-Danlos syndromes are rare. There have been several cases of the hypermobility form of Ehlers-Danlos syndrome with significantly slow gastric emptying times (personal experience), but it is not clear whether individuals with Ehlers-Danlos syndrome are at higher risk for this than the general population. Hiatal hernia has been widely reported in adults with Ehlers-Danlos syndrome (Steinman et al., 1993).

Development and Behavior

Motor delay can sometimes be seen in patients with very lax joints due to Ehlers-Danlos syndrome. This appears to be caused by inability to stabilize the joints.

Cognitive development is no different from that in the general population. There are no behavior problems specific to the Ehlers-Danlos syndromes.

Evaluation

- Standard pediatric developmental assessment is adequate for evaluation of motor delays.
- Occasionally, referral for physical therapy evaluation will be indicated.

Treatment

- Physical therapy to improve the strength of muscles surrounding lax joints can improve attainment of joint stability

Musculoskeletal

Joint dislocations are a relatively frequent complication of any form of Ehlers-Danlos syndrome. The joints most commonly affected are the shoulders, patellae, temporomandibular joints, and digits. Congenital dislocation of the hip is a hallmark of the arthrochalasia form (Ehlers-Danlos syndrome VIIA, VIIB), and occurs in the classical form (Ehlers-Danlos syndrome I) and the vascular form (Ehlers-Danlos syndrome IV) as well.

Chronic pain is a major manifestation of the Ehlers-Danlos syndrome. Although it is seen in all forms, it is most common and most debilitating in the hypermobility form (Ehlers-Danlos syndrome III) [personal experience]. The origin of this pain is not well understood. There is acute pain from dislocations and subluxations and from soft tissue injury. Many individuals with Ehlers-Danlos syndrome present with significant joint pain; many have been previously evaluated for inflammatory arthritis. However, the pain is not associated with erythema or point tenderness and only rarely with swelling.

More study is needed to evaluate the pain and the effectiveness of different pain control interventions. Two studies have been published that address the experience of chronic pain in Ehlers-Danlos syndrome and other psychosocial effects of living with the disorder (Lumley et al., 1994; Sacheti et al., 1997). Both studies relied on a convenience sample composed primarily of individuals attending the Ehlers-Danlos National Foundation educational meetings in 1992 and 1995 or seen in a clinic setting. Although the data are clearly collected from a subset of patients who are motivated to attend a meeting hosted by a national voluntary support organization, it is clear that moderate to severe pain is a common daily occurrence for many patients. The pain starts early in life and intensifies over time. The average number of pain locations per patient is eight. Most respondents reported that their chronic pain began in at least one location during childhood. Large numbers of respondents (70%) reported that pain interfered with their sleep and physical activity. Slightly less than half (45%) reported interference with school or job, social relations, and sexual activity. Chronic pain is frequently compounded by secondary depression (Lumley et al., 1994).

Evaluation

- A medical history that excludes systemic signs such as fever and weight loss and lack of focal signs such as erythema and point tenderness in specific joints is usually sufficient to exclude inflammatory arthritis. If necessary, an erythrocyte sedimentation rate can help exclude inflammatory arthritis.

- X rays of joints are rarely useful in evaluating chronic pain associated with Ehlers-Danlos syndrome.

- It can be very useful to consult a psychiatrist in cases where long-term chronic pain is compounded by an affective component, provided that the matter is discussed diplomatically with the patient and there is the understanding that the affective component is secondary to chronic pain.

Treatment

- With the exception of congenital dislocation of the hip, joint dislocation in Ehlers-Danlos syndrome either spontaneously resolves or usually can be corrected by closed reduction.

- Surgical procedures to correct dislocation have involved primary reduction of congenital dislocation of the hip or reduction of joint laxity to prevent chronic dislocations of other joints.

- For congenital dislocation of the hip, the best result requires open reduction. Badelon and co-workers reported a series of 9 patients with Ehlers-Danlos syndrome (8 with Ehlers-Danlos syndrome type VII, 1 with Ehlers-Danlos syndrome type I) with congenital hip dislocation (Badelon et al, 1990). All nine patients achieved ambulation after open reduction, although resolution of the dislocation by radiographic criteria was modest.

- Orthopedic procedures designed to reduce ligamentous laxity and therefore prevent recurrent dislocations have been generally unsatisfactory. Shoulder surgery has been particularly unsuccessful (Jerosch and Castro, 1990). Surgery to prevent patellar dislocation is also rarely successful (personal experience). Procedures to reduce temporomandibular dislocation may be more successful.

- The most productive avenue of therapy involves anticipatory guidance. It is useful to take an environmental history to determine whether conditions of employment or home life exacerbate symptoms (personal observation). For example, work that requires standing for long periods of time will often result in foot and hip pain. This can be alleviated somewhat by wearing supportive, well-cushioned shoes, but it may require reassignment of job duties. At home, hard flooring such as concrete or ceramic tile should be avoided in high-use areas such as the kitchen. It is often not appreciated that wood flooring is substantially more forgiving than stone or concrete. Wherever possible, carpeting makes a significant difference in symptoms by the end of the day.

- Many different interventions have been utilized for pain management. Generally, none of these has been completely effective, and there are no published studies or guidelines concerning the management of the pain associated with Ehlers-Danlos syndrome. Nonsteroidal anti-inflammatory drugs (NSAIDs) are often tried, but long-term use may lead to gastrointestinal and hematologic problems. Other medications that may be used include fixed combination products (NSAID/opioid) or single-entity opioids and tricyclic antidepressants. There is too little experience with the new class of cox-2 inhibitors to determine whether they are a significant improvement over earlier NSAIDS. The relevant issue may be the significant decrease in gastrointestinal complications versus a much higher cost. Physical therapy, hydrotherapy, and behavioral and/or cognitive coping strategies may also be tried to improve pain. Some patients utilize orthopedic devices such as orthotics and braces.

- A regular exercise program may be helpful for strengthening muscles, helping to stabilize the joints and relieve stress. We have found that physical therapy directly aimed at strengthening the shoulder girdle has lowered the frequency of shoulder dislocations in individuals with chronic or recurrent dislocation. Swimming is an ideal choice for many patients, but they may require physical therapy for the shoulder girdle beforehand.

- Patients have found it useful to have a pain problem list in their medical chart for tracking purposes.

Cardiovascular

There have been numerous reports of cardiac and aortic abnormalities in the Ehlers-Danlos syndromes, including aortic and mitral valve incompetence, mitral valve prolapse, aortic dilatation, and aortic dissection/rupture (Leier et al., 1980; Wenstrup et al., 1989; Beighton, 1992; Steinmann et al., 1993; Tiller et al., 1998). Table 8.2 lists the type of cardiac abnormalities reported with the various Ehlers-Danlos syndrome subtypes (1988 classification). Although it is highly likely that the prevalence of these complications is substantially greater than in the general population, their prevalence within the Ehlers-Danlos syndromes in general and within each Ehlers-Danlos syndrome subtype is unknown.

TABLE 8.2. Aortic Complications Reported in Various Ehlers-Danlos Syndrome Subtypes

Aortic Complication	EDS I	EDS II	EDS III	EDS IV	EDS VI	EDS untyped
Aortic valve incompetence, dilatation, rupture of ascending aorta and arch	H,K,L	L	L		B	C,D,I
Dilatation, rupture of descending aorta				A,E,F,G		
Dilated sinus of Valsalva	H,J		H			

A; Beighton, 1992; B; Wenstrup et al., 1989; C; Hata et al., 1988, D; Nicholls et al., 1996; E; Barabas, 1967; F; Kuivaniemi et al., 1990; G; Kontusaari et al., 1990; H; Leier et al., 1980; I; Serry et al., 1988; J; Tucker et al., 1963; K; McKusick et al., 1966; L; Tiller et al., 1998. EDS, Ehlers-Danlos syndrome.

As shown in Table 8.2, some patterns regarding the relative prevalence of cardiovascular abnormalities within some Ehlers-Danlos syndrome subtypes may be inferred from the literature. Aortic abnormalities in patients with the classical form (Ehlers-Danlos syndrome I and II) and the hypermobility form (Ehlers-Danlos syndrome III) nearly always involve the ascending aorta and extend distally. In these Ehlers-Danlos syndrome forms, aortic rupture or dissection is preceded by dilatation (Tiller et al., 1998; personal observation). A prevalence study of aortic root dilatation has recently been completed in 50 individuals with types I, II, and III; approximately 20% have measurements greater than 2 standard deviations above the mean (personal observation). The rate of progression and the likelihood of rupture or dissection are still unknown. At present, the data are still too preliminary to justify routine screening of Ehlers-Danlos syndrome patients for aortic root dilatation. Specifically, the rate of severe complication, such as dissection and rupture, and the rate of progression of aortic root dilatation have not been determined yet.

Patients with the vascular form (Ehlers-Danlos syndrome IV) and the kyphoscoliotic form (type VI) of Ehlers-Danlos syndrome also have increased incidence of mitral valve prolapse and aortic abnormalities. The aortic disease in these forms may be more prevalent than that found in the other forms of Ehlers-Danlos syndrome and is different in its location. Rupture and/or dissection of the aorta, when it occurs, is usually more distal than that found in the classical forms (Ehlers-Danlos syndrome I and II) and the hypermobility form of (Ehlers-Danlos syndrome III). Although it can occur anywhere along the aorta, dissection or rupture usually occurs at or distal to the midaortic arch and extends distally. For the vascular form of Ehlers-Danlos syndrome, there is no good evidence that dissection and rupture of the aorta — or any vessel, for that matter — is preceded by dilation, as is nearly always true for Marfan syndrome and the other forms of Ehlers-Danlos syndrome (Tiller et al., 1998; personal observation). Therefore, the prudent clinician should assume that all patients with the vascular form of Ehlers-Danlos syndrome are equally at risk for vascular and aortic catastrophe.

Surgical complications and intraoperative problems have been widely reported in the Ehlers-Danlos syndrome, but their prevalence is most common in the classical forms (Ehlers-Danlos syndrome I and II) and the vascular form (Ehlers-Danlos syndrome IV), and they are comparatively uncommon for individuals with the hypermobility form (Ehlers-Danlos syndrome III).

Individuals with the vascular form of Ehlers-Danlos syndrome face great risks at surgery. The surgical literature is rife with case reports of operative "nightmares" in patients diagnosed with this form or in whom the diagnosis was postoperatively made.

Patients with this form have a high baseline risk for rupture of medium-sized arteries and aorta, both spontaneously and following relatively minor trauma. Patients may present to the surgeon with any one of these emergent problems that can quickly spiral out of control in the operating room. Spontaneous perforations of the bowel occur as well.

The main problems during surgery are related to fragility of tissues, and vascular tissues in particular. The initial incision may widen spontaneously (see **Dermatologic** section below), and internal tissues may fall apart. Sutures may fail in internal tissues, bleeding may be severe, and ligation of friable vessels is extremely difficult. Death may occur from exsanguination.

Freeman et al. (1996), in a compilation of 45 published cases of the vascular form of Ehlers-Danlos syndrome, noted that vascular complications were diverse and were grouped as hemorrhages (22), aneurysms (17), arterial dissections (5), and arterioveous fistulas (1). Vascular complications in this series are comparable in location and type to those in other, smaller series. Twelve patients (30%) died of vascular complications: four presented in shock and died during resuscitation efforts, and five died intraoperatively during repair of ruptured aorta or iliac artery or innominate artery. Three of these deaths resulted from transection of the aorta when a cross-clamp was applied. One other patient died of disseminated intravascular coagulation in the immediate postoperative period following repair of a ruptured iliac artery aneurysm, and one patient died of angiography complication. In this series, angiography had morbidity and mortality rates of 16.7% and 5.6%, respectively. Treatment methods for patients with vascular complications included operative therapy (28): simple vessel ligation (8), arterial reconstruction (20); nonoperative supportive care (11); and therapeutic angiography (2). Angiography was performed in 18 patients (40%). Four patients

had a major complication from angiography, with 3 peripheral artery dissections and one aortic perforation (the latter one resulted in death). Of the 7 patients who survived initial resuscitation efforts and angiography and then died, all were in the reconstruction group—no deaths occurred in the simple vessel ligation or observation treatment groups.

Evaluation

- Aortic size should be monitored by echocardiogram during initial evaluation of new patients with Ehlers-Danlos syndrome, as with patients with Marfan syndrome.

- For patients with normal echocardiograms at the initial exam, follow-up is problematic because there are no good cross-sectional or longitudinal data on prevalence and progression of aortic root dilatation in Ehlers-Danlos syndrome. At present, we recommend repeating echocardiograms at 3-year intervals; patients with normal echocardiograms who are involved in competitive athletics (junior high school and beyond) are evaluated more frequently. Our impression is that the prevalence is lower and the rate of progression is slower than the corresponding aortic dilatation seen in Marfan syndrome (Roman et al., 1993).

- Patients with aortic diameters greater than +2 SD for body surface area (Roman et al., 1989) should be followed yearly, or occasionally at 6-month intervals, depending on the apparent rate of increase.

Treatment

- Patients with truly enlarged aortic root diameter (> +3 SD) can be placed empirically on beta blockers, but at present the limited number of patients on beta blockers preclude drawing any conclusions regarding efficacy or length of treatment. At present, there is no evidence that beta blockers delay or reduce the risk of aortic disease in the vascular form of Ehlers-Danlos syndrome.

- Management of these patients also includes exercise limitation; we encourage casual exercise and discourage competitive sports. It is also useful to distinguish between low-repetition, high-resistance activities (discouraged) and the kind of high-repetition, low-resistance activities that help maintain some level of aerobic fitness.
- In Ehlers-Danlos syndrome types IV and VI, medical management is limited to diligent prevention of and aggressive treatment of hypertension.
- During cardiovascular surgery, the application of hemostats is risky.
- Electric cautery may be helpful in controlling bleeding intraoperatively.
- On the basis of their review of vascular complications, Freeman and co-workers (1996) made a number of treatment recommendations:
  - Vascular complications are best treated noninvasively, when possible. Bed rest with external compression and careful monitoring are appropriate in patients with peripheral vascular hemorrhage who are hemodynamically stable.
  - Angiography should only be used if dynamic CT, magnetic resonance angiography, or digital subtraction angiography using IV infusion do not suffice.
  - When operative therapy is required, minimal vessel dissection with balloon catheter or tourniquet occlusion should be used. Vessel loops and vascular clamps often produce unrepairable injuries.
  - Standard vascular anastamoses often fail because of poor tensile strength of the vessels.

- Primary arterial repair, if attempted, should be tensionless, using interrupted horizontal mattress sutures reinforced with pledgets. Vessel ligation with umbilical tapes may be the safest; bypass grafting is then performed only if distal ischemia develops.

Gastrointestinal

In 1996, Freeman et al. compiled the 44 published cases of gastrointestinal complications of Ehlers-Danlos syndrome type IV in an effort to determine whether superior treatment options were available. Many of the surgical complications discussed in the **Cardiovascular** section also apply to the bowel. Large bowel perforations were the most common gastrointestinal complication reported (41); nearly all were spontaneous, and 80% occurred in the sigmoid colon. The overall mortality rate for patients experiencing a gastrointestinal complication was 23.3% — lower than isolated case reports might suggest. The mortality rate did not differ significantly by patient age or technique of operative therapy or in patients who experienced a second or third colonic perforation. Anastamotic leak was also less frequent than previously suggested but had a 66% mortality rate. Two-thirds of the patients with bowel resection were initially treated with a resection and diversion procedure, and two-thirds of these eventually had intestinal continuity re-established. However, 55% had a subsequent reperforation. Some patients had initial treatment with total abdominal colectomy, whereas others underwent this procedure after one or more reperforations.

Evaluation

- Individuals with Ehlers-Danlos syndrome type IV (vascular Ehlers-Danlos syndrome) or a clinical phenotype compatible with it who experience significant abdominal pain should be evaluated quickly for bowel perforation and for rupture of the superior mesenchymal artery.

- Diverticulitis commonly occurs in all forms of Ehlers-Danlos syndrome, and suggestive symptoms should lead to evaluation.

Treatment

- Because of the high incidence of bowel reperforations, Freeman et al (1996) recommended that perforations of the colon be treated with total abdominal colectomy with end ileostomy. This procedure eliminates the possibility of recurrent colon perforation and avoids the mortality associated with an anastomotic leak when it occurs.

Dermatologic

The dermal fragility associated with the severe classical form of Ehlers-Danlos syndrome presents special problems. When the skin splits from trauma, it is relatively painless and does not bleed excessively, but the wounds tend to gape. The wound margins tend to retract and heal slowly. Dehiscence is common, and complete wound breakdown may require repeated suturing. Alternatively, the skin may appear to hold the stitches well initially, but the wound may fall apart after sutures are removed. Wide, thin papyraceous scars develop, with eventual stretching of scars over several months. Thin, atrophic, darkly pigmented scars form because of intradermal or subdermal hematomata and occur mainly at pressure points.

Failure of dermal sutures prevents close apposition of wound edges. There may be continued oozing from small vessels. This, together with the general tissue laxity, predisposes the patient to formation of postoperative hematomas in the wound. These may be a factor in wound dehiscence and may require exploration, drainage, and transfusion. Healing is slow, and wound dehiscence is common. An increased frequency of infection accompanies this slow healing.

Scars may darken, and gradual stretching and widening may take place over a long period of time.

Evaluation

- Accidental or operative wounds should be closely monitored for dehiscence and inadequate scar formation.

Treatment

- During the initial healing, adhesive tapes and steri strips may help support the skin, but they will not be able to prevent spreading of scars, which occurs over many months.
- Retention sutures tied at a distance from the incision may help, and adhesive strips may be used to support the skin during scar formation.
- A plastic surgeon should be employed for closure of facial wounds or other aesthetically significant areas.
- A significant number of patients will eventually present to plastic surgeons for scar revision; excision of hyperpigmented scars from elbows and knees is the most common cosmetic operation. In some cases, skin grafts may be necessary to repair extensive scarring on the shin. Early adolescence is probably the best time for this surgery, because additional traumatic events are less likely.
- Pseudotumors are easily removed from the elbows and knees, but those related to bursae over the heels are often diffusely involved with the underlying tissues and may be difficult to excise.
- Subcutaneous spheroids should be left alone.

RESOURCES

The Ehlers-Danlos National Foundation

6399 Wilshire Blvd., Ste 510
Los Angeles, CA 90048

Phone (323) 651-3038
www.ednf.org
This organization is devoted to education and support for patients with Ehlers-Danlos syndrome and/or their parents. They have several up-to-date educational pamphlets, publish a quarterly newsletter, *Loose Connections*, and sponsor an annual education and support meeting.

REFERENCES

Arneson MA, Hammerschmidt DE, Furcht LT, King RA (1980) A new form of Ehlers-Danlos syndrome. Fibronectin corrects defective platelet function. *JAMA* 244:144–147.

Badelon O, Bensahel H, Csukonyi Z, Chaumien JP (1990) Congenital dislocation of the hip in Ehlers-Danlos syndrome. *Clin Orthoped* 138–143.

Barabas AP (1967) Heterogenity of the Ehlers-Danlos syndrome: Description of three clinical types and a hypothesis to explain the basic defect. *Br Med J* 2:612–613.

Beighton P (1992) The Ehlers-Danlos Syndromes. In: *McKusick's Heritable Disorders of Connective Tissue*, edited by Beighton, P. St. Louis, MO: Mosby, p. 189–251.

Beighton P, De Paepe A, Danks D, Finidori G, Gedde-Dahl T, Goodman R, Hall JG, Hollister DW, Horton W, McKusick VA (1988) International nosology of heritable disorders of connective tissue, Berlin, 1986. *Am J Med Genet* 29:581–594.

Beighton P, De Paepe A, Steinmann B, Tsipouras P, Wenstrup RJ (1998) Ehlers-Danlos syndromes: revised nosology, Villefranche, 1997. Ehlers-Danlos National Foundation (USA) and Ehlers-Danlos Support Group (UK). *Am J Med Genet* 77:31–37.

Beighton P, Grahame R, Bird H (1989) *Hypermobility of Joints*, 2nd ed. London: Springer.

Burrows NP, Nicholls AC, Yates JR, Gatward G, Sarathachandra P, Richord A, Pope FM (1996) The gene encoding collagen alpha1(V) (*COL5A1*) is linked to mixed Ehlers-Danlos syndrome type I/II. *J Invest.Dermatol* 106: 1273–1276.

Byers PH (1995) Disorders of collagen biosynthesis and structure. In: *The Metabolic Basis of Inherited Diseases*, edited by Schriver, CR, Beaudet, AL, Sly, WS and Valle, D. New York: McGraw-Hill, p. 4029–4078.

Byers PH, Siegel RC, Holbrook KA, Narayanan AS, Bornstein P, Hall JG (1980) X-linked cutis laxa: Defective collagen crosslink formation due to decreased lysyl oxidase activity. *N Engl J Med* 303: 61–65.

Colige A, Sieron AL, Li SE, Schwarze U, Petty E, Wertelecki W, Wilcox W, Krakow D, Cohn DH, Reardon W, Byers PH, Lapiere CM, Prockop DJ, Nusgens BV (1995) Human Ehlers-Danlos syndrome type VII C and bovine dermatosparaxis are caused by mutations in the procollagen I N-proteinase gene. *Am J Hum Genet* 65(2):308–317.

Chessler SD, Wallis GA, Byers PH (1993) Mutations in the carboxyl-terminal propeptide of the pro alpha 1(1) chain of type I collagen result in defective chain association and produce lethal osteogenesis imperfecta. *J Biol Chem* 268:18218–18225.

De Paepe A (1994) Ehlers-Danlos syndrome type IV. Clinical and molecular aspects and guidelines for diagnosis and management [review]. *Dermatology* 189, Suppl 2:21–25.

De Paepe A, Nuytinck L, Hausser I, Anton-Lamprecht I, Naeyaert J-M (1997) Mutations in the *COL5A1* gene are causal in the Ehlers-Danlos syndromes I and II. *Am J Hum Genet* 60:547–554.

Eyre DR, Glimcher MJ (1972) Reducible crosslinks in hydroxylysine-deficient collagens of a heritable disorder of connective tissue. *Proc Natl Acad Sci USA* 69:2594–2598.

Freeman RK, Swegle J, Sise MJ (1996) The surgical complications of Ehlers-Danlos syndrome. *Am Surg* 62:869–873.

Greenspan DS, Northrup H, Au KS, McAllister KA, Francomano CA, Wenstrap RJ, Marchuk DA, Kwiatkowski DJ (1995) *COL5A1*: fine genetic mapping and exclusion as candidate gene in families with nail-patella syndrome, tuberous sclerosis 1, hereditary hemorrhagic telangiectasia, and Ehlers-Danlos syndrome type II. *Genomics* 25:737–739.

Hata R, Kurata S, Shinkai H (1988) Existence of malfunctioning pro alpha2(I) collagen genes in a patient with a pro alpha 2(I)-chain-defective variant of Ehlers-Danlos syndrome. *Eur J Biochem* 174:231–237.

Hautala T, Heikkinen J, Kivirikko KI, Myllyla R (1993) A large duplication in the gene for lysyl hydroxylase accounts for the type VI variant of Ehlers-Danlos syndrome in two siblings. *Genomics* 15:399–404.

Heikkinen J, Hautala T, Kivirikko KI, Myllyla R (1994) Structure and expression of the human lysyl hydroxylase gene (*PLOD*): Introns 9 and 16 contain Alu sequences at the sites of recombination in Ehlers-Danlos syndrome type VI patients. *Genomics* 24:464–471.

Heikkinen J, Toppinen T, Yeowell H, et al. (1997) Duplication of seven exons in the lysyl hydroxylase gene is associated with longer forms of a repetitive sequence within the gene and is a common cause for the type VI variant of Ehlers-Danlos syndrome. *Am J Hum Genet* 60:48–56.

Ihme A, Krieg T, Nerlich A, Feldman U, Rauterberg J, Glanvitle RW, Edel G, Muller PK (1984) Ehlers-Danlos syndrome type VI: Collagen type specificity of defective lysyl hydroxylation in various tissues. *J Invest Dermatol* 83:161–165.

Jaffe AS, Geltman EM, Rodey GE, Uitto J (1981) Mitral valve prolapse: A consistent manifestation of type IV Ehlers-Danlos syndrome. *Circulation* 64:121–125.

Jerosch J, Castro WH (1990) Shoulder instability in Ehlers-Danlos syndrome. An indication for surgical treatment? *Acta Orthoped Belg* 56:451–453.

Kontusaari S, Tromp G, Kuivaniemi H, Ladda RL, Prockop DJ (1990) Inheritance of an RNA splicing mutation (G+ 1 IVS20) in the type III procollagen gene (*COL3A1*) in a family having aortic aneurysms and easy bruisability: Phenotypic overlap between familial arterial aneurysms and Ehlers-Danlos syndrome type IV. *Am J Hum Genet* 47:112–120.

Kuivaniemi H, Kontusaari S, Tromp G, Zhao MJ, Sabol C, Prockop DJ (1990) Identical G+1 to A mutations in three different introns of the type III procollagen gene (*COL3A1*) produce different patterns of RNA splicing in three variants of Ehlers-Danlos syndrome. IV. An explanation for exon skipping some mutations and not others. *J Biol Chem* 265:12067–12074.

Leduc L, Wasserstrum N (1992) Successful treatment with the Smith-Hodge pessary of cervical

incompetence due to defective connective tissue in Ehlers-Danlos syndrome. *Am J Perinatol* 9:25–27.

Leier CV, Call TD, Fulkerson PK, Wooley CF (1980) The spectrum of cardiac defects in the Ehlers-Danlos syndrome, types I and III. *Ann Int Med* 92:171–178.

Lumley MA, Jordan M, Rubenstein R, Tsipouras P, Evans MI (1994) Psychosocial functioning in the Ehlers-Danlos syndrome. *Am J Med Genet* 53:149–152.

McDonald A, Pogrel MA (1996) Ehlers-Danlos syndrome: An approach to surgical management of temporomandibular joint dysfunction in two cases. *J Oral Maxillofac Surg* 54:761–765.

McKusick VA, Larsen AL, Wilson R (1966) The Ehlers-Danlos syndrome and "congenital" aterio-venous fistulae, a clinicopathologic study of a family. In: *Heritable Disorders of Connective Tissue*, edited by Royce PM and Steinmann B. St. Louis, MO: Mosby, p. 292–371.

Michalickova K, Susic M, Willing MC, Wenstrup RJ, Cole WG (1998) Mutations of the alpha2(V) chain of type V collagen impair matrix assembly and produce Ehlers-Danlos syndrome type I. *Hum Mol Genet* 7:249–255.

Nicholls AC, Oliver JE, McCarron S, Harrison JB, Greenspan DS, Pope FM (1996) An exon skipping mutation of a type V collagen gene (*COL5A1*) in Ehlers-Danlos syndrome. *J Med Genet* 33:940–946.

Pasqual M, Dembure PP, Still MJ, Elsas LJ (1994) Urinary pyridinium cross-links: A noninvasive diagnostic test for Ehlers-Danlos syndrome type VI (letter). *N Engl J Med* 331:132–133.

Pepin M, Schwarze U, Superti-Furga A, Byers PH (2000) Clinical and genetic features of Ehlers-Danlos syndrome type IV, the vascular type. *N Engl J Med* 342(10):673–680.

Pinnell, SR, Krane SM, Densora JE, Glimcher MJ (1972) A heritable disorder of connective tissue: Hydroxylysine-deficient collagen disease. *New Engl J Med* 286:1013–1020.

Richards AJ, Martin S, Nicholls AC, Harrison JB, Pope FM, Burrows NP (1998) A single base mutation in *COL5A2* causes Ehlers-Danlos syndrome type II. *J Med Genet* 35:846–848.

Rochelson B, Caruso R, Davenport D, Daelber A (1991) The use of prophylactic desmopressin in labor to prevent hemorrhage in a patient with Ehlers-Danlos syndrome. *NY State J Med* 91:268–269.

Roman MJ, Devereux RB, Kramer-Fox R, O'Loughlin J (1989) Two-dimensional echocardiographic aortic root dimensions in normal children and adults. *Am J Cardiol* 64:507–512.

Roman MJ, Rosen SE, Kramer-Fox R, Devereux RB (1993) Prognostic significance of the pattern of aortic root dilation in the Marfan syndrome. *J Am Col Cardiol* 22:1470–1476.

Sacheti A, Szemere J, Bernstein B, Tafas T, Schechter N, Tsipouras P (1997) Chronic pain is a manifestation of the Ehlers-Danlos syndrome. *J Pain Symptom Manage* 14:88–93.

Schwarze U, Atkinson M, Hoffman GG, Greenspan DS, Byers PH (2000) Null alleles of the *COL5A1* gene of type V collagen are a cause of the classical forms of Ehlers-Danlos syndrome (types I and II). *Am J Hum Genet* 66(6):1757–1765.

Serry C, Agomuoh OS, Goldin MD (1988) Review of Ehlers-Danlos syndrome. Successful repair of rupture and dissection of abdominal aorta. [review]. *J Cardiovasc Surg* 29:530–534.

Steinmann B, Royce PM, Superti-Furga A (1993) The Ehlers-Danlos syndrome. In: *Connective Tissue and its Heritable Disorders*, edited by Royce PM and Steinmann B. New York: Wiley-Liss, p. 351–408.

Steinmann B, Eyre DR, Shao P (1995) Urinary pyridinoline cross-links in Ehlers-Danlos syndrome type VI [letter]. *Am J Hum Genet* 57:1505–1508.

Tiller GE, Cassidy SB, Wensel C, Wenstrup RJ (1998) Aortic root dilatation in Ehlers-Danlos syndrome types I, II and III. A report of five cases. *Clin Genet* 53:460–465.

Toriello HV, Glover TW, Takahara K, Byers PH, Miller DE, Higgins JU, Greenspan DS (1996) A translocation interrupts the *COL5A1* gene in a patient with Ehlers-Danlos syndrome and hypomelanosis of Ito. *Nat Genet* 13:361–365.

Tucker DH, Miller DE, Jacoby WJ Jr. (1963) Ehlers-Danlos syndrome with sinus of Valsalva aneurysm and aortic insufficiency simulating rheumatic heart disease. *Am J Med* 35:715–720.

Wenstrup RJ, Langland GT, Willing MC, D'Souza VN, Cole WG (1996) A splice-junction mutation in the region of proα1(V) chains results in the gravis form of the Ehlers-Danlos syndrome (type I). *Hum Mol Genet* 5:1733–1736.

Wenstrup RJ, Murad S, Pinnell SR (1989) Ehlers-Danlos syndrome type VI: Clinical manifestations of collagen lysyl hydroxylase deficiency. *J Pediatr* 115:405–409.

Wenstrup RJ, Florer JB, Wiling MC, Giunta C, Steinmann B, Young F, Susic M, Cole WG (2000) *COL5A1* halopinsufficiency is a common molecular mechanism underlying the classical form of EDS. *Am J Hum Genet* 66(6):1766–1776.

CHAPTER 9

FETAL ALCOHOL SYNDROME

STERLING K. CLARREN AND SUSAN J. ASTLEY

INTRODUCTION

Incidence

Fetal alcohol syndrome is found in a subset of individuals affected by ethanol teratogenesis. An accurate and accepted incidence of fetal alcohol syndrome has not been fully established. The few methodologically sound prospective studies have found the incidence to be in the range of 1–3 in 1000 live births (Sampson et al., 1997). Analysis of passive birth defect surveillance systems suggests that the incidence is 1–3 in 10,000 live births (Abel 1995). There is reason to believe that this second figure is an underestimate caused by a general difficulty in recognition of the syndrome at birth. The number of individuals exposed to alcohol in utero and affected with physical anomalies and/or brain alterations, but without the characteristic and recognizable pattern of fetal alcohol syndrome, is not known. Many authors have stated that the frequency is at least the same as fetal alcohol syndrome, but it is potentially far greater.

Diagnostic Criteria

The cardinal features of fetal alcohol syndrome were established in the late 1970s. The condition has been typified by a specific facial appearance, evidence of organic brain damage, and growth deficiency in the presence of alcohol exposure during gestation (Clarren and Smith, 1978). The problem with the criteria for the diagnosis of fetal alcohol syndrome, as so often occurs in dysmorphology, is the lack of precision in both the definition and the measurement of each component. How many facial features must be present, how severe must the features be, and what scale of measurement should be used to judge their severity? What is the minimal definition of organic brain damage? How small must a patient be in height and/or weight to be called "growth deficient"? What is acceptable confirmation of alcohol exposure during pregnancy? How much alcohol exposure is considered necessary to place the embryo or fetus "at risk"? When fetal alcohol syndrome is defined by specific abnormalities in face, growth, and brain, no other single organ of the body seems to be regularly affected. Heart defects, renal anomalies, palatal clefts, minor bony anomalies, and possibly malformation of the retina and inner ear occur, apparently at increased rates above background level.

Management of Genetic Syndromes, Edited by Suzanne B. Cassidy and Judith E. Allanson
ISBN 0-471-31286-X   Copyright © 2001 by Wiley-Liss, Inc.

Another problem is how to diagnose individuals who present with physical and/or cognitive problems and prenatal alcohol exposure but do not have fetal alcohol syndrome. These adverse outcomes are frequently diagnosed as fetal alcohol-effects, alcohol-related birth defects, and alcohol-related neurodevelopmental disorders (Aase et al., 1995; Stratton et al, 1996). These terms inappropriately imply that alcohol is causally associated with the adverse outcomes, nor an association that can neither be confirmed nor ruled out in an individual patient. Adverse outcomes like growth deficiency and central nervous system dysfunction are not specific to alcohol exposure; they can be caused by a myriad of prenatal and postnatal risk factors.

In the absence of specific measurement techniques and case definitions, the specific clinical criteria used to make the diagnosis of fetal alcohol syndrome will continue to vary widely from clinic to clinic. From a clinical perspective, diagnostic misclassification leads to inappropriate patient care, increased risk for secondary disabilities (Streissguth and Kanter, 1997), and missed opportunities for primary prevention. From a public health perspective, diagnostic misclassification leads to inaccurate estimates of incidence and prevalence. Inaccurate estimates thwart efforts to allocate sufficient social, educational, and health care services to this high-risk population and preclude accurate assessment of primary prevention and intervention efforts. From a clinical research perspective, diagnostic misclassification reduces the power to identify meaningful contrasts between groups. Nonstandardized diagnostic methods prevent comparison of results between studies from different research centers.

One approach to overcoming these measurement and diagnostic limitations has been proposed by Astley and Clarren (1996, 1997, 1999) in the *Diagnostic Guide for Fetal Alcohol Syndrome and Related Conditions*. The *Guide* introduces a comprehensive, quantitative, case-defined approach to diagnosis

called the "4-digit diagnostic code." The four digits of the diagnostic code reflect the magnitude of expression of four key diagnostic features of fetal alcohol syndrome in the following order: (1) growth deficiency, (2) the fetal alcohol syndrome facial phenotype, (3) brain dysfunction, and (4) gestational alcohol exposure. The magnitude of expression of each feature is ranked independently on a 4-point Likert scale with 1 reflecting complete absence of the fetal alcohol syndrome feature and 4 reflecting a strong "classic" presence of the fetal alcohol syndrome feature. Each Likert rank is specifically case defined. A 4-digit code of 4444 reflects the most severe expression of fetal alcohol syndrome. A code of 1111 reflects a complete absence of fetal alcohol syndrome features and alcohol exposure. All codes in between reflect the broad spectrum of outcome and exposure combinations. A standardized nomenclature system is presented to construct clinically meaningful names for all combinations of 4-digit codes. For example, a 4-digit code of 4144 reflects severe growth deficiency, absence of fetal alcohol syndrome facial features, severe organic brain damage, and confirmed exposure to teratogenic levels of alcohol. This code would receive the clinical name, "sentinel physical findings, static encephalopathy, alcohol exposed." It should be noted that alcohol exposure is reported without implying causality. The terms "fetal alcohol syndrome" and "atypical fetal alcohol syndrome" are retained in the nomenclature system. The terms "fetal alcohol effects," "alcohol-related birth defects," and "alcohol-related neurodevelopmental disorders" are not retained. This diagnostic system has been used successfully for several years across multiple clinical sites (Astley and Clarren, 2000).

Etiology, Pathogenesis and Genetics

Ethanol is clearly a teratogen that can cross the placenta and interrupt development at any time in pregnancy. It is less clear whether it can impact development before embryonic implantation and placentation. Whether alcohol is a mutagen affecting the human ova or sperm before conception remains unknown. A growing body of evidence suggests that preconceptional alcohol usage by the father diminishes infant birth weight, although by an unknown mechanism, in small laboratory animals (Passaro et al., 1998).

Although evidence of dose-response relationships between maternal alcohol levels and fetal impact exist, predicting outcome from exposure in an individual is far from precise. Heavy exposure is not uniformly teratogenic, and light exposure is not uniformly harmless (Jacobson and Jacobson, 1994). In general, patients who have the full features of the fetal alcohol syndrome have been subjected to high-dose exposures (estimated blood alcohol concentrations to ≥ 150 mg/dl) delivered at least weekly for at least several weeks in the first trimester. In general, individuals exposed to light or moderate amounts of alcohol cannot be identified individually as falling physically, cognitively, or behaviorally outside of the normal range. However, population-based studies demonstrate that chronic low-dose exposures with average consumption in the range of 15 cc of absolute alcohol per day can be associated with lower intelligence score and increased rates of attention and learning problems. The U.S. Surgeon General's conclusion that zero exposure to alcohol equals zero risk remains the only defensibly true statement (U.S. Public Health Service, 1981).

Timing plays an important role in adverse outcomes associated with alcohol exposure. Facial dysmorphology is related to first-trimester exposures. Some features such as the characteristic premaxillary anomalies may be related to a very short window in development during the period of gastrulation on day 19 or 20 in a human pregnancy (Sulik, 1984; Astley et al., 1999). Features like short palpebral fissures, which may reflect decreased size of the optic globe,

seemingly have a longer first-trimester period of vulnerability, although the specific timing is not established. Growth deficiency appears to be related to exposure in the second half of pregnancy. Women who stop drinking by the fifth to sixth month of gestation are generally reported to have normally grown infants (Rosett and Weiner, 1982). The brain seems uniquely vulnerable to alcohol and can be altered in a wide variety of ways. Presumably, these variations in abnormality are due to the dose, frequency, and timing of exposure as well as genetic factors, including metabolic pathways in mother and fetus, and, potentially, other environmental factors. The first trimester seems to be the period of maximum brain vulnerability, although the brain could be damaged by alcohol at any time in gestation (West, 1986).

Animal models and human neuropathologic investigations have demonstrated the wide-ranging damage ethanol can do to the central nervous system. Ethanol can be neurotoxic and lead to decreased numbers of neuroblasts and/or glioblasts, resulting in a generalized reduction in brain size (microcephaly). Ethanol can interrupt normal patterns of neuronal migration, leading to heterotopias. There can be reductions in white matter. Animal models have demonstrated that virtually every neurotransmitter can be decreased or increased utilizing some methodological approach. There have been recent reports of magnetic resonance images in patients with fetal alcohol syndrome. Common specific abnormalities have included thinning or absence of the corpus callosum and cerebellar vermis hypoplasia. The experimental studies in humans and animals, when taken as a whole, suggest that ethanol does not produce any specific focal pattern of brain lesions but rather causes diffuse lesions that vary in severity within and among affected persons (Roebuck et al., 1998).

Therefore, current understanding would suggest that the full fetal alcohol syndrome would be expected in pregnancies in which women drink voluminously enough and frequently enough to disrupt a large number of separate embryological and fetal developmental steps in receptive conceptuses.

Diagnostic Testing

At present there is no wholly reliable clinical test to determine whether a woman is an alcoholic or whether she is likely to produce a child with fetal alcohol syndrome or a related condition if she drinks during pregnancy. Similarly, there is no test in her offspring to prove that there was alcohol exposure in pregnancy or that the malformations that are present were conclusively caused by alcohol exposure.

The face of fetal alcohol syndrome is the most "alcohol-specific" component of fetal alcohol syndrome. Computer modeling has determined that the face can be distinguished from normal with 100% sensitivity and specificity by analyzing the length of palpebral fissures, the thinness of the upper lip vermillion, and the flatness of the philtrum. The lip and philtrum are measured using a 5-point Likert lip-philtrum pictorial guide (Fig. 9.1). Such facial anomalies can be used for photographic screening of high-risk populations (Astley and Clarren, 1996; 2000). In addition to short palpebral fissure length, smooth philtrum, and thin upper lip, individuals with prenatal alcohol exposure are at increased risk for a number of minor and major anomalies including ptosis, epicanthal folds, and mild hypoplasia of the mandible or maxilla. Identifying the face as

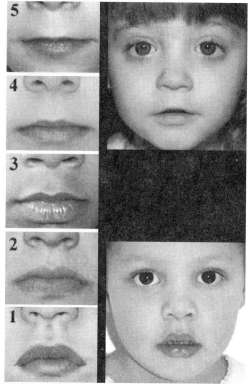

FIGURE 9.1. The 5-point Likert lip-philtrum pictorial guide (*left*) is used to measure upper lip thinness and philtrum smoothness. The child in the top right photo has the classic fetal alcohol syndrome facial phenotype. Her thin upper lip and smooth philtrum would both receive Likert ranks of 5. In contrast, the child in the bottom right photo has a normal facial phenotype. Her full upper lip and deep philtral groove would both receive Likert ranks of 1.

compatible with fetal alcohol syndrome does not mean, of course, that the patient has fetal alcohol syndrome. A clinical assessment is still required after facial screening to evaluate the patient for the other components of the condition necessary for diagnosis.

Evaluation of the brain for evidence of organic brain damage is the most important part of the diagnostic process because it leads to understanding of the problems faced by the patient and is necessary for treatment planning. Organic brain damage can be discussed structurally, neurologically, or psychometrically. The firmest evidence for organic brain damage is through physical findings such as microcephaly. A head circumference more than 2–3 standard deviations below the mean is clearly beyond the normal growth range and, in fetal alcohol syndrome, is due to decreased brain growth. Imaging studies that identify anomalies produced during brain formation, such as an absent corpus callosum, small cerebellar vermis, cerebral heteropias, etc., are other clear indicators of brain malformation. Childhood epilepsy and hard neurologic signs that are present from an early age without alternate explanation also support the conclusion of underlying organic brain damage.

A high percentage of patients exposed to substantial amounts of alcohol in gestation who have the sentinel physical stigmata of fetal alcohol syndrome in growth and face do not necessarily have evidence of organic brain damage detectable at the current level of brain imaging or through a clinical neurological examination (personal observation). However, these patients have significant behavioral and cognitive defects that can be quantified and understood through an age-appropriate comprehensive battery of psychometric tests, generally when performed after the age of 5 years. Such a battery, when taken as a whole, will often suggest diverse and inconsistent brain processing abilities most likely based in microcellular or neuroclinical abnormalities. This type of battery is not only helpful in establishing the diagnosis but also essential in organizing a treatment plan — even when the diagnosis of brain damage can be established through the physical examination or an imaging study.

The final fetal alcohol syndrome diagnosis combines a psychological assessment with appropriate physical findings and a thorough prenatal history. This nearly always requires the team effort of a diagnostician like a clinical geneticist and the assessment skills of clinical psychologists, language pathologists, occupational therapists, and possibly educational psychologists and neuropsychologists. No one specialty can bring all the necessary skills to the evaluatory process. The diagnosis is likely often missed because a full-team assessment either has not been done or has not been coherently organized.

Differential Diagnosis

Glue and solvent sniffing can produce a euphoric state. The primary volatile compound is toluene. Recent reports demonstrate that women who sniff toluene throughout pregnancy can have children who look strikingly like children with fetal alcohol syndrome (toluene embryopathology). Because toluene is metabolized to benzyl alcohol, it is possible that this syndrome and fetal alcohol syndrome are pathogenetically as well as phenotypically similar, and the study of these conditions together may lead to clues to pathogenesis (Wilkins-Haug, 1997).

Hydantoin, valproic acid, phenobarbital, and other seizure medications can produce syndromes that feature anomalies of face and growth and organic brain damage. The "classic" facial features of these disorders are somewhat different than fetal alcohol syndrome, but all involve the shape and size of the eyes and subtle defects in the frontonasal region (nose, philtral region, and premaxilla). In some individuals the phenotypic appearance may overlap with fetal alcohol syndrome.

A wide variety of syndromes present with some of the typical features of fetal alcohol syndrome. Conditions often said to potentially resemble fetal alcohol syndrome would include Aarskog syndrome, Bloom syndrome, Dubowitz syndrome, Opitz-Frias syndrome, Noonan syndrome (see Chapter 15), and Williams syndrome (see Chapter 30). In each of these syndromes, the additional anomalies typical of those disorders and not typically part of fetal alcohol syndrome help to establish the correct diagnosis.

The behavior of children with alcohol-related brain damage is discussed below. Cognitive and behavioral overlap with other conditions that are not necessarily physically similar to fetal alcohol syndrome occurs in velocardiofacial syndrome (see Chapter 29) and fragile X syndrome (see Chapter 10).

MANIFESTATIONS AND MANAGEMENT

The management of a patient with fetal alcohol syndrome or related conditions can best be accomplished through a team approach (personal observation). Management starts with diagnosis. The diagnosis helps the caretakers and systems that are working with the patient to understand that the patient is disabled with a complex pattern of cognitive and behavioral problems. This leads to a crucial paradigm shift in management from assuming that the patient is deliberately choosing to be noncomplaint ("she won't") to understanding that the patient has a real disability ("she can't"). The team members who did the testing that led to the compilation of physical and psychometric abnormalities can then use those data as the basis for specific ideas about interventions in education, vocation, social service needs, mental health (including drug therapy, intellectual counseling, behavior management, and family support and counseling), and the legal system.

The manifestations of ethanol teratogenesis can largely be considered in four areas: manifestations of organic brain damage, growth, specific dysmorphic features, and associated major malfunctions (Stratton et al., 1996). Because virtually any and every malformation has been reported in someone with fetal alcohol syndrome, careful and repeated complete physical examinations are needed in early childhood.

Growth and Feeding

Assessing growth deficiency in the context of alcohol teratogenesis is complex. An impact on growth is apparently related to a different time frame in gestation than facial anomalies and to the more severe forms of brain damage, so growth deficiency has not proven to be a good "proxy" measure for alcohol teratogenesis generally. Sometimes the impact of alcohol on growth leads to a small-for-gestational age infant, with catch-up growth in early childhood. In other affected infants, birth size is within the normal range but the child falls below the curves in the first 12–18 months of life. Often, growth after 1 year is stable and parallel to the normal curves. Curiously, there is often a robust growth spurt in early puberty leading to a final height within the normal range. The growth deficit must be considered relative to the genetic potential for height within the family. Growth deficiency can be confounded by a wide variety of other prenatal or postnatal causes. In general, any pattern of episodic growth deficiency, or a significant loss in growth centiles after 18–24 months of age, should be viewed as "alcohol related" only as a final diagnosis of exclusion. The specific patient's history and physical exam should guide the diagnostic search for alternative explanations.

Evaluation

- Growth should be carefully monitored by plotting on growth charts at regular pediatric visits. No growth charts specific for alcohol teratogenesis exist.

Treatment

- No specific treatment for alcohol-related growth deficiency is available because the condition appears to be constitutional.
- In extremely small children with fetal alcohol syndrome and no alternate explanation for growth failure, growth hormone therapy has been proposed. Results of case series are not available.

Development and Behavior

As noted above, ethanol leads to structural alterations of the brain at intracellular, intercellular, microcellular, and/or macrocellular levels. There are additional neurochemical impacts. The types and degrees of resulting cognitive and behavioral dysfunction are protean in diversity and severity, and they are often compounded by other teratogenic or genetic factors of prenatal origin as well as difficult or destructive early postnatal environments. Mental retardation is only one measure of such brain dysfunction, and it is not present in many of the patients. Brain problems can best be summarized as "complex." Some patients have microcephaly, epilepsy, or hard neurological signs. Most show subtle neurological problems of clumsiness, difficulties with visual-motor integration, and increased soft neurological signs. Some patients complain of subtle sensory discomfort to bright light, loud noises, or coarse fabrics. There may be sleep regulation difficulty. Clinical features of attention deficit hyperactivity disorder are frequently found. Psychometric testing often demonstrates wide variations on subtest scales, irregular patterns of academic achievement, language processing difficulties, and problems with attention. These abnormalities lead to learning problems at school and at home and poor intersocial relationships. Parents are often at a loss to guide, discipline, and otherwise manage these children.

Frequently, in children older than age 6–8 years, there are additional problems of emotional response to chronic poor performance and lack of encouragement as well as emotional response to early environmental problems like abuse, neglect, and multiple moves and caretakers (Streissguth, 1997). Children often show signs of depression and/or anxiety and may meet the clinical criteria for reactive attachment disorder, oppositional defiant disorder, or posttraumatic stress disorder.

Evaluation

- Alcohol-affected individuals frequently seem to need multiple interventions in the mental health arena. Psychological and psychiatric assessment is needed to evaluate attention, impulsivity, and distractibility that may be related to attention deficit disorder with hyperactivity but could also be signs of depression or anxiety as well as secondary emotional reaction conditions.
- A development evaluation battery would generally include a test of intelligence, tests of academic achievement, tests of expressive and receptive language, tests of higher-order language usage (as in storytelling), tests of adaptation, and neuropsychological tests.

Treatment

- The profiling of the cognitive and behavioral deficits in children exposed to alcohol would suggest that fetal alcohol syndrome-"specific" interventions could be/should be developed. Caution is advised. Although mild to moderate diffuse brain damage should lead to "themes" in cognitive and behavioral performance, marked differences in individuals' abilities coupled with a wide range of exposures to other prenatal and postnatal cofactors that can alter brain performance lead to varied problem lists specific to each individual patient. Many "common problems" in this patient population like inattention, poor social skills, or poor memory retention can have a neurochemical source in one patient, a neurocognitive source in another, and an emotional source in another (personal observation). These patients would deserve very different interventions for the same descriptive problem.

- To date, no intervention therapies have been rigorously evaluated using the scientific method to assess habilitating individuals with fetal alcohol syndrome and related conditions. Management recommendations are based solely on anecdotal experience.

- Careful drug selection and drug monitoring is often necessary. Patients with organic brain damage may require typical or atypical dosing regimes utilizing typical drugs (i.e., methylphenidate for attention deficit disorder with hyperactivity) or may have symptoms due to a less common cause (i.e., hyperactive behavior due to depression or anxiety), potentially requiring an alternative medication. The use of any medications should be carefully supervised by physicians highly skilled and experienced with psychotropic management.

- Individual interpretive counseling has usually not been reported as helpful by patients and their families (personal experience). Language processing difficulties may be related to this lack of success.

- Play therapy, art therapy, and therapeutic work with animals are reported to be helpful.

- Behavioral management and careful structuring of the environment will often reduce situations that lead to punishment and will result in enhanced self-esteem. "Structure" can lead to "overcontrol" that is adversive. Families need supervision and help to establish the right balance.

- Family therapy is almost always helpful. Parents (be they biologic, foster, or adoptive) need to deal with their anger toward the gestational events that caused the problems, guilt about their inevitable mismanagement of the patient before recognition of the true disability, and anxiety about the future.

- Finally, patients often develop secondary disability caused by postnatal experiences and poor processing of those experiences. They may meet the diagnostic criteria for oppositional defiant disorder, posttraumatic stress disorder, reactive attachment disorder, and others. Older patients may have their own problems with substance abuse (Streissguth et al., 1996). These conditions need very sophisticated management by mental health experts who can work with alternative therapies for brain-damaged individuals who cannot bring the normal degree of memory, reasoning, or judgment to the therapeutic process.

- Schools must provide appropriate academic help. Patients with fetal alcohol syndrome and related conditions are generally found to be doing poorly in school and often can be qualified for special education in one or more of the following categories: mental retardation, learning disabled, traumatic brain injury (prenatal), neurologically impaired, or otherwise health impaired. However, families report that the schools do not have programs in place for the type of diffuse, complex learning problems faced by these students. Individual schools and school districts have shown extreme variability in flexibly developing programs to meet the individual needs of this brain-damaged population.

- Students with fetal alcohol syndrome and related conditions generally have difficulty with increasing independent behavior with increasing grade level and with delayed internal integration of school rules and social norms. Asking these students continuously to behave and organize themselves at a level beyond their abilities only increases secondary disabilities and disrupts academic achievement. Schools often punish these students for these "deficiencies," which are actually "disabilities." Schools must appropriately lower expectations for these students.

- Increased patient recognition will be the first step in developing large enough groups of patients with specific cognitive profiles for evaluative studies of specific intervention strategies.

Ophthalmologic

Malformation of the retina appears to occur more frequently in fetal alcohol syndrome than in the general population. Anomalies of the periorbital region such as ptosis, epicanthal folds, and short palpebral fissures are common clues to the diagnosis of fetal alcohol syndrome.

Evaluation

- A thorough ophthalmologic evaluation should be obtained at age 3 years or at time of initial diagnosis.

Treatment

- Treatment is specific to the abnormalities found. The diagnosis of fetal alcohol syndrome or related conditions is not known to change the general approach to care.

Ears and Hearing

Malformation of the inner ear may be more common in fetal alcohol syndrome than in the general population.

Evaluation

- Routine audiological evaluation is recommended at diagnosis, with follow-up determined by the anomalies found.

Treatment

- Treatment is specific to the abnormalities found. The diagnosis of fetal alcohol syndrome or related conditions is not known to change the general approach to care.

Cardiovascular

Although no single major malformation occurs in a majority of patients with fetal alcohol syndrome, there appears to be an increased rate of cardiac defects, with septal defects being most common.

Evaluation

- A careful clinical evaluation of cardiovascular function is recommended at the time of diagnosis and in routine check-ups. No study has documented the cost effectiveness of routine echocardiography.

Treatment

- Treatment does not differ from that in the general population.

Genitourinary

Renal anomalies are reported to occur at increased frequency. Renal hypoplasia, hydronephrosis, and duplex systems have been the most common problems reported.

Evaluation

- Renal ultrasound is recommended in all patients who have had a urinary tract infection or enuresis after age 7 or 8 years.

Treatment

- Treatment does not differ from that in the general population.
- No study has documented the cost effectiveness of routine renal ultrasound or radiographic studies.

Musculoskeletal

Vertebral defects occur at increased frequency, but dangerous abnormalities like cervical subluxation are not known to be particularly problematic in this population. Scoliosis without hemivertebrae is also a commonly reported finding. Patients often have mild to moderate clinodactyly of the fourth and fifth fingers, and a few have elbow limitation caused by radioulnar synostosis. Generally, there is no significant compromise in hand or arm function.

Evaluation

- Patients should have a careful clinical evaluation for spinal curvature at the time of diagnosis and as part of their annual check-up.
- No study has demonstrated a cost-effective need for a spinal radiograph series without clinical signs or symptoms.

Treatment

- Treatment does not differ from that in the general population.

Socioeconomic Problems

The term "fetal alcohol syndrome" actually identifies both the biologic mother and her child as "the patient." If these biologic mothers continue to abuse alcohol, they are at high risk for serious health problems, frequently have difficulty rearing their children or protecting them from abuse by others, and often produce other affected children. Follow-up studies of patients diagnosed with fetal alcohol syndrome in the 1970s suggested that over half of the biologic mothers of individuals with fetal alcohol syndrome were missing or dead within 5 years of the birth of the index case. Although such numbers are probably somewhat high, it remains likely that the biologic mothers of affected individuals are at high risk to die from traumatic or medical conditions related to their drug and alcohol use. The diagnosis in the child should lead to immediate concern for the birth mother's health and well-being. Only 20% of children brought to the University of Washington Fetal Alcohol Syndrome Clinic for consideration of an alcohol-related condition live with their biologic mothers, and 50% are in foster or adoptive care (Clarren and Astley, 1998). Generally, the reasons for final separation were abuse and neglect, and separation was only finalized after the child had endured much adversity. This pattern of prenatal and postnatal harm can then be repeated with subsequent children. These women constitute the group with the highest risk in the community to have other children with fetal alcohol syndrome and related conditions. Mechanisms must be developed so that the birth mothers can be identified and helped even when they no longer are directly caring for their child(ren).

Given the amount of information that is widely available in the media to warn women not to drink alcohol during pregnancy, it would seem unlikely that women would not know that alcohol could be dangerous to the fetus. It would seem irrational for women to ignore such information. Women do not drink during pregnancy to harm their fetuses, but rather, as a group, they have a high rate of major mental illness, live lives of abuse, have limited financial resources, often live with men who do not want them to go into recovery, and often are phobic. Some have fetal alcohol syndrome or a related condition themselves (Astley et al., 2000). Alcohol appears to be a self-medication, and babies appear to be a partial solution to the above problems. Nevertheless, this is not a hopeless or unsolvable problem. When these women can be helped to identify the major problems in their lives and are helped to marshal the resources necessary to effect change, the secondary gains from alcohol use in pregnancy are diminished (Astley et al., 2000). Women who are helped to deal with the major problems in their lives, as they see them, have a more effective and substantial alcohol recovery and make better pregnancy planning decisions (personal experience).

Evaluation

- Social services evaluation should be considered for every parent of a patient with fetal alcohol syndrome.

Treatment

- The social workers, public health nurses, or advocates who can find the biologic mothers and help them are not traditionally linked to most clinical genetics or neurodevelopmental diagnostic centers. Such linkages are critically needed at this time.

RESOURCES

Newletters

Iceberg
An educational newsletter written principally by professionals in the field for the general public
P.O. Box 95597
Seattle, WA 98145-2597

Fetal Alcohol Syndrome Times
A parent-to-parent newsletter written by the Fetal Alcohol Syndrome Family Resource Institute. Distributed through

Washington PAVE
DASA — Fetal Alcohol Syndrome Project
6316 S. 12th Street
Tacoma, WA 98465-1900

Support Groups

Support groups are increasing nationwide. This list is by no mean exhaustive.

ALASKA
Anchorage Parent Education Group
Contact: Carolyn, (907) 694-6644, or Cheri, (907) 345-4808

CANADA
Peer Support Group for Women Parenting Children with Fetal Alcohol Syndrome/NAS
Contact: YWCA Crabtree Corner,
(604) 689-2808, Vancouver, B.C.
Yellowknife, Northwest Territories
Contact: Helen White, (403) 873-5785

CALIFORNIA
Contact: Liz Zemke, PHN, MS,
(209) 432-6035 or FAX (209) 432-8942

COLORADO
Fetal Alcohol and Substance Abuse Coalition
Contact: Karen Riley, (303) 764-8361

IDAHO
Idaho Support Group
Contact: Hilary O'Loughlin,
(208) 634-3449, Donnelly, ID

ILLINOIS
Contact: Kelly King-Shaw,
(309) 691-3800, or Colleen Matarelli,
(309) 682-2024, Peoria

INDIANA
Fetal Alcohol Network (FAN),
Contact: Tara, (317) 542-7128
or Lisa, (317) 737-6430

IOWA
Fetal Alcohol Syndrome/FAE
Prime Time Two Support Group
Contact: Leslie Schmalzried,
(515) 961-8830, Indianola, IA

MICHIGAN
Catholic Human Services
Contact: Martie Manty, MA, CSW,
(616) 947-8110, Traverse City, MI

Parents Supporting Parents
Contact: Barbara Wybrecht,
(313) 662-7231;
Betsy Soden, (313) 662-2906,
Ann Arbor, MI

Fetal Alcohol Parent Support Group
Contact: Janet Dunning, (616) 532-3689,
Kentwood, MI Nancy Halberstadt,
(616) 874-8735, Rockford, MI
Flint, MI
Contact: Pam O'Briant, (810) 736-8099

MINNESOTA
ARC Duluth
Contact: Addie Jesswein, (218) 290-9920

Thunderspirit Lodge Support Group
Contact: Joyce Glass, (612) 726-4725

MISSOURI
The Family Information Network
Contact: Peggy Oba, (816) 361-7589,
Kansas City, MO Jenni Loynd,
(314) 993-4882

NEW JERSEY
Support Network for Adoptive
and Foster Parents
Contact: Ronnie Jacobs, (201) 261-2183,
Paramus, NJ

Tri-County Fetal Alcohol Syndrome/FAE
Educational Support Group
Contact: Linda Tunick, (201) 383-4787,
Newton, NJ

OHIO
Columbus Central Area Ohio Fetal
Alcohol Syndrome/FAE Support Group
10 Contact: Philipa Petrosky,
(614) 755-4803

Double ARC Parent Support Group
Contact: Debbie Cichocki, Sr. Suzzette
Fisher, or Sr. Joselyn Weenman at
(419) 479-3060, Toledo, OH

N. Kentucky/S. Ohio Support Group
Contact: Marge Schaim, (513) 931-2116
or Bonnie Shuman, (513) 825-1269
for South Ohio; or Mary Jo Theis,
(606) 261-2802 for North Kentucky.
Group alternates sites each month.

OREGON
Oregon Family Support Network
1-800-323-8521

PENNSYLVANIA
Special Kids Network
Contact: Diane Lawton, (717) 327-8140 or
(717) 893-8196

TEXAS
Dallas, TX
Contact: ARC, Sandy Shidler,
(214) 317-1206

WASHINGTON
Bellevue, WA

Contact: Marceil Ten Eyck,
(206) 827-1773

Bellingham Caregiver Support Group
Contact: Catholic Community Service's
Children's Hospital Alternative Program,
(360) 676-2164

Eastern Washington Biological
Mothers Support Group
Contact: Kathy Dunham, P.O. Box 2343
Walla Walla, WA, 99362; home
(509) 337-6911, or work (509) 522-0622

Eastern Washington Fetal Alcohol
Support Group
Contact: Janet Vernon, (509) 684-3772

Tri-Cities Support Group
Contact: Kathy Dodson, (509) 545-2207;
Karin Reep, (509) 627-6104; Neurological
Center, (509) 943-8455

Olympia, WA, Fetal Alcohol Syndrome
Parents/Families Group
Contact: Diane Bailey, (360) 943-0582
Seattle, WA
Contact: Roberta Wright, (206) 546-6226
Southwest Washington
Contact: Joanne Roberts, (360) 896-6147
or (360) 696-8444, Vancouver, WA

Snohomish County fetal alcohol syndrome
Parent Group
Contact: June Ettestad, (206) 793-7895
Tacoma, WA

FAS FRI
Parent support for families and parent
training
Contact: Vickie McKinney,
(800) 999-3429

VIRGINIA
Fetal Alcohol Syndrome/FAE
Kid Connection
Group for parents and their children
Contact: Mary Ann Lee, (804) 520-2201,
Chester, VA

WISCONSIN
National Family Empowerment Network
Contact: Moira Chamberlain,
(800) 462-5254, Madison, WI

Family Empowerment Network-North
Contact: Richard Walker, EdD.,
(714) 394-6909;
or Judith Walker, PhD, RN,
(715) 395-1494, Superior, WI

Internet

fetal alcohol syndromelink@list.ccsa.ca

http://weber.u.washington.edu/~fetal alcohol syndromedpn

http://mirconnect.com/specificnational/fetal alcohol syndrome.html

http://www.irsc.org/fetal alcohol syndrome .htm

http://www.azstarnet.com/~tjk/fetal alcohol syndromehome.htm

REFERENCES

Aase JM, Jones KL, Clarren SK (1995) Do we need the term "FAE"? *Pediatrics* 95:428–430.

Abel EL (1995) An update on incidence of fetal alcohol syndrome: Fetal alcohol syndrome is not an equal opportunity birth defect. *Neurotoxicol Teratol* 17:427–443.

Astley SJ, Bailey D, Talbot C, Clarren SK (2000) FAS primary prevention through FAS diagnosis part I. Identification of high-risk birth mothers through the diagnosis of their children and Part II. A comprehensive profile of 80 birth mothers of children with FAS. Alcohol + Alcoholism (in press).

Astley SJ, Clarren SK (1996) A case definition and photographic screening tool for the facial phenotype of fetal alcohol syndrome. *J Pediatr* 129:33–41.

Astley SJ, Clarren SK (1997) *Diagnostic Guide for Fetal Alcohol syndrome and Related Conditions*; The 4-Digit Diagnostic Code. Seattle, WA; University of Washington Press (93 pages).

Astley SJ, Clarren SK (1999) *Diagnostic Guide for Fetal Alcohol Syndrome and Related Conditions. The 4-Digit Diagnostic Code*, 2nd ed, Seattle, WA; University of Washington Press (111 pages).

Astley SJ, Clarren SK (2000) Diagnosing the full spectrum of fetal alcohol exposed individuals: Introducing the 4-Digit Diagnostic Code. *Alcohol + Alcoholism* 35:400–410.

Astley SJ, Magnuson SI, Omnell LM, Clarren SK (1999) Fetal alcohol syndrome: Changes in craniofacial form with age, cognition and timing of ethanol exposure in the Macaque. *Teratology.* 59:163–172.

Clarren SK, Astley SJ (1998) Identification of children with fetal alcohol syndrome and opportunity for referral of their mothers for primary prevention — Washington (1993–1997). *Morbid Mortality Weekly Rep* 47: 861–864.

Clarren SK, Smith DW (1978) The fetal alcohol syndrome. *New Engl J Med* 298:1063–1067.

Ebrahim SH, Luman LT, Floyd RL, Murphy CC, Bennett EM, Boyle CA (1998) Alcohol consumption by pregnant women in the United States during 1988–1995. *Obstet Gynecol* 92: 187–192.

Jacobson JL, Jacobson SW (1994) Prenatal alcohol exposure and neurobehavioral development: Where is the threshold? *Alcohol Health Res World* 18:30–36.

Passaro KT, Little RE, Savitz DA, Noss J, ALSPAC study team (1998) Effects of paternal alcohol consumption before conception on infant birth weight. *Teratology* 57:294–301.

Roebuck TM, Mattson SN, Riley EP (1998) A review of the neuroanatomical findings in children with fetal alcohol syndrome or prenatal exposure to alcohol. *Alcoholism: Clinical and Experimental Research* 22:339–344.

Rosett HL, Weiner L (1982) Prevention of fetal alcohol effects. *Pediatrics* 69:813–816.

Sampson PD, Streissguth AP, Bookstein FL, Little RE, Clarren SK, Dehaene P, Hanson JW, Graham JM (1997) The incidence of fetal alcohol syndrome and the prevalence of alcohol-related neurodevelopmental disorder. *Teratology* 56:317–326.

Stratton K, Howe C, Battaglia FC, (editors) (1996) *Fetal Alcohol Syndrome: Diagnosis, Epidemiology, Prevention, and Treatment.* Institute of Medicine, Washington DC; National Academy Press.

Streissguth AP, Barr HM, Kogan J, Bookstein FL (1996) Understanding the occurrence of secondary disabilities in clients with fetal alcohol syndrome and FAE. Final report submitted to

Centers for Disease Control, Seattle, University of Washington Press.

Streissguth AP (1997) *Fetal Alcohol Syndrome: A Guide for Families and Communities*. Seattle, WA; University of Washington Press.

Streissguth AP, Kanter J (eds.) (1997) *The Challenge of Fetal Alcohol Syndrome*. Seattle, WA University of Washington Press.

Sulik, KK (1984) Critical periods for alcohol teratogenesis in mice, with special reference to the gastrulation stage of embryogenesis. Mechanisms of alcohol damage in utero. *Ciba Found Symp* 105:124–141.

U.S. Public Health Service (1981) Surgeon General's Advisory on Alcohol and Pregnancy,: *FDA Bull* 11:9–10.

West J, Editor (1986) *Alcohol and Brain Development*. Oxford; Oxford University Press.

Wilkins-Haug L (1997) Teratogen update. *Toluene Teratol* 55:145–151.

CHAPTER 10

FRAGILE X SYNDROME

RANDI J. HAGERMAN

INTRODUCTION

Incidence

Fragile X syndrome is the most common inherited cause of mental retardation known. Lubs identified the first patients with fragile X syndrome in 1969 when the fragile site at the bottom end of the X chromosome was noted in cytogenetic studies. Individuals were diagnosed throughout the 1970s and 1980s with the use of cytogenetic studies with tissue culture medium that was deficient in folic acid, which allowed the fragile site to be visible. In 1991, the gene for fragile X syndrome was identified and sequenced by an international collaborative effort (Verkerk et al., 1991).

Fragile X is caused by a trinucleotide repeat expansion $(CGG)_n$ that occurs in the fragile X mental retardation 1 gene (*FMR1*) at Xq27.3. A small expansion, or pre-mutation, has approximately 50–200 CGG repeats and is usually not associated with cognitive deficits. However, a larger expansion greater than 230 CGG repeats, the full mutation, is associated with fragile X syndrome, including typical physical features such as a long face, prominent ears, and macroorchidism, in addition to intellectual deficits. When a full mutation is present, the gene becomes methylated and is not expressed.

The so-called premutation, or predisposition mutation for fragile X syndrome, is relatively common, and it has been identified in 1 in 259 females in the general population and 1 in 700 males in the general population (Rousseau et al., 1995; Rousseau et al., 1996). Molecular studies have found that the prevalence rate of fragile X syndrome associated with mental retardation is approximately 1 in 4,000 in the general population in Australia and in England (Turner et al., 1996) and approximately 1 in 6,000 males in the Netherlands (de Vries et al., 1997). These prevalence studies, however, have not screened individuals who may demonstrate milder degrees of cognitive deficits, such as learning disabilities, which are common, particularly in females. With more thorough population studies that include mild manifestations of fragile X, the overall prevalence in males and females may be as high as 1 in 2,000 to 1 in 3,000.

Diagnostic Criteria

The spectrum of clinical involvement of fragile X syndrome is quite broad. It includes mild emotional problems or learning disabilities for individuals with a normal

Management of Genetic Syndromes, Edited by Suzanne B. Cassidy and Judith E. Allanson
ISBN 0-471-31286-X Copyright © 2001 by Wiley-Liss, Inc.

IQ through all levels of mental retardation. The classical physical features include large or prominent ears, a long face, high-arched palate, prognathism (mainly in older individuals), hyperextensible finger joints, subluxable thumbs, mitral valve prolapse, macroorchidism (large testicles), flat feet, and soft, velvetlike skin. Many of these features relate to a mild connective tissue disorder. Orthopedic complications, such as congenital hip dislocation or patellar dislocation, in addition to scoliosis and pes planus, are caused by connective tissue dysplasia. Individuals who are less affected cognitively will have fewer physical features.

Prominent ears are perhaps the most common physical feature of this disorder, but approximately 20–25% of young children will not demonstrate this manifestation (Figs. 10.1 and 10.2). Macroorchidism typically begins at approximately 9 years of age, and testicles will increase in size throughout puberty, with a mean testicular volume in adulthood of approximately 50 ml. Macroorchidism is therefore usually not present in early childhood. Because many young children may look absolutely normal, the behavioral features including language deficits, motor incoordination, and hyperactivity are important clues for consideration of this diagnosis.

Females are less affected by fragile X than males because they have two X chromosomes, and the normal X is producing variable amounts of *FMR1* protein (FMRP), depending on the X inactivation ratio. The level of FMRP correlates with the degree of cognitive involvement in both males and females (Tassone et al., 1999).

The clinician should have a high index of suspicion for fragile X syndrome when evaluating any individual with significant cognitive deficits. Fragile X syndrome represents approximately 30% of all cases of X-linked mental retardation, and it is the most common inherited cause of mental retardation known (Sherman, 1996).

Etiology, Pathogenesis and Genetics

In the full mutation, the CGG repeat range is from 200 to approximately 2,000 repeats. Within the premutation range (50–200 repeats), the size of the CGG repeat expansion correlates with the risk of passing on a full mutation from a mother to the next generation. For instance, women with more than 90–100 CGG repeats have approximately 100% risk for expansion to the full mutation when that X chromosome is passed on to the next generation (Nolin et al., 1996). There is a low likelihood (<1%) of contraction of the CGG repeat to the normal range (Nolin et al., 1996). Males with the premutation will pass on the premutation to 100% of their daughters but to none of their sons, because the sons receive the Y chromosome. Both small contractions and small expansions can be seen when the premutation is passed on by a male, but the CGG repeat number will remain within the premutation range. On rare occasions, individuals with a premutation may be clinically affected with learning disabilities or cognitive deficits, although the vast majority of individuals with the premutation have an IQ in the normal range (Hagerman et al., 1996; Tassone et al., 2000).

It is the absence or deficiency of FMRP that causes the clinical features of fragile X. There is some correlation between the degree of expression of the *FMR1* gene, as reflected in the extent of methylation, and the clinical expression and severity. An example of this relates to intelligence and is discussed below under **Development and Behavior**.

Once FMRP is made, it travels from the cytoplasm into the nucleus, where it picks up RNA messages and then moves back to the cytoplasm, where it binds to the 60S segment of the ribosome (Imbert et al., 1998). FMRP appears to regulate translation of multiple messages in conjunction with two other fragile X-related proteins, FXR1 and FXR2 (Imbert et al., 1998). The amino acid sequences of FMR1, FXR1, and FXR2 are

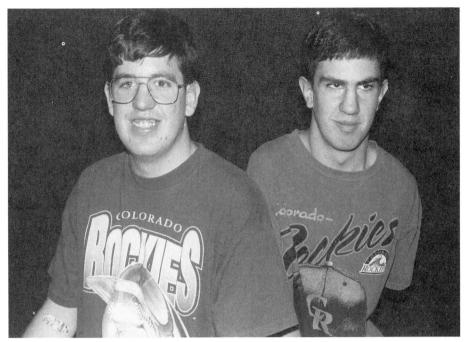

FIGURE 10.1. Two young adult brothers with fragile X syndrome. Note long face and mildly prominent ears with cupping of the upper pinnae, particularly for the brother on *right*.

very similar, including the presence of a KH domain and an RGG box, which relates to their mRNA binding abilities (Holden et al., 1999). FMRP binds to approximately 4% of human fetal brain messages, and the lack of FMRP apparently leads to dysfunction in the translation of the messages to which it binds (Imbert et al., 1998).

The presence of a point mutation within *FMR1*, as opposed to the usual triplet expansion, has been described in 3 patients, leading to an abnormally functioning FMRP. A deletion of the *FMR1* gene will also lead to a typical phenotype of fragile X syndrome. A deletion of a larger segment of DNA that removes the *FMR1* gene and additional genes will have a more severe phenotype than just fragile X alone. For example, Quan et al., (1995) described a patient with anal atresia in addition to fragile X syndrome, because of a large deletion that removed FMR1 and a region proximal to *FMR1*.

The etiology of the connective tissue problems presumably is related to a connective tissue gene(s) that is regulated by FMRP, such that the lack of FMRP causes a deficiency in translation of this gene(s).

Genetic counseling in fragile X syndrome is very complex, and inheritance generally cannot be expected to follow a standard X-linked inheritance pattern. For instance, expansion of a triplet repeat may not occur with every pregnancy in a carrier female, and there are males and females with the premutation who may have significant clinical involvement (Tassone et al., 2000). Recurrence risks and who is at risk vary considerably with the sex of the individual in question. A complete discussion of genetic counseling is beyond the scope of this book. It is suggested that families with an individual who has fragile X syndrome should be referred to a geneticist or genetic counselor to identify those at risk of having affected children and should be provided an explanation of the options available for reproductive decision making (Cronister 1996).

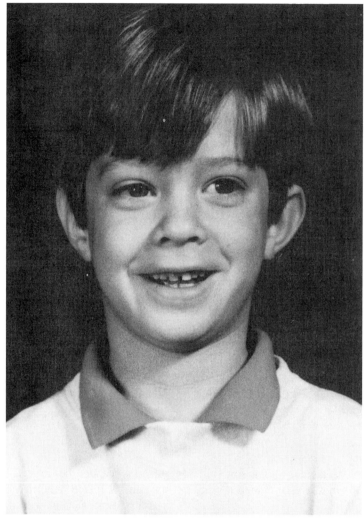

FIGURE 10.2. Young boy with a full mutation that is partially unmethylated. He presents with learning disabilities, not mental retardation, and his facial features are normal except for slight prominence of his left ear.

Diagnostic Testing

The diagnosis of fragile X syndrome can be made either by DNA testing or by cytogenetic testing using tissue culture media that will facilitate expression of the fragile site at Xq27.3. Standard cytogenetic testing will generally not detect the fragile site, even if the individual is affected. Cytogenetic testing in special medium is occasionally used when the etiology for mental retardation is unknown and other cytogenetic causes must be ruled out in addition to fragile X. However, some higher-functioning individuals may be negative on cytogenetic testing and positive on DNA testing. If a fragile site at Xq27.3 is identified, subsequent DNA testing is necessary to confirm the diagnosis.

The diagnosis of fragile X is confirmed by DNA studies using Southern blot analysis, which demonstrates the CGG repeat number within the *FMR1* gene. PCR testing will give a more exact CGG repeat number within the premutation range (Brown, 1996). Individuals who are diagnosed by cytogenetic studies should undergo DNA studies to confirm the CGG expansion. On rare occasions, individuals who are cytogenetically positive may be negative on DNA testing, because the cytogenetic fragile site can be elicited with a mutation at the *FRAXE* or *FRAXF* loci, which are more distal to *FRAXA*, where the *FMR1* gene lies (Nelson, 1998).

Once a proband with fragile X syndrome has been identified in a family, further workup of family members should take place with DNA testing only. This is because DNA testing will demonstrate an abnormality in all individuals who are carriers or have the premutation for fragile X, whereas premutation carriers will not be positive on cytogenetic testing.

Direct genomic Southern blot analysis using a probe that flanks the CGG repeat region is the standard methodology used in individuals with the full mutation. Use of a methylation sensitive enzyme (EagI) that cuts nonmethylated DNA at the CpG island but leaves methylated DNA uncut allows an analysis of the methylation status of *FMR1*. Higher-functioning males usually have a full mutation that is partially nonmethylated. Therefore, analysis of the methylation status may give helpful prognostic information.

Differential Diagnosis

The typical features of fragile X, including mental retardation, attention deficit hyperactivity disorder (ADHD), and autistic like features such as poor eye contact, hand flapping, hand biting, and perseverative speech, can be seen in a number of disorders, including nonspecific mental retardation, autism, Asperger syndrome, fetal alcohol syndrome (see Chapter 9), and pervasive developmental disorder not otherwise specified (PDD). DNA *FMR1* testing should be considered in all individuals who present with mental retardation or autism when the etiology

for these problems is not known. Individuals who present with just hyperactivity or ADHD are not routinely tested for fragile X, unless typical physical features, cognitive deficits, or behavioral problems that are reminiscent of fragile X syndrome are present or there is a family history of mental retardation compatible with an X-linked inheritance pattern. Typically, the DNA testing of individuals with mental retardation and no family history will lead to a 2–5% positive rate for the *FMR1* abnormality. In addition, a similar rate of other cytogenetic abnormalities will be found in individuals with mental retardation who are studied cytogenetically.

Some individuals suspected of having Sotos syndrome (see Chapter 23), Prader-Willi syndrome (see Chapter 18), FG syndrome, or Pierre Robin sequence (see Chapter 19) will instead be positive for fragile X on DNA testing (Hagerman, 1996b). In addition, fragile X syndrome has been seen in conjunction with a variety of common chromosomal aneuploidy syndromes, such as Klinefelter syndrome (XXY) (see Chapter 12), Turner syndrome and XXX (see Chapter 27), and Down syndrome (see Chapter 7). Therefore, patients with these disorders should have fragile X testing when typical features of fragile X are seen. There is also a variety of X-linked disorders that have physical features reminiscent of fragile X, such as Coffin-Lowry syndrome, with prominent ears, coarse features, and hypotonia; Lujan-Fryns syndrome, with marfanoid habitus and macroorchidism; and Atkin syndrome, with large ears, short stature, and macroorchidism.

MANIFESTATIONS AND MANAGEMENT

Individuals with fragile X syndrome require careful follow-up by the physician, who usually orchestrates the intervention of multiple professionals. An intensive treatment program will help the affected person achieve his or her potential and find a productive role in our society.

Growth and Feeding

There may be a mild overgrowth syndrome associated with fragile X syndrome. Individuals usually have a normal to increased birth weight, and the head circumference may be large at the time of birth, because the overall brain size, particularly the hippocampus, caudate, and thalamus, is increased in patients with fragile X syndrome (Kates et al., 1997). Growth in childhood is usually slightly enhanced in both males and females with fragile X syndrome, although the timing of puberty is normal (Loesch et al., 1995). The growth spurt that occurs during puberty is somewhat diminished in patients with fragile X syndrome compared to controls, and therefore final height may be shorter than average.

Feeding problems are common in infancy, and recurrent emesis is usually associated with gastroesophageal reflux (Hagerman, 1996a). Usually, feeding problems and emesis improve with age.

Evaluation

- If feeding problems are severe, an esophageal pH probe study should be done to assess for gastroesophageal reflux.
- A barium swallow can be used to assess reflux treatment.

Treatment

- Thickening of feedings and upright positioning after meals are usually sufficient for treatment of reflux.
- No treatment is needed for growth abnormalities.

Development and Behavior

Some infants with fragile X syndrome may be irritable in the first year because of sensory integration problems and tactile defensiveness. Hypotonia and mild motor delays

are relatively common. The loose connective tissue and the hyperextensibility of the joints may further interfere with the achievement of normal motor milestones. Tantrum behavior and hyperactivity may begin in the second year, particularly after children learn to walk. The tantrums commonly occur during times of transition, such as coming home after a busy day, or in environments with excessive stimulation, such as shopping in a grocery store. These tantrums are often related to excessive sensory stimulation.

Language delays are usually noted by $2\frac{1}{2}$ to 3 years of age, and unusual autisticlike features such as hand flapping, hand biting, poor eye contact, and social anxiety or shyness in groups are usually noted by the family when they are specifically questioned on these issues.

In males with the full mutation that is fully methylated (and therefore not expressed), little or no FMRP is produced. The average IQ in adulthood for a male with a full mutation that is fully methylated is approximately 41. Less affected or higher-functioning males usually have incomplete methylation, causing incomplete inactivation of *FMR1*, or the presence of mosaicism (some cells with the premutation and some cells with the full mutation). The cells with the premutation should be producing FMRP, in contrast to the cells with the full mutation that are fully methylated. The average IQ in adulthood of males who have a full mutation with greater than 50% of the cells unmethylated is approximately 88, and the average IQ of individuals with a mosaic pattern is 60 (Hagerman, 1996b). Approximately 70% of females with the full mutation will have cognitive deficits, that is, an IQ in the borderline range (70–84) or in the mildly retarded range. An occasional female with the full mutation will be moderately or severely retarded.

Hyperactivity persists throughout childhood in approximately 70–80% of males and 30–50% of females with fragile X syndrome. The attentional problems and impulsivity may be severe, even when hyperactivity is not present. Hyperactivity tends to improve in adolescence and adulthood (Hagerman, 1996b).

Anxiety, particularly social anxiety, is present in both males and females with fragile X syndrome, and it is more common in individuals who do not demonstrate hyperactivity or impulsivity. The social anxiety may be severe even in females with fragile X syndrome who have an IQ in the normal range. In males, anxiety or uncertainty can lead to aggressive outbursts in a new situation or when meeting someone unfamiliar. The treatment of anxiety may improve the aggression, as described below.

Obsessive and compulsive behavior is quite common in individuals affected by fragile X syndrome, and it blends into perseverative, or repetitive, behavior. For instance, an individual may obsess on a person or on an activity and ask questions about this issue over and over again. The treatment of obsessive-compulsive behavior with selective serotonin reuptake inhibitors (SSRIs) as described below may improve perseveration at times.

Usually, psychopharmacological intervention combined with other treatment modalities, including counseling and sensory integration occupational therapy, in addition to language intervention and special education support in school, can be very beneficial for significant behavior problems in children, adolescents, and adults with fragile X syndrome.

Psychosis or psychotic features may occur on occasion in individuals with fragile X who are severely disorganized in their thinking or who have regressed in their level of functioning. Aging, severe stress, or other disruptive factors in the environment can precipitate episodes of psychotic thinking.

Evaluation

- A speech and language evaluation should be done on all affected individuals at the time of diagnosis.

- An occupational therapy or motor evaluation should be done with an assessment of sensory integration abilities.

- A complete psychological evaluation that includes IQ testing is an essential part of the evaluation of cognitive deficits.

- An emotional assessment should take place to look at the degree of attention and concentration problems, in addition to anxiety, obsessive-compulsive behavior, aggression, depression, and other psychopathology.

- A learning disability evaluation by a special education teacher is essential to assess academic status and learning strengths and weaknesses. A computer evaluation is a desirable component of the evaluation, to assess computer software technology that can enhance learning and language abilities.

- The medical evaluation should include an assessment of connective tissue problems, hypotonia, and the degree of attention and concentration problems and hyperactivity.

- Children who are treated with psychotropic medication require periodic physical assessment, including blood pressure, cardiac examination, an ECG in certain circumstances as described below, and an assessment of behavior, including anxiety and obsessive-compulsive features.

- The use of behavior checklists, such as the Child Behavior Checklist by Achenbach or the Connors Rating Scale with a specific focus on attention deficit/hyperactivity disorder symptoms, is helpful in the medical follow-up of psychopharmacological medication.

Treatment

- Parents should become aware of the need to avoid excessive sensory stimulation whenever possible. The avoidance of large crowds and loud noises or shielding the child from stimuli, for example, by using earphones so that the child can listen to a favorite tape or calming music while shopping, can be helpful (Scharfenaker et al., 1996).

• Children who are diagnosed with fragile X syndrome in infancy require early developmental services, which may include a home program with parent training to enhance language and motor development or an infant stimulation program, often carried out on a group basis.

• Developmental preschools usually begin at age $2\frac{1}{2}$ and include speech and language therapy, motor therapy either by an occupational therapist or a physical therapist, and special education support by a special education teacher. Many of these programs are in an integrated setting with both developmentally disabled children and normal children. Whenever possible, children with fragile X syndrome should be incorporated in a mainstreamed situation, because they model normal children very well (Scharfenaker et al., 1996; Hagerman, 1999).

• By approximately 5 years of age, children are usually placed in a kindergarten program, but they qualify for special education services, which should include speech and language therapy, occupational therapy or physical therapy, and support from the special education teacher.

• Even in the preschool period, computer technology with software programs that can enhance language skills and early academic skills, including reading and math, can be incorporated into the special education program (Hagerman, 1999).

• Most individuals with fragile X can be mainstreamed in a school situation and mainstreamed in a working situation in the community with appropriate support (Scharfenaker et al., 1996).

• The use of vocational intervention in high school can lead to appropriate placement in the community in a job situation that can utilize the best of the individual's abilities.

• Children with significant behavior problems, such as tantrums, oppositional behavior, or severe hyperactivity, usually benefit from work with a psychologist, either through school or on a private basis.

• Behavioral intervention techniques that emphasize the importance of decreasing excessive sensory stimulation and the use of positive behavior reinforcement with the setting of specific goals and the use of behavioral charting are described by Braden (1997).

• The use of psychopharmacological interventions to help with specific behavior problems can be very beneficial to many children, adolescents, and adults with fragile X syndrome. One of the presenting problems for young children with fragile X syndrome is hyperactivity, with a short attention span and impulsivity. The use of stimulant medication is helpful for approximately 60–70% of children who are of school age (Hagerman, 1996a). Typically, a low dose of methylphenidate two or three times a day, Adderall once or twice a day, or a dextroamphetamine Spansule once or twice a day is effective (Hagerman, 1996a, Hagerman, 1999). Sometimes when stimulants are used for children under 5 years of age, an increase in irritability or even hyperactivity is seen. If this occurs, clonidine, which is an antihypertensive medication that has an overall calming effect, can improve hyperactivity and hyperarousal (Hagerman, 1999). For children between the ages of 3 and 5 years, a very low dose is required, because sedation is a significant side effect. For these preschool children, $\frac{1}{4}$ of a 0.1-mg tablet can be tried twice a day. This dose can be increased somewhat if tolerated and if sedation is not a problem. Clonidine may also slow cardiac conduction, and therefore an ECG should be undertaken in follow-up to make sure the conduction is normal. A rare case of dysrhythmia has been reported with clonidine use, and the combination of clonidine with other medications, such as stimulants, requires careful follow-up (Hagerman, 1999). Clonidine also comes in a patch form, which can be placed in the mid-back area, preferably where the child cannot reach. It provides a continuous level of clonidine in the bloodstream for approximately 5 days, after which the patch typically requires changing to a new location on the back. In approximately 30% of cases the patch can be irritating to the skin, so a topical steroid can be sprayed on the skin and allowed to dry before placing the clonidine patch. One must be careful with the use of the clonidine patch in young children, who may rip off the patch and eat it, leading to an overdose. Such an overdose can cause coma, and it will require intensive care. Clonidine is also often used in the school-aged child to calm down hyperactivity and to decrease tantrums and aggression. Appropriate medical follow-up, including periodic ECG, is important if clonidine is combined with stimulant medication.

- Pemoline has been previously used for treatment of attention deficit/hyperactivity disorder symptoms; however, the recent reports of liver failure in rare incidences of pemoline use has made this medication a less popular alternative. If it is used as a second-line medication for treatment of attention deficit/hyperactivity disorder, liver function studies should be followed carefully (Hagerman, 1999).
- For treatment of anxiety, social phobia, obsessive-compulsive disorder, depression, and aggression, the use of an SSRI

can be safe and often effective. The first SSRI that became available was fluoxetine; however, at times fluoxetine has a significant activation effect that may exacerbate hyperactivity. A typical dose of fluoxetine for the young child between the ages of 3 and 6 years would be 5 mg per day. For the school-aged child, the dose can be increased to 10 mg per day, which is usually given once in the morning. An adolescent or adult dose begins at 20 mg per day and may go as high as 60 mg per day if tolerated. In approximately 20–30% of cases, use of an SSRI may lead to an increase in hyperactivity, agitation, or manic symptoms. If an increase in aggression occurs with the use of an SSRI, it should be discontinued. In general, SSRI agents should be tapered off when discontinued, or a flulike syndrome may occur in a limited percentage of patients. Usually, SSRIs do not require monitoring of blood levels, blood counts, or liver function studies; nor do they require follow-up ECGs. Other SSRI agents include sertraline, paroxetine, and fluvoxamine (Leonard et al., 1997). The SSRI agents have been found to be particularly helpful in females with fragile X syndrome, or even in females with the premutation who are experiencing anxiety, depression, or mood lability, in addition to males and females with fragile X syndrome who are aggressive (Hagerman, 1996a). However, controlled studies have not been published regarding the efficacy of SSRIs in patients with fragile X syndrome.

- If severe mood instability and/or aggression occur and do not respond to an SSRI or clonidine, the use of a mood stabilizer such as lithium, valproic acid, or carbamazepine can be helpful. These medications require more careful medical follow-up, including regular blood testing to check blood levels, electrolytes, liver function studies, and, in the case of lithium, renal function studies (Hagerman, 19996a). The long-term use of valproic acid is associated with the onset of polycystic ovarian disease in adolescence and adulthood in some women.

- Valproic acid and carbamazepine are also anticonvulsant medications. If seizures or spike wave discharges on the EEG are associated with severe behavior problems, these medications are the treatment of choice.

- In approximately 10% of patients with fragile X syndrome, psychotic symptoms may occur, often associated with severe paranoia, which may lead to significant problems with aggression. The treatment of choice for psychotic thinking is an atypical antipsychotic medication. The atypical antipsychotics have a decreased risk for extrapyramidal symptoms and tardive dyskinesia. This is because atypical antipsychotics block both serotonin receptors and dopamine receptors, and when the dose is kept relatively low, the long-term motor side effects are rare (Kapur et al., 1996). The atypical antipsychotics include risperidone and olanzapine. Often, an evaluation by a psychiatrist can be helpful in consultation for the assessment of psychotic symptoms and for medication recommendations. In our personal experience, risperidone, olanzapine, or quietiapine can be helpful in approximately 50% of patients with fragile X syndrome who have indications for their use.

Neurologic

Studies by Reiss and colleagues have shown an increase in the size of certain regions of the brain, particularly the hippocampus, caudate, thalamus, and lateral ventricles, in patients with fragile X syndrome. However, the cerebellar vermis is smaller in size compared to controls (Kates et al., 1997, Reiss et al., 1995). These size differences in CNS structures are reported in group studies of patients with fragile X syndrome compared to controls and are usually not seen in an individual MRI that is ordered clinically. Therefore, routine MRI studies are not usually recommended in these patients. The CNS research findings, however, are important clinically because they relate to the cognitive strengths and weaknesses reported in fragile X syndrome, including attention deficit/hyperactivity disorder, enhanced sensitivity to stimuli, frontal deficits, and enhanced memory (Hagerman, 1996b).

Seizures are an important clinical feature found in approximately 20% of individuals with fragile X syndrome (Musumeci et al., 1999). They usually present in early childhood, and may include generalized tonic-clonic seizures, staring spells or absence seizures, partial motor seizures, and temporal lobe seizures. Usually the seizures respond well to anticonvulsant medication (Musumeci et al., 1999). The seizures usually resolve by adolescence, although on occasion they may persist into adulthood.

Evaluation

- A careful medical history must include questions regarding possible seizure episodes.
- An EEG should be obtained if seizures are suspected by medical history. The EEG should include a waking and a sleep record, because spike wave discharges are more likely to appear in drowsiness or during a sleep study.
- Neurological consultation can be obtained to guide the evaluation or treatment of seizures.
- If focal abnormalities are seen on neurological exam, an MRI should be done.

Treatment

- If spike wave discharges are seen on the EEG or if there is strong clinical evidence for seizures, treatment with an anticonvulsant is usually indicated. The most commonly used anticonvulsants are valproic acid or carbamazepine. Both of these medications require careful medical follow-up, including blood testing for serum levels, complete blood count and platelet count, electrolytes, and liver function studies. The presence of neutropenia is common with the use of both anticonvulsants, and white blood cell count should be monitored regularly. Valproic acid can cause severe hepatic toxicity and pancreatitis, and hepatic failure can occur in 1 in 500 young patients who are treated with multiple drugs (Hagerman, 1996a). Carbamazepine can cause a hypersensitivity reaction in approximately 3% of patients, and this usually presents with fever and rash. Patients must be monitored closely on anticonvulsant medication. These medications can also be used to stabilize mood, as mentioned above.

- Newer anticonvulsants such as gabapentin (Neurontin) may be used as an adjunct for treatment of seizures or mood stabilization when carbamazepine or valproic acid are not sufficient as single therapy. Phenobarbital should be avoided, because it typically increases hyperactivity.
- The use of folic acid may exacerbate a seizure disorder, and it is often avoided in individuals with seizures (Hagerman, 1996a).

Ophthalmologic

Ophthalmologic problems, including strabismus and refractive errors, particularly hyperopia and astigmatism, can be seen in 25–56% of individuals with fragile X (Hagerman, 1999; Holden et al., 1999).

Evaluation

- Children diagnosed with fragile X syndrome should be evaluated carefully for strabismus, nystagmus, and even ptosis (American Academy of Pediatrics, 1996). If these problems are found, referral to an ophthalmologist is indicated.
- If no abnormality is seen on clinical examination, then a routine assessment by an ophthalmologist or an optometrist should occur before 4 years of age (Hagerman, 1996a).

Treatment

- The treatment for ophthalmologic problems depends on the abnormalities seen. Refractive errors or astigmatism are usually treated with glasses. Strabismus may require surgical intervention, although before this, patching, eye exercises, or lenses are often used to strengthen the weak eye.

Craniofacial

The facial structural changes in patients affected by fragile X syndrome include a long face, a high forehead, a high-arched palate, and prominent ears. Cleft palate occurs occasionally, but dental crowding and malocclusion are common. The most common medical complication associated with the facial structural changes is recurrent otitis media, seen in approximately 60–80% of patients. This usually begins in the first year of life and is associated with a persistent conductive hearing loss. Approximately 23% of individuals with fragile X syndrome have recurrent sinus infections, again most likely related to facial structural changes and, perhaps, the connective tissue dysplasia and hypotonia. A rare patient has been documented to have transient hypogammaglobulinemia with IgG subclass deficiencies, although this may be secondary to the recurrent otitis and sinusitis (Hagerman, 1996b). Recurrent ear infections and recurrent sinusitis usually resolve by 5–6 years of age.

The rare patient with isolated IgG subclass immunoglobulin deficiency usually also improves with time.

An occasional patient has been reported with obstructive sleep apnea, and this may relate to facial structural changes, enlarged adenoids, connective tissue dysplasia, or hypotonia of facial and pharyngeal muscles. A history of snoring and obstruction during sleep should be elicited.

Evaluation

- On all visits to the physician, the tympanic membranes should be visualized to assess for infection or persistent serous otitis media (American Academy of Pediatrics, 1996).
- Referral to an otolaryngologist is appropriate for recurrent otitis media.
- Audiometric evaluations and/or tympanograms should be obtained at the end of otitis media treatment to assess hearing and possible persistence of middle ear fluid.

Treatment

- Recurrent ear infections should be treated aggressively to normalize hearing. The use of prophylactic antibiotic therapy and/or the insertion of ventilation tubes are recommended for recurrent infections.
- On occasion, parents request ear pinning surgery if the pinnae are excessively large, leading to social problems.
- If obstructive sleep apnea is found, adenoidectomy is usually carried out, and this typically alleviates the problems. Persistent sleep apnea may require the use of continuous positive airway pressure (CPAP) with nasal prongs during sleep.

Cardiovascular

The most common cardiac problem in fragile X syndrome is mitral valve prolapse. Although this is rarely seen in childhood, it may be present in approximately 50% of adult patients, including females with fragile X syndrome (Hagerman, 1996b). Mild dilation of the aortic root has also been seen in adults with fragile X syndrome, although it does not appear to progress with age. Sudden death secondary to an arrhythmia, perhaps precipitated by mitral valve prolapse, is very rare, but it has been seen twice by this author and rarely by others (Hagerman, 1996a; Loesch, 1998 personal communication). The role of FMRP in the heart has not been clarified in normal individuals, so the effect of absence of FMRP on cardiac function in individuals with fragile X syndrome is also not well defined.

Hypertension is relatively common in adult patients with fragile X syndrome (personal experience), although this may relate to anxiety in clinic, which is a significant problem for most patients (Hagerman, 1996a). It is possible that the connective tissue problems, specifically abnormal elastin fibers in the vessels, may affect the resilience of the vessel wall and predispose individuals with fragile X syndrome to hypertension.

Evaluation

- Auscultation of the heart should be carried out at all clinical visits (American Academy of Pediatrics, 1996). The presence of a murmur or a click requires an evaluation by a cardiologist to clarify the presence of mitral valve prolapse or other problems. The cardiology evaluation should include an ECG and an echocardiogram.
- Blood pressure should also be monitored at all clinical visits, and this should be measured at least once a year in all adults.

Treatment

- Hypertension can be initially treated with diuretics. Other antihypertensive medication, such as clonidine, may be helpful.

- If mitral valve prolapse is severe or associated with mitral regurgitation, prophylactic antibiotics for surgical or dental procedures that involve the contamination of the bloodstream with bacteria are usually recommended (Hagerman, 1996a).

Genitourinary

Macroorchidism is the most common genital anomaly in males with fragile X syndrome. It is present in 80–90% of affected adolescent and adult males. It is usually not associated with other complications, although the weight of the testicle in combination with connective tissue problems may predispose patients to inguinal hernias. A hernia is present in approximately 15% of patients with fragile X syndrome and may occur in childhood, adolescence, or adulthood.

Males and females with fragile X syndrome are fertile.

Enuresis and delays in toilet training are common in both males and females with fragile X syndrome. Although children are not considered to be at an increased risk for recurrent urinary tract infections, the connective tissue dysplasia may predispose to dilation of the ureters with reflux. Four cases of significant and persistent ureteral reflux have been seen among 350 patients with fragile X syndrome (personal experience). In three cases, this has led to nephrectomy because of renal complications including hypertension.

Evaluation

- Testicular volume should be measured with an orchidometer.
- Patients should be assessed for the presence of a hernia.
- Urinary tract infection should be evaluated with a cystourethrogram and renal ultrasound.
- Referral to nephrology or urology is recommended for patients with recurrent urinary tract infections, abnormalities in renal structure, or reflux on the cytourethrogram.

- Hypertension should be followed closely, and the presence of persistent hypertension requires a more detailed work-up, including studies of the kidney.

Treatment

- Delays in toilet training can be helped by behavioral interventions, including the use of a music video developed by Duke University to facilitate toilet training for individuals with development disabilities (1-800-23-POTTY) (Luxem and Christopherson, 1994).
- Treatment of enuresis includes the use of behavior modification techniques, including monitoring enuretic episodes with a star chart, in addition to an enuretic alarm system such as the Potty Pager (Ideas for Living, Boulder, CO, 1-800-497-6573), the Nytone alarm, which utilizes a clip to the underwear (801-973-4090), or the Wet-Stop alarm, which uses Velcro fasteners (Palco labs, 1-800-346-4488).
- Medications can also be helpful for the treatment of enuresis, and they include imipramine at bedtime, oxybutynin, an anticholinergic that is also a muscle relaxant, or desmopressin acetate (DDAVP), which is an analog of antidiuretic hormone (Tietjen et al., 1996). Only occasional patients require medication for this problem.
- In addition, decreasing fluids after dinner, urination at bedtime, and waking the child to urinate again when the parents go to bed can help to decrease the frequency of enuresis.
- Bladder musculature and volume can be increased by intermittently stopping urine flow in an exercise program and reinforcing urination of larger and larger volumes.
- Macroorchidism will be maintained throughout adult life and does not require intervention.

Musculoskeletal

The most common orthopedic complication in fragile X syndrome is hyperlaxity or hyperextensibility. This appears to be related to connective tissue dysplasia, although the biochemical abnormality for the connective tissue problems has not been clarified. Hyperextensible finger joints are seen in over 70% of children, but only 30% of adults have this problem. Flat feet, or pes planus, is also related to joint laxity, and approximately 80% of younger patients and 60% of older patients have this finding (Hagerman, 1996b). Most patients do not have significant pain associated with flat feet, although it can cause uneven shoe wear. Approximately 3% of patients with fragile X syndrome have joint dislocations, particularly congenital hip dislocation identified at birth, recurrent patellar dislocation, or shoulder dislocation. The joint hyperextensibility usually improves with age, perhaps related to ligament tightening with time.

Three cases of clubfoot deformity were identified in 150 males with fragile X syndrome (personal experience), and there may be a slight predisposition to this problem because of hypotonia in utero and the connective tissue dysplasia. Scoliosis is seen in less than 20% of individuals with fragile X, and it is typically mild and does not require treatment.

Evaluation

- The regular physical examination of patients with fragile X syndrome should include an assessment of joint hyperextensibility in addition to asking for a history of joint dislocation.
- All patients should be assessed for the presence of scoliosis with flexion of the back by having the patient lean forward and touch his fingers to the floor.
- If scoliosis is present, it should be documented with baseline spine films and followed clinically by either the general physician or an orthopedist.

Treatment

- The majority of cases with joint hyperextensibility do not require treatment. Patients with joint dislocations, however, require an orthopedic evaluation and follow-up. Recurrent joint dislocations may require surgery. Severe joint hyperlaxity, particularly in association with hypotonia, may require physical therapy intervention in early childhood.
- Flat feet are frequently treated with a shoe insert or orthosis, which may improve shoe wear and gait patterns.
- Scoliosis should be treated as in the general population.

Endocrine

Several females with the full mutation have been reported to have precocious puberty (reviewed in Hagerman, 1996b). The cause of this problem is unknown, although hypothalamic dysfunction, which can lead to growth abnormalities in fragile X syndrome, may also cause precocious puberty and perhaps macroorchidism (Hagerman, 1996b). Women with the full mutation usually have a cognitive deficit, and on occasion this can lead to promiscuous sexual behavior. These individuals may require more detailed counseling for birth control and may be unable to reliably take medication or birth control pills on a daily basis.

Women with the premutation have been found to have a higher incidence of premature menopause compared to normal women. Approximately 24% of women with the premutation undergo premature menopause, and this may occur as early as the 20s. There is also an increased twinning rate in women with the premutation, reported to be three times the rate of the general population. Increased twinning and premature menopause may also be related to hypothalamic dysfunction. Poor ovarian reserve has also been reported in women with the premutation, and this can complicate the harvesting of eggs for *in vitro* fertilization.

All women with the *FMR1* mutation should be offered prenatal diagnosis with pregnancies. In addition, both women with the premutation and women with the full mutation are at higher risk for emotional problems compared to the general population, particularly at times of hormonal changes or estrogen deficiencies, such as menopause, postpartum, and even during their monthly periods. Some women suffer from severe premenstrual syndrome (PMS).

Evaluation

- Signs of precocious puberty should be sought in the periodic clinical examination of females with the full mutation.
- Questions regarding the emotional status of both girls and women with the premutation or the full mutation should be addressed at each clinical evaluation, including questions regarding anxiety, depression, and mood lability.
- All women at risk to be a carrier or affected with fragile X syndrome should undergo DNA testing as described above.

Treatment

- Girls who present with features of precocious puberty should be referred to an endocrinologist for evaluation and treatment. The use of Lupron to block precocious puberty may be necessary.
- Problems related to emotional dysfunction associated with menstruation should be discussed with the parents, so that such clinical problems can be addressed in treatment. The use of SSRIs as described above is usually helpful for severe premenstrual syndrome and the depression associated with menopause or postpartum states. Most of the emotional problems seen in females with the premutation or full mutation can be treated effectively with the combination of medication

and counseling. The prognosis is usually good with appropriate intervention (Hagerman et al., 1998).

- The use of Depo Provera injections, monthly or every three months for birth control may be beneficial in women with a cognitive deficit who may forget to take daily pills.
- All females who have the premutation or the full mutation should be referred for genetic counseling and a discussion of reproductive alternatives, including new reproductive strategies such as *in vitro* fertilization and prenatal diagnosis techniques (Cronister, 1996).
- The risks of premature menopause should be explained to carriers of the premutation so that appropriate adjustments can be made in reproductive planning.

RESOURCES

Foundations

National Fragile X Foundation
  P.O.Box 190488
  San Francisco, California, 94119-0488
  Phone: (510) 763-6030 toll free:
  1-800-688-8765
  Fax: (510) 763-6223
  web page: *http://www.fragile X.org*
  email: *natlfx@sprintmail.com*

FRAXA Research Foundation
  P.O. Box 935
  West Newbury, MA 01985-0935
  Phone: (978) 462-1866
  Fax: (978) 463-9985
  web page: *http://www.fraxa.org*
  email: *info@fraxa.org*

Fragile X syndrome listserv sponsored by FRAXA — to be added to the listserv, email "SUBSCRIBE FRAGILEX-L" to LISTSERV@LISTSERV.CC.EMORY.EDU

Fragile X Research Foundation of Canada
  167 Queen Street West
  Brampton, Ontario

Canada, L6Y 1M5
Phone: (905) 453-9366
email: *FXRFC@ibm.net*
web page: *http://dante.med.utoronto.ca/
fragile X-X/linksto.htm*

The Fragile X Society (England)
53 Winchelsea Lane
Hastings, East Sussex TN35 4LG
United Kingdom
Phone: 011-424-813147

The International Fragile X Alliance
(Australia)
263 Glen Elra Rd.
Nth Caulfield 3161, Melbourne
Australia
Phone: (03) 9528-1910
Fax: (03) 9532-9555
email: *jcohen@netspace.net.au*

Fragile X Association of Australia, Inc.
15 Bowen Close
Cherrybrook, NSW
Australia
Phone: (019) 987012
email: *fragilex@ozemail.com.au*

Reading For Families

Braden M (1997) Fragile X, Handle With
Care: Understanding Fragile X Syndrome.
Chapel Hill: Avanta.

Dykens EM, Hodapp RM, Leckman JF (1994)
Behavior and Development in Fragile X
Syndrome. Thousand Oaks, CA: Sage.

*Educating Children with Fragile X Syn-
drome: A Guide for Parents and Professionals.* Copies can be obtained by calling
Gail Spiridigliozzi at (919) 684–5513.

Hagerman RJ and Cronister A (eds) (1996)
*Fragile X Syndrome: Diagnosis, Treatment
and Research*, 2nd ed. Baltimore, MD:
The Johns Hopkins University Press.

Schopmeyer BB and Lowe F (1992) *The
Fragile X Child*. San Diego, CA: Singular.

Finucane B, McConkie-Rosell A, and Croni-
ster-Silverman A (1993) *The Fragile X
Syndrome: A Handbook for Parents and
Professionals*. National Fragile X Foundation, San Francisco, California.

Tranfaglia MR (1996) *A Parent's Guide to
Drug Treatment of Fragile X Syndrome.*
West Newbury, MA: FRAXA Research
Foundation.

Weber JD *Transitioning "Special" Children
into Elementary School.* Books Beyond
Borders, Inc. 1881 4th Street, #108, Boulder, CO 80302 (1-800-347-6440).

Wilson P, Stackhouse T, O'Connor R, Scharfenaker S, and Hagerman R (1994) *Issues
and Strategies for Educating Children
with Fragile X syndrome: a Monograph.*
National Fragile X Foundation San Francisco, California.

Newsletters

National Fragile X Foundation Newsletter.
Call the National Fragile X Foundation at
800-688-8765.

FRAXA Research Foundation Newsletter.
Subscriptions through FRAXA, P.O. Box
935, West Newbury, MA 01985

*National Fragile X Advocate: Quarterly
Magazine for Parents and Professionals.*
1-800-434-0322. Avanta Media Corpora-
tion, P.O. Box 17023, Chapel Hill, NC
27516-1702.

Reading for Children

O'Connor R (1995) *Boys with Fragile X Syndrome.* Can be obtained from the National
Fragile X Foundation at 1-800-688-8765.

Steiger C (1998) *My Brother has Fragile X
Syndrome.* Chapel Hill: Avanta Publishing,
800-434-0322.

Internet Resources

The National Fragile X Foundation,
http://www.fragileX.org

FRAXA Research Foundation Home Page,
http://www.fraxa.org

Descriptions of fragile X syndrome issues,
http://TheArc.org/faqs/fragqa.html

Molecular Genetic Testing (DNA): Frequently asked questions
http://www.givf.com/molgen1.html

Audio/Visual Aids

Fragile X Syndrome: Medical and Educational Approaches to Intervention — Cassette: This 90-minute audio cassette is a tool for families and educators as they develop appropriate educational programs for children with fragile X syndrome. Speakers include Lois Hickman OTR, Sarah Scharfenaker SLP-CCC, Tracy Stackhouse OTR, Randi Hagerman MD, and Phil Wilson PhD. Available from The National Fragile X Foundation.

Educational Strategies and Issues for Children with Fragile X Syndrome — Video: In this 59-minute video, Dr. Randi Hagerman, Elizabeth Holder, Sarah Scharfenaker, Tracy Stackhouse, and numerous teachers present tactics for educating children with fragile X syndrome. The video, which includes molecular information and medication therapies, follows one child through a multidisciplinary evaluation. It then looks into the school day of a kindergartner, a fifth grader, and a freshman in high school, all of whom have fragile X syndrome. Available from The National Fragile X Foundation.

The National Fragile X Foundation Medical Video, "Diagnosis and Treatment": This concise video explains the medical diagnosis and treatments in a very informative way for professionals and families. Available from The National Fragile X Foundation.

General Family Support-Internet

The Family Village
http://www.familyvillage.wisc.edu
This site was organized by the Waisman Center of the University of Wisconsin-Madison.

The Family Village integrates resources and communication opportunities on the Internet for people with disabilities, their families, and those who support and serve them. Selections include: Library (information re: disabilities), Coffee Shop (connections with other families), Hospital (links re: health care concerns), Shopping Mall (assistive technology suppliers), and others.

REFERENCES

American Academy of Pediatrics (1996) Health supervision for children with fragile X syndrome. *Pediatrics* 98:297–300.

Braden ML (1997) *Fragile X, Handle with Care: Understanding Fragile X Syndrome*-2nd Edition. Avanta Publishing, Chapel Hill.

Brown WT (1996) The Molecular Biology of the Fragile X Mutation. In: *Fragile X Syndrome: Diagnosis, Treatment, and Research*. Hagerman RJ, Cronister A. (eds) 2nd. The Johns Hopkins University Press, Baltimore, pp 88–113.

Cronister AJ (1996) Genetic Counseling. In: *Fragile X Syndrome: Diagnosis, Treatment, and Research*. Hagerman RJ, Cronister, A. (eds) 2nd. The Johns Hopkins University Press, Baltimore, pp 251–282.

de Vries BB, van den Ouweland AM, Mohkamsing S, Duivenvoorden HJ, Mol E, Gelsema K, van Rijn M, Halley DJ, Sandkuijl LA, Oostra BA, Tibben A, Niermeijer MF (1997) Screening and diagnosis for the Fragile X syndrome among the mentally retarded: An epidemiological and psychological survey. Collaborative Fragile X Study Group. *Am J Hum Gene* 61(3):660–7.

Hagerman RJ (1996a) Medical Follow-up and Pharmacotherapy. In: *Fragile X Syndrome: Diagnosis, Treatment, and Research*. Hagerman RJ, Cronister A (eds) 2nd. The Johns Hopkins University Press, Baltimore, pp 283–331.

Hagerman RJ (1996b) Physical and Behavioral Phenotype. In: *Fragile X Syndrome: Diagnosis, Treatment and Research*, 2nd edition. Hagerman RJ, Cronister A (eds) 2nd. The Johns Hopkins University Press, Baltimore, pp 3–87.

Hagerman RJ (1999) Fragile X Syndrome. In: *Selected Neurodevelopmental Disorders: Diagnosis and Treatment*. Oxford University Press, New York.

Hagerman RJ, Kimbro LT, Taylor AK (1998) Fragile X syndrome: a common cause of mental retardation and premature menopause. *Contemporary OB/GYN* 43(1):47–70.

Hagerman RJ, Staley LW, O'Conner R, Lugenbeel K, Nelson D, McLean SD, Taylor A (1996) Learning-disabled males with a Fragile X CGG expansion in the upper premutation size range. *Pediatrics* 97(1):122–6.

Holden JA, Percy M, Allingham-Hawkins D, Brown WT, Chiurazzi P, Fisch G, Gane L, Gunter C, Hagerman R, Jenkins E, Kooy F, Lubs HA, Murray A, Neri G, Schwartz C, Tranebjaerg L, Villard L, Willems P (1999) Conference report: Eighth international workshop on the fragile X syndrome and X-linked mental retardation. *Am J Med Genet* 83:221–236.

Imbert G, Feng Y, Nelson DL, Warren ST, Mandel J-L (1998) FMR1 and mutations in fragile X syndrome: Molecular biology, biochemistry, and genetics. In: *Genetic Instabilities and Hereditary Neurological Diseases*. Wells RD, Warren ST, Sarmiento M (eds). Academic Press, San Diego, pp 27–53.

Kapur S, Remington G (1996) Serotonin-dopamine interaction and its relevance to schizophrenia. *Am J Psychiatry* 153(4): 466–476.

Kates WR, Abrams MT, Kaufmann WE, Breiter SN, Reiss AL (1997) Reliability and validity of MRI measurement of the amygdala and hippocampus in children with fragile X syndrome. *Psychiatry Res: Neuroimaging Section* 75:31–48.

Leonard HL, March J, Rickler KC, Allen AJ (1997) Pharmacology of the selective serotonin reuptake inhibitors in children and adolescents. *J Am Acad Child* and *Adolescent Psychiatry* 36(6):725–736.

Loesch DZ, Huggins RM, Hoang NH (1995) Growth in stature in fragile X families: a mixed longitudinal study. *Am J Med Genet* 58(3):249–56.

Luxem M, Christopherson E (1994) Behavioral toilet training in early childhood: Research practice and implications. *J Develop* and *Behavioral Pediatrics* 15:370–378.

Musumeci SA, Hagerman RS, Ferri R, Bosco P, Dalla Bernardine B, Tassinari CA, Desarro GB, Elia M (1999) Epilepsy and EEG findings in males with fragile X syndrome. Epilepsia 40(8):1092–1099.

Nelson DL (1998) *FRAXE* mental retardation and other folate-sensitive fragile sites. In: *Genetic Instabilities and Hereditary Neurological Diseases*. Wells RD, Warren ST, Sarmiento M (eds). Academic Press, San Diego, pp 65–74.

Nolin SL, Lewis FA, 3rd, Ye LL, Houck GE, Jr., Glicksman AE, Limprasert P, Li SY, Zhong N, Ashley AE, Feingold E, Sherman SL, Brown WT (1996) Familial transmission of the *FMR1* CGG repeat. *Am J Hum Genet* 59(6):1252–61.

Quan F, Zonana J, Gunter K, Peterson KL, Magenis RE, Popovich BW (1995) An atypical case of fragile X syndrome caused by a deletion that includes the *FMR1* gene. *Am J Hum Genet* 56(5):1042–51.

Reiss AL, Abrams MT, Greenlaw R, Freund L, Denckla MB (1995) Neurodevelopmental effects of the *FMR-1* full mutation in humans. *Nat Med* 1(2):159–67.

Rousseau F, Morel M-L, Rouillard P, Khandjian EW, Morgan K (1996) Surprisingly low prevalence of FMR1 premutation among males from the general population. *Am J Hum Genet* 59, Suppl:1069.

Rousseau F, Rouillard P, Morel ML, Khandjian EW, Morgan K (1995) Prevalence of carriers of premutation-size alleles of the *FMR1* gene — and implications for the population genetics of the fragile X syndrome (see comments). *Am J Hum Genet* 57(5):1006–18.

Scharfenaker S, O'Connor R, Stackhouse T, Braden M, Hickman L, Gray K (1996) An Integrated Approach to Intervention. In: *Fragile X Syndrome: Diagnosis, Treatment, and Research*. Hagerman RJ, Cronister A (eds) 2nd. The Johns Hopkins University Press, Baltimore, pp 349–411.

Sherman S (1996) Epidemiology. In: *Fragile X Syndrome: Diagnosis, Treatment, and Research*. Hagerman RJ, Cronister A (eds) 2nd. The Johns Hopkins University Press, Baltimore, pp 165–192.

Tassone F, Hagerman RJ, Ikle D, Dyer PN, Lampe M, Willemsen R, Oostra BA, Taylor AK (1999) FMRP expression as a potential prognostic indicator in fragile X syndrome. *Am J Med Genet* 84:250–261.

Tassone F, Hagerman RJ, Taylor AK, Mills JB, Harris SW, Gane LW, Hagerman PJ (2000) Clinical involvement and protein expression in individuals with *FMR1* permutation *Am J Med Genet* 91:144–152.

Tietjen DN, Husmann DA (1996) Nocturnal enuresis: a guide to evaluation and treatment. *Mayo Clin Proc* 71:857–862.

Turner G, Webb T, Wake S, Robinson H (1996) Prevalence of fragile X syndrome. *Am J Med Genet* 64(1):196–7.

Verkerk AJ, Pieretti M, Sutcliffe JS, Fu YH, Kuhl DP, Pizzuti A, Reiner O, Richards S, Victoria MF, Zhang FP, et al. (1991) Identification of a gene (*FMR-1*) containing a CGG repeat coincident with a breakpoint cluster region exhibiting length variation in fragile X syndrome. *Cell* 65(5):905–14.

CHAPTER 11

INCONTINENTIA PIGMENTI

DIAN DONNAI

INTRODUCTION

Incidence

Familial incontinentia pigmenti is sometimes referred to as incontinentia pigmenti 2 and should be distinguished from incontinentia pigmenti 1, the disorder observed in females with X:autosome translocations involving Xp11. Incontinentia pigmenti 2 was first described in 1906 by Garrod (Garrod, 1906), although others defined the condition further. There have been many anecdotal reports and small series in the literature. In 1976, Carney reviewed the literature and, from published reports and his own series, derived incidence figures for both cutaneous and noncutaneous features (Carney, 1976). Carney's series may have been biased because ascertainment was by publication, and the series may be etiologically heterogeneous. A review of clinical features from the literature and from a large study was published in 1993 (Landy and Donnai, 1993), and a review of male cases of incontinentia pigmenti was published in 1998 (Scheuerle, 1998). Incidence figures are not available.

Incontinentia pigmenti is a multisystem disorder affecting predominantly females, although rare male cases have been described. Pedigree analysis supports X-linked dominant inheritance, and 50% of the female offspring of an affected woman will inherit the condition and manifest it to a variable extent. Affected women have an increased risk of miscarriage, most likely representing male lethal conceptions. It is likely that many mild cases are not diagnosed. Often, an affected mother and female relatives are only diagnosed after the birth of a female with more severe manifestations.

Diagnostic Criteria

The cutaneous manifestations of incontinentia pigmenti are diagnostic and classically occur in four stages: vesicular, verrucous, hyperpigmented, and atrophic (Fig. 11.1). These skin lesions occur in the distribution of Blaschko's lines. These were described in 1901 by Blaschko and reviewed by Jackson (Jackson, 1976). This distribution most likely represents the migrational pathways of cells derived from the neural crest. Curth and Warburton suggested that pigmentation following Blaschko's lines in incontinentia pigmenti 2 reflects functional X chromosome mosaicism due to Lyonization (X-inactivation) (Curth and Warburton, 1965). In addition to these cutaneous manifestations, there may be a variety of dental, ocular, neurological, and developmental

Management of Genetic Syndromes, Edited by Suzanne B. Cassidy and Judith E. Allanson
ISBN 0-471-31286-X   Copyright © 2001 by Wiley-Liss, Inc.

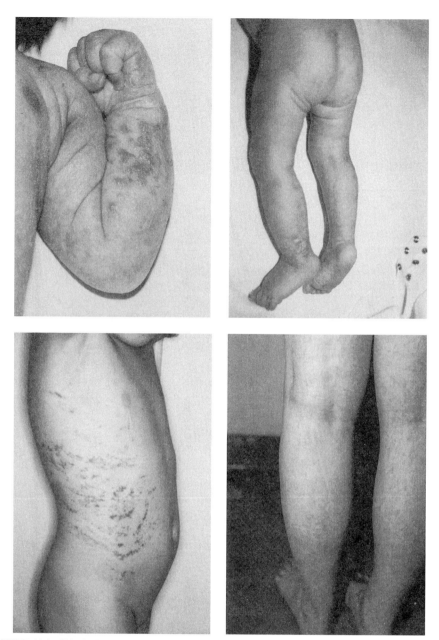

FIGURE 11.1. Skin lesions seen in incontinentia pigmenti 2 *Top left*, blistering lesions; note linear distribution. *Top right*, verrucous lesions over ankles. *Bottom left*, hyperpigmented lesions around trunk. *Bottom right*, atrophic lesion on back of lower limbs.

abnormalities (Fig. 11.2). Diagnostic criteria for incontinentia pigmenti 2 have been suggested (Landy and Donnai, 1993). The skin manifestations (vesicular, verrucous, pigmentary, and atrophic lesions in Blaschko's lines) represent major criteria, and minor criteria are typical retinal findings, dental abnormalities, alopecia, woolly hair, and abnormal nails, and a history of multiple male miscarriages. In the absence of a

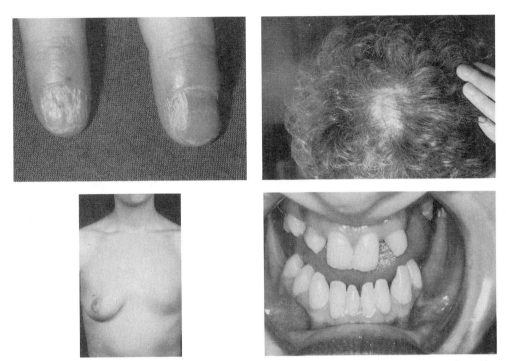

FIGURE 11.2. Non-skin manifestations of incontinentia pigmenti 2 *Top left*,. nail dystrophy in a 2 yr old child. *Top right*, alopecia on vertex of adult female. *Bottom left*, breast and nipple hypoplasia. *Bottom right*, missing and small teeth.

family history of affected female relatives, at least one major criterion should be present together with one or more minor criteria. Where there is a first-degree female relative with incontinentia pigmenti, the diagnosis should be suspected if there are skin manifestations or any minor criteria. To these clinical criteria can be added evidence from X-inactivation studies (Parrish et al., 1996, Woffendin et al., 1997).

Etiology, Pathogenesis, and Genetics

Pedigree analysis of familial incontinentia pigmenti is consistent with X-linked dominant inheritance with lethality in affected males. This mode of inheritance is supported by the high female-to-male ratio, by female-to-female transmission, and by the increased incidence of miscarriage in affected females. In the study of familial incontinentia pigmenti (Landy and Donnai, 1993), 53 of 111

affected females were adults who had been pregnant at least once. They had in total 158 pregnancies, of which 40 ended in miscarriage, 32 in normal males, 56 in affected females, and 30 in normal females (personal data). Father-to-daughter transmission has been reported, but in these instances the father was the first affected member of the family and is thought to have been a somatic mosaic. The half-chromatid mutation model and post-zygotic mutation, genetic mechanisms in which the mutation occurred in one strand of the X chromosome before division or in one cell after initial division resulting in a mixture of mutated and normal cells, have been suggested to explain the survival of occasional sporadic males. Incontinentia pigmenti has been reported in males with Klinefelter syndrome (47,XXY). There have been occasional affected males born to apparently typically affected females. It has been suggested that either these families have a phenocopy of incontinentia pigmenti 2 or the gene mutation in such families does not result in male lethality. Using genetic linkage analysis, it has been shown that incontinentia pigmenti 2 is caused by mutation of a single gene that lies close to the locus for factor VIII in the Xq28 region of the X chromosome (Jouet et al., 1997).

The gene for NEMO (NF-*k*B essential modulator) has been mapped to this region and 80% of cases with incontinentia pigmenti have a mutation which is a genomic rearrangement within this gene. This mutation results in defective NF-*k*B activation. NF-*k*B is a transcription factor which is central to many immune, inflammatory and apoptotic pathways. (The International Incontinentia Pigmenti Consortium, 2000)

In the early vesicular cutaneous stage of incontinentia pigmenti 2, there is massive infiltration of eosinophils into the epidermis. There is also marked peripheral blood eosinophilia. Hyperkeratosis, papillomatosis, and mild dyskeratosis are seen in the verrucous stage, and the pigmentary stage shows degeneration of the basal cells and melanin-loaded macrophages in the dermis, giving the condition its name. In time, the hyperpigmentation fades. In the atrophic phase, Moss and Ince (1987) noted that, although the lesions are described as hypopigmented, the contrast with normal skin is probably due to reduced vascularity and the lack of hair follicles. The sweat glands are probably also affected in these lesions, and a linear arrangement of sweating and nonsweating skin was demonstrated.

Diagnostic Testing

Diagnosis is mainly made by clinical evaluation and follow-up to observe the cutaneous manifestations and associated features. In families in which there are sufficient numbers of affected individuals, genetic linkage analysis may be possible using markers from the Xq28 region. Following reports of skewed X-inactivation in affected females (Parrish

et al., 1996), it has been suggested that an X-inactivation assay can be used to investigate the status of females in incontinentia pigmenti 2 families (Woffendin et al., 1997). Mutation testing of the gene for NEMO is now possible and 80% of cases will have the common mutation (the International Incontinentia Pigmenti Consortium, 2000). In typical incontinentia pigmenti 2 there is no evidence of genetic heterogeneity.

Differential Diagnosis

Any condition with skin manifestations in Blaschko's lines may be confused with incontinentia pigmenti 2. Strict diagnostic criteria and examination of first degree female relatives are essential to confirm the diagnosis of incontinentia pigmenti 2.

Incontinentia pigmenti 1 is the name given to the condition observed in females with an X:autosome translocation that has a breakpoint at Xp11. The vesicular and verrucous lesions are not seen in such patients, and the whorled pigmentation or hypopigmentation is observed from infancy. Most of these individuals have more severe developmental problems than those with incontinentia pigmenti 2. Not all such individuals have exactly the same breakpoint, and, recently, studies by Hatchwell (Hatchwell et al., 1996) have demonstrated random X-inactivation in uncultured fibroblasts, lending support to the hypothesis that in incontinentia pigmenti 1 the phenotype is a manifestation of mosaicism, with some cells expressing genes from both copies of the X chromosome and other cells expressing genes from just one X chromosome. They suggest that there is no evidence that the effects are caused by the disruption of a single genetic locus.

Hypomelanosis of Ito (incontinentia pigmenti achromians) is the skin phenotype associated with various forms of genetic mosaicism. Vesicular and verrucous phases of incontinentia pigmenti 2 are not observed, and there may be hypo- or hyper-pigmented lesions in Blaschko's lines. Happle has suggested that a more appropriate name would be pigmentary mosaicism (Happle, 1993). Males and females can be affected, and chromosomal mosaicism has been demonstrated in about one-third of such cases. The reports claiming familial occurrence of hypomelanosis of Ito are not convincing. Histological features are relatively nonspecific. The diagnosis of hypomelanosis of Ito should be considered in individuals without the preceding vesicular and verrucous skin lesions and should be further investigated by skin biopsy and chromosome analysis of cultured fibroblasts, because the chromosomal mosaicism is rarely demonstrated in lymphocytes.

Goltz focal dermal hypoplasia (Temple et al., 1990) also has lesions in Blaschko's lines and is also likely to be an X-linked dominant condition with male lethality. The skin lesions of Goltz syndrome are quite distinct and consist of focal absence of dermis in the distribution of Blaschko's lines, with herniation of fat and with multiple papillomas of the mucous membranes around the mouth, anus, and genitalia. There is no vesicular or verrucous phase, but there can be linear hyper- and hypo-pigmented lesions, particularly visible in children from ethnic groups with darker skin. Skeletal and ocular abnormalities are common in Goltz syndrome and may be severe.

The early stages of X-linked dominant chondrodysplasia punctata can be confused with incontinentia pigmenti 2 because the ichthyosiform erythroderma observed can be mistaken for the verrucous phase of incontinentia pigmenti 2. This phase is followed by linear scarring with follicular pitting. Alopecia can be a major problem, as can severe skeletal abnormalities and cataracts.

Linear epidermal nevi also occur in Blaschko's lines and may be confused with the verrucous lesions of incontinentia pigmenti 2, as can the lesions of mosaic congenital ichthyosiform erythroderma. In the latter condition, there is no prior history of vesicular or pigmentary lesions and no family history.

MANIFESTATIONS AND MANAGEMENT

Growth and Feeding

There is no impact on growth in this disorder.

Development and Behavior

In general, females with incontinentia pigmenti 2 make normal developmental progress, and the frequency of neurological and developmental problems is unlikely to be as high as suggested in the Carney review (Carney, 1976). In one series of 111 patients, only 6% had persistent seizures (personal data). These individuals and a further 3% had some learning difficulties, but only 3% of the total group had severe deficiencies.

Evaluation

- At the first sign of delayed development, a full evaluation should be initiated.

Treatment

- Intervention for learning difficulties and developmental delay is the same as in the general population.

Skin

The cutaneous manifestations of incontinentia pigmenti 2 are diagnostic (Fig. 11.1). Classically, the features are described in four stages; all stages do not necessarily occur and several stages may overlap; stage 1: erythema, vesicles, pustules; stage 2: papules, verrucous lesions; hyperkeratosis; stage 3: hyperpigmentation; stage 4: pallor, atrophy and scarring.

Stage 1. The lesions of the first stage develop within the first few days or weeks of life. They tend to appear in crops in the distribution of Blaschko's lines and clear within weeks and may or may not be replaced by new crops at the same or differing sites. The lesions are blisters that can be preceded by erythema. The author has observed transient erythema toxicum neonatorum in Blaschko's lines in an affected female hours after birth, which preceded the typical vesicles. The lesions occur in a linear distribution along the limbs and circumferentially around the trunk. Lesions often occur on the head, typically at the vertex, but rarely on the face. The inflammatory phase is accompanied by massive infiltration of eosinophils into the epidermis and marked peripheral blood leukocytosis with up to 65% eosinophils. In most children, the vesicular stage has cleared completely by four months, but milder, short-lived eruptions might occur during the first year of life, often accompanying an acute febrile illness.

Stage 2. The typical lesions are hyperkeratotic, warty appearing lesions occurring in Blaschko's lines and often appearing in the lower legs. They may be present in the first few weeks but usually develop after several weeks as the blisters are healing. These warty lesions are less common on the trunk and face but may occur on the scalp. Most of these warty lesions have disappeared by 6 months. In one large series, 80% of those in whom the lesions occurred were clear by 6 months (personal data).

Stage 3. Although it is this stage that gives the condition its name, its presence and extent are very variable. The hyperpigmentation is more often apparent on the trunk than the limbs and occurs in streaks or whorls in Blaschko's lines. The nipples are frequently involved, but the regions that are most often affected are the axilla and groin. The distribution of these lesions is often unrelated to the distribution of the previous stages. The pigmented lesions remain static for several years but then begin to fade, and by the age of 16 the majority of pigmented lesions, which may be brown or slate gray, have faded.

Stage 4. This atrophic phase is classically seen in affected adult females and most frequently is observed on the posterior aspect of the upper and lower legs and over the shoulders and upper arms. In the author's series these pale linear lesions were observed in many girls under the age of 10 years, concurrent with hypopigmented or even vesicular and verrucous lesions (Landy and Donnai, 1993). They perhaps become more obvious with age and with the resolution of the lesions of the first three stages. Studies have demonstrated that hair follicles and sweat glands are reduced in number in these atrophic lesions and that there is decreased vascularity rather than true hypopigmentation.

Evaluation

- Affected females should be frequently assessed during the first few months, and indeed years, and the type and distribution of the skin lesions carefully documented.
- Photographic records are very useful.
- Skin biopsy and/or analysis of vesicular fluid for eosinophilia may be considered, although the macroscopic appearance is usually sufficient to establish the diagnosis.
- X-inactivation studies can provide supportive evidence for the diagnosis.
- Mutation testing will reveal the common genomic rearrangement in 80% of cases.
- Genetic counseling and examination of first-degree female relatives should be offered.

Treatment

- During the neonatal period, and whenever the blisters are present, strict attention should be paid to hygiene to prevent secondary infection.
- There is no specific treatment to hasten the healing of the vesicular or verrucous phases, except that the lesions should be kept dry.

- Families should be reassured that the lesions will improve with time.

Ophthalmologic

The incidence of ocular abnormalities is high, and in one series of 111 patients it was greater than 30% (personal data). The characteristic lesion involves abnormalities of the developing retinal vessels and the underlying pigmented cells (Goldberg and Custis, 1993). New vessel proliferation is stimulated in areas of retinal ischemia with resulting bleeding and fibrosis. The process is similar to that found in retinopathy of prematurity. Although signs of this process are present in many patients with incontinentia pigmenti, it is generally limited. In only 10% does it present as gross intraocular scarring with a degree of visual loss. Retinal detachment has been described (Wald et al., 1993). In one family, a mother and her daughter both had enucleation of one eye because of a suspicion of retinoblastoma (personal experience). It was only after the atrophic skin lesions and alopecia were noted in the mother that the diagnosis of incontinentia pigmenti 2 was made. Strabismus is common, often in association with refractive errors. Occasional patients have microphthalmos or cataract. In a series of 111 patients only three females had complete visual loss in one eye, the two patients who had enucleation (see above) and an additional woman from a large pedigree (personal experience). Despite the high frequency of ophthalmic complications, over 90% of patients have normal vision.

Evaluation

- Because ocular abnormalities are so frequent, it is recommended that all people diagnosed with incontinentia pigmenti 2 have an ophthalmologic evaluation and follow-up.

Treatment

- If retinal abnormalities are detected, early photocoagulation or cryotherapy

might be helpful in promoting regression of new vessel formation.

Neurologic

Carney's review found a high frequency of neurological abnormalities (Carney 1976). However, the reports of patients analyzed may well have been biased because they were literature cases and more likely to be published if there were severe manifestations. In this review, many of the reports contained insufficient detail to make a definite diagnosis of incontinentia pigmenti 2, and it is likely that there was etiological heterogeneity with some cases representing hypomelanosis of Ito (pigmentary mosaicism). More recent studies, in which strict diagnostic criteria were applied, suggest a much lower incidence of CNS abnormalities (Landy and Donnai, 1993). Fourteen percent of patients had seizures, but only six percent had persistent seizures with a degree of mental retardation, with the rest having transient seizures with no associated mental retardation. In those with persistent seizures the first seizure occurred before 12 weeks of age, often in the first week of life. Of the 111 patients studied, just under 10% (including those with persistent seizures) had mental retardation, although in only one third of these could it be classified as severe. CNS involvement in the neonatal period is a poor prognostic sign, and potential long-term problems should be discussed.

Evaluation

- Full neurological assessment should be part of the initial management of females with incontinentia pigmenti.
- Electroencephalography and cranial imaging studies may be indicated in those with seizures or other neurological signs.
- In those infants in whom there are no neurological features and no seizures, the child should be kept under careful review and the parents reassured.

Treatment

- For those with recurrent seizures, anti-convulsant medication may be indicated.

Hair and Nails

Nail dystrophy (Fig. 11.2, *top left*) is frequent, occurring in approximately 40% of affected individuals. Manifestations range from mild ridging or pitting to severe nail dystrophy resembling onychomycosis. Nail dystrophy may be a transient phenomenon, and complete resolution may occur. Particularly in those infants with severe verrucous lesions, there may be subungual keratotic lesions.

Alopecia is common (Fig. 11.2, *top right*), especially at the vertex and often after blistering or verrucous lesions at this site. Hair is often described as sparse early in childhood and later as lustreless, wiry, or coarse. Although hair abnormalities are very common, it is rare for females to have a major cosmetic problem with this, unlike X-linked dominant chondrodysplasia punctata, in which major alopecia may occur.

Evaluation

- Inspection of the nails and hair should be part of the regular evaluation and follow-up of people with incontinentia pigmenti 2.

Treatment

- Unless there is infection, surgical treatment of nail dystrophy is not indicated and resolution of severe lesions often occurs.

Dental

Over 80% of females with incontinentia pigmenti 2 have dental abnormalities (Fig. 11.2, *bottom right*). Deciduous or permanent dentition or both may be affected. Deciduous teeth may be retained into adult life, and abnormalities include missing teeth, small teeth, delayed eruption, impaction and malformation of the crowns, particularly conical forms, and accessory cusps.

Evaluation

- Because dental abnormalities are so frequent, regular dental checks should be part of the ongoing care of affected individuals.
- Dental features can be of diagnostic value in first-degree female relatives and can support the diagnosis in those with skin signs that are very mild or atypical.

Treatment

- Orthodontic treatment with braces, surgical removal, crowns, and prostheses may be necessary in affected individuals.

Breast Abnormalities

Although breast anomalies have been rarely reported in patients with incontinentia pigmenti 2, in the author's series (Landy and Donnai, 1993) breast anomalies occurred in 10% of affected females. Most of these were supernumerary or hypoplastic nipples (Fig. 11.2, *bottom left*), but one woman had unilateral breast and nipple aplasia.

Evaluation

- The thorax should be examined to determine the presence of supernumerary nipples

Treatment

- Most individuals with supernumerary nipples have no major problems.
- The development of a supernumerary breast at puberty may necessitate surgical removal.
- In women with breast aplasia or hypoplasia, surgical reconstruction may be indicated.

Miscellaneous

There are anecdotal reports of skeletal abnormalities, limb asymmetry, talipes, and cleft lip and palate in patients with incontinentia pigmenti 2. Similarly, there have been reports of patients with recurrent infections, and an immune deficiency has been suggested. However, in the author's series, all structural abnormalities observed were associated with severe neurological deficit and included contractures, dislocations, and scoliosis. It is likely that the other malformations reported in previous cases have occurred by chance or that the patients have been misdiagnosed as having incontinentia pigmenti 2. It should be noted that structural malformations including clefting, polydactyly, and syndactyly have been often associated with hypomelanosis of Ito (pigmentary mosaicism).

RESOURCES

National Incontinentia Pigmenti Foundation

30 East 72nd Street, New York NY 10021, Telephone 212 452-1231, Fax 212 452-1406, Email NIPF@PIPELINE.COM, Website *http:\\www.medhelp.org\www\nipf.htm*

REFERENCES

Carney RG (1976) Incontinentia pigmenti: a world statistical analysis. *Arch Dermatol* 112:535–542.

Curth HO, Warburton D (1965) The genetics of incontinentia pigmenti. *Arch Dermatol* 92:229–235.

Garrod AE (1906) Peculiar pigmentation of the skin of an infant. *Trans Clin Soc Lond* 39:216.

Goldberg MF, Custis PH (1993) Retinal and other manifestations of incontinentia pigmenti (Bloch-Sulzberger syndrome). *Ophthalmology* 100:1645–1654.

Happle R (1993) Mosaicism in human skin. Understanding the patterns and mechanisms. *Arch Dermatol* 129:1460–1470.

Hatchwell E, Robinson D, Crolla JA, Cockwell AE (1996) X-inactivation analysis in a female with hypomelanosis of Ito associated with a balanced X;17 translocation: Evidence for functional disomy of Xp. *J Med Genet* 33:216–220.

Jackson R (1976) The lines of Blaschko: A review and reconsideration. *Br J Dermatol* 95:349–360.

Jouet M, Stewart H, Landy S, Yates J, Yong SL, Harris A, Garrett C, Hatchwell E, Read A, Donnai D, Kenwrick S (1997) Linkage analysis in 16 families with incontinentia pigmenti. *Eur J Hum Genet* 5:168–170.

Landy SJ, Donnai D (1993) Incontinentia pigmenti (Bloch-Sulzberger Syndrome). *J Med Genet* 30:53–59.

Moss C, Ince P (1987) Anhydrotic and achromians lesions in incontinentia pigmenti. *Br J Dermatol* 116:839–850.

Parrish JE, Scheuerle AE, Lewis RA, Levy ML, Nelson DL (1996) Selection against mutant alleles in blood leukocytes is a consistent feature in incontinentia pigmenti type 2. *Hum Mol Genet* 5:1777–1783.

Sheuerle AE (1998) Male cases of incontinentia pigmenti: Case report and review. *Am J Med Genet* 77:201–218.

Temple IK, MacDowall P, Baraitser M, Atherton DJ (1990) Focal dermal hypoplasia (Goltz syndrome). *J Med Genet* 27:180–187.

The International Incontinentia Pigmenti (IP) Consortium (2000) Genomic rearrangement in NEMO impairs NF-κB activation and is a cause of incontinentia pigmenti. *Nature* 405:466–472.

Wald KJ, Mehta MC, Katsumi O, Sabates NR, Hirose T (1993) Retinal detachments in incontinentia pigmenti. *Arch Ophthalmol* 111:614–617.

Woffendin H, Jouet M, Landy S, Donnai D, Read A, Kenwrick S (1997) Use of an X-inactivation assay to investigate the affected status of females in incontinentia pigmenti families. *J Med Genet* 34:521.

CHAPTER 12

KLINEFELTER SYNDROME

ARTHUR ROBINSON, BRUCE G. BENDER, AND MARY G. LINDEN

INTRODUCTION

Klinefelter syndrome is the most common sex chromosome abnormality and the most common cause of male hypogonadism and infertility. The term "Klinefelter syndrome" describes a group of disorders characterized by the addition of at least one extra X chromosome to a 46,XY male karyotype. It usually presents as a 47,XXY karyotype; other forms include 48,XXXX, 48,XXYY, 49,XXXXY, and mosaicism for 47,XXY. A rare form has a 46,XX chromosome complement with Y sequences due to X-Y interchange at paternal spermatogenesis. Klinefelter syndrome is usually described as the presence of at least two X chromosomes and one Y chromosome in combination with male hypogonadism, but the presentation and prognosis are quite variable. It should be noted that most descriptions of Klinefelter syndrome refer to individuals with a 47,XXY karyotype; those with mosaicism or other chromosome complements may have a different prognosis.

The original description of male adults by Dr. Klinefelter in 1942 included a constellation of features: testicular dysgenesis, elevated urinary gonadotropins, microorchidism, eunuchoidism, azoospermia, and gynecomastia. This phenotype is not present in newborns or children with 47,XXY, and not all features may be fully expressed in adulthood. Many affected individuals do not have gynecomastia, some may have normal gonadotropins, and others may fulfill the clinical criteria but have normal chromosomes and another disorder.

Because the clinical features of Klinefelter syndrome are not present until mid to late adolescence, it is technically correct to refer to fetuses, newborns, and children as having 47,XXY and to reserve the term Klinefelter syndrome for affected adolescents and adults.

Incidence

The incidence of 47,XXY is estimated to be 1 in 600 male births, which is equivalent to a prevalence of 8–9 births per day or 3000 male births per year in the United States alone (Robinson et al., 1998). Lifespan is normal, and mortality is similar to that in men with normal chromosomes. Most individuals with Klinefelter syndrome are identified in one of two ways: a karyotype as part of a work-up for infertility, or prenatal diagnosis of an affected fetus detected by amniocentesis performed for other indication. The majority are probably never diagnosed.

Management of Genetic Syndromes, Edited by Suzanne B. Cassidy and Judith E. Allanson
ISBN 0-471-31286-X   Copyright © 2001 by Wiley-Liss, Inc.

Diagnostic Criteria

An individual is diagnosed as having Klinefelter syndrome through a karyotype analysis. The presence of small testes or gynecomastia may alert a practitioner to the possible diagnosis, but confirmation is dependent the presence of at least one extra X chromosome.

Etiology, Pathogenesis, and Genetics

Nondisjunction of the sex chromosomes during the first or second meiotic division of gametogenesis in either parent is thought to be responsible for the chromosomal aneuploidy. The extra X chromosome is contributed only slightly more frequently by the mother than the father, and there are no apparent differences in the phenotype or imprinting effects.

Advanced maternal age is slightly associated with the presence of the extra X chromosome, but the effect is less than that associated with Down syndrome. There is no paternal age effect.

There are no predisposing or preventive factors. The occurrence of the 47,XXY karyotype is sporadic and considered "an accident of nature." Parents of such boys need to understand that none of their actions could cause or prevent the occurrence of the extra X chromosome (Linden et al., 1990).

Diagnostic Testing

A karyotype analysis of peripheral blood lymphocytes, skin fibroblasts, amniocytes, or chorionic villi can establish the diagnosis.

Differential Diagnosis

Because the manifestations of Klinefelter syndrome are variable, there are many phenotypic abnormalities that may suggest the possible presence of an extra X chromosome. When some of the following features are present in an undiagnosed boy, adolescent, or man, a karyotype analysis may be indicated:

Learning disabilities
Language difficulties
Attention deficits
Psychosocial problems
Small testes
Infertility

Another syndrome that can present with one or more similar physical features is Kallman syndrome. This condition is characterized by hypogonadotrophic hypogonadism and anosmia.

MANIFESTATIONS AND MANAGEMENT

Growth and Feeding

Infants with 47,XXY are in the normal range at birth for height, weight, and head circumference. Height velocity is increased by 5 years of age, and by grade school these boys are often the tallest in their class. By adolescence most are at or above the 80th percentile. Leg length is generally increased such that the upper segment-to-lower segment ratio is decreased.

Evaluation

- Monitoring of growth during childhood is the same as that in the general population.

Treatment

- No treatment is necessary.

Development and Behavior

The appearance and development of most 47,XXY infants are unremarkable, and seldom does a pediatrician request chromosome studies because of unusual presentation or delayed early development. Nevertheless, there is a tendency toward slightly delayed motor and language milestones. Infants with 47,XXY have been noted to be somewhat placid and hypotonic, although these findings can be subtle enough that they are missed on physical examination. Approximately two-thirds of boys with 47,XXY are slightly delayed in the age at which they begin walking. The age of key language milestones, including first words and sentences, falls slightly behind that of siblings. Delayed language development can be seen in approximately half of boys with 47,XXY (Robinson et al., 1979). It is important to note, however, that development is variable; some affected boys experience no developmental delays.

By school age, mild sensorimotor integration problems may arise, manifesting as hypotonia, apraxia, primitive reflex tension, and problems with bilateral coordination and visual perceptual motor integration (Salbenblatt et al., 1987).

Language skills can be an area of particular difficulty for boys with 47,XXY. Early language milestones, such as the age of first words, can be slightly delayed but are generally within normal limits. By age 4 years verbal-intellectual skills on average lag significantly behind nonverbal skills. Language deficits frequently take the form of reduced processing speed. Word retrieval and verbal fluency skills are often less than those of siblings, with the consequence that communication is sometimes impeded. Although the rate of verbal information processing may be diminished, verbal comprehension is not.

On average, intellectual skills are slightly diminished in boys with 47,XXY, and learning problems are increased. However, intellectual skills vary widely, with some boys with 47,XXY having above average intelligence and no learning difficulties. In a report summarizing six separate studies around the world, the combined group of 73 boys with 47,XXY demonstrated a verbal IQ of 90 and a performance IQ of 103, in contrast to a group of chromosomally normal male controls with verbal and performance IQs of 102 and 104, respectively (Netley, 1986). These results indicate again that the cognitive difficulty experienced by some boys with 47,XXY is largely limited to the area of verbal skills.

Reading skills, which are highly dependent upon other verbal abilities, are the area of academic progress most problematic for boys with 47,XXY. Slightly more than half of the boys with 47,XXY included in the combined report demonstrated a reading disability. For most affected boys, specific remediation in reading is typically sufficient to maintain academic progress while remaining in a regular education classroom.

The most frequently observed personality characteristics among boys with 47,XXY are shyness, nonassertiveness, and immaturity. The language difficulty experienced by these boys undoubtedly contributes to the pattern of reluctance in interpersonal interactions. Additionally, sensorimotor integrative problems, also prevalent in this group, further add to their apparent social immaturity when these boys are unable to demonstrate success in physical achievements relative to their male peers. Occasional instances of aggressive behavior sometimes occur as a result of repeated and prolonged frustrations but are not, by and large, characteristic of this group. Some investigators have reported an increased occurrence of attention deficit/hyperactivity disorder (ADHD), whereas others have not.

In adolescence, males with 47,XXY are frequently reticent and lacking in confidence. Many struggle through adolescence with limited athletic and academic success, continued learning difficulties, many frustrations, and, in a few instances, serious emotional and behavioral difficulties. Signs of psychological distress, such as depression, loss of interests, decline in schoolwork, or suspected substance abuse, may signify a need to seek individual counseling or psychotherapy, just as they would among chromosomally normal adolescents. Although such problems may occur, most do not have serious psychiatric problems, and many boys with 47,XXY move toward full independence from their families, although their emancipation tends to be later than that of their male siblings. Although affected boys are likely to have friends, many date less frequently or begin dating later than their peers.

Reports on the adult adaptation of unselected men with 47,XXY are few. For the most part, these men separate from their families, obtaining competitive employment and developing their individual adult identity. Many marry, although probably less frequently than among their siblings. Sexual functioning is typically normal, although sexual drive is often low if supplemental testosterone therapy is not utilized. Although educational achievements tend to lag behind those of siblings, some men with 47,XXY complete college and pursue professional careers.

The incidence of psychiatric difficulty is increased in adults with 47,XXY but does not appear to be greater than the incidence identified in adolescence (Bender et al., 1999). Severe psychopathology is seldom reported in this group.

Thus the development and behavior of boys with 47,XXY are variable; on average, they are mildly impaired. Motor skill development may be delayed, and although boys with 47,XXY frequently enjoy physical activities, few are accomplished athletes. Reading difficulties are the most common learning problem found in this group. Behavioral development is often characterized by reluctance and hesitancy, a tendency that is increased where language skills are lagging. In adolescence and adulthood, frank psychopathology is rare, but educational and vocational success and personal independence sometimes arrive more slowly than for chromosomally normal siblings.

All of the aforementioned tendencies, however, are just that. Individual boys and men with 47,XXY have a wide range of skills, problems, successes, and failures. The developmental prognosis for any newborn baby with 47,XXY is unknown and is subject to all of the factors, genetic and environmental, that guide and shape all developing children.

Evaluation

- Developmental milestones in early childhood should be evaluated using standard pediatric office measures.
- Evidence of developmental delay or impairment may prompt evaluation by a developmental specialist such as a developmental pediatrician or child development clinic.
- Any evidence of learning problems should be pursued with a comprehensive educational evaluation.
- Evidence of behavioral or emotional problems with which the parents have difficulty in dealing should prompt referral to a behavior specialist for further assessment.
- In the absence of any developmental concerns, some boys will require no evaluations other than routine childhood care.

Treatment

- Enrollment in programs providing early developmental stimulation for significant delays is seldom necessary in this group of boys.
- Treatment by a pediatric physical therapist may occasionally be indicated for mild sensorimotor integration problems. Although most boys with 47,XXY do not present with obvious motor awkwardness, many have slight difficulty mastering new motor skills, and few compete successfully in group sports. Many affected boys find satisfaction in pursuing less competitive sports, such as hiking, camping, and bicycling for personal pleasure. Noncompetitive mastery of such skills promotes a sense of confidence and personal competence, as well as good health. The fine motor skills of many boys with 47,XXY are

quite good, and many find pleasure in art, craft, and mechanical pastimes.

- For those boys who demonstrate significant language delays, early speech and language intervention is recommended. The techniques of such intervention are no different than those provided for chromosomally normal children and are prescribed in accordance with the particular problems demonstrated by the individual child. However, prompt intervention will lead to greater success.

- Early intervention is strongly recommended for learning problems. In most instances, there is no need to disclose the 47,XXY karyotype to teachers or therapists because therapy is identical to that for chromosomally normal boys with similar learning problems. In many cases, the boys read adequately but somewhat more slowly than others. Writing and spelling can also be difficult for some. For these individuals, providing extra time to take tests and to complete assignments can be very helpful. Additionally, provision of the opportunity to complete written assignments on a computer, including the use of spell check programs, can aid progress. For other skills, including arithmetic computation, clear and repetitious presentation of information along with intensive practice will frequently assure age-appropriate mastery.

- Every attempt should be made by parents to facilitate successful experiences and to build self-esteem and self-confidence. The variability in behavioral adaptation is traced in part to stability in family life (Bender et al., 1987), underscoring the importance of ample nurturing and consistent support from parents.

- Regardless of whether risk for attention deficit/hyperactivity disorder is increased in 47,XXY, decisions about treatment options, including environmental change or medication, are made using the same criteria that are employed in chromosomally normal children.

- Psychopathology should be treated as in the general population, keeping in mind the problems with self-esteem more commonly noted in males with 47,XXY.

Endocrine

The sexual development of males with 47,XXY is normal in infancy and during childhood. Penile length and testicular volume are generally in the normal range, as are the levels of testosterone, follicle-stimulating hormone (FSH), and luteinizing hormone (LH). Pubertal boys initially experience normal pituitary-gonadal function and normal development. There is an adolescent elevation of testosterone that begins to plateau around age 14 years. Serum levels then remain in the low to low normal adult range. By midpuberty the boys are hypergonadotropic, with FSH and LH levels 5–10 times the normal range (Salbenblatt et al., 1985).

Concurrent with these endocrine changes, testicular growth is arrested. Adolescent mean testicular volume is 3 ml, and testicular size is usually <3 cm length ×1.5 cm width. These measurements remain constant throughout adulthood. The testes are firm, and there is progressive hyalinization and fibrosis of the seminiferous tubules. The number of Leydig cells (testosterone-secreting cells) is decreased, and they are hyperplastic with a decreased capacity to synthesize testosterone. As a result of these changes, azoospermia and infertility are present. Sexual function is normal, but the ejaculate contains no sperm. The mechanism by which the extra X chromosome causes these abnormalities is unknown.

Infertility is a classic feature of Klinefelter syndrome caused by primary testicular failure characterized by small gonads, elevated

FSH and LH levels, low testosterone levels, and azoospermia. A few cases of fertility have been reported in the literature, but it is thought that cryptic mosaicism may be present in some of these men. Men on testosterone therapy will not attain fertility. Elevated levels of FSH and LH may not normalize.

Gynecomastia is associated with Klinefelter syndrome in about 15% of cases. Although an increase in size of breast tissue is common in adolescent males, it may not always regress in some adolescents with 47,XXY. If the condition produces anxiety regarding body image for the teenager or adult, a simple mastectomy can be performed. It has been suggested that gynecomastia may be related to an increased secretion of estrogen and a decreased secretion of testosterone, but this has not been proven. Supplemental testosterone does not usually prevent or diminish gynecomastia.

Facial hair, axillary hair, and pubic hair all increase during puberty, but this may occur to a lesser degree than in males with normal chromosome constitutions. Untreated adolescent and adult males may shave only once a week. Hair pattern is male. A typical 47,XXY male does not have a female distribution of fat, as described in older literature. There is no evidence for increased aberrant sexual behavior. There is normal gender orientation.

Evaluation

- At early adolescence, a careful physical examination should be performed to document the development of secondary sex characteristics and other findings related to Klinefelter syndrome.
- Repeat physical examinations and documentation should be conducted annually.
- Obtain baseline testosterone, FSH, and LH levels at 12–13 years of age or at diagnosis if it is later.

Treatment

- Adolescents and adults with Klinefelter syndrome are generally unable to produce normal quantities of testosterone. Supplemental testosterone can raise and subsequently maintain their levels in the normal range. This enables them to stimulate and maintain androgen-dependent processes and in most cases promotes an increased sense of well-being. Testosterone helps to maintain secondary sex characteristics including facial and body hair. In many cases, it can increase and maintain muscle mass and promote weight gain. It can also contribute to increased energy and drive. Libido is generally increased. It can also lower cholesterol levels.

- One of the most important functions of testosterone is to maintain bone density. In Klinefelter syndrome there is decreased bone formation and increased bone resorption caused by testosterone deficiency. As a result, there is a risk for osteoporosis including spinal compressions and fractures of the femur and radius. Treatment with testosterone reduces the rate of bone resorption and increases calcium absorption to stimulate bone mineralization. If bone density has already diminished before testosterone is initiated, the damage will not be reversed, but testosterone can prevent further loss of bone mass.

- Males who receive supplemental testosterone report positive psychological effects. Some of these include feeling less tired, less depressed, and more alert and having a better ability to work and to concentrate. The mood lability associated with adolescence may also decrease. There is an improvement in psychosocial adjustment, and many describe "just feeling better about myself" (personal experience). Because many of the boys with 47,XXY experience learning difficulties or have learning disabilities, they often reach adolescence with poor self-esteem. Testosterone can increase their sense of well-being and promote a more positive self-image. In these individuals, it is particularly important to begin testosterone therapy before symptoms worsen.

- Testosterone therapy is usually considered in mid to late adolescence. Because serum testosterone levels do not plateau until about age 14–15 in most affected males, there is no need for supplementation during the pubertal process, but therapy can be started as early as age 12. Low doses of testosterone may have no effect on the physical habitus or behavior. Excess testosterone can occasionally lead to inappropriate sexual behavior, and there are some reports of aggressiveness when higher concentrations are administered. Therefore, serum testosterone levels should be carefully monitored during the initiation process. When testosterone therapy is started in adolescence, it is often helpful for the boy or his parents to keep a chart or daily record of the effects of the medication, especially as the dosage is being adjusted. As the boys mature, the amount of testosterone can be gradually adjusted to the normal adult dose. There is generally no need to regularly monitor serum levels once the adult dose has been successfully established.

- For most males, the best indication of the effectiveness of testosterone is their clinical status. Initial changes generally affect level of energy, libido, and muscle strength. Physical changes may occur after a few months of therapy. The goal of the therapy is to bring the serum testosterone levels into the midrange of normal, but adjustments may need to be made on an individual basis, depending on the response of the patient.

- Intramuscular injections of testosterone enanthate or cypionate have historically been the most common method of testosterone replacement. An injection is usually given approximately every 10–14 days. Testosterone levels initially rise to normal or supranormal levels during the first few days and then slowly decrease to the preinjection level of low normal to below normal until the next injection is administered. Most males report positive responses during the first few days, but they usually return to their preinjection symptoms of decreased activity and fatigue for a week to 10 days before the next injection. Because this method does not mimic normal physiologic production there may be fluctuations in mood and physical functioning. The preparations are usually injected into deep muscle in the thighs or buttocks. Because the testosterone ester is dissolved in an oil base, the injections can often be slow and painful. For some males, a dose of ibuprofen before the injection can be helpful.

- The standard intramuscular adult dose is 200 mg of testosterone enanthate or cypionate every 10–14 days. In an adolescent, the initial dose is considerably lower, usually 100 mg every 4 weeks. After a few weeks or months, the dose is generally increased to 150 mg every 3 weeks and then, eventually, to the adult dose. The dose and frequency of injection should be individualized for each patient according to age, body size and weight, and metabolism of the drug. Serum testosterone should be measured at days 1, 7, and 14.

- Adolescents who begin intramuscular injections should be followed by a nurse or physician for a few months, both to receive the injection and to be assessed for the efficacy of the dose. Over time, a parent or a school nurse can assume the responsibility of the injections. Eventually, most adult men learn to self-inject.

- Transdermal testosterone patches provide a more normal physiological availability of testosterone (Meikle et al.,

1998). After the patch is applied, the serum testosterone concentration rises to mid-normal range and slowly decreases to the low end of the normal range during a 24-hour period. The androgen levels produced by the transdermal system mimic the physiological circadian rhythm. At the end of the 24-hour period, the patch is discarded and a new one applied. Transdermal testosterone is available for two types of application areas, scrotal and nonscrotal. The scrotal patch is effective in postpubertal males, but adolescents in one study were resistant to daily application to their genitalia and compliance was low (Robinson et al., 1990). The scrotal patch may result in elevated serum dihydrotestosterone, most likely caused by the conversion of testosterone to dihydrotestosterone by 5-α reductase in the scrotal skin. A nonscrotal patch has more recently become available that can be worn on the thighs, abdomen, trunk, or upper arm (Meikle et al., 1998). There is no elevation of dihydrotestosterone. Side effects of either transdermal system are rare but may include acne, leg edema, breast tenderness, and local skin reactions. Many males who have traditionally used intramuscular injections now prefer the transdermal patches. These are available in different sizes, and the dose should initially be monitored and adjusted. Symptoms of hypogonadism may decrease in 2–4 weeks but may take longer.

- Development of long-lasting or alternative forms of testosterone is promising. Because it is degraded by the liver, testosterone must be provided in a chemically altered state to be utilized effectively by the body. Oral testosterone derivatives must be taken several times a day and may result in poor bioavailability. Some preparations can also cause hepatotoxicity. Oral testosterone is not generally available in the United States. New formulations of testosterone currently being investigated include implantable pellets, sublingual tablets, gels, and long-lasting injections.

- Some recent reports in the literature offer promise of biological fatherhood to a select group of men with Klinefelter syndrome by using testicular sperm extraction and intracytoplasmic sperm injection (ICSI). Some men with 47,XXY have been shown to have a few sperm in their testes, even when no sperm are present in ejaculate, but there is no way to predict which of these males will have testicular sperm. After a course of testosterone therapy and testicular biopsy, sperm have been recovered and utilized in the ICSI procedure to achieve pregnancy and birth (Palermo et al., 1998). It has been hypothesized that 47,XXY germ cells are able to complete meiosis and produce mature spermatozoa, but there is a significant risk for chromosomal abnormalities in these sperm. Preimplantation/prenatal diagnosis is necessary to rule out chromosomal aneuploidy. The process of testicular sperm extraction, ICSI, and preimplantation diagnosis is not routinely offered at this time. For most 47,XXY males, the most realistic prospects for fatherhood are achieved by the utilization of artificial insemination by donor or through adoption.

Neoplasia

There is no overall increased incidence of cancer in 47,XXY males (Hasle et al., 1995). However, an association between extragonadal germ cell tumors, usually in the mediastinum, has been documented. Studies have shown that 8–22% of males with primary mediastinal germ cell tumors have 47,XXY, which is 30–50 times the expected frequency. Thus the relative risk is high, but because of the rarity of these tumors, the lifetime risk is about 1%. Klinefelter syndrome is thought to be a predisposing factor to the aberrant migration of primordial germ cells, but the reason for this is uncertain. Affected males may present with respiratory symptoms due to the mass size. The ages of susceptibility are early adolescence to age 30.

Some cases of precocious puberty in boys with 47,XXY have been caused by germ cell tumors in the mediastinum or elsewhere that secrete human chorionic gonadotropin (hCG). Not enough data have accumulated to establish risk figures, but any boy with 47,XXY exhibiting signs of precocious puberty should be carefully examined for neoplasia.

There is an increased risk for breast cancer in men with 47,XXY. Some studies have estimated the incidence to be equivalent to that in females, but current reports indicate the risk to approach 3%. This represents a 20-fold increase over the normal male population, but the overall incidence does not warrant routine screening or prophylactic surgery.

There is no increased risk with 47,XXY for leukemia, lymphoma, or other forms of cancer.

Evaluation

- Persistent unexplained respiratory symptoms should be investigated with chest X-ray.
- All cases of precocious puberty should be evaluated for possible neoplasia.
- Breast examinations should be performed in adult men with 47,XXY with routine medical visits and self-examination should be taught.

Treatment

- Treatment is identical to that for testicular germ cell tumors in the general population: resection and chemotherapy.

Immunologic

Adults with Klinefelter syndrome are at a slightly increased risk for susceptibility to certain autoimmune disorders including systemic lupus erythematosis, diabetes mellitus, and thyroid disorders (Robinson and de la Chapelle, 1997).

It has been suggested that sex hormones may be involved in the pathogenesis and in modulation of autoimmune diseases.

Evaluation

- An annual physical examination should include an assessment of symptoms relating to autoimmune disorders.

Treatment

- Treatment is identical to that provided to those in the general population with autoimmune disorders.
- Some of the features of these immunological disorders may benefit from testosterone treatment.

Cardiovascular

Mitral valve prolapse has been reported in several patients with a 47,XXY karyotype. There is also a risk for cardiovascular disease associated with elevated cholesterol levels. Untreated adult males have low testosterone and elevated high-density cholesterol levels.

Chronic leg ulcers are occasionally reported in men with 47,XXY. The frequency is estimated to be 6–13%. The underlying cause may be associated with androgen deficiency or a vascular abnormality. In young men with chronic leg ulcers, a diagnosis of 47,XXY should be considered.

Evaluation

- Auscultation of the heart should occur at routine annual medical evaluations.
- A baseline cardiac echo is not warranted.
- Cholesterol levels should be obtained with routine medical visits.

Treatment

- Mitral value prolapse should be treated in the standard way.
- Testosterone treatment tends to lower high-density cholesterol levels.
- Some reports indicate leg ulcer healing after the administration of testosterone.

Dental

Taurodontism is an abnormality of the teeth in which the tooth size is enlarged and the root size is decreased. It is occasionally associated with Klinefelter syndrome and does not usually cause functional abnormalities. Early tooth decay may occur.

Evaluation

- Regular semiannual dental visits should be encouraged.

Treatment

- The treatment of dental decay is no different than in the general population.

OTHER MALE X CHROMOSOME ANEUPLOIDY

Over 50% of males with Klinefelter syndrome have a 47,XXY karyotype, whereas the remainder have variations of the karyotype. The natural history of individuals with chromosome variants of 47,XXY is not known because few cases have been followed prospectively. Most information has been assimilated from case reports of abnormal individuals. It is possible that the features of some of the variants are milder than such cases would indicate because of the bias of ascertainment (Linden et al., 1995).

Mosaicism

46,XY/47,XXY mosaicism is the most common form of 47,XXY mosaicism. The presence of the normal cell line modifies the risks for developmental delay. Fertility may be possible. A semen analysis in late adolescence can predict reproductive competency. Testosterone supplementation is probably not indicated. Other mosaic karyotypes include 46,XX/47,XXY and 46,XX/46,XY/47,XXY and other 47,XXY combinations. The phenotype may reflect features of more than one cell line.

48,XXYY

48,XXYY is the most common variant of Klinefelter syndrome. The physical phenotype is similar, but these males are taller and have disproportionately longer lower extremities. There may be an increased risk for leg ulcers or varicose veins. IQ is typically reduced and ranges from 60 to 80; however, at least 10% of reported cases had IQs ranging from 80 to 111. Speech and motor delays are common, and behavior may be shy or impulsive and aggressive. Hypergonadotrophic hypogonadism is similar to that in males with 47,XXY, and testosterone treatment is the same. Genitalia may be small.

48,XXXY

48,XXXY is the result of the addition of an extra X chromosome to a 47,XXY karyotype. It often produces a more abnormal phenotype, including facial anomalies such as hypertelorism, epicanthal folds, simplified ears, and mild prognathism. Tall stature is common, and there may also be skeletal abnormalities such as clinodactyly, elbow abnormalities, and radioulnar synostosis. Generally, there is mild to moderate mental retardation (IQ 40–60), and behavior is usually passive and cooperative. Genitalia may be small, and gynecomastia is frequently reported.

49,XXXXY

A further additional X results in 49,XXXXY and causes the most severe variant of

Klinefelter syndrome. Abnormal facial features include hypertelorism, epicanthal folds, broad nasal bridge, low-set and malformed ears, and prognathism. The neck is short and broad, whereas the thorax is narrow. Cardiac defects, usually patent ductus arteriosus, are present in 15–20% of cases. These males have short stature, radioulnar synostosis, genu valgus, pes cavus, and hyperextensible joints. Genitalia are hypoplastic, and cryptorchidism is often present at birth. The range of mental retardation is broad (IQ generally 20–70), with speech and motor skills severely impaired. Behavior ranges from placid to aggressive.

47,X,i(Xq)Y

Individuals with a 47,X,i(Xq)Y karyotype (Xp monosomy and Xq trisomy) demonstrate typical manifestations of 47,XXY, except that stature is not increased and intelligence is normal.

46,XX males

Males with the clinical features of Klinefelter syndrome but who appear to have a normal female karyotype occur in about 1 in 20,000 male births. These individuals are shorter than males with 47,XXY, and their extremities are not disproportionately long. Genitalia are usually normal male, but there is an increased risk for hypospadias or ambiguous genitalia. Testes are small, and azoospermia is present. Testosterone therapy is indicated. IQ is generally higher than with 47,XXY, and the risk for learning disabilities and behavior problems is lower.

Over 90% of 46,XX males have a portion of Yp containing the *SRY* (sex determining region Y) gene translocated to the paternally derived X chromosome. This Y material is not always cytogenetically visible but can be detected using fluorescence in situ hybridization (FISH) probes. The remaining 10% of 46,XX males are thought to be the result of an autosomal or X chromosome mutation. These males are more likely to have genital abnormalities.

RESOURCES

Support Groups

Klinefelter Syndrome and Associates, P.O. Box 119, Roseville, CA 95678-0119. Phone and Fax: 916-773-1449.

Brochures

Klinefelter Syndrome and Association of Canada, 1001 Queen Street West, Unit 3, 2nd floor. Toronto ON M6J 1H4 Canada.

Klinefelter Syndrome. Klinefelter Syndrome and Associates, P.O. Box 119, Roseville, CA 95678-0119. There is no charge for this pamphlet.

Klinefelter Syndrome, The X-tra Special Boy, by Diane Plumridge, Christine Barkost, and Stephen La Franchi (1982) Oregon Health Sciences Center, CDRC, P.O. Box 574, Portland, OR 97207. This pamphlet can be ordered for $3.50.

Klinefelter Syndrome, For Boys Only, A Supplement, by Diane Plumridge, Christine Barkost, and Stephen La Franchi (1982) Oregon Health Sciences Center, CDRC, P.O. Box 574, Portland, OR 97207. This pamphlet can be ordered for $1.25.

Understanding Klinefelter Syndrome, A Guide for XXY Males and Their Families, by Robert Bock (1993) National Institutes of Health, P.O. Box 29111, Washington, DC 20040; 301-496-5133. There is no charge for this booklet.

On-Line Agencies

Klinefelter Syndrome and Associates web site: *www.genet.org/KS*

Klinefelter Syndrome and Associates e-mail: *KS47XXY@ix.netcom.com*

World listing of Klinefelter Syndrome Societies
http://hometown.act.com/kscuk/index.html.

REFERENCES

Bender BG, Harmon RJ, Linden MG, Bucher-Bartelson B, Robinson A (1999) Psychosocial competence of unselected young adults with sex chromosome abnormalities. *Neuropsychiatr Genet* 88:200–206.

Bender BG, Linden MG, Robinson A (1987) Environment and developmental risk in children with sex chromosome abnormalities. *J Am Acad Child Psychiatry* 26:499–503.

Hasle H, Mellemgaard A, Nielsen J, Hansen J (1995) Cancer incidence in men with Klinefelter syndrome. *Br J Cancer* 71: 416–420.

Linden MG, Bender BG, Robinson A (1990) Clinical manifestations of sex chromosome anomalies. *Compr Ther* 16(5):3–10.

Linden MG, Bender BG, Robinson A (1995) Sex chromosome tetrasomy and pentasomy. *Pediatrics* 96:672–682.

Linden MG, Bender BG, Robinson A (1996) Intrauterine diagnosis of sex chromosome abnormalities. *Obstet Gynecol* 87:468–475.

Mandoki MW, Sumner GS, Hoffman RP, Riconda DL (1991) A review of Klinefelter syndrome in children and adolescents. *J Am Acad Child Adolesc Psychiatry* 30:167–172.

Meikle AW, Dobs AS, Arver S, Caramelli KE, Sanders SW, Mazer NA (1998) Androgen replacement in the treatment of Klinefelter's syndrome: Efficacy and safety of a nonscrotal permeation-enhanced testosterone transdermal system. *Endocr Pract* 4:17–22.

Netley C (1986) Summary overview of behavioral development in individuals with neonatally identified X and Y aneuploidy. In: *Prospective Studies on Children with Sex Chromosome Aneuploidy*, Ratcliffe SG, Paul N, eds., *Birth Defects* 22(3):293–306.

Palermo GD, Schlegel PN, Sills ES, Veeck LL, Zaninovic N, Menendez S, Rosenwaks Z (1998) Births after intracytoplasmic injection of sperm obtained by testicular extraction from men with nonmosaic Klinefelter's syndrome. *N Engl J Med* 338:588–590.

Robinson A, Bender BG, Linden M (1992) Prognosis of prenatally diagnosed children with sex chromosome aneuploidy (SCA). *Am J Med Genet* 44:365–368.

Robinson A, Bender BG, Linden M (1998) Prenatal diagnosis of sex chromosome abnormalities. In: *Genetic Disorders and the Fetus: Diagnosis, Prevention, and Treatment*, 4th ed., Milunsky A, ed., Baltimore: Johns Hopkins University Press, p. 249–285.

Robinson A, Bender BG, Linden MG, Salbenblatt JA (1990) Sex chromosome aneuploidy: The Denver prospective study. In: *Children and Young Adults with Sex Chromosome Aneuploidy: Follow-up, Clinical, and Molecular Studies*, Evans JA, Hamerton JL, Robinson A, eds., *Birth Defects* 26:225–228.

Robinson A, de la Chapelle A (1997) Sex chromosome abnormalities. In: *Emery and Rimoin's Principles and Practice of Medical Genetics*, 3rd ed., Rimoin DL, Connor JM, Pyeritz RE, eds., New York: Churchill Livingstone, p. 973-998.

Robinson A, Linden MG (1993) Sex chromosome anomalies. In: *Clinical Genetics Handbook*, 2nd ed., Robinson A, Linden MG, eds., Boston: Blackwell Scientific p. 109–117.

Robinson A, Puck M, Pennington B, Borelli J, Hudson M (1979) Abnormalities of the sex chromosomes: A prospective study on randomly identified newborns. In: *Sex Chromosome Aneuploidy: Prospective Studies on Children*, Robinson A, Lubs HA, Bergsma D, eds., Birth Defects 15(1):203–241.

Salbenblatt JA, Bender BG, Puck MH, Robinson A, Faiman C, Winter JSD (1985) Pituitary-gonadal function in Klinefelter syndrome before and during puberty. *Pediatr Res* 19:82–86.

Salbenblatt JA, Meyers DC, Bender BG, Linden MG, Robinson A (1987) Gross and fine motor development in 47,XXY and 47,XYY males. *Pediatrics* 80:240–244.

CHAPTER 13

MARFAN SYNDROME

IRIS SCHRIJVER, DEBORAH M. ALCORN, AND UTA FRANCKE

INTRODUCTION

Incidence

In 1896, Dr. Antoine Marfan first presented a patient with features of the syndrome that would later bear his name. Although disproportionately long fingers and limbs, scoliosis, and chest asymmetry were recognized features around the turn of the last century, the full range of manifestations in the ocular, cardiovascular, pulmonary and other connective tissue systems has only been delineated in recent decades.

The Marfan syndrome is inherited in an autosomal dominant fashion. Even though variability in clinical manifestations between and within families can be considerable, the syndrome is fully penetrant. The estimated incidence is 1–2 per 10,000 individuals without gender or ethnic biases. The prevalence of spontaneous mutations approximates 25%.

Diagnostic Criteria

The diagnosis of Marfan syndrome is almost exclusively based on clinical criteria. The first international diagnostic consensus was established in 1986, resulting in the Berlin nosology (Beighton et al., 1988). According to these criteria, Marfan syndrome can be diagnosed if two organ systems are involved

in the presence of an unequivocally affected first-degree family member. In the absence of such a positive family history, involvement of the skeleton and two or more organ systems is required, as well as the presence of at least one major criterion. Major criteria are aortic dilatation or dissection, ectopia lentis, and dural ectasia.

The identification of mutations in the fibrillin-1 (*FBN1*) gene as a cause of the Marfan syndrome has led to the possibility of including molecular evidence in the diagnostic patient evaluation. At the same time, mutation analysis in families showed that a fraction of relatives who met diagnostic criteria of the Berlin nosology did not carry the disease-causing mutation. This finding underlines the fact that features such as joint hypermobility and myopia are common in the general population. In an effort to achieve more diagnostic specificity, the Berlin nosology was revised in 1996 (de Paepe et al., 1996). The resulting Ghent nosology takes into consideration the presence of a disease-causing *FBN1* mutation, and, where a mutation has not yet been identified, the presence of a 15q21 marker haplotype that segregates with unequivocally diagnosed Marfan syndrome in members of the same family. In addition, clinical features have been divided into major and minor criteria, depending on diagnostic specificity (Table 13.1). Major

Management of Genetic Syndromes, Edited by Suzanne B. Cassidy and Judith E. Allanson
ISBN 0-471-31286-X   Copyright © 2001 by Wiley-Liss, Inc.

TABLE 13.1. Ghent Nosology: Revised Diagnostic Criteria for Marfan Syndrome

Index case

    Major criteria in two different organ systems *and* involvement of a third system

    or Mutation present *and* one major criterion *and* involvement of a second organ system

Relative of index case

    One major criterion provided by family history *and* one major criterion in an organ system *and* involvement of a second organ system

Skeletal

    Major (presence of at least 4 of the following)

        Pectus carinatum

        Pectus excavatum requiring surgery

        Reduced upper to lower segment ratio* *or* arm span to height ratio >1.05

        Wrist† *and* thumb signs‡

        Scoliosis of >20° *or* spondylolisthesis

        Reduced extension at the elbows (<170°)

        Medial displacement of the medial malleolus causing pes planus

        Protrusio acetabuli of any degree (ascertained on radiographs)

    Minor

        Pectus excavatum of moderate severity

        Joint hypermobility

        High-arched palate with crowding of teeth

        Facial appearance (dolichocephaly, malar hypoplasia, enophthalmos, retrognathia, down-slanting palpebral fissures)

    Involvement: Two of the components of major criteria *or* one major and two minor

Ocular

    Major

        Ectopia lentis

    Minor

        Flat cornea

        Increased axial length of globe (>23.5 mm, measured by ultrasound)

        Hypoplastic iris *or* hypoplastic ciliary muscle causing decreased miosis

    Involvement: Two minor criteria

Cardiovascular

    Major

        Dilatation of the ascending aorta with or without aortic regurgitation and involving at least the sinuses of Valsalva *or* Dissection of the ascending aorta

    Minor

        Mitral valve prolapse with or without mitral valve regurgitation

        Dilatation of the main pulmonary artery, in the absence of valvular or peripheral pulmonic stenosis before the age of 40 years

        Calcification of the mitral annulus before the age of 40 years

        Dilatation or dissection of the descending thoracic or abdominal aorta before 50 years of age

    Involvement: One minor criterion

Pulmonary

    Minor (only)

        Spontaneous pneumorthorax

        Apical blebs

    Involvement: One minor criterion

TABLE 13.1. (*continued*)

Skin
  Minor (only)
    Striae atrophicae
    Recurrent or incisional hernia
  Involvement: One minor criterion
Dura
  Major (only)
    Lumbosacral dural ectasia by CT or MRI
Family history/genetic laboratory data
  Major (only)
    First-degree relative who independently meets the diagnostic criteria
    Presence of mutation in FBN1
    Presence of haplotype around FBN1 inherited by descent and unequivocally associated with
      diagnosed Marfan syndrome in the family

Data from De Paepe A, Devereux RB, Dietz H, et al: Revised diagnostic criteria for the Marfan syndrome. *Am J Med Genet* 62:417–426, 1996.
*Hall JG, Froster-Iskenius UG, Allanson JE; Handbook of Normal Physical Measurements. Oxford University Press, 1989, pp. 270–275.
†Wrist sign: Thumb overlaps the distal phalanx of the fifth digit when grasping the contralateral wrist.
‡Thumb sign: Entire nail of the thumb projects beyond the ulnar border of the hand when the hand is clenched without assistance.

criteria include features that are rarely seen in other disorders, such as ectopia lentis and dilatation of the ascending aorta. Most systems can be affected by manifestations that are considered major features or they can be merely involved. The musculoskeletal system, for example, qualifies as a major criterion only if at least four major manifestations are present. It is considered involved but not severely affected when at least two major features, or one major feature and two minor manifestations, are present. Features in the pulmonary system or skin and integument are only considered for system involvement and are not regarded as major characteristics. According to these proposed guidelines, an index case without an unequivocally affected first-degree relative meets diagnostic criteria when major criteria are present in at least two organ systems and a third organ system is involved. One major criterion in an organ system and involvement of a second organ system are required in the presence of an unequivocally affected first-degree relative, an *FBN1* mutation that is known to cause Marfan syndrome in others, or a disease-associated 15q21 haplotype.

Although the Ghent criteria have improved diagnostic specificity, their applicability in practice has serious limitations (personal observation). The first limitation concerns the age of onset for typical manifestations. Although children affected with the severe neonatal form of Marfan syndrome who represent new mutations will easily meet the Ghent criteria, affected children with inherited mutations may not meet diagnostic criteria because some features may not become apparent until the teenage years or later. In particular, the onset of dilatation of the ascending aorta is variable between families and may not be detectable before adulthood. Lens subluxation and scoliosis may only become manifest during adolescence. Implementation of β-blocker therapy during childhood may further delay notable dilatation of the aorta and, thus, the diagnosis of Marfan syndrome.

Second, the Ghent diagnostic criteria contain requirements that are not part of the diagnostic work-up in most health care institutions. For example, ultrasonic axial length measurements of the eye are not routinely performed. There are normal standards dependent on age (Gordon and Donzis, 1985), yet a single value of axial length is cited as a cut-off for diagnosis in the Ghent critera. Because enlargement of the globe leads to myopia, the authors propose to replace the required length measurement with the presence of moderately high- to high-grade myopia as a minor criterion for ocular involvement, although we recognize that myopia can occur for other reasons. Likewise, the presence of protrusio acetabuli and apical blebs must be ascertained by radiographic evaluations that are difficult to justify in the absence of clinical symptoms involving the lung or hip joint. Lumbosacral dural ectasia was an accidental discovery in Marfan syndrome patients, and CT or MRI scanning is required to determine its presence. The frequency of asymptomatic dural ectasia in patients with ascending aortic aneurysms or other isolated features of the Marfan spectrum, as well as in the general population, is currently unknown. Therefore, the diagnostic specificity and sensitivity of this finding have not yet been established, and its designation as a major criterion for Marfan syndrome appears premature. The cost and effort required to assess its presence are difficult to justify unless back or abdominal pain provide an indication. In contrast, debilitating orthostatic headache due to chronic leakage of cerebrospinal fluid through dural lesions may be an underrecognized manifestation of Marfan syndrome that is treatable (see below).

Finally, the clinical features may be modified in different racial and ethnic groups. For example, dolichostenomelia cannot be assessed accurately in individuals of ethnicities other than Caucasian or African because standards for skeletal measurements have not been established in these populations. We have diagnosed Asian individuals with Marfan syndrome whose skeletal measurements were well within the normal range for Caucasians.

These issues are of great concern because individuals who may not meet the Ghent diagnostic criteria, because of age, ethnicity, or limited access to diagnostic imaging technology, may still be at risk for serious complications such as dissection of the ascending aorta. The authors propose that children of affected individuals receive periodic evaluation by a cardiologist, ophthalmologist, and geneticist and be monitored like children with unequivocal Marfan syndrome in the event that this diagnosis is suspected but criteria are not (yet) met. In individuals of Asian descent, we recommend flexibility in the application of the musculoskeletal criteria. Dolichostenomelia may not be present according to the Caucasian standard, but patients are often much taller than their relatives and others of the same ethnic extraction (personal experience). Clearly, anthropometric standards must be developed for all ethnic groups. In all other instances in which individuals do not meet criteria with readily available diagnostic means, the stigma of the Marfan syndrome diagnosis must be weighed on an individualized basis against the necessity for clinical follow-up to minimize risk of serious complications. Realizing that the clinical features of Marfan syndrome belong to a wide spectrum of connective tissue phenotypes, many of which are associated with mutations in the *FBN1* gene, the authors have proposed the term "fibrillinopathy" to include all those individuals whose fibrillin metabolism is clearly abnormal but who cannot currently be diagnosed with established connective tissue disease diagnoses (Aoyama et al., 1995).

Etiology, Pathogenesis, and Genetics

In the 1980's, linkage studies of multigenerational Marfan syndrome families failed to identify linkage to known candidate genes for connective tissue components such as elastin, fibronectin, and collagens. When linkage analysis was expanded to random, genomewide genetic markers, most of the 22 autosomes could be excluded. Finally in 1990, linkage of Marfan syndrome was established to markers in chromosome band 15q21 (Kainulainen et al., 1990; Dietz et al., 1991).

At the same time, a monoclonal antibody against an extracellular microfibril component, named fibrillin, was used for immunofluorescence assays of fibroblast cultures from individuals with and without Marfan syndrome. Patterns of immunofluorescence in affected subjects were substantially decreased, suggesting a primary defect in microfibril formation. Fibrillin, a 350 kDa cysteine-rich glycoprotein, is the major component of the largest class of microfibrils in the extracellular meshwork of elastic as well as nonelastic tissues (Sakai et al., 1986). Subsequently, the gene that encodes the fibrillin protein (*FBN1*) was isolated, mapped

to band 15q21, and screened for mutations in Marfan patients (reviewed in Francke and Furthmayr, 1993).

The efforts of detection and analysis of *FBN1* mutations is a continuing process. At this time, more than 100 individual mutations including missense and nonsense mutations, nucleotide deletions and insertions, and mutations leading to abnormal mRNA splicing have been reported and are collected in an international database (Collod-Beroud et al., 1998). Very few of these have been observed in more than one family.

The *FBN1* gene (Fig. 13.1) spans more than 110 kilobases and is composed of 65 exons. The most common motif, the epidermal growth factor (EGF)-like domain, is encoded by individual exons and occurs 47 times. Each of these domains contains six conserved cysteine residues that form three disulfide bonds. In 43 EGF-like domains a consensus sequence for calcium binding is present, which facilitates intra- as well as

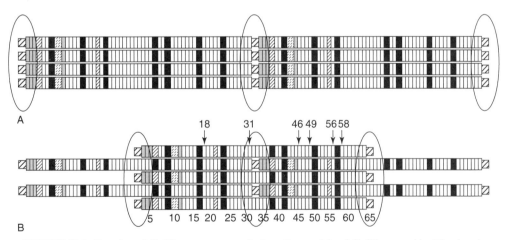

FIGURE 13.1. Domains of fibrillin monomers and alternative models of fibrillin assembly. The domain structure of the fibrillin monomer is deduced from the cDNA sequence. Black boxes: 8-cysteine domains; white boxes: calcium-binding EGF-like (6-cysteine) domains; gray boxes: non-cb EGF-like domains; hatched boxes: hybrid domains; stippled area: proline-rich region; the unique N- and C-terminal regions are boldly crosshatched and narrow. Ovals symbolize the location of the globular beads seen by electronmicroscopy of isolated microfibrils. *A*: Parallel alignment of head-to-tail interacting monomers with 1 bead per monomer. *B*: Staggered alignment with overlap of monomers leading to 2 beads per monomer in the microfibril structure. This model is favored by recent NMR solution structure analysis of a pair of calcium-binding EGF-like fibrillin domains. The EGF-like domains deleted by the exon skipping mutations are indicated by arrows and the numbers refer to the exons skipped (from Liu et al., 1996).

intermolecular interactions. Mutations that affect either one of the highly conserved cysteine residues or an amino acid of the consensus sequence for calcium binding generally lead to classic Marfan syndrome (Schrijver et al., 1999). Another motif in *FBN1*, the transforming growth factor binding protein (TGFbp)-like domain, contains eight conserved cysteines and is proposed to play an important role in the lateral alignment of individual fibrillin monomers (Fig. 13.1). The consequences of disease-causing *FBN1* mutations on the production and stability of mutant mRNA and protein have been studied. Increasing evidence supports the notion of a dominant-negative mechanism, by which the presence of structurally abnormal (truncated, misfolded, or internally deleted) fibrillin molecules interferes with microfibril assembly and stability. Heterozygosity for a null mutation is not likely to produce a Marfan syndrome phenotype, because individuals with stop codons leading to preferential degradation of the mutant mRNA are among the least severely affected people (personal observation). On the basis of the amount of fibrillin synthesis and deposition in cultured fibroblasts, affected individuals can be divided into four protein groups. The degree of reduction of extracellular microfibril formation, as measured by the incorporation of newly synthesized labeled fibrillin molecules, correlates with the clinical phenotype and disease progression (Aoyama et al., 1994; 1995).

Because fibrillinopathies are connective tissue disorders transmitted as autosomal dominant traits, affected individuals have a 50% chance of passing on the mutant allele in each pregnancy, regardless of whether the child is male or female. Prenatal detection by direct DNA analysis is only possible in those families in which the mutation has been identified previously. In families for which the disease-causing mutation is not known, prenatal diagnosis by linkage analysis can be done if linkage of the phenotype to 15q21 markers has been established

in the family. Likewise, direct mutation or indirect linkage analysis can be applied to relatives of probands with Marfan syndrome. To fully evaluate the clinical phenotype and to determine whether diagnostic criteria are met, however, detailed clinical examination of each individual is imperative.

Diagnostic Testing

The diagnosis of Marfan syndrome and related connective tissue disorders is strongly based on the clinical manifestations (Fig. 13.2). Because *FBN1* mutations have also been detected in individuals with other fibrillinopathies, the presence of a mutation does not by itself confirm the diagnosis. In addition, mutations have not been detected in at least 25% of research subjects with unequivocal Marfan syndrome, even when the most advanced methods of mutation detection were employed (Liu et al., 1997/98). Therefore, the possibility that the Marfan syndrome phenotype may be produced by mutations in at least one other gene cannot be excluded. For these reasons, a definitive DNA-based test does not exist, nor is it likely that a test specific for Marfan syndrome will be available in the near future. On the other hand, automated (DNA microchip based) screening for mutations is expected to further define the spectrum of fibrillinopathies and possibly allow the development of a subclassification system that will make the term "Marfan syndrome" obsolete.

If a specific mutation is unknown, an intragenic *FBN1* marker haplotype that cosegregates with the disease in the family can be determined as an alternative tool in diagnosis of affected family members. Given the likelihood of genetic heterogeneity, this approach is limited to families large enough to unequivocally establish linkage of the phenotype to *FBN1* markers.

Immunofluorescence studies of extracellular microfibrils with fibrillin antibodies have

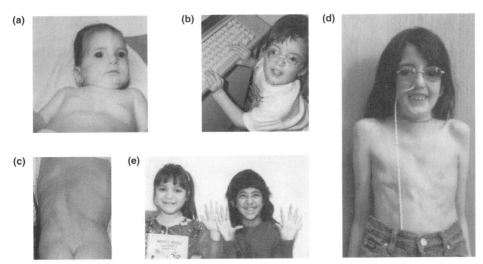

FIGURE 13.2. a: Patient 1 with Marfan syndrome at 4 months of age. Note typical facies and pectus excavatum. b: Patient 1 at 2 years. Note arachnodactyly and correction for severe myopia. c: Patient 1 at 2 years: severe progressive left thoracolumbar scoliosis. d: Patient 1 at 7 years: status post pectus repair and spinal fusion. Note aphakic correction for bilateral dislocated lenses and nasogastric tube for nightly feeding in preparation for cardiovascular surgery for aortic aneurysm and severe mitral valve regurgitation. e: Patient 2 with Marfan syndrome at 7 years (*right*) and her unaffected sister at 8.5 years (*left*). Note deep-set eyes, narrow elongated face, and arachnodactyly.

been offered as diagnostic aids. Skin biopsies from affected individuals show a deficiency in microfibrillar content, and cultured skin fibroblasts produce a reduced amount of microfibrillar meshwork (Godfrey et al., 1990). The qualitative nature of this test makes it easy to recognize the effects of severe types of dominant negative mutation, which are usually found in patients who independently meet the Ghent criteria. This test is of limited use, however, in the less severely affected cases who do not meet diagnostic criteria and are caused by *FBN1* (or other microfibrillar gene) mutations whose effects on microfibril formation are less obvious (Brenn et al., 1996).

In contrast, quantitation of fibrillin synthesis and extracellular matrix deposition, as determined by pulse-chase analysis in cultured skin fibroblasts, has been shown to have high specificity, sensitivity, and possibly even prognostic value (Aoyama et al., 1994; 1995). The current methodology, however, requires high levels of technical expertise, time, and cost that preclude it from routine diagnostic application. In summary, a reliable and conclusive diagnostic test is not currently available, and diagnosis must be based mainly on clinical findings.

Differential Diagnosis

Most phenotypes that overlap with the clinical features of the Marfan syndrome are related fibrillinopathies (Fig. 13.3). *FBN1* mutations as well as abnormal fibrillin metabolism have been demonstrated in affected individuals (reviewed in Furthmayr and Francke, 1997).

Neonatal Marfan syndrome is the most severe disorder in the spectrum of fibrillinopathies (Milewicz and Duvic, 1994). It overlaps with classic Marfan syndrome as well as congenital contractural arachnodactyly but is distinguished by sporadic occurrence and poor prognosis. The features, which are present at birth, include a characteristic progeric face, crumpled ears or simple helices, redundant skin, congenital hernias, flexion contractures, arachnodactyly,

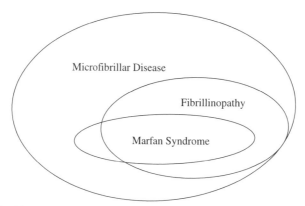

FIGURE 13.3. Classification of disorders involving connective tissue microfibrils. This concept, first proposed by Aoyama et al., (1995), defines Marfan syndrome as a major component of the fibrillinopathies but extending beyond the boundaries, because *FBN1* mutations have not been detected in more than 20% of clinically defined Marfan syndrome. Fibrillinopathies outside of the Marfan circle include individuals with documented *FBN1* mutations who do not meet clinical criteria for Marfan syndrome as well as individuals with congenital contractural arachnodactyly and *FBN2* mutations. The largest circle further encompasses connective tissue disorders caused by mutations in other genes involved in microfibril formation.

ectopia lentis, cardiomegaly with severe aortic regurgitation, multivalvular cardiac insufficiency, aortic root dilatation, pulmonary emphysema, chest deformities, and pes planus. Neonatal Marfan syndrome is often fatal within the first year of life because of congestive heart failure. *FBN1* mutations that lead to this severe disorder tend to cluster in a central region of the gene, between exons 24 and 32 (Fig. 13.1). This region is likely to be important for intermolecular interactions and stabilization of the extracellular matrix microfibrils (for discussion see Liu et al., 1996). Because neonatal Marfan syndrome results from spontaneous mutations, the family history is usually negative and the recurrence risk for a couple with an affected child should be negligible, except for the remote possibility of germline mosaicism in one of the parents. Conversely, adults with Marfan syndrome should be counseled that they are unlikely to have offspring with the neonatal lethal form of Marfan syndrome.

The MASS phenotype (*m*itral valve prolapse, mild *a*ortic dilatation, *s*keletal and *s*kin involvement) is a fibrillinopathy characterized by mild features that can be part of

Marfan syndrome. The aortic root diameter does not increase more than 2 standard deviations above the normal mean diameter. Skin involvement is limited to striae distensae, and skeletal features are generally minor by the Ghent classification (see Table 13.1).

Many individual features of Marfan syndrome can be inherited as autosomal dominant traits, such as isolated ascending aortic aneurysm/dissection, isolated ectopia lentis, and isolated skeletal features. Although these fall within the spectrum of fibrillinopathies, the molecular basis for isolated familial funnel chest has not yet been identified.

Outside of the fibrillinopathies, familial joint hypermobility can be interpreted as a normal variant when there are few clinical consequences. Joint instability is a feature of the hypermobility type of Ehlers-Danlos syndrome (formerly type III), an autosomal dominant disorder (see Chapter 8). The skin may be smooth and hyperextensible, but scarring is normal. Joint dislocations occur frequently, especially of the patellae, temporomandibular joints, and shoulders.

Congenital contractural arachnodactyly (also known as Beals syndrome) is a connective tissue disorder caused by mutations in the fibrillin-2 (*FBN2*) gene, located on chromosome 5 (Viljoen, 1994). The domain organization of *FBN1* and that of *FBN2* are nearly identical, and 80% of amino acids are conserved. Both proteins are structural components of the microfibrils. Fibrillin-2, however, is enriched in cartilaginous structures, which offers an explanation for the crumpled shape of the external ear and predominant involvement of the skeletal system in congenital contractural arachnodactyly. Children with this disorder display camptodactyly and congenital flexion contractures that generally improve in childhood. Contractures are less prominent in Marfan syndrome, most often affecting the elbows and toes (hammer toes). The remaining skeletal features in congenital contractural arachnodactyly resemble those seen in Marfan syndrome, whereas ocular and cardiovascular manifestations are less prevalent and variable.

Shprintzen-Goldberg syndrome (Greally et al., 1998) is a rare sporadic condition that resembles Marfan syndrome in its skeletal features but also includes craniosynostosis and neurodevelopmental defects. Mental retardation is a common feature. Craniofacial abnormalities that distinguish Shprintzen-Goldberg syndrome include low-set or malformed ears, ptosis, and strabismus. A cysteine substitution in *FBN1* has been detected in one patient (Sood et al., 1996) whereas the other mutation reported, a proline-to-alanine change, was found to be a polymorphism (Schrijver et al., 1997).

The trisomy 8 mosaicism syndrome (Kurtyka et al., 1988) shares some connective tissue features with Marfan syndrome. Notably, these include deep set-eyes, high-arched palate, joint contractures, narrow body habitus, and tall stature. In trisomy 8 syndrome, however, it is the trunk that is relatively elongated — because of the presence of extra thoracic vertebrae — rather than the extremities. This chromosomal imbalance syndrome also includes mental retardation and deep creases on the palms and soles but does not share any ocular or cardiovascular manifestations

with Marfan syndrome. Karyotyping of lymphocytes and, if necessary, skin fibroblasts, establishes the diagnosis.

Stickler syndrome is a pleiotropic disorder defined by craniofacial and ophthalmologic abnormalities (Temple, 1989) (see Chapter 24). Features overlapping the Marfan syndrome include joint hypermobility, high-grade myopia, and retinal detachment. Furthermore, this disorder is characterized by midface hypoplasia, progressive deafness, vitreoretinal degeneration with an optically empty anterior vitreous, and arthropathies. Mutations in collagen genes (*COL2A1*, *COL11A1*, and *COL11A2*) have been reported in families with this disorder.

Homocystinuria was first identified in institutionalized individuals thought to be affected with the Marfan syndrome. Although mental retardation is an occasional feature in homocystinuria, the intellect of individuals with Marfan syndrome is unaffected. Ectopia lentis, on the other hand, is a prominent feature in both disorders, though much more progressive in homocystinuria (Cross and Jensen, 1973; Nelson and Maumenee, 1982). Approximately 40% of the homocystinuric patients develop mild ectopia lentis by age 5, and almost all of them have ectopia lentis in their mid-twenties. Although in both diseases the lenses may be displaced in any direction, ectopia lentis occurs earlier in life and is predominantly superior and temporal in Marfan syndrome, whereas it is mostly inferior in homocystinuria. Lenses of homocystinuric patients may dislocate totally, often into the anterior chamber, and may cause pupillary block and glaucoma. These patients present with a red eye and cloudy cornea. The appearance of the lens zonular fibers may be an additional characteristic helpful in distinguishing homocystinurics from individuals with Marfan syndrome. In homocystinuria, the zonules often break completely and create a "fringe " by scrolling onto the anterior lens capsule. With detachment or degeneration of the lens zonules, the lens assumes a more globular configuration as the diameter is reduced, called spherophakia, and high lenticular myopia may develop. The cardiovascular involvement in Marfan syndrome is generally limited to the cardiac valves and dilatation and dissection of the ascending aorta, although dissection of the arch and descending aorta extending into the renal arteries may occur in later stages of the disease. In homocysteinuria, cardiovascular involvement is characterized by thrombotic events. Homocystinuria (De Franchis et al., 1998) is an autosomal recessive disorder occurring at a frequency of 1 in 200,000 newborns. It is caused by mutations in the gene for cystathionine-β-synthase leading to deficiency of the enzyme. Homocystinuria can be diagnosed by a positive cyanide-nitroprusside test of the urine, but the more reliable diagnostic assay is documentation of an elevated homocysteine level in blood.

Lujan-Fryns syndrome (Lacombe et al., 1993) is an X-linked dominant disorder characterized by mental retardation with a marfanoid body habitus. Features include a long, narrow face and a high-arched palate, a small mandible, and a hypernasal voice. Although these features can also be part of the Marfan syndrome spectrum, mental retardation and psychotic behavior are not. Only a dozen cases of Lujan-Fryns syndrome have been reported, and the underlying defect is not known.

MANIFESTATIONS AND MANAGEMENT

Comprehensive health management of persons with the Marfan syndrome and related connective tissue disorders requires involvement of many different medical specialists and an individualized approach throughout life. Therefore, a multidisciplinary setting with access to a geneticist for initial diagnosis and counseling, a cardiologist for regular cardiac evaluation, an ophthalmologist experienced in recognizing and treating ocular manifestations of connective tissue disorders, an orthopedist, a physical therapist, and psychosocial counseling opportunities is best suited for optimal care. The American Academy of Pediatrics has established guidelines for health supervision in children with Marfan syndrome, categorized by stages of development (American Academy of Pediatrics, 1996).

In infants with classic Marfan syndrome, increased length, arachnodactyly, pectus abnormalities, and ectopia lentis may already be apparent at birth. Growth parameters will generally be above the 95th percentile but must be interpreted with ethnicity and parental heights in mind. In addition, newborns may be mildly hypotonic and may display scoliosis and joint laxity on examination. Psychosocial development is completely normal.

Growth and Feeding

Tall stature and long, slender limbs and digits are cardinal features of Marfan syndrome. Children with Marfan syndrome are generally taller than their classmates, and affected adults are taller than unaffected family members. Preliminary growth curves for Marfan syndrome compared to normal Caucasian controls were constructed for approximately 200 patients (Pyeritz, 1985).

The majority of children and young adults affected with the Marfan syndrome have a weight below the 50th centile and a reduction in the amount of subcutaneous fat.

Evaluation

- All individuals with Marfan syndrome should be measured periodically, noting height, arm span-to-height ratio, and upper-to-lower body segment ratio.
- Dolichostenomelia (disproportionately long limbs) should be assessed in the correct manner. Norms exist for both Caucasian and African-American populations (Fig. 13.4). The lower

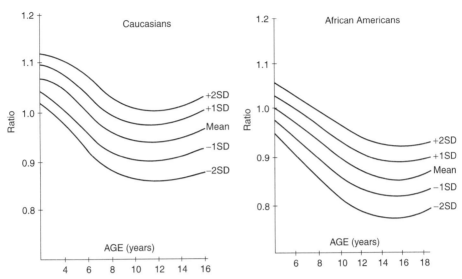

FIGURE 13.4. Upper-to-lower segment ratios for Caucasians (*left*) and African Americans (*right*). The data were collected from 2104 Baltimore school children in 1959. (Adapted from McKusick, 1972).

segment is measured from the middle of the upper rim of the symphysis pubis to the floor. The feet must be aligned and the heels must touch the wall. The upper segment measurement is obtained by subtraction of the lower segment from the height. The range of normal for the upper-to-lower segment ratio changes with age (Fig. 13.4). In adults, an upper-to-lower segment ratio of 0.85 or lower is considered significant, as the average value in unaffected adults is 0.93. The arm span-to-height ratio is an additional means to assess a disproportionate body habitus. In the Ghent criteria, the ratio is considered increased if it is greater than 1.05 (de Paepe et al., 1996). Average differences of span from height have been published for children of both sexes (see Fig. 8.2 in Hall et al., 1989). As discussed above, these measurement ratios may also be influenced by ethnicity.

Treatment

- In prepubertal girls with excessively tall stature due to Marfan syndrome,

final adult height can be reduced by initiation of high-dose estrogen therapy, combined with progesterone to prevent endometrial hyperplasia.

- Girls receiving hormone treatment to prevent excessive height are predicted to have a final height that is the average of the calculated final height before treatment and the height at the beginning of treatment. Therefore, if treatment is started around the age of 8 or 9 years, final results may be better than when treatment is postponed to early puberty. On the other hand, premature induction of puberty has the potential of bringing about additional psychological strain (Binder et al., 1997).

- Although requests for endocrine therapy are not often made for boys, accelerated bone maturation can be accomplished by treatment with testosterone.

Development and Behavior

Cognitive development is unaffected by Marfan syndrome. Motor development may be somewhat delayed by joint hyperextensibility.

The psychosocial impact of having a disorder that includes increased risk for aortic rupture and death is a significant one.

Evaluation

- Developmental milestone achievement should be assessed at each routine childhood medical visit.
- If significant delays occur in cognitive development, this is likely due to an unrelated cause and should be evaluated as in the general population.
- Motor delays can be assessed in more detail by a physical therapy evalution.

Treatment

- Physical therapy is of value in promoting motor skill development.
- Psychosocial counseling is important for family adjustment to the diagnosis and for support when complications arise. Families should be advised regarding the existence of support groups and literature, and intrafamilial interactions should be evaluated to stimulate full integration of the affected individuals in normal life activities.

Musculoskeletal

In people with Marfan syndrome, the musculoskeletal features are the most conspicuous (Fig. 13.2). Although skeletal abnormalities may not be pronounced in the first few years, they are the key to early diagnosis for observant physicians. Tall stature with disproportionately long limbs and digits, a long and narrow face with deep-set eyes, and a high, narrow palate are often combined with joint hypermobility and pectus deformities.

Chest deformities such as pectus excavatum or carinatum are related to overgrowth of the ribs, pushing the sternum outward or inward. The deformity is not limited to the chest bone and can also present as asymmetric prominence of costosternal junctions. Chest asymmetry and asymmetric placement

of the scapulae also occur secondary to scoliosis. Pectus excavatum occurs in 8 in 1,000 live births but in two-thirds of people with Marfan syndrome (Scherer et al., 1988). In adolescence, chest deformities are commonly perceived as the most disturbing physical feature.

Scoliosis is a feature in approximately 60% of children with Marfan syndrome (Sponseller et al., 1995), and the frequency is higher in adults. Individuals with a spinal curvature of less than 30 degrees have an excellent long-term prognosis, whereas moderate progression of at least 10 degrees can be expected with a curve between 30 and 50 degrees. Marked progression occurs if the curve exceeds 50 degrees (Sponseller et al., 1995). Untreated, significant spinal deformity can lead to chronic back pain and restrictive lung disease. There is a correlation between scoliosis and back pain, which occurs with greater frequency in adults with Marfan syndrome than in the general population (Sponseller et al., 1995).

Joint laxity can be pronounced in young children and may lead to delayed gross motor development. Joint dislocations are rare occurrences. When adult patients are evaluated for Marfan syndrome, it is important to keep in mind that joint hyperextensibility lessens with increasing age.

Mild contractures of elbows, knees, or toes are present in a small fraction of children and adults with Marfan syndrome. Typically, the first toe is longer than the others and there may be a wide space between the first and second toe (personal observations). Over time, pes planus and laxity of ligaments and joints can lead to painful joints and feet.

Adults often have an asthenic body habitus, and crowding of the teeth because maxilla and mandible are narrow.

Protrusio acetabuli is present in approximately half of adults with Marfan syndrome. This finding is often concurrent with deformities of the spine.

Evaluation

- On clinical suspicion, kyphosis and scoliosis should be evaluated by radiography to determine the degree of spinal curvature.

- Scoliosis must be followed, because it progresses during childhood and may undergo a rapid increase during growth spurts. Scoliosis is likely to progress if the curvature exceeds 20 degrees during childhood and adolescence and 30–40 degrees in adulthood.

- Arachnodactyly (long, slender digits) is objectively assessed by hand measurements. The ratio of middle finger to total hand length is increased compared to normal standards (Hall et al., 1989). Arachnodactyly in conjunction with small joint hypermobility results in the characteristic wrist, thumb, and thumb-to-arm signs. The wrist sign is positive when the thumb can overlap the nail of the fifth digit when the two fingers are wrapped around the wrist. The thumb sign is considered positive when the whole thumb nail extends beyond the ulnar side of the palm when folded into a fist. If the thumb can touch the forearm when the wrist is passively flexed, the thumb-to-arm sign is positive.

- Asking about hypermobility during childhood should be part of the medical history taking.

- Evaluation of the skeletal system should also include assessment of long/narrow face, prominent supraorbital ridges, deep-set eyes, high, narrow palate and dental crowding, limited elbow extension, cubitus valgus, genu recurvatum, and pes planus or cavus.

Treatment

- Delays in gross motor development caused by joint hypermobility can be ameliorated with physical therapy and orthopedic braces as needed.

- The treatment of scoliosis and kyphosis depends on the severity of the curvature and rate of progression over time. In children with Marfan syndrome, pediatric orthopedists will often treat even minor spinal curvatures with a brace to prevent progression (Sponseller et al., 1995). In the most seriously affected individuals spinal arthrodesis may be warranted.

- Pectus excavatum or carinatum need be repaired only in severe cases to prevent cardiac or pulmonary compromise, and preferably after growth has been completed. Surgical intervention for chest deformities before growth has ceased often results in recurrence due to continuing bone overgrowth.

- In addition, severe pectus excavatum interferes with the interpretation of echocardiographic studies and can lead to intra- or postoperative complications in aortic valve/root replacement surgery. Therefore, surgical correction of the pectus deformity before elective cardiovascular surgery is often recommended.

Cardiovascular

The cardiovascular manifestations of Marfan syndrome are potentially life-threatening and must be monitored closely. In childhood, the most frequently observed abnormalities are mitral valve prolapse (>60%) and mitral regurgitation. Dilatation of the ascending aorta is diagnosed in approximately half of the children with Marfan syndrome and is the most common indication for cardiovascular surgery in childhood, followed by mitral regurgitation (Gillinov et al., 1997). Aortic root dilatation generally progresses over a period of years. Because the sinuses of Valsalva are often the first part of the aortic root to dilate in Marfan syndrome, the aorta attains a characteristic flasklike shape. In adults, secondary aortic regurgitation is a common feature. If aortic complications are left untreated, the life expectancy of patients with classic Marfan syndrome is considerably reduced, but with the advances in cardiovascular pharmacotherapy and aortic root replacement surgery Marfan syndrome has become one of the more manageable genetic disorders. Medical therapy and cardiovascular surgical techniques have greatly increased life expectancy for individuals with Marfan syndrome. The average life expectancy was 70 years in 1995 (Silverman et al., 1995) but may be higher for individuals who undergo cardiovascular surgery on an elective rather than an emergency basis.

Evaluation

- Cardiology evaluation is recommended in every patient suspected of having Marfan syndrome (Moodie, 1997). Echocardiographic examination is the method of choice to establish baseline aortic root dimensions and to assess mitral valve prolapse or regurgitation. The 95% confidence interval for aortic root dimensions in children and adults has been determined by comparison of body surface area to the aortic diameter at the sinuses of Valsalva (Fig. 13.5) (Roman et al., 1989). Progression of aortic root diameter and development of mitral and aortic valve regurgitation and subacute dissection should be monitored on a regular basis throughout life. Annual cardiology evaluations are appropriate in most cases, but more frequent evaluations may be advisable if disproportionate increases in aortic root size or changes in valvular function are diagnosed.

Treatment

- β-Adrenergic blockade has been demonstrated to slow progression of the aortic root dilatation by decreasing the stress on the aortic wall and the most pervasively affected tunica media (Shores et al., 1994). Thereby, negative inotropic therapy can prevent complications such as aneurysm formation and dissection and should be implemented at the first signs of aortic enlargement or when the aortic root reaches the 95th percentile for body surface area (Salim et al., 1994). Because aortic dilatation in individuals with Marfan syndrome may progress throughout life, β-blockade is continued indefinitely.

- Lifelong β-blockade therapy is generally well tolerated. Side effects depend on the dose and type of medication and can often be alleviated by changing pharmacological agents. In individuals with asthma, calcium channel blockers can be substituted.

- Even though aortic dissection and rupture are rare in children (Moodie, 1997), advanced aortic dilatation with aortic regurgitation requires composite graft replacement surgery in a substantial fraction of untreated young adults. Although β-blocker therapy may increase the interval between initial stages of dilatation and elective surgery in many patients, aortic graft surgery may be necessary in childhood if there is a rapid increase of aortic diameter leading to aortic regurgitation. There is great individual variability in aortic root diameter at the time of dissection. Although previous guidelines recommended aortic root replacement surgery at an aortic diameter of 50–60 mm, recent observations underscore the importance of family history of dissection and/or rupture. Furthermore, the ratio between the size of the dilated aortic segment and the diameter of the aorta with normal appearance downstream should be taken into account. Also fairly common during childhood is the need for mitral valve repair.

- Cardiovascular surgery can be delayed significantly by appropriate β-adrenergic blockade. However, most adults with Marfan syndrome will eventually

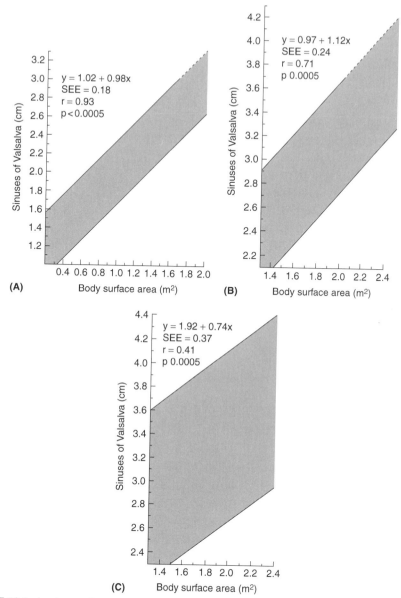

FIGURE 13.5. Aortic root dimensions in relation to body surface area for infants and children (A), adults less than 40 years old (B), and adults age 40 years and older (C). The gray area represents the 95% confidence interval (from Roman et al., 1989).

need replacement of a dilated aortic root and leaking aortic valve. Aortic root replacement has an operative risk of under 5%. Valve-sparing procedures are not recommended because the fibrillin abnormalities in the aortic valve leaflets render them prone to further weakening (Gott et al., 1996).

- If mitral valve prolapse is diagnosed, standard prophylaxis against bacterial endocarditis is recommended for all dental procedures.

- Even though individuals with Marfan syndrome can enjoy an almost normal activity level, certain guidelines should be observed to prevent excessive strain on the cardiovascular system, joints, and ligaments. Physical activity supports motor development and increases muscle strength, but contact sports such as football, basketball, hockey, volleyball, boxing, and wrestling are contraindicated because of the risk of trauma to the chest and aorta. The risk for retinal detachment (discussed below) is another good reason to evade blows to the head. Heavy lifting should also be avoided because of the acute increase of pressure on the ascending aorta. Noncompetitive aerobic activity such as swimming, bicycling, hiking, and general physical conditioning are encouraged.

Ophthalmologic

The most characteristic ocular manifestation of the Marfan syndrome is ectopia lentis, which is caused by the microfibrillar weakness of the ciliary zonules. As an early hallmark of the disorder, ectopia lentis is detected in 50–80% of individuals with Marfan syndrome (Cross and Jensen, 1973; Maumenee 1981; Nelson and Maumenee, 1982). It is usually bilateral and typically superotemporal, although it may occur in any direction. Most often, ectopia lentis becomes evident in young children and is slowly progressive, particularly in childhood and the early teenage years (Alcorn and Maumenee, 1989). Severity varies from very mild to total ectopia lentis, but — in contrast to homocystinuria — dislocation into the anterior chamber is uncommon. Most children and adults with classic Marfan syndrome have myopia, albeit at varying degrees. Individuals with Marfan syndrome also develop cataracts 10–20 years earlier than the general population.

Retinal detachment is a leading cause of visual loss in these patients. Retinal detachment is a complication related to elongation of the globe and frequently even occurs in younger individuals. Retinal detachment has an increased incidence after intraocular surgery.

The prognosis of ocular involvement in Marfan syndrome is excellent with appropriate evaluations and treatment of possible complications as they arise. Over 90% of patients who start treatment in early childhood retain a visual acuity of at least 20/40 in both eyes (Alcorn and Maumenee, 1989).

Evaluation

- Annual eye examination by an ophthalmologist who has experience with the ocular manifestations of Marfan syndrome and related connective tissue disorders is strongly recommended. Visual acuity, refraction, and fundoscopic findings must be assessed at diagnosis and regularly thereafter to maximize vision. It is important to keep in mind that patients do not need to be verbal to undergo an ophthalmologic evaluation.

- Evaluation for strabismus is also important, because it can lead to amblyopia and loss of binocularity. The incidence of strabismus in Marfan syndrome (19%) is increased compared with that in the general population (5%), presumably because ectopia lentis as well as mechanical and craniofacial factors contribute to its development (Izquierdo et al., 1994). Exotropia (outward deviation) is the most common type of strabismus in Marfan syndrome.

- During the general ophthalmic examination, ectopia lentis can be suspected when iridodonesis, or a "wobbly" iris, is observed. When the iris loses its posterior support of the lens and zonules, it may appear to shimmer or be tremulous. This phenomenon is called iridodonesis and is most easily detected on rapid lateral eye movement or blinking.

- Slit lamp examination may also reveal a smooth surface of the iris with lack of crypts and furrows, giving it a "velvety appearance".

- Ectopia lentis is best appreciated by retroillumination using the slit lamp biomicroscope, direct ophthalmoscope, or retinoscope or, in cases of posterior dislocation, by having the patient look downward, which may reveal a gap between the pupillary margin and the lens. Ectopia lentis is more evident with increasing amounts of lens displacement. Small degrees of ectopia lentis, however, can only be detected when pupils are maximally dilated. Because the dilator muscle of the iris is hypoplastic, pupils are small and may be difficult to dilate. Minor ectopia lentis may manifest as a slight notch or crenated edge, most commonly inferiorly (Nelson and Maumenee, 1982; Ruttum, 1995; Speedwell and Russell-Eggitt, 1995).

- The degree of ectopia lentis should be monitored. Generally, it is only gradually progressive, most often in childhood and early adolescence (Alcorn and Maumenee, 1989).

- Individuals with Marfan syndrome must be monitored for glaucoma that can occur because of various etiologies: anatomical, mechanical, and/or vascular. For example, angle abnormalities may cause open angle glaucoma, or dislocation of the lens into the anterior chamber of the eye can cause obstruction (Izquierdo et al., 1992).

- High-grade myopia is often associated with increased axial globe length, which can be assessed by ophthalmologic ultrasound examination (Gordon and Donzis, 1985). These enlarged globes also carry an increased risk for retinal detachment, and the retina should always be examined for early signs.

- Children and adults need to be informed of the symptoms and signs of a retinal detachment. They are advised to routinely check their own vision monocularly. If they experience flashes, floaters, visual field changes, or a "curtain or shadow" over their visual field, they should see a retinal specialist immediately. Dilated fundoscopic examinations are essential, particularly in the myopic individuals who are at greater risk of retinal detachment if they have increased axial lengths.

Treatment

- Corrective lenses should be prescribed as necessary. Lenses will also prevent the development of amblyopia. Aphakic correction is needed in cases of severely dislocated lenses.

- Adequate optical correction must be prescribed and worn. Meticulous assessment of refraction must be performed regularly to maximize visual acuity. Patients should be tried in both their phakic and aphakic corrections to assess their best vision. The use of mydriatic eyedrops may be required to dilate pupils to maximize visual space, particularly if asymmetric lens subluxation is present.

- β-Blocker therapy, often initiated to delay cardiovascular disease progression, is also beneficial from an ocular standpoint. β-Blockers decrease intraocular pressure by diminishing aqueous fluid production and are used topically as antiglaucoma medication.

- Amblyopia must be treated aggressively, in standard fashion.

- The so-called "presenile" cataract of Marfan syndrome is a true indication for lens extraction.

- Lens removal for optical reasons is not recommended (Nelson and Maumenee, 1982; Ruttum, 1995; Speedwell and Russell-Eggitt, 1995).

- When the ectopia lentis is progressive and leads to secondary complications such as iritis, glaucoma, vitreal compromise, or cataract, surgical lens removal may be indicated. These complications are rare in childhood.

- Because individuals with Marfan syndrome are prone to spontaneous retinal detachment, contact sports should be avoided. The incidence of retinal detachment increases after intraocular surgery. If retinal detachment occurs, time is of the essence. Good visual results after retinal detachment are dependent upon reattachment of the retina either by laser or scleral buckling procedures and/or vitrectomy. Success is dependent on the location, extent, and duration of the detachment.

Neurologic

The widening and weakness of the spinal cord sac can result in leakage of spinal fluid and intractable orthostatic headaches when the tear does not heal spontaneously. Prognosis after surgical hernia repair is good, although the underlying connective tissue defect may lead to recurrence. Although episodes of orthostatic headache resulting from cerebrospinal fluid leakage are not uncommon in the third or fourth decade, these symptoms are usually transient and benign. Dural ectasia is reported to occur in 63% of adults with Marfan syndrome (Pyeritz et al., 1988). It is probably infrequent in children.

Evaluation

- Dural ectasia can be evaluated only by MRI or CT scan. Because the evaluation is not commonly performed for diagnostic purposes, the precise frequency of this manifestation and its clinical significance are currently unknown.

Treatment

- Orthostatic headache resulting from cerebrospinal fluid leakage is often transient. Treatment with bed rest may

be sufficient in most cases, because the intracranial hypotension will subside in the recumbent position. If leakage of the spinal fluid persists, however, treatment with corticosteroids or epidural patches can be effective.

- Neurosurgical repair may be considered in patients with recurring or severe complaints, if the location of the leak can be identified and the area can be approached with low risk (Schievink et al., 1996).

Respiratory

Marfan syndrome is associated with pulmonary manifestations, including apical blebs and spontaneous pneumothorax. In individuals with Marfan syndrome who have an asthenic body habitus, spontaneous pneumothorax occurs more frequently than in other body types. These events occur in males more often than in females. They are rare in childhood, with an adult estimated frequency of 4.4% (Hall et al., 1984) but are more frequently seen in adolescents. Patients will present with acute dyspnea and chest pain, secondary to intrapleural air accumulation. Chest radiography is generally conclusive.

Evaluation

- The medical history regarding manifestations in the respiratory system should be explored at each evaluation.
- Apical blebs can be observed on chest radiography but do not require special evaluation because their presence is inconsequential unless their thin wall ruptures, leading to spontaneous pneumothorax.

Treatment

- Spontaneous pneumothorax is treated by evacuation of the intrapleural air and restoration of the negative pleural pressure by insertion of a drainage chest tube.

- In individuals with Marfan syndrome, there is an increased risk for repeated rupture of an apical bleb. Therefore, pleurodesis is recommended after recurring pneumothorax (Hall et al., 1984).

Dermatologic

Involvement of the integument is seen in Marfan syndrome. Features include inguinal as well as incisional hernias and striae distensae. The skin may be soft and thin in appearance, and stretch marks are often present, especially after the adolescent growth spurt. Such striae distensae are common in the general population but have a different distribution in persons with Marfan syndrome. Most frequently, they develop on the shoulders, axilla, chest, lower back, hips, thighs, and dorsum of the knee.

Evaluation

- Congenital inguinal hernia as well as hernias of later onset require timely surgical correction to prevent intestinal strangulation and further weakening of the surrounding connective tissue.
- The presence or absence of inguinal or femoral hernias should be assessed at the first examination and throughout childhood, because they may be congenital and often recur. Hernias manifest in at least 50% of affected individuals. Incisional hernias may develop after abdominal surgery.

Treatment

- For striae, neither prevention nor effective treatment is available.
- Hernias should be treated as in the general population.

Pregnancy

Although the chance for aortic dissection is somewhat elevated in all pregnant women (Simpson et al., 1997), women with Marfan syndrome clearly have an increased risk of cardiovascular complications during gestation and labor. In women with minimal cardiovascular involvement of Marfan syndrome, pregnancy can be tolerated safely with adequate management of the aortic status. If the aortic root diameter exceeds 40 mm, or if it has shown a recent increase in diameter, pregnancy carries a significant risk for dissection and aortic rupture not limited to the third trimester and labor (Lipscomb et al., 1997).

Evaluation

- To achieve a favorable outcome, it is preferable to start cardiovascular evaluation and stabilization before pregnancy.
- The preconceptional aortic root diameter is the single most important parameter that determines the degree of safety of undergoing pregnancy. This measurement is not necessarily correlated with patient age, and the risk must be determined on an individual basis, taking into account the absolute diameter as well as the aortic diameter at the time of dissection in other family members.
- Pregnant women affected with the Marfan syndrome need to receive continuing prenatal care because of the possibility of accelerating aortic root dilatation and aortic dissection. Serial monthly echocardiography is highly recommended, and every pregnancy should be treated as a high-risk event (Lipscomb et al., 1997).

Treatment

- A combined approach involving cardiology, clinical genetics, and maternal/fetal medicine is pivotal in women considering pregnancy.
- In pregnant women, β-blocker therapy can have adverse effects on the fetus, such as intrauterine growth retardation, and on the mother, such as hypoglycemia, bradycardia, and apnea. By decreasing pressure on the ascending aorta, however, these drugs may reduce

the risk for aortic dilatation and dissection. Therefore, the benefits of β-blocker therapy throughout pregnancy are likely to outweigh the risks (Simpson et al., 1997).

- Pregnancy-induced hypertension poses an additional risk factor for aortic dissection and must be treated aggressively.
- Vaginal delivery with epidural anesthesia is preferred over cesarean section except for women with obstetric complications or with progressive aortic dilatation and a very high chance of dissection (Rossiter et al., 1995).
- All women with mitral valve prolapse should receive bacterial endocarditis prophylaxis before delivery.

RESOURCES

National Marfan Foundation

382 Main Street
Port Washington, NY 11050
Telephone: 1-800-8-MARFAN
(1-800-862-7326) and 516-883-8712

Canadian Marfan Association

Centre Plaza Postal Outlet
128 Queen St. South
P.O. Box 42257
Mississauga, Ontario, L5M 4Z0, Canada
Telephone: (905) 826-3223

Marfan Association UK

Rochester House
5 Aldershot Road
Fleet, Hampshire
GU13 9NG, England
Telephone: (0)1252 810472

Internet

National Marfan Foundation
http://www.marfan.org/on-line.html
Email: *staff@marfan.org*

Stanford University Center for Marfan Syndrome and Related Connective Tissue Disorders: *http://marfan.stanford.edu*

The Canadian Marfan Association:
http://www.marfan.ca
Email: *info@marfan.ca*

Marfan Association UK:
http://www.thenet.co.uk/~marfan/Default.htm
Email: *marfan@thenet.co.uk*

The Elastic Fiber Homepage:
http://ef.wustl.edu
Email: *tritty@cellbio.wustl.edu*

REFERENCES

Alcorn D and Maumenee I (1989) Optical correlation and visual acuity in patients with the Marfan syndrome and dislocated lenses. *Am J Med Genet* 32:249.

American Academy of Pediatrics, Committee on Genetics (1996) Health supervision for children with Marfan syndrome. *Pediatrics* 98:978–982.

Aoyama T, Francke U, Dietz HC, Furthmayr H (1994) Quantitative differences in biosynthesis and extracellular deposition of fibrillin in cultured fibroblasts distinguish five groups of Marfan syndrome related patients and suggest distinct pathogenetic mechanisms. *J Clin Invest* 94:130–137.

Aoyama T, Francke U, Gasner C, Furthmayr H (1995) Fibrillin abnormalities and prognosis in Marfan syndrome and related disorders. *Am J Med Genet* 58:169–176.

Beighton P, dePaepe A, Danks D, Finidori G, Gedde-Dahl T, Goodman R, Hall JG, Hollister DW, Horton W, McKusick VA, Opitz JM, Pope FM, Pyeritz RE, Rimoin DL, Sillence D, Spranger JW, Thompson E, Tsipouras P, Viljoen D, Winship I, Young I (1988) International nosology of heritable disorders of connective tissue, Berlin, 1986. *Am J Med Genet* 29:581–594.

Binder G, Grauer ML, Wehner AV, Wehner F, Ranke MB (1997) Outcome in tall stature. Final height and psychological aspects in 220 patients with and without treatment. *Eur J Pediatr* 156:905–910.

Brenn T, Aoyama T, Francke U, Furthmayr H. (1996) Dermal fibroblast culture as a model system for studies of fibrillin assembly and pathogenetic mechanisms: defects in distinct groups of individuals with Marfan's syndrome. *Lab Invest* 75:389–402.

Collod-Beroud G, Béroud C, Ades L, Black C, Boxer M, Brock DJH, Holman KJ, de Paepe A, Francke U, Grau U, Hayward C, Klein H-G, Liu W, Nuytinck L, Peltonen L, Alvarez Perez AB, Rantamäki T, Junien C, Boileau C (1998) Marfan database (third edition): New mutations and new routines for the software. *Nucleic Acids Res* 26:229–233.

Cross HE, Jensen AD (1973) Ocular manifestations in the Marfan syndrome and homocystinuria. *Am J Ophthalmol* 75:405–420.

De Franchis R, Sperandeo MP, Sebastio G, Andria GM (1998) Clinical aspects of cystathionine synthetase deficiency: How wide is the spectrum? *Eur J Pediatr* 157, Suppl 2: S67–S70.

de Paepe A, Devereux RB, Dietz HC, Hennekam RCM, Pyeritz RE (1996) Revised diagnostic criteria for the Marfan syndrome. *Am J Med Genet* 62:417–426.

Dietz HC, Pyeritz RE, Hall BD, Cadle RG, Hamosh A, Schwartz J, Meyers DA, Francomano CA (1991) The Marfan syndrome locus: Confirmation of assignment to chromosome 15 and identification of tightly linked markers at 15q15-q21.3. *Genomics* 9:355–61

Francke U, Furthmayr H (1993) Genes and gene products involved in Marfan syndrome. *Semin Thorac Cardiovasc Surg* 5:3–10.

Furthmayr H, Francke U (1997) Ascending aortic aneurysm with or without features of Marfan Syndrome and other fibrillinopathies: New insights. *Semin Thorac Cardiovasc Surg* 9:191–205.

Gillinov A, Zehr K, Redmond JM, Gott VL, Dietz HC, Reitz BA, Laschinger JC, Cameron DE (1997) Cardiac operations in children with Marfan syndrome: indications and results. *Ann Thorac Surg* 64:1140–1144.

Godfrey M, Menashe V, Weleber RG, Koler RD, Bigley RH, Lovrien E, Zonana J, Hollister DW (1990) Cosegregation of elastin-associated microfibrillar abnormalities with the Marfan phenotype in families. *Am J Hum Genet* 46:652–660.

Gordon RA, Donzis PB (1985) Refractive development of the human eye. *Arch Ophthalmol* 103:785–789.

Gott V, Laschinger J, Cameron DE, Dietz HC, Greene PS, Gillinov AM, Pyeritz RE, Alejo DE, Fleischer KJ, Anhalt GJ, Stone CD, McKusick VA (1996) The Marfan syndrome and the cardiovascular surgeon. *Eur J Cardiothor Surg* 10:149–158.

Greally MT, Carey JC, Milewicz DM, Hudgins L, Goldberg RB, Shprintzen RJ, Cousineau AJ, Smith WL Jr, Judisch GF, Hanson JW (1998) Shprintzen-Goldberg syndrome: A clinical analysis. *Am J Med Genet* 76:202–212.

Hall JG, Pyeritz JE, Dudgeon DL, Haller JA Jr (1984) Pneumothorax in the Marfan syndrome: Prevalence and therapy. *Ann Thorac Surg* 37:500–504.

Hall JG, Froster-Iskenius UG, Allanson JE (1989) *Handbook of Normal Physical Measurements*. Oxford: Oxford University Press.

Izquierdo NJ, Traboulsi EI, Enger C, Maumenee IH (1992) Glaucoma in the Marfan syndrome. *Trans Am Ophthalmol Soc* 90:111–122.

Izquierdo NJ, Traboulsi EI, Enger C, Maumenee IH (1994) Strabismus in the Marfan syndrome. *Am J Ophthalmol* 117:632–635.

Kainulainen K, Pulkkinen L, Savolainen A, Kaitila I, Peltonen L (1990) Location on chromosome 15 of the gene defect causing Marfan syndrome. *N Engl J Med* 323:935–939.

Kurtyka ZE, Krzykwa B, Piatkowska E, Radwan M, Pietrzyk JJB (1988) Trisomy 8 mosaicism syndrome. *Clin Pediatr* 27:557–564.

Lacombe D, Bonneau D, Verloes A, Couet D, Koulischer L, Battin J (1993) Lujan-Fryns syndrome (X-linked mental retardation with marfanoid habitus): Report of three cases and review. *Genet Counseling* 4:193–198.

Lipscomb KJ, Smith JC, Clarke B, Harris R (1997) Outcome of pregnancy in women with Marfan's syndrome. *Br J Obstet Gynaecol* 104:201–206.

Liu W, Qian C, Comeau K, Brenn T, Furthmayr H, Francke U (1996) Mutant fibrillin-1 monomers lacking EGF-like domains disrupt microfibril assembly and cause severe Marfan syndrome. *Hum Mol Genet* 5:1581–1587.

Liu W, Oefner P, Qian C, Odom R, Francke U (1997/98) Denaturing HPLC identified novel FBN1 mutations, polymorphisms and sequence variants in Marfan syndrome and related connective tissue disorders. *Genetic Testing* 1: 237–242.

Maumenee I (1981) The eye in the Marfan syndrome. *Trans Am Ophthalmal Soc* 79:684–733.

McKusick VA (1972) *Heritable Disorders of Connective Tissue*. S Louis, MO: CV Mosby.

Milewicz DM, Duvic M (1994) Severe neonatal Marfan syndrome resulting from a de novo 3-bp insertion into the fibrillin gene on chromosome 15. *Am J Hum Genet* 54:447–453.

Moodie DS (1997) American Academy of Pediatrics: Health supervision for children with Marfan syndrome. *Clin Pediatr (Phila)* 36:489.

Nelson LB, Maumenee IH (1982) Ectopia lentis. *Surv Ophthalmol* 27:143–160.

Pyeritz RE (1985) Growth and anthropometrics in the Marfan syndrome. In: *Endocrine Genetics and Genetics of Growth* New York: Liss p.135–140. .

Pyeritz RE, Fishman EK, Bernhardt BA, Siegelman SS (1988) Dural ectasia is a common feature of the Marfan syndrome. *Am J Hum Genet* 43:726–732.

Roman M, Devereux R, Kramer-Fox R, O'Ranghlin J (1989) Two dimensional aortic root dimensions in normal children and adults. *Am J Cardiol* 64:507–512.

Rossiter JP, Repke JT, Morales AJ, Murphey EA, Pyeritz RE (1995) A prospective longitudinal evaluation of pregnancy in the Marfan syndrome. *Am J Obstet Gynecol* 173:1599–1606.

Ruttum MS (1995) Managing situations involving children with ectopia lentis. *J Pediatr Ophthalmol Strabismus* 32:94–97.

Sakai LY, Keene DR, Engvall E (1986) Fibrillin, a new 350-kD glycoprotein, is a component of extracellular microfibrils. *J Cell Biol* 103: 2499–2509.

Salim M, Alpert B, Jewell CW, Pyeritz RE (1994) Effect of beta-adrenergic blockade on aortic root rate of dilation in the Marfan syndrome. *Am J Cardiol* 74:629–633.

Scherer L, Arn P, Dressel DA, Pyeritz DM, Haller JA (1988) Surgical management of children and young adults with Marfan syndrome and pectus excavatum. *J Pediatr Surg* 23:1169–1172.

Schievink WI, Meyer FB, Atkinson JLD, Mokri B (1996) Spontaneous spinal cerebrospinal fluid leaks and intracranial hypotension. *J Neurosurg* 84:598–605.

Schrijver I, Liu W, Francke U (1997) The pathogenicity of the Pro1148Ala substitution in the *FBN1* gene: Causing or predisposing to Marfan syndrome and aortic aneurysm, or clinically innocent? *Hum Genet* 99: 607–611.

Schrijver I, Liu W, Brenn T, Furthmayr H, Francke U (1999) Cysteine substitutions in EGF-like domains of fibrillin-1: Distinct effects on biochemical and clinical phenotypes. *Am J Hum Genet* 65:1007–1020.

Shores J, Berger KR, Murphy EA, Pyeritz RE (1994) Progression of aortic root dilatation and the benefit of long-term beta-adrenergic blockade in Marfan's syndrome. *N Engl J Med* 330:1335–1341.

Silverman DI, Burton KJ, Gray J, Bosner MS, Kouchoukos NT, Roman MJ, Boxer M, Devereux RB, Tsipouras P (1995) Life expectancy in the Marfan syndrome. *Am J Cardiol* 72:157–160.

Simpson L, Athanassious A, D'Alton ME (1997) Marfan syndrome in pregnancy. *Curr Opin Obstet Gynecol* 9:337–341.

Sood S, Eldadah ZA, Krause WL, McIntosh I, Dietz HC (1996) Mutation in fibrillin-1 and the Marfanoid-craniosynostosis (Shprintzen-Goldberg) syndrome. *Nat Genet* 12:209–211.

Speedwell L, Russell-Eggitt I (1995) Improvement in visual acuity in children with ectopia lentis. *J Pediatr Ophthalmol Strabismus* 32: 94–97.

Sponseller P, Hobbs W, Riley LH 3rd, Pyeritz RE (1995) The thoracolumbar spine in Marfan syndrome. *J Bone Joint Surg Am* 6:867–876.

Temple I (1989) Stickler's syndrome. *J Med Genet* 26:119–126.

Viljoen D (1994) Congenital contractural arachnodactyly. *J Med Genet* 31:640–643.

CHAPTER 14

NEUROFIBROMATOSIS TYPE 1

DAVID VISKOCHIL

INTRODUCTION

The clinical management of neurofibromatosis type 1 (also called neurofibromatosis 1 or NF1) involves recognition and treatment of myriad features associated with congenital anomalies and age-related abnormal tissue proliferation. Like many genetic disorders covered in this text, the molecular biology of neurofibromatosis 1 has outpaced the treatment of this condition. Presumably, this is a temporary hiatus, because, as our knowledge of the biochemical pathways involved in neurofibromatosis 1 expands, practitioners will be able to progress from the "watchful waiting" mode of surgical intervention toward a more directed medical management approach. While waiting for specific medical protocols to be developed for treatment of neurofibromatosis 1-related abnormalities, there are clear reasons to diagnose and counsel individuals and families who have this disorder. Furthermore, it is also important for primary care providers to familiarize themselves both with indications and contraindications for the application of therapies performed by subspecialists who may not themselves consistently evaluate the specific and unique complications of neurofibromatosis 1 in the context of the whole condition and the whole person.

Incidence

Neurofibromatosis 1, also known as peripheral neurofibromatosis or von Recklinghausen disease, was first described in modern medical literature in 1882. There are now a number of historical perspectives, reviews, and textbooks devoted to the various manifestations of this condition (Crowe et al., 1956; Rubenstein and Korf, 1990; Riccardi, 1992; Huson and Hughes, 1994; Upadhyaya and Cooper 1998; Friedman et al., 1999). It is an autosomal dominant condition with a high degree of variability of clinical expression. Although it is fully penetrant in adults, there is an age-related penetrance for a number of the individual clinical signs. Neurofibromatosis 1 affects approximately 1 in 3,500 individuals worldwide (Carey et al., 1986), and, in general, diagnosis can be made before age 10 by straightforward clinical evaluation.

Diagnostic Criteria

The variability in clinical expression and age-related penetrance of a number of clinical manifestations sometimes makes neurofibromatosis 1 a difficult condition to diagnose with confidence, especially in children who are sporadic cases. The autosomal dominant inheritance pattern and full penetrance

Management of Genetic Syndromes, Edited by Suzanne B. Cassidy and Judith E. Allanson
ISBN 0-471-31286-X   Copyright © 2001 by Wiley-Liss, Inc.

TABLE 14.1. NIH Diagnostic Criteria for Neurofibromatosis 1

Neurofibromatosis 1 is present in an individual who has two or more of the following signs:

Six or more café au lait macules >5 mm in greatest diameter in prepubertal individuals or >15 mm in greatest diameter after puberty

Two or more neurofibromas of any type, or one or more plexiform neurofibroma

Freckling in the axilla or inguinal regions (Crowe's sign)

A tumor of the optic pathway

Two or more Lisch nodules (iris hamartomas)

A distinctive osseous lesion, such as sphenoid wing dysplasia or long-bone bowing (with or without pseudarthrosis)

A first-degree relative with neurofibromatosis 1 by the above criteria

in adults facilitates diagnosis. It should be noted that diagnostic criteria established in 1988 (National Institutes of Health Consensus Development Conference, 1988) and reviewed in 1997 (Gutmann et al., 1997) serve as guidelines only, through the incorporation of 7 characteristic features of neurofibromatosis 1 into a list of diagnostic criteria (see Table 14.1). The presence of any two features satisfies the diagnostic criteria and enables one to diagnose this condition on clinical grounds. The diagnostic criteria do not provide insight into severity of the disorder or prognosis. Cutaneous manifestations of café au lait spots, freckling, and dermal neurofibromas were selected for their high prevalence in almost all adults with neurofibromatosis 1. Other signs, including Lisch nodules, skeletal dysplasia, optic pathway tumor, and plexiform neurofibroma, were selected for their specificity. There is a role for clinical judgment, and the use of imaging studies to determine the presence or absence of a feature, simply for diagnostic purposes, is rarely indicated (Gutmann et al., 1997).

It is necessary to consider age in the application of diagnostic criteria. Each of the diagnostic features has a distinctive age of presentation. The café au lait spots (Fig. 14.1) tend to arise in the first year of life and approximately 80% of those who have neurofibromatosis 1 will demonstrate over 5 café au lait spots by age 1 year. This is typically the first sign of the condition. Axillary or groin freckling (Fig. 14.2) is the second

diagnostic sign noted in approximately three-fourths of individuals with neurofibromatosis 1 (Korf, 1992). The subtlety of Crowe's sign (intertriginous freckling) can make it difficult for practitioners to feel confident in diagnosing neurofibromatosis 1 in sporadic cases where nonpigmentary manifestations are absent. Dermal neurofibromas and Lisch

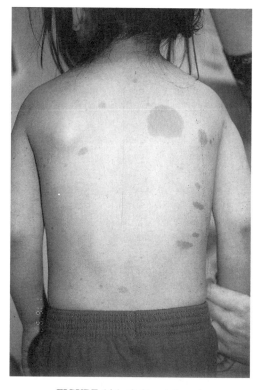

FIGURE 14.1. Café au lait spot.

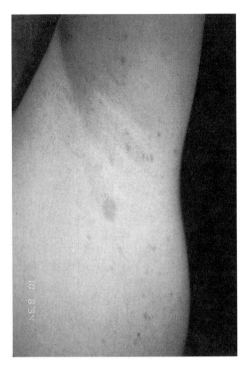

FIGURE 14.2. Axillary freckling.

nodules are usually detected in the teenage years, whereas optic gliomas, skeletal dysplasias, and plexiform neurofibromas tend to present in the early childhood years. It is important to use care in applying the affected status of a first-degree relative as one of the diagnostic criteria. A parent of an index case who has neurofibromatosis 1 should not be diagnosed with generalized neurofibromatosis 1 if such parent has only one of the six physical signs of neurofibromatosis 1. For example, a parent with 8 café au lait spots who has a child with unequivocal neurofibromatosis 1 should not be designated as "affected" based on satisfying a second criterion of having a first degree relative (the child) with neurofibromatosis 1. Such a parent could either be unaffected or mosaic for neurofibromatosis 1 with germ line involvement. It is important to make this distinction because the recurrence risk for siblings of this hypothetical index case would be much lower than the 50% risk for a clear autosomal dominant pattern of inheritance.

Some multidisciplinary team clinics for patients with neurofibromatosis 1 routinely perform imaging studies in asymptomatic individuals. This could serve as a baseline screen to identify both optic pathway tumors and T2-weighted intense signals (UBOs, or unidentified bright objects) which could help make the diagnosis. Practitioners who are familiar with the diagnostic criteria and follow many families with neurofibromatosis 1 rarely need such studies as a diagnostic aid. The lack of consistent correlation of the number and location of UBOs with learning problems and mental retardation diminishes the clinical indication to perform brain MRI in the absence of symptoms. The parental anxiety induced by the finding of UBOs in an otherwise normal brain MRI scan may not be easily diffused by counseling about the relative insignificance of these ill-defined and benign lesions. Sometimes, the MRI scans can invoke management decisions that are based on incidental findings rather than symptoms. For example, an initial finding of an apparent low-grade glioma on brain MRI in an asymptomatic individual may lead to sequential scanning without a medically defined endpoint for surveillance. Finally, sedation in infants and toddlers for MRI scanning and their exposure to enhancing dyes carry some, albeit small, risks to the child. As a general guideline, the use of ancillary imaging for diagnostic purposes in neurofibromatosis 1 is not warranted without symptoms.

There are other common features of neurofibromatosis 1 that can be considered in the diagnostic evaluation, even though they are not very specific. Short stature, relative macrocephaly, learning and speech problems, and hyperintense T2-weighted signals on brain MRI are commonly seen. When clinical suspicion is high in children, it may be reasonable to provisionally diagnose neurofibromatosis 1 and counsel families about possible associations and medical complications that may otherwise be overlooked in standard health care. This is especially true in toddlers who have classical multiple café au lait spots as their only manifestation. A provisional diagnosis of neurofibromatosis 1 could guide practitioners to modify their clinical evaluations to detect complications associated with neurofibromatosis 1. Annual reevaluation of the diagnostic criteria and ophthalmology evaluations are indicated in those who carry a provisional diagnosis of neurofibromatosis 1.

To provide effective anticipatory guidance, it is important to be aware of the incidence of neurofibromatosis 1-related complications. There are a number of published reports that have recorded the incidence of various neurofibromatosis 1 features (Riccardi, 1992; Huson and Hughes, 1994), and presently there is an ongoing collection of neurofibromatosis 1-related manifestations recorded through the International Clinical Database of Neurofibromatosis located in Vancouver, British Columbia (Friedman and Birch, 1997). Table 14.2–14.4 list a number of manifestations associated with neurofibromatosis 1 and the incidences of some less common findings and the ages at which they occur. It is important to keep these incidence figures in mind in the evaluation of unusual complications of neurofibromatosis 1. As a primary care provider for someone with neurofibromatosis 1, the question, "Could this manifestation be caused by neurofibromatosis 1?" is an important one to address at each encounter. Having some knowledge of the incidence of neurofibromatosis 1-associated manifestations helps the practitioner with the diagnostic work-up when confronted with a rare medical condition.

Etiology, Pathogenesis, and Genetics

Neurofibromatosis 1 has been genetically mapped to the centromeric region of the long arm of chromosome 17 (Barker et al., 1987). The *NF1* gene was cloned and characterized as a Ras-GAP protein (reviewed in Viskochil et al., 1993). Its encoded product, neurofibromin, is a 240-kDa peptide (reviewed in Sherman et al.,

TABLE 14.2. Manifestations of Neurofibromatosis 1 and available frequencies (modified from Riccardi, 1992; Huson and Hughes, 1994; Friedman and Birch, 1997)

Cutaneous

Multiple café au lait spots
Intertriginous freckling
Dermal neurofibromas
Xanthogranulomas (2–5%)
Hemangiomas (5–10%)

Ophthalmologic

Optic pathway tumor
Lisch nodules
Glaucoma (rare)

Musculoskeletal

Sphenoid wing dysplasia (5–10%)
Long-bone bowing (2–5%)
Scoliosis (20–30%)
Short stature (25–35%)
Relative macrocephaly

Cardiovascular

Hypertension (2–5%)
Congenital heart defect (2%)

Neurological

Hydrocephalus (5%)
Seizures (6–7%)
Educational difficulty (40–60%)
Sensorineural hearing loss (5%)
Precocious puberty (2–5%)

Tumors

Plexiform neurofibromas (25%)
Malignant peripheral nerve sheath tumors (2–5%)
CNS glioma (2%)
Pheochromocytoma, rhabdomyoma, neuroblastoma (all rare)
Myelogenous leukemia (rare)

1998) that stimulates the intrinsic hydrolysis of guanosine triphosphate (GTP) bound to Ras (Martin et al., 1990) (Fig. 14.3). Ras is a small intracellular protein attached to the inner membrane of the cell that, when bound to GTP, transduces both growth signals to the cell's nucleus by the mitogen-activated protein kinase (MAPK) pathway and antiapoptotic signals. The conversion

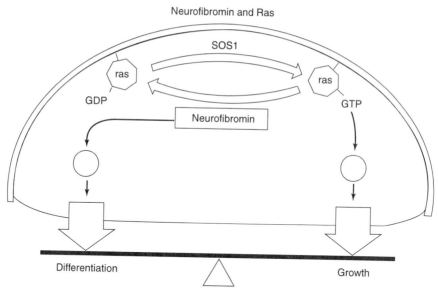

FIGURE 14.3. The interaction between ras and neurofibromin. A simplified cartoon showing the balance between activated, GTP-bound Ras, which is loaded with GTP and guanine nucleotide exchange factors, and inactive, GDP-bound Ras that is generated by neurofibromin action. GDP, guanosine diphosphate; GTP, guanosine triphosphate; SOS1, guanine nucleotide exchange factor.

of normal Ras-GTP to Ras-guanosine diphosphate (GDP) terminates intracellular signaling; thus neurofibromin acts as a negative regulator of the Ras-mediated signal transduction pathway (reviewed in Bernards, 1995). Inactivating mutations of *NF1* lead to increased intracellular signaling through Ras (Fig. 14.3). *RAS* was the first protooncogene identified in the early 1980s, and a specific missense mutation that prevents the conversion of Ras-GTP to Ras-GDP is associated with a large number of cancers.

Mutations in the *NF1* gene (Upadhyaya et al., 1995) generally predict inactivation of its gene product, neurofibromin, which results in cells that are haploinsufficient, i.e., they have half the normal amount of intracellular neurofibromin. Complete loss of neurofibromin by somatic mutation of the normal *NF1* allele is seen in neurofibromatosis 1-associated tumors. Given these findings, the *NF1* gene is classified as a "tumor suppressor." This "tumor suppressor" activity results in downregulation of the Ras signal transduction pathway.

The pathogenesis of neurofibromatosis 1 is not completely understood. The tumor phenotype likely arises as a consequence of abnormal regulation of Ras signaling; however, the other features of neurofibromatosis 1 are not easily explained by the neurofibromin-Ras interaction. A common theme in neurofibromatosis 1 is the apparent neural crest derivation of cells that are most affected by *NF1* mutations. Melanocytes, peripheral sensory nerves, and anterior cranial facial bones fit this paradigm. However, other cell types are clearly affected in neurofibromatosis 1. The skeletal dysplasias, tibial pseudarthrosis, scoliosis, short stature, macrocephaly, and learning disabilities are difficult to reconcile with a neural crest origin. It is likely that neurofibromin plays additional, as yet undefined, biological roles in different cell types. Insight for such roles may come from animal model systems. For example, the *Drosophila* homolog for *NF1* encodes a protein that interacts with a cAMP-adenylate cyclase pathway (Bernards, 1998), and this pathway, in fruit flies, has been implicated in learning problems. Along these lines, bony abnormalities and even café au lait spots, as seen in the overlapping clinical features of the McCune-Albright syndrome, which is caused by mutations in the *GNAS1* gene encoding a G protein, could arise by dysregulation of G protein-cAMP pathways that have yet to be linked to the human *NF1* gene product. Future work may clarify the pathogenesis of the pleiotropic manifestations of neurofibromatosis 1, but presently strategies for the development of rational medical treatment protocols focus on the Ras-neurofibromin signal transduction pathway.

Neurofibromatosis 1 is an autosomal dominant condition. Approximately half of all individuals diagnosed in North American and European neurofibromatosis clinics do not have a family history, which supports the observation that the *NF1* gene has a high germ line mutation rate. This characteristic likely applies to the somatic *NF1* mutation rate and may partially explain the high variability of clinical expression. Somatic mutation leading to double inactivation of *NF1* and loss of intracellular neurofibromin could lead to variable manifestations depending on the timing and cell types harboring both somatic *NF1* mutations and constitutional *NF1* mutations. Likewise, even though neurofibromatosis 1 is almost always fully penetrant in the adult population, those individuals who either have signs of neurofibromatosis 1 localized to body segments or who demonstrate incomplete penetrance could represent cases of mosaicism. It is important to identify such individuals because genetic counseling for individuals who manifest mosaicism must include an estimation of the number of cells affected by an *NF1* mutation and the likelihood of germ line involvement. For example, the chance of a parent who is mosaic for neurofibromatosis 1 to have offspring with generalized neurofibromatosis 1 is much lower than the expected 50% incidence for autosomal dominant disorders.

Diagnostic Testing

Neurofibromatosis 1 is a clinical diagnosis. Strict application of the diagnostic criteria allows practitioners to make the diagnosis in the vast majority of cases. In cases where presymptomatic or prenatal diagnosis is desired, either linkage analysis or direct gene mutation analysis has been helpful. Families with two or more affected individuals can use linkage analysis to confidently identify carriers of the abnormal *NF1* gene. The intragenic markers are highly informative and can usually establish the affected chromosome within pedigrees. Sporadic cases would require direct mutation analysis if presymptomatic testing were desired. There are only rare instances where clinical judgment cannot determine the affected status of an individual. In such cases, a protein truncation test has been applied to screen for an *NF1* mutation (Heim et al., 1995). The protein truncation test uses RNA from the patient's white blood cells to amplify segments of the expressed gene that serve as the template for in vitro transcription and translation of peptide products that reflect the genetic code of expressed *NF1* alleles. The peptides are screened for premature truncation of translation by polyacrylamide gel electrophoresis. Those peptides that migrate abnormally indicate an underlying mutation in the *NF1* gene. Presently, this is performed as a screening test, and it identifies variant peptide bands in approximately 70% of individuals with known neurofibromatosis 1 by application of the diagnostic criteria. The test itself does not determine the actual DNA mutation, only the observation of abnormally migrating peptide bands by the protein truncation test. Other protocols must be applied to ascertain the *NF1* mutation at the genomic DNA level. Even though the protein truncation test is the best molecular screening test available, it is not clear what percentage of mutations are detected in those who do not fulfill the diagnostic criteria for neurofibromatosis 1. Prenatal screening using the protein truncation test is not currently available in the United States, although one of the most common requests for molecular testing is for prenatal diagnosis of a fetus conceived by a parent who is a sporadic case. Thus the utility of diagnostic testing by molecular means in the clinical setting is somewhat limited (Viskochil, 1999). As preimplantation selection of in vitro blastocysts becomes available in medical practice, there may be an increased demand for direct DNA analysis in parents with neurofibromatosis 1.

In addition to the protein truncation test, fluorescence *in situ* hybridization (FISH) has been applied to screen individuals with neurofibromatosis 1 for a microdeletion of chromosome 17q11.2. If an affected individual is cognitively impaired, practitioners should consider the possibility that the *NF1* mutation is a deletion of the entire *NF1* gene and contiguous genes (Carey and Viskochil, 1999). This may carry implications for clinical management because individuals with large submicroscopic deletions tend to have mental retardation and an increased tumor burden. Approximately 5% of individuals with neurofibromatosis 1 have whole-gene deletions. A microdeletion can be detected by high-resolution banding karyotype analysis followed by FISH using an assortment of well-defined intragenic *NF1* probes.

Differential Diagnosis

There are a number of clinical conditions that should be considered as part of the diagnostic evaluation of neurofibromatosis 1. Overlap of neurofibromatosis 1 with other conditions primarily lies in cutaneous features, especially café au lait macules. Café au lait spots are commonly seen in Russell-Silver (see Chapter 20), Bloom, Noonan (see Chapter 15), Watson, multiple lentigines/LEOPARD, Sotos (see Chapter 23) and Proteus syndromes and less frequently in Dubowitz, Klippel-Trenaunay-Weber, ataxia-telangiectasia, and Carney syndromes. The cutaneous manifestations of epidermal nevus and bathing trunk nevus syndromes, including

elements of schwannoma and/or neurofibroma on biopsy, can overlap with segmental (or mosaic) neurofibromatosis 1. The pigmentary changes in McCune-Albright syndrome can be difficult to distinguish from the café au lait spots of neurofibromatosis 1. In general, neurofibromatosis 1 café au lait spots have uniform and regular borders that typically involve the flanks in addition to other sites in the body. The café au lait spots in McCune-Albright syndrome tend to be more pigmented and irregular in shape, and they tend to be arrayed centrally in a patchy configuration. A history of long-bone fractures or endocrine anomalies should alert one to the possibility of McCune-Albright syndrome, and endocrine studies plus skeletal survey radiographs should enable one to distinguish McCune-Albright syndrome from neurofibromatosis 1. Other cutaneous manifestations that are difficult at times to sort out from neurofibromatosis 1 include lentigines or wide-spread freckling patterns, especially in individuals with fair complexions, urticaria pigmentosa, and multiple xanthogranulomas.

The neurofibromatosis 1 tumor phenotype overlaps with a number of hamartomatous syndromes including Bannayan-Riley-Ruvalcaba syndrome, Carney syndrome, Proteus syndrome, Maffucci syndrome, multiple endocrine neoplasia 2B, von Hippel-Lindau syndrome, multiple lipomatosis, Gardner (familial adenomatous polyposis) syndrome, and schwannomatosis. As part of the evaluation of these hamartomatous conditions, histological identification of tumor biopsy specimens can be invaluable as an aid to the syndrome diagnosis. This is especially true when evaluating the likelihood that a relative with "bumps" has neurofibromatosis 1. A rare condition that has few neurofibromatosis 1 features and is allelic to *NF1* in some pedigrees is familial spinal neurofibromatosis (Pulst et al., 1991; Poyhonen et al., 1997; Ars et al., 1998). Individuals have multiple paraspinal neurofibromas but lack the other, more common features of neurofibromatosis

1. Care must be used in determining whether these paraspinal tumors are neurofibromas versus schwannomas, which are a major feature of neurofibromatosis type 2 and multiple schwannomatosis.

Few conditions have overlap with skeletal manifestations of neurofibromatosis 1. There are case reports of individuals with McCune-Albright syndrome who have poor healing of long-bone fractures that fit a similar pattern to pseudarthrosis in neurofibromatosis 1. Patients with Jaffe-Campanacci syndrome have multiple nonossifying fibromas and café au lait spots; however, they do not have other specific neurofibromatosis 1 manifestations. Dysplastic scoliosis and sphenoid wing dysplasia are somewhat unique to neurofibromatosis 1.

There are a few families that have multiple café au lait macules that are inherited as an autosomal dominant trait with no other manifestations of neurofibromatosis 1. Some of these families are linked to the *NF1* locus and presumably carry an *NF1* mutation, whereas in a few families linkage to *NF1* has been excluded (Abeliovich et al., 1995; Charrow et al., 1993; Brunner et al., 1993). Watson syndrome (Watson, 1967) is characterized by pulmonic stenosis, multiple café au lait spots, and low normal intelligence. Other manifestations of neurofibromatosis 1 such as Lisch nodules, short stature, neurofibromas, and axillary freckling occur less frequently (Allanson et al., 1991). *NF1* mutations have been identified in Watson and LEOPARD syndrome patients (Tassabehji et al., 1993; Wu et al., 1996). Likewise, a family with multiple café au lait spots, short stature, pulmonic stenosis, and Noonan syndrome-like facial features has been shown to harbor a 3-bp deletion in the *NF1* gene (Carey et al., 1998). The overlap of café au lait spots, pulmonary valve dysplasia, and developmental delay seen in Watson and Noonan syndromes, combined with the variability of clinical expression of neurofibromatosis 1, suggests that biological pathways may share components that are encoded by the Noonan syndrome and *NF1* genes.

Finally, the differential diagnosis of neurofibromatosis 1 also includes neurofibromatosis 2 and segmental neurofibromatosis. The distinction between neurofibromatosis 1 and neurofibromatosis 2 was first recognized by Gardner & Frazier (1930) and fully separated as central as opposed to peripheral neurofibromatosis in 1981 (Eldridge, 1981). Lisch nodules and axillary freckling are never seen in neurofibromatosis 2. The café au lait spots sometimes seen in neurofibromatosis 2 are usually less than 6 in number and tend to be more plaque-like. Small dermal tumors are occasionally seen in neurofibromatosis 2 and, without biopsy, are sometimes interpreted as neurofibromas. The intracranial tumors of neurofibromatosis 2 are usually easily differentiated from neurofibromatosis 1-related findings, although optic nerve meningiomas are sometimes confused with optic pathway tumors. The distinct features of neurofibromatosis 2 include hearing loss associated with vestibular schwannomas, multiple intraspinal schwannomas, posterior lenticular cataracts, and multiple meningiomas. There is minimal clinical overlap between neurofibromatosis 1 and neurofibromatosis 2, and there should be no confusion about the appropriate diagnosis. Furthermore, a confusing issue for many families with an affected family member with neurofibromatosis 1 is the question regarding the progression of neurofibromatosis 1 to neurofibromatosis 2. Neurofibromatosis 1 never progresses to neurofibromatosis 2. These are two very distinct conditions whose genes map to different loci, chromosomes 17q and 22q, respectively, and encode proteins that are involved in two distinct intracellular biochemical pathways.

Segmental neurofibromatosis likely represents a mosaic pattern of neurofibromatosis 1, whereby only localized expression of neurofibromatosis 1 manifestations is seen (Viskochil and Carey, 1994; Hager et al., 1997). Parents of children with generalized neurofibromatosis 1 should be closely evaluated for signs of segmental neurofibromatosis, which, if present, would indicate potential germ line involvement and an increased recurrence risk for subsequent children (Zlotogora, 1998). The empiric recurrence risk for a sibling of an affected child from a parent who has localized expression of neurofibromatosis has not been firmly established but is likely below 3%.

MANIFESTATIONS AND MANAGEMENT

Anticipatory guidance counseling in neurofibromatosis 1 is important for a number of reasons. Individuals with neurofibromatosis 1 should be placed on a surveillance program for related manifestations that are not otherwise obvious. An example of the effectiveness of this surveillance program lies in the diagnosis of optic pathway tumors. The recognition of neurofibromatosis 1 signifies a need for periodic ophthalmologic evaluations that may not otherwise be performed. Clearly, the benefits of anticipatory guidance counseling also encompass manifestations that are not included in the diagnostic criteria. Table 14.3 lists the age-related concerns of neurofibromatosis 1 that need to be woven into the anticipatory guidance process (Table 14.4). Even if a diagnosis of neurofibromatosis 1 has not been conclusively

established, recognition of its possibility may affect clinical management decisions. Thus anticipatory guidance should be provided in all circumstances, even where the diagnosis of neurofibromatosis 1 is only suspected.

Growth and Feeding

In general, there are no consistent prenatal complications associated with neurofibromatosis 1. Fetuses of mothers with neurofibromatosis 1 could suffer consequences of high blood pressure because of pregnancy-induced hypertension. Otherwise, no complications would be expected. Neonates with neurofibromatosis 1 are generally delivered at term and have normal intrauterine growth. Postnatal growth retardation is seen in approximately one-third of children with neurofibromatosis 1, and relative macrocephaly is common. The etiologies of relative macrocephaly and short stature are not understood. A few individuals with neurofibromatosis 1 have large stature. Precocious puberty and large stature are usually associated with optic pathway tumors involving the chiasm. Disproportionate growth of the extremities is generally associated with plexiform neurofibromas; however, some individuals with a large gene deletion have somewhat large and fleshy distal extremities. Feeding is not an issue in this condition and usually weight-to-height ratios are normal.

TABLE 14.3. List of Manifestations of Neurofibromatosis 1 That Have Age-Dependent Clinical Expression

Café-au-lait macules	Infancy to early childhood
Intertriginous freckling	Childhood
Dermal neurofibromas	Late childhood and adolescence through adulthood
Plexiform neurofibroma	Infancy through adulthood
Lisch nodules	Late childhood through adulthood
Optic pathway tumors	Early childhood
Sphenoid wing dysplasia	Infancy
Long-bone bowing	Infancy
Scoliosis	Childhood
Hypertension	Childhood through adulthood
Learning disabilities	Early childhood through adolescence
Nerve sheath tumors	Adolescence through adulthood

TABLE 14.4. Anticipatory Guidance for Neurofibromatosis 1

Newborn to 2 years

Café-au-lait spots for diagnosis
Long-bone bowing
Plexiform neurofibromas
Optic pathway tumor
Development delay assessment

2–10 years

Optic pathway tumors
Plexiform neurofibromas
Scoliosis
Hypertension
Freckling patterns
Learning problems

10 years to Adulthood

Onset of dermal neurofibromas
Learning problems
Self-esteem
Scoliosis
Plexiform neurofibromas
Reproductive decisions
Hypertension

Adult

Offspring
Progression of dermal neurofibromas
Malignant peripheral nerve sheath tumors
Hypertension
Plexiform neurofibromas

Evaluation

- Growth charts specifically for neurofibromatosis 1 (Friedman et al., 1999; Clementi et al., 1999) prove helpful in determining the etiology of short stature. An increase or decrease in growth velocity should alert practitioners to an intracranial process that should be addressed.

Treatment

- Presently, there is no approved treatment for short stature in neurofibromatosis 1. Growth hormone treatment trials have not been conducted. There is some concern that growth hormone could affect Ras-signal transduction, and additional stimulatory signals in cells that are haploinsufficient for a "tumor suppressor," neurofibromin, could lay the foundation for increased tumor burden in neurofibromatosis 1. This unaddressed biologic concern precludes the administration of growth hormone until more information is available.

- Precocious puberty and large stature are routinely treated with luteinizing hormone releasing hormone analogs.

Development and Behavior

Mental retardation is not a common finding in neurofibromatosis 1, yet the incidence of frank mental retardation (full scale IQ < 70) is estimated between 4 and 8% (North et al., 1997), which is higher than the background population. Those individuals with a large *NF1* deletion (~5% of the screened neurofibromatosis 1 population) seem to be more developmentally delayed than expected. This association could represent a significant component of the increased incidence of intellectual impairment associated with this condition. The size of the deletion is usually 1.2 megabases and likely contains contiguous genes that, when deleted, contribute to the clinical manifestations, including cognitive impairment. Genes immediately bordering *NF1* have not been characterized; however, like many contiguous gene syndromes, expression of such genes will likely be found in brain. If so, haploinsufficiency could play a major role in the developmental delay seen in individuals with the microdeletion.

In contrast to mental retardation, learning disabilities are very common and affect approximately 40–60% of individuals with neurofibromatosis 1 (North et al., 1997; Ozonoff, 1999). The nature of learning difficulties experienced by children with neurofibromatosis 1 is not unique. There is no well-characterized learning disability profile that can be used to establish a broad-based and consistent approach for educators who are working with affected individuals. Affected children have a mixed pattern of learning difficulties including impairment of both verbal and nonverbal skills.

The management of potential learning problems is one of the primary reasons to consider the diagnosis of neurofibromatosis 1 in early childhood, before many other age-dependent signs arise. The lack of a diagnosis of neurofibromatosis 1 may hinder access to specialized neuropsychometric testing and school services. A provisional diagnosis, based solely on multiple café au lait spots or another singular manifestation of neurofibromatosis 1, may be helpful for some families to obtain services. Clearly, individuals with neurofibromatosis 1 can, and do, have normal intellectual function, which requires no intervention; however, there is a significant portion of adults with neurofibromatosis 1 who easily recall the school performance problems they faced in their formative education. Although not substantiated, a number of adults have stated that their learning problems improve with age (personal observation). This is in contrast to diminished cognitive function in other genetic conditions that often worsen rather than improve with age. For individuals with neurofibromatosis 1, age-related improvements in learning problems can generally be expected; however, those who have a large deletion have a more guarded prognosis for cognitive development.

A consistent behavioral pattern has not been firmly established in individuals with neurofibromatosis 1. However, some individuals may be impulsive and misinterpret social cues. Failure to recognize problems with either behavior or self-esteem may interfere with their full achievement of potential abilities.

Evaluation

- Preschool developmental and behavioral testing may help both in school placement and in teacher awareness for children who do not have mental retardation but, by virtue of having neurofibromatosis 1, are at risk for school achievement problems.

- Each affected individual seems to have a unique cognitive profile; therefore, it is imperative that complete batteries of neuropsychological testing be performed for educational purposes. Important considerations for testing include visual-spatial-perceptual skills, language function, neuromotor skills, phonological decoding skills and lexical retrieval for reading disability, and achievement testing for nonverbal learning disability. In addition, executive function skills associated with planning, attention, organization, and self-monitoring behaviors deserve more assessment in the identification of educational needs of children with neurofibromatosis 1 (Ozonoff 1999).

- For those individuals with neurofibromatosis 1 who appear cognitively impaired, the primary care provider should consider the possibility of deletion of the entire gene and order karyotype analysis with a FISH study for a gene deletion.

Treatment

- Appropriate school placement for the disabilities identified should be ensured, with aides if necessary.

- Self-esteem issues should be dealt with in childhood, even if physical manifestations are minimal. As teenagers develop physically distinctive signs of neurofibromatosis 1, they are potentially more vulnerable than their peers, especially if they are struggling in school with learning problems. It is incumbent on primary care providers to prepare the family and the child for this possibility.

- An educational environment developed within a structured organizational framework that has consistent rules and reinforcement of socialization skills may be extremely beneficial.

- Medication for impulsivity, distractibility, and mood disorders is not contraindicated by virtue of the child having neurofibromatosis 1, and judicious medical management of attention deficit and hyperactivity conditions is recommended. Presently, treatment strategies should be the same as for individuals in the general population with similar problems.

- Support groups and camp experiences are two options that families may wish to consider in the mobilization of services that may be beneficial in the social management of affected adolescents.

Tumors

Neurofibromas. Neurofibromas are one of the hallmark findings of neurofibromatosis 1. They usually develop by adulthood, and they are progressive in number and size. The progressive nature has been well-documented in a population study conducted in southeast Wales, which scored individuals with neurofibromatosis 1 for the number of dermal neurofibromas by age in decades (Huson et al., 1989). There were few neurofibromas in children less than 10 years, whereas individuals older than 50 years invariably had hundreds. As benign cellular proliferations, they are comprised of Schwann cells and fibroblasts, and there is a generous amount of extracellular matrix, mostly comprised of collagen. Neurofibromas originate from the cutaneous sensory nerves, large motor nerve sheaths, spinal nerve roots and ganglia, and spinal cord plexi. They are exclusively found in the peripheral nervous system.

There are two major neurofibroma tumor categories, dermal neurofibromas and plexiform neurofibromas. Dermal neurofibromas are either cutaneous or subcutaneous, and the cutaneous tumors can be sessile or pedunculated. They tend to be relatively small, dis-

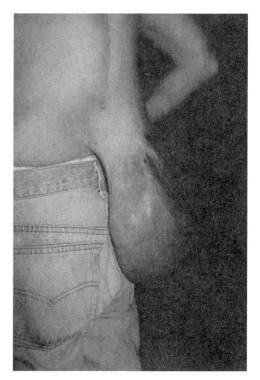

FIGURE 14.4. Plexiform neurofibroma.

crete nodules that are easily defined by virtue of a fibrous capsule and skin surface presentation. Plexiform neurofibromas tend to be large, amorphous tumors that arise from large nerve sheaths (Fig. 14.4). They can originate from anywhere in the peripheral nervous system and tend to have spurts of growth that do not always coincide with overall body growth. Because many of the plexiform neurofibromas arise from nerve sheaths, they tend to remain below the skin surface and are initially identified by palpation or visual recognition of asymmetry and unusual overlying pigmentary and hair patterns. The etiology and pathogenesis of neurofibromas are not understood; however, a large percentage of tumors have been shown to harbor somatic *NF1* mutations (Serra et al., 1997). This implies that lower levels of intracellular neurofibromin are likely a necessary, albeit insufficient, step in the development of neurofibromas.

Dermal neurofibromas are found in virtually all adults with neurofibromatosis 1. They typically arise in the teenage years and progressively increase in number throughout life. Even though they are usually asymptomatic, some tumors tend to itch and they can be painful if located at sites of irritation or pressure, such as belt or bra lines. Dermal neurofibromas are always benign. They never transform to a malignant phenotype. To some extent, dermal neurofibromas are of cosmetic concern; however, they rarely cause medical problems unless they enlarge as pedunculated tumors or become infected and/or inflamed. Spurts of neurofibroma growth, both in size and numbers, coincide with puberty and pregnancy; however, intermittent growth persists as dermal neurofibromas progressively arise throughout life. The hormonal milieu that causes these growth spurts is not known, but estrogen effects do not seem to account for the pathological growth because there is not a significant change in neurofibroma development or growth for individuals who are either on low-dose birth control medication or are postmenopausal.

Plexiform neurofibromas are found in approximately 25% of all individuals with neurofibromatosis 1, and they tend to present earlier in life, even at birth. These tumors are usually solitary and tend to become somewhat quiescent in older age. Periods of rapid tumor growth are followed by long periods of no growth; however, it is not clear what promotes their cellular proliferation. Plexiform neurofibromas can be a cause of morbidity by virtue of their location and size. Facial and orbitotemporal plexiform neurofibromas affect approximately 1–5% of individuals with neurofibromatosis 1, and they tend to involve the skin surface and underlying vascularity. As space-occupying lesions, internal plexiform neurofibromas can impinge on vital organs. They are also associated with bony overgrowth, hemihyperplasia, and scoliosis.

Plexiform neurofibromas purportedly have the capacity to undergo malignant transformation. This is most notable in long-standing, benign-appearing plexiform tumors that undergo rapid growth with associated pain. Malignant peripheral nerve sheath tumors (sometimes inappropriately called neurofibrosarcomas or malignant schwannomas) arise in approximately 2–4% of individuals with neurofibromatosis 1, and almost half of these tumors reported in the United States are found in patients with neurofibromatosis 1. This propensity for malignant transformation of a small percentage of plexiform neurofibromas warrants diligence in monitoring the growth and associated symptoms of these tumors. Because plexiform neurofibromas are unpredictable, the decision to surgically excise a tumor is one for a soft-tissue tumor oncology team to determine. A currently ongoing natural history study by volumetric MRI of different plexiform neurofibromas in different age groups over a 3-year period might provide more details regarding prognosis (personal communication, B Korf, 1999). Plexiform neurofibromas that undergo malignant transformation portend a poor prognosis with a 5-year survival of less than 50%.

Optic Nerve Pathway Tumors. Approximately 15% of individuals with neurofibromatosis 1 have a glioma involving the optic nerve pathway, and half of these tumors are symptomatic. They tend to arise in the toddler or early childhood years. Symptoms include loss of visual acuity, decreased field of view, agitation, and behavioral changes. Signs of optic pathway glioma include proptosis, strabismus, optic nerve pallor, and increased optic disk fullness. These tumors are always low grade; however, this cellular proliferation of type II astrocytes can impinge on the optic nerve as well as interfere with the hypothalamic-pituitary axis. A unique observation of neurofibromatosis 1-associated optic pathway gliomas is the lack of invasiveness as compared with non-neurofibromatosis 1 gliomas.

Optic nerve pathway tumors in neurofibromatosis 1 are not malignant; however, there may be loss of vision and/or precocious puberty. Secondary effects of radiation therapy, if administered to control tumor growth, can be very pronounced with fibrotic changes involving the hypothalamic-pituitary axis. Optic pathway tumors rarely develop after the childhood years, and a lower incidence in African-American and Asian populations suggests that there may be significant ethnic differences with respect to optic pathway tumors.

Cancer. The actual incidence of cancer in individuals with neurofibromatosis 1 is not available because of bias of ascertainment. In a Danish cohort study (Sorenson et al., 1986), an increased relative risk for malignancy in individuals with neurofibromatosis 1 was ascertained in a hospital-based setting (relative risk = 4.0) versus their relatives with neurofibromatosis 1 who were ascertained by virtue of their relationship to the proband (relative risk = 1.5). Other surveys of cancer in children with neurofibromatosis 1 also indicate an elevated relative risk for extremely rare tumors that are likewise quite rare in the neurofibromatosis 1 population. The major tumor types associated with neurofibromatosis 1 include gliomas, malignant peripheral nerve sheath tumors, rhabdomyosarcomas, myeloproliferative and myelodysplastic leukemia, and pheochromocytoma. There are a smattering of other case reports of rare malignancies, but, clearly, patients with neurofibromatosis 1 do not have a higher likelihood of developing the more common cancers of the prostate, breast, and colon. Melanoma and basal cell carcinomas are also not increased.

The link with oncogenic Ras would suggest that patients with neurofibromatosis 1 should be predisposed to other cancers that have *RAS* mutations; however, the only shared tumor type between inactivating *NF1* and activating *RAS* mutations is the relatively rare juvenile chronic myelogenous leukemia. Even though few children with neurofibromatosis 1 develop juvenile chronic myelogenous leukemia, there is a clear association. Approximately 10% of children who have this leukemia also have neurofibromatosis 1, and boys who inherit neurofibromatosis 1 from their mothers appear at highest risk. This malignancy clearly demonstrates the important role of the Ras-neurofibromin pathway in specific myelogenous stem cells. Individuals who have juvenile chronic myelogenous leukemia but not neurofibromatosis 1 generally have an oncogenic *RAS* mutation, whereas those individuals with neurofibromatosis 1 have inactivation of both *NF1* alleles with concomitant deregulation of Ras signaling in myelocytic stem cells (Side et al., 1997). This observation does not hold true for other tumors that harbor oncogenic *RAS* mutations. One might predict that either activation of *RAS* or inactivation of *NF1* could lead to tumor development; however, tumors with the highest incidence of *RAS* mutations (i.e., bladder cancer) are not typically seen in neurofibromatosis 1. This implies that the "tumor suppressor" function of neurofibromin is more complex than simply downregulating Ras.

The prognosis for low-grade central nervous system glioma in neurofibromatosis 1 is predictably good. In general, low-grade gliomas in individuals with neurofibromatosis 1 tend to grow at a slower pace than histologically similar tumors from individuals without neurofibromatosis 1. Sequential scans can be very helpful in determining treatment. Neurosurgery teams are inclined to follow such tumors in asymptomatic individuals with neurofibromatosis 1 rather than recommending surgical intervention.

Low-grade malignant peripheral nerve sheath tumors have a relatively good prognosis, which is even better if the surgical margins are clear of malignancy. On the other hand, high-grade malignant peripheral nerve sheath tumors harbor a poor prognosis. Individuals with juvenile chronic myelogenous leukemia, with and without monosomy 7, also have a poor prognosis. Risk for second malignancies in those treated with radiation and/or chemotherapy (especially alkylating agents) may be higher in the neurofibromatosis 1 population; therefore long-term surveillance is indicated.

Evaluation

- Dermal neurofibromas are visible on skin surfaces and can be monitored for size, vascularity, and inflamation. Dermal neurofibromas do not require imaging.
- Plexiform neurofibromas should be suspected if there is soft tissue asymmetry or unusual skin pigmentary or hair growth patterns. Magnetic resonance imaging is optimal for determination of the extent and position of plexiform neurofibromas. Sequential examinations may be required to gain knowledge about cellular proliferation.
- Vascularity may be important in evaluating plexiform neurofibromas; therefore, magnetic resonance angiography may be beneficial in determining the vascular supply. In surgical cases, embolization of major feeder vessels before surgery has been helpful.
- Ophthalmologic evaluation should occur annually in childhood for both known neurofibromatosis 1 and those provisionally diagnosed with neurofibromatosis 1. This should include field of vision, visual acuity, color vision, direct and indirect fundoscopic exam, slit-lamp examination, and consideration of visual evoked potential (VEP) testing (Listernick et al., 1997).
- Any suspicion of an optic nerve pathway glioma warrants a brain MRI study. The need for intervention should be carefully assessed with the oncology team and includes sequential MRI scans.
- If an optic pathway tumor is asymptomatic, watchful observation and generously spaced brain MRI scans through the teenage years are appropriate.
- If an optic pathway tumor is symptomatic and nonprogressive, appropriate management includes repeating the scan in 3 months, in association with a visual evoked potential study, and ophthalmologic evaluation.
- Precocious puberty in neurofibromatosis 1 is almost always associated with an optic nerve glioma that involves the optic chiasm; therefore, a brain MRI should always be performed when this condition is present.
- Many children with gliomas extensively involving radiation of the optic nerve tract seem to have learning and behavior disabilities (personal observation); therefore, detailed neuropsychometric testing is indicated before, during, and after radiation therapy.
- Clinical history of pain and/or increasing size of a mass is an indication for radiological imaging, usually with MRI, for any tumor. Use of enhancement may help in discerning whether a solid tumor is benign or malignant. Sequential scans should be used to assess interval growth.
- Biopsy of solid tumors that are painful or growing should be obtained. If benign, one should not be reassured but continue close follow-up by imaging and palpation.
- Blood smear and bone marrow study should be used to evaluate those suspected of having juvenile chronic myelogenous leukemia.

Treatment

- Dermal neurofibromas should be surgically resected if they are symptomatic.

Resection should be performed through deep excision by an experienced dermatologist or general surgeon to take the entire neurofibroma. Shave excisions are not recommended.

- If plexiform neurofibromas are symptomatic, or if there is concern about malignant transformation, then they should be widely excised with full knowledge that the entire tumor is likely not resectable without resultant neurological deficit. Embolization of the tumor by arterial injection is sometimes helpful to decrease the vascularity. Ketotofin has also been used as a preoperative medication to decrease bleeding in the surgical field. This agent is not FDA-approved in the United States. Pathological evaluation of the tumor, including inked margins, is essential for all tumors to determine the malignant potential.

- Pathological evaluation of the excised tissue by those experienced in peripheral nerve sheath tumor diagnosis is paramount in decisions regarding treatment protocol selection, specifically, decisions regarding chemotherapy and local radiation therapy. If it is malignant, as noted by cell atypia, necrosis, or elevated mitotic index, then surgical resection can be planned accordingly. Without this information, some presumed benign peripheral nerve sheath tumors could be excised with narrow margins, and, after pathological review, a second surgical procedure may be needed to obtain wider margins around the tumor.

- Early surgical resection for plexiform neurofibromas in the orbitotemporal region should be considered. This may subsequently entail numerous surgical procedures over time; however, this is sometimes preferred to an extensive operation on a large facial plexiform tumor. Referral to plastic surgery and/or ENT subspecialists in reconstructive surgery is recommended.

- There are pilot studies to treat plexiform neurofibromas by chemotherapy. Interferon, retinoic acid, and carboplatin have been used with minimal efficacy. Other agents are under development, and they include antiangiogenesis compounds to decrease new blood vessel formation in an enlarging but nonmalignant tumor and farnesyltransferase inhibitors to decrease Ras signaling.

- Radiation therapy for plexiform neurofibromas is not of proven benefit and may be detrimental.

- If an optic pathway tumor is symptomatic and progressive, current recommendations include implementation of the Pediatric Oncology Group/Childhood Cancer Group (POG/CCG) approved single-drug chemotherapy protocol of carboplatin.

- If an optic pathway tumor progresses on therapy and the affected individual is older than 6 years, external radiation beam therapy is the current recommended treatment.

- Given that neurofibromatosis 1 fits the paradigm of a cancer predisposition syndrome, and the *NF1* gene is considered a "tumor suppressor", there is some concern that children who are treated for malignancies with radiation or chemotherapy may be at higher risk for second tumors. The decision to treat low-grade malignant peripheral nerve sheath tumors or rapidly growing plexiform neurofibromas with other nonsurgical modalities should include recognition of the potential for second malignancies.

- For solid malignant tumors associated with neurofibromatosis 1, especially peripheral nerve sheath tumors, wide surgical excision is recommended. Adjuvant therapy should be determined by grade, stage, and surgical field.

- Low-grade gliomas of the central nervous system can be treated with single-agent chemotherapy instead of surgical excision. Otherwise, surgical resection is the protocol of choice.
- Juvenile chronic myelogenous leukemia may require bone marrow transplant.

Musculoskeletal

Pseudarthrosis. Long bone pseudarthrosis affects approximately 5% of individuals with neurofibromatosis 1 registered with the International Clinical Database of Neurofibromatosis (Stevenson et al., 1999). The tibia is the most common site, and the pseudarthrosis is heralded by a distinctive anterior-lateral bowing infancy (Fig. 14.5). The pseudarthrosis represents a failure of union after fracture. The incidence of fracture is higher in males than females, and the affected status of parents is not prognostic. The bone abnormality that leads to bowing and subsequent fracture is not understood. It is not associated with neurofibroma growth and appears to be a dysplastic process. It is always unilateral, which suggests that somatic mutation plays a role, and the sex difference implies that there may be a biochemical link to embryonic androgen

exposure. The critical time for fracture and poor healing is infancy to early childhood. Bone remodeling and strengthening seems to improve with age, yet fractures beyond the middle childhood years do occur. Fractures that are independent of the dysplastic long bone bowing tend to heal easily. There is no known genotype-phenotype correlation for pseudarthrosis.

Scoliosis. Individuals with neurofibromatosis 1 experience both idiopathic scoliosis and dystrophic scoliosis (Crawford and Schorry, 1999). Dystrophic scoliosis is a short, angular lordotic form that typically spans 4 to 6 vertebral segments. The incidence of scoliosis in neurofibromatosis 1 ranges between 10 and 30%. The dystrophic form can be debilitating.

Even though some cases of dystrophic scoliosis are associated with neurofibromas, both spinal and plexiform, the link to tumor growth is overstated. There appears to be an intrinsic abnormality of bone that is poorly understood. Dystrophic scoliosis presents in early childhood and is progressive, causing significant rotation of the thoracic cage with variable degrees of pulmonary compromise. Evolution of the curvature may take place over a short period of time and requires close monitoring. The idiopathic form of scoliosis

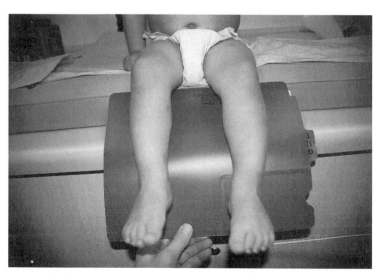

FIGURE 14.5. Anterolateral bowing of the tibia (pseudarthrosis).

in neurofibromatosis 1 is not different from that in the general population; however, it may be difficult at times to distinguish dystrophic segments at an early stage. These segments might account for the poor healing of surgically treated cases of neurofibromatosis 1-associated idiopathic-type long lordoscoliosis. This "induction" of spine worsening by surgical manipulation implies that there is a dysplastic feature of the vertebral bodies in neurofibromatosis 1. In general, orthopedic surgeons recognize the difficulties in managing scoliosis in the context of neurofibromatosis 1, and making the diagnosis before surgical intervention is important (Crawford and Schorry, 1999).

It is difficult to determine the response to therapy in the management of neurofibromatosis 1-associated scoliosis. Each center has only a few cases, each of which is very distinct, and it is difficult to compare procedures between patients. The variability in progression of scoliosis makes prognostic counseling difficult, and one should balance the optimism of surgical correction with the knowledge of the dynamic nature of the neurofibromatosis 1 spine abnormalities.

Evaluation

- A primary concern relating to pseudarthrosis is the early recognition of tibial bowing. The presence of anterolateral bowing on physical examination requires radiologic examination with comparison films of the contralateral limb. Orthopedic referral for long bone bowing management is essential.

- An essential part of the physical examination in neurofibromatosis 1 is assessment for curvature of spine, even in early childhood. Initial spine radiographs, AP and lateral, should be performed in any suspected case of scoliosis. Serial examination is imperative, with close monitoring for dystrophic segments.

- Referral to an orthopedist with proven experience in neurofibromatosis 1 is highly recommended for individuals who are suspected of having scoliosis. Before surgical correction, an MRI of the spine should be performed to identify neurofibromas.

Treatment

- Management of pseudarthrosis is one of the most difficult aspects of neurofibromatosis 1 care and is complex. Standardized orthopedic protocols have not been established (Crawford and Schorry, 1999).

- Early recognition of long bone bowing with the implementation of bracing to prevent fracture is imperative. Bracing is effective and may enable bone to mature to a point at which subsequent fracture is less likely.

- Once there is a fracture, a number of orthopedic procedures can be implemented; however, few are consistently effective. Most protocols focus on stability and provision of adequate blood supply and normal bone transplantation at the site of the fracture (Coleman et al., 1995). Multiple surgeries are typical, and long recuperation periods including use of orthopedic devices can be extremely stressful for families and deleterious for normal development in the child.

- In the event a stable union cannot be maintained, below-the-knee amputation becomes a viable, and sometimes preferred, therapeutic option. Prosthetics for below-the-knee amputations are relatively easy to implement, and they enable children to remain in school and fully engaged in recreational activities. Sometimes the therapeutic option of amputation is not presented by orthopedists; therefore, the primary care provider should review the "whole child," presenting this as an option to consider when multiple surgical procedures for long-term management of lower leg pseudarthrosis are anticipated.

- Conventional bracing is indicated for idiopathic scoliosis.

- The dystrophic form of scoliosis does not respond to back bracing and usually requires early fusion, generally before overall growth is complete. Depending on the degree of kyphosis, there is some operative risk for distal nerve dysfunction and poor union in addition to the possibility of loss of correction. Complete correction is usually not possible; therefore, defining successful outcomes should be clear before surgery.

- Surgical procedures for dystrophic scoliosis involve fusion, both anterior and posterior. Postoperative care, especially pain management and treatment of hypertension, requires close monitoring that can be coordinated between primary care providers and orthopedists.

- Psychosocial stressors in dystrophic scoliosis management should be recognized and addressed. Rehabilitation is a long, arduous process that affects ambulation, recreational participation, and school activities. Even though scoliosis is not unique to neurofibromatosis 1, families should recognize that neurofibromatosis 1-related scoliosis is very different than non-neurofibromatosis 1 scoliosis. Fostering independence, even by providing a wheelchair, is an important activity for the primary health care provider.

Hypertension

There are three primary causes of neurofibromatosis 1-associated hypertension; renovascular disease, tumors that secrete vasoactive compounds, and coarctation of the aorta. However, essential hypertension is still the most common cause of high blood pressure in patients with neurofibromatosis 1, as it is in the general population. Among neurofibromatosis 1-related causes, renovascular disease is the most common etiology, affecting approximately 4% of all patients. The major site of involvement is the renal artery, where it can present either as a fusiform arterial narrowing or an aneurysm. In addition to involving the afferent renal arteries, there can be intrarenal vascular lesions that are difficult to detect by angiography. The pathophysiology of hypertension in renovascular disease in neurofibromatosis 1 manifests as abnormal regulation of the renin-angiotensin pathway. The perception of decreased blood flow to one kidney leads to increased renin secretion, which is usually measurable only by renal vein sampling. The presenting sign of renovascular disease is hypertension; therefore, the success of surgical correction is dependent on the site and degree of involvement. Surgical procedures may not always effectively treat hypertension caused by renovascular disease.

Tumors that cause neurofibromatosis 1-related hypertension include pheochromocytoma and ganglioneuroma. Although these are rare in neurofibromatosis 1, an evaluation of hypertension should, nonetheless, include a complete history addressing headache patterns, tachycardia and palpitations, and gastrointestinal abnormalities. The presence of symptoms of catechol-secreting tumors should direct further diagnostic workup.

Finally, although it is rare, some patients with neurofibromatosis 1 have coarctation of the thoracic aorta that can present with hypertension. Physical examination of pulses and four-limb blood pressures, if abnormal, should lead to a more detailed evaluation for a vascular cause of hypertension.

Long-term prognosis for neurofibromatosis 1-related hypertension is dependent on the underlying etiology and surgical outcome.

Evaluation

- Routine history and physical with blood pressure monitoring should be a part of every visit to the physician and should be performed at least once a year for individuals who either have, or are suspected of having, neurofibromatosis 1. Four-limb blood pressures should be obtained on at least one occasion.

- Abdominal MRI or MRA should be obtained both to pursue suspected vascular abnormalities involving the kidneys and for visualization of adrenal glands in those cases presenting with persistent elevated blood pressure readings or malignant hypertension.
- A 24-hour urine collection should be obtained for catecholamines, homovanillic acid (HVA) and vanillylmandelic acid (VMA), and creatinine to assess secretion by a tumor. Abdominal CT scan is sensitive in identifying some pheochromocytomas. It is not clear how often this study should be performed; however, in cases of persistent hypertension, the likelihood of discovering a catechol-secreting tumor on subsequent urine collections when hypertension was present on initial testing is low.
- Primary consideration should be given to evaluating renovascular disease with angiography in cases where MRA/MRI fails to detect renal vessel anomalies.

Treatment

- Treatment of hypertension depends on the etiology. Consideration should be given to surgical management for vascular and tumor etiologies. The surgical team should include a vascular surgeon, a general surgeon, a radiologist, and a nephrologist.
- Medical therapy is directed at the presumed etiology.
- There should be close monitoring of progression and response to medical management.

RESOURCES

Textbooks and Articles

Ablon J (1999) Living with a genetic disorder. The impact of neurofibromatosis 1. Westport, CT: Auburn House.

Carey JC (1992) Health supervision and anticipatory guidance for children with genetic disorders (including specific recommendations for trisomy 21, trisomy 18, and neurofibromatosis). Pediatr Clin North AM 39:25–53.

Crowe F, Schull W, Neel J (1956) *A Clinical, Pathological, and Genetic Study of Multiple Neurofibromatosis*. Springfield, IL: Thomas, p 1–181.

Friedman JM, Gutmann DH, MacCollin M, Riccardi VM (1999) *Neurofibromatosis: Phenotype, Natural History, and Pathogenesis*. 3rd ed. Baltimore, MD: Johns Hopkins Press.

Huson SM, Hughes RAC (1994) *The Neurofibromatoses: A Pathogenetic and Clinical Overview*. London: Chapman and Hall Medical.

Riccardi V (1992) *Neurofibromatosis: Phenotype, Natural History, and Pathogenesis*. Baltimore, MD: Johns Hopkins University Press.

Rubenstein AE, Korf BR, eds (1990) *Neurofibromatosis: Handbook for Patients, Families, and Health-Care Professionals*. New York: Thieme Medical, 256 pp.

Upadhyaya M, Cooper D (1998) *Neurofibromatosis Type 1: From Genotype to Phenotype*. Oxford: Bios Scientific.

Support Organizations
National Neurofibromatosis Foundation, Inc.

95 Pine St., 16th Floor
New York, NY 10005
Phone: 1-800-323-7938
Fax: 212-747-0004
Web page: *www.nf.org*

Neurofibromatosis, Inc.

8855 Annapolis Road, Suite #110
Lanham, MD 20706-2924
Phone: 1-800-942-6825
Web page: *www.nfinc.org*

The Neurofibromatosis Foundation

United Kingdom
Phone: 0181-547-1636
Web page: *www.nfa.zetnet.co.uk*

Neurofibromatosis Association of Australia, Inc.

Phone: 02 9628 5044
Email: *R.Pynor@echs.usyd.edu.au*

There are numerous local support groups that are affiliated with national organizations. Likewise, many neurofibromatosis multidisciplinary clinics are located in many academic institutions worldwide. Educational materials have been published from many of the organizations, and neurofibromatosis summer camps have been sponsored by national and international organizations, including the Belgium support organization (Association Belge pour personnes atteintes de la neurofibromatose, phone: 32.3.766.13.41), the National Neurofibromatosis Foundation, and the Texas NF Foundation.

REFERENCES

Abeliovich D, Gelman-Kohan Z, Silverstien S, Lerer I, Chemke J, Merin S, Zlotogora J (1995) Familial café au lait spots: A variant of neurofibromatosis type 1. *J Med Genet* 32:985–386.

Allanson JE, Upadhyaya M, Watson G, Partington M, MacKenzie A, Lahey D, Macleod H, Sarfarazi M, Broadhead W, Harper P, Huson SH (1991) Watson syndrome: Is it a subtype of type 1 neurofibromatosis? *J Med Genet* 28:752–356.

Ars E, Kruyer H, Gaona A, Casquero P, Rosell J, Volpini V, Serra E, Lazaro C, Estivill X (1998) A clinical variant of neurofibromatosis type 1: Familial spinal neurofibromatosis with a frameshift mutation in the *NF1* gene. *Am J Hum Genet* 62:834–341.

Barker D, Wright E, Nguyen K, Cannon L, Fain P, Goldgar D, Bishop D, Carey J, Baty B, Kivlin J, Willard H, Waye J, Greig G, Leinwald L, Nakamura Y, O'Connell P, Leppert M, Lalouel J,

White R, Scolnick M (1987) Gene for von Recklinghausen neurofibromatosis is in the pericentric region of chromosome 17. *Science* 236:1100–3102.

Bernards A (1995) Neurofibromatosis type 1 and Ras-mediated signaling: Filling in the GAPs. *Biochim Biophys Acta* 1242:43–59.

Bernards A (1998) Evolutionary comparisons. In: *Neurofibromatosis Type 1: From Genotype to Phenotype,* Upadhyaya M and Cooper DN, eds. Oxford: Bios Scientific.

Brunner HG, Hulsebos T, Stiejlen PM, der Kinderen DJ, Steen A, Hamel BCJ (1993) Exclusion of the neurofibromatosis 1 locus in a family with inherited café au lait spots. *Am J Med Genet* 46:472–374.

Carey J, Viskochil D (1999) Neurofibromatosis type 1: A model condition for the study of the molecular basis of variable expressivity in human disorders. *Am J Med Genet* 89:7-13.

Carey JC (1992) Health supervision and anticipatory guidance for children with genetic disorders (including specific recommendations for trisomy 21, trisomy 18, and neurofibromatosis). *Pediatr Clin North AM* 39:25–53.

Carey J, Baty B, Johnson J, Morrison T, Skolnick M, Kivlin J (1986) The genetic aspects of neurofibromatosis. *Ann NY Acad Sci* 486:45–52.

Carey JC, Stevenson DA, Ota M, Neil S, Viskochil DH (1998) Is there a NF/Noonan syndrome? II. Documentation of the clinical and molecular aspects of an important family. *Proc Greenwood Genet Ctr* 17:52–53.

Charrow J, Listernick R, Ward K (1993) Autosomal dominant multiple café au lait spots and neurofibromatosis-1: Evidence of non-linkage. *Am J Med Genet* 45:606–608.

Clementi M, Milani S, Mammi I, Boni S, Monciotti C, Tenconi R (1999) Neurofibromatosis type 1 growth charts. *Am J Med Genet* 87:317–323.

Coleman S, Coleman D, Biddulph G (1995) Congenital pseudarthrosis of the tibia: Current concepts of treatment. *Adv Operative Orthop* 3:121–145.

Crawford A, Schorry E (1999) Neurofibromatosis in children: The role of the orthopaedist. *J Am Acad Orthop Surg* 7:217–230.

Crowe F, Schull W, Neel J (1956) *A Clinical, Pathological, and Genetic Study of Multiple Neurofibromatosis.* Springfield IL: Thomas, p 1–181.

Eldridge R (1981) Central neurofibromatosis. *Adv Neurol* 29:57–65.

Friedman JM, Birch PH (1997) Type 1 neurofibromatosis: A descriptive analysis of the disorder in 1,728 patients. *Am J Med Genet* 70:138–143.

Friedman JM, Gutmann DH, MacCollin M, Riccardi VM (1999) *Neurofibromatosis: Phenotype, Natural History, and Pathogenesis*, 3rd ed. Baltimore, MD: Johns Hopkins Press.

Gardner WJ and Frazier GH (1930) Bilateral acoustic neurofibromas: A clinical study and field survey of a family of five generations with bilateral deafness in 28 members. *Arch Neurol Psychiatry* 23:266–300.

Gutmann DH, Aylsworth A, Carey J, Korf B, Marks J, Pyeritz RE, Rubenstein A, Viskochil D (1997) The diagnostic evaluation and multi-disciplinary management of neurofibromatosis 1 and neurofibromatosis 2. *JAMA* 278:51–57.

Hager CM, Cohen PR, Tschen JA (1997) Segmental neurofibromatosis: Case reports and review. *J Am Acad Dermatol* 37:864–869.

Heim RA, Kam-Morgan LNW, Binnie CG, Corns DD, Cayouette MC, Farber RA, Aylsworth AS, Silverman LM, Luce MC (1995) Distribution of 13 truncating mutations in the neurofibromatosis 1 gene. *Hum Mol Genet* 4:975–981.

Huson S, Clark D, Compston D, Harper P (1989) A genetic study of von Recklinghausen neurofibromatosis in South East Wales. I. Prevalence, fitness, mutation rate and effect of parental transmission on severity. *J Med Genet* 26:704–711.

Huson SM, Hughes RAC (1994) *The Neurofibromatoses: a Pathogenetic and Clinical Overview.* London: Chapman and Hall Medical.

Korf BR (1992) Diagnostic outcome in children with multiple café au lait spots. *Pediatrics* 90:924–927.

Korf BR (1999) Plexiform neurofibromas. *Am J Med Genet* 89:31–37.

Listernick R, Louis D, Packer R, Gutmann D (1997) Optic pathway gliomas in children with neurofibromatosis 1: Consensus statement from the NF1 optic pathway glioma task force. *Ann Neurol* 41:143–149.

Martin G, Viskochil D, Bollag G, McCabe P, Cosier W, Haubruck H, Conroy L, Clark R, O'Connell P, Cawthon R, Innis M, McCormick F (1990) The GAP-related domain of the *NF1* gene product interacts with ras p21. *Cell* 63:843–849.

National Institute of Health Consensus Development Conference (1988) Neurofibromatosis: Conference statement. *Arch Neurol* 45:575–578.

North KN, Riccardi V, Samango-Sprouse C, Ferner R, Moore B, Legius E, Ratner N, Denckla MB (1997) Cognitive function and academic performance in neurofibromatosis 1: Consensus statement from the NF1 cognitive disorders task force. *Neurology* 48:1121–1127.

Ozonoff S (1999) Learning disorders in neurofibromatosis type 1 (NF1). *Am J Hum Genet* 89:45–52.

Poyhonen M, Leisti E-L, Kytölä S, Leisti J (1997) Hereditary spinal neurofibromatosis: A rare form of NF1? *J Med Genet* 34:184–187.

Pulst S, Riccardi V, Fain P, Korenberg J (1991) Familial spinal neurofibromatosis: Clinical and DNA linkage analysis. *Neurology* 41:1923–1927.

Riccardi V (1992) *Neurofibromatosis: Phenotype, Natural History, and Pathogenesis.* Baltimore, MD: Johns Hopkins University Press.

Rubenstein AE, Korf BR, eds (1990) *Neurofibromatosis: Handbook for Patients, Families, and Health-Care Professionals.* New York: Thieme Medical, 256 pp.

Serra E, Otero D, Gaona A, Kruyer H, Ars E, Estivill X, Lazaro C (1997) Confirmation of a double-hit model for the *NF1* gene in benign neurofibromas. *Am J Hum Genet* 61:512–519

Sherman L, Daston M, Ratner N (1998) Neurofibromin: Distribution, cell biology, and role in neurofibromatosis type 1. In: *Neurofibromatosis Type 1: From Genotype to Phenotype,* Upadhyaya M and Bios Scientific. Cooper DN, eds. Oxford.

Side L, Taylor B, Cayoutte M, Connor E, Thompson P, Luce M, Shannon K (1997) Homozygous inactivation of *NF1* in the bone marrows of children with neurofibromatosis type1 and malignant myeloid disorders. *New Eng J Med* 336:1713–1720.

Sorenson SA, Mulvihill JJ, Nielsen A (1986) Long-term follow-up of von Recklinghausen neurofibromatosis: Survival and malignant neoplasms. *New Engl J Med* 314:1010–1015.

Stevenson DA, Birch PH, Friedman JM, Viskochil DH, Balestrazzi P, Boni S, Buske A, Korf BR, Niimura M, Pivnick EK, Schorry EK, Short MP, Tenconi R, Tonsgard JH, Carey JC (1999) Descriptive analysis of tibial pseudarthrosis in patients with neurofibromatosis 1. *Am J Med Genet* 84:413–419.

Tassabehji M, Strachan T, Sharland M, Colley A, Donnai D, Harris R, Thakker N (1993) Tandem duplication within a neurofibromatosis type 1 (*NF1*) gene exon in a family with features of Watson syndrome and Noonan syndrome. *Am J Hum Genet* 53:90–95.

Upadhyaya M, Cooper D, eds. (1998) *Neurofibromatosis Type 1: From Genotype to Phenotype.* Oxford: Bios Scientific.

Upadhyaya M, Maynard J, Osborn M, Huson S, Ponder M, Ponder B, Harper P (1995) Characterization of germline mutations in the neurofibromatosis type 1 (*NF1*) gene. *J Med Genet* 32:706–710.

Viskochil D and Carey J (1994) Alternate and related forms of the neurofibromatoses. In: *The Neurofibromatoses: A Pathogenetic and Clinical Overview,* Huson SM & Hughes RAC, eds. London: Churchill & Hall Medical.

Viskochil D, White R, Cawthon R (1993) The neurofibromatosis type 1 gene. *Ann Rev Neurosci* 16:183–205.

Viskochil D (1999) In search of the Holy Grail: *NF1* mutation analysis and genotype-phenotype correlation. *Genet Med* 1:245–247.

Watson GH (1967) Pulmonic stenosis, café au lait spots, and dull intelligence. *Arch Dis Child* 42:303–307.

Wu R, Legius E, Robberecht W, Dumoulin M, Cassiman J-J, Fryns J-P (1996) Neurofibromatosis type I gene mutation in a patient with features of LEOPARD syndrome. *Hum Mutat* 8:51–55.

Zlotogora J (1998) Germ line mosaicism. *Hum Genet* 102:381–386.

CHAPTER 15

NOONAN SYNDROME

JUDITH E. ALLANSON

INTRODUCTION

Incidence

Noonan syndrome, a common autosomal dominant multiple congenital anomaly syndrome, was first described over 30 years ago (Noonan and Ehmke, 1963), although historical evidence of the phenotype dates back to the late 19th century. Many of the features of Noonan syndrome are similar to those seen in Turner syndrome (see Chapter 27), and this disorder has sometimes mistakenly been called "male Turner syndrome." However, Noonan syndrome occurs in both males and females with equal frequency. Good reviews are available (Mendez and Opitz, 1985; Allanson, 1987; Sharland et al., 1992a; Noonan, 1994). The incidence of Noonan syndrome is reported to be between 1 in 1000 and 1 in 2500, although mild expression is said to occur in 1 in 100 (Mendez and Opitz, 1985). Average age at diagnosis is 9 years (Sharland et al., 1992a).

Diagnostic Criteria

Despite a lack of defined diagnostic criteria, the cardinal features of Noonan syndrome are well delineated. These include short stature, congenital heart defect, broad or webbed neck, chest deformity with pectus carinatum superiorly and pectus excavatum inferiorly, developmental delay of variable degree, cryptorchidism, and characteristic facies (Allanson, 1987). Various coagulation defects and lymphatic dysplasias are common findings.

The facial appearance of Noonan syndrome is well established and shows considerable change with age, being most striking in the newborn period and middle childhood and most subtle in the adult (Allanson et al., 1985a). In the neonate, the main features are a tall forehead, hypertelorism with downslanting palpebral fissures (95%), lowset, posteriorly rotated ears with a thickened helix (90%), a deeply grooved philtrum with high, wide peaks to the vermillion border of the upper lip (95%), and a short neck with excess nuchal skin and low posterior hairline (55%). In infancy, the head appears relatively large with a small face tucked beneath a large cranium. Eyes are prominent, with horizontal fissures, hypertelorism, and thickened or ptotic lids. The nose has a depressed root, a wide base, and a bulbous tip (Fig. 15.1). In childhood, facial appearance is often lacking in affect or expression, resembling a myopathy (Fig. 15.2). By adolescence, facial shape is an inverted triangle, wide at the forehead and tapering to a pointed chin (Fig. 15.3). Eyes are less prominent, and features are sharper. There is a

Management of Genetic Syndromes, Edited by Suzanne B. Cassidy and Judith E. Allanson
ISBN 0-471-31286-X   Copyright © 2001 by Wiley-Liss, Inc.

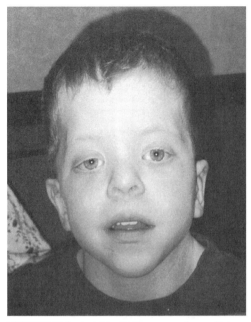

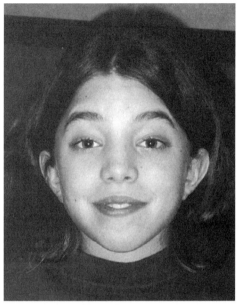

FIGURE 15.3. The adolescent with Noonan syndrome showing finer facial features and an inverted triangular face shape.

FIGURE 15.2. A child with Noonan syndrome demonstrating thickened droopy eyelids, epicanthal folds, short nose, and small, pointed chin.

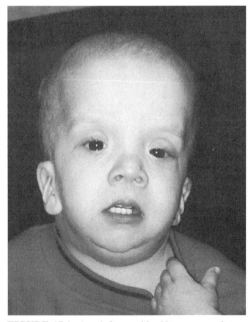

FIGURE 15.1. An infant with Noonan syndrome showing the tall, boxy forehead, thick and hooded eyelids, epicanthal folds, small upturned nose, small chin, and short neck.

pinched nasal root with a thin bridge. The neck lengthens, accentuating skin webbing or prominence of the trapezius muscle. In the older adult, nasolabial folds are prominent, and the skin appears transparent and wrinkled (Fig. 15.4).

Hair may be wispy in the toddler, whereas it is often curly or wooly in the older child and adolescent. Regardless of age, eyes are frequently pale blue or blue-green and much lighter in color and pigmentation than expected for family background; eyebrows are diamond shaped; ears are low set and posteriorly rotated with a thickened helix (Allanson, 1987).

Because of the evolution of phenotype and subtlety of features in the adult, an assessment of the family after diagnosis in a child should include a thorough review of serial photographs of both parents.

Etiology, Pathogenesis, and Genetics

In 1994, linkage analysis in one large Dutch family and 20 smaller families allowed mapping of a Noonan syndrome gene to 12q

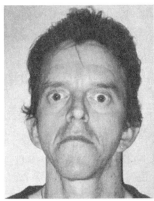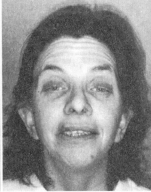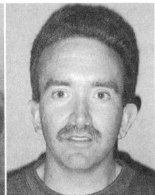

FIGURE 15.4. Three adults with Noonan syndrome demonstrating marked variability of the phenotype at this age. The face may be an inverted triangular shape with few unusual features (*right*) or may share many of the individual features shown in the younger children (*center*).

(van der Burgt et al., 1994). No candidate gene has yet been identified, although more detailed mapping has been done. Absence of linkage of some families suggests heterogeneity (Jamieson et al., 1994).

Pathogenesis may in part be associated with jugular lymphatic obstruction. The morphological consequences of lymphatic obstruction or dysfunction may remain long after the actual pathological process has subsided. Webbing of the neck and prominence of the trapezius may be secondary to tissue distension caused by a cystic hygroma. Cryptorchidism, wide-spaced nipples, low-set and angulated ears, hypertelorism, ptosis, and dermatoglyphic abnormalities are postulated to be the result of tissue disruption or displacement by lymphedema during development. Lymphatic dilatation at the base of the developing heart has been shown to alter blood flow and account for left-sided cardiac defects in Turner syndrome (Witt et al., 1987). This mechanism may be germane in Noonan syndrome, although there are no data to support a statistical association between webbed neck and structural anomalies of the heart in Noonan syndrome (Brady and Patton, 1996).

Because Noonan syndrome is an autosomal dominant single-gene disorder, an affected individual has a 50% chance to pass the abnormal gene to each of his or her children. Direct transmission from parent to child is reported in between 14% and 75% of cases (Mendez and Opitz, 1985; Allanson, 1987), and predominantly mothers, not fathers, transmit the gene (3:1 ratio). This is likely to be related to cryptorchidism and consequent reduced fertility in males (Allanson, 1987).

Diagnostic testing

Because the gene has not been identified, laboratory-based diagnostic testing is not yet available. The diagnosis rests on the pattern of clinical findings. Particularly in females, a karyotype should be done to assure that the constellation of findings is not caused by Turner syndrome.

Differential Diagnosis

The most difficult differential diagnosis clinically is between Turner syndrome and Noonan syndrome in a female. However, obtaining a karyotype and identifying deficiency of a sex chromosome distinguishes Turner syndrome.

Trisomy 8p, trisomy 22 mosaicism, sex chromosome rearrangement, in utero exposure to alcohol or primidone, and Williams, Aarskog, Baraitser-Winter, and Costello syndromes all share some phenotypic features with Noonan syndrome. There is also considerable overlap with other cardiocutaneous syndromes, such as multiple lentigines/LEOPARD, cardiofaciocutaneous, and Watson syndromes. Multiple lentigines/LEOPARD syndrome and Noonan syndrome both can be associated with pulmonary valve dysplasia and cardiomyopathy, short stature, hypertelorism, pectus deformity, hearing loss, and developmental delay (Allanson, 1987; Sharland et al., 1992a).

Watson syndrome and Noonan syndrome share pulmonary valve stenosis, short stature, mild intellectual handicap, and café-au-lait patches (Allanson et al., 1991). The Watson syndrome phenotype also overlaps with that of neurofibromatosis type 1 (see Chapter 14), although only axillary freckling and café-au-lait spots show equal incidence in the two conditions; Lisch nodules and neurofibromata are less frequently seen in Watson syndrome, whereas short stature, cardiac defects, and mild intellectual handicap are more common in Watson syndrome. Linkage of Watson syndrome to the neurofibromatosis type 1 locus was described in 1991 (Allanson et al., 1991) and mutations in neurofibromin were subsequently found, confirming that the two conditions are allelic.

Cardio-facio-cutaneous syndrome exhibits the greatest overlap with Noonan syndrome, and there has been considerable controversy about whether it is a separate condition (Neri et al., 1991; Fryer et al., 1991). The cardiac and lymphatic abnormalities in both conditions are very similar. Mental retardation in cardio-facio-cutaneous syndrome is usually more severe, with a higher likelihood of structural central nervous system anomalies, autistic-like behaviour, and seizures. Skin abnormalities in cardio-faciocutaneous syndrome are more florid, particularly hyperkeratosis, keratosis pilaris, ichthyosis, absent eyebrows, and sparse, thin, straight or curly hair. Gastrointestinal problems in cardio-facio-cutaneous syndrome are more severe and longlasting. A bleeding diathesis is very rarely found in cardio-faciocutaneous syndrome. No one feature appears to be pathognomonic of either Noonan syndrome or cardio-facio-cutaneous syndrome and there is no feature that perfectly discriminates between the two conditions.

The face in cardio-facio-cutaneous syndrome shares many features with Noonan syndrome, including a tall forehead with narrowing at the temples, ptosis, a short nose with relatively broad base, a well-grooved philtrum with cupids-bow lip and small chin. This is particularly true of the younger child. Even in this age range, however, features tend to be a little more coarse than those seen in Noonan syndrome. At older ages, the face is broad and coarse and lacks the typical inverted triangular shape. Head shape is more likely to be dolichocephalic than round as in Noonan syndrome. In cardio-facio-cutaneous syndrome there is a high likelihood of absent eyebrows with hyperkeratosis. The eyes are rarely the characteristic blue or blue-green of Noonan syndrome and a lateral gaze is frequently seen. The typical ear finding in Noonan syndrome, oval shape with a thickened helix, low-set and posteriorly rotated, is very uncommon. Earlobe creases, rarely described in Noonan syndrome, appear quite frequent in cardio-facio- cutaneous syndrome.

Initially, cardio-facio-cutaneous syndrome was felt to be sporadic, thus facilitating separation from Noonan syndrome, however, there are at least four reports in the literature of dominant inheritance of this syndrome. One putative family (Legius et al., 1998) is said to show linkage to chromosome 12q, however the phenotype of this family is much more in keeping with Noonan syndrome. Determination as to whether or not Noonan syndrome and cardio-faciocutaneous syndrome are allelic will await molecular diagnosis of these two overlapping conditions.

A rare case of Noonan syndrome has been diagnosed as 3C (cranio-cerebellocardiac) syndrome because of the accompanying brain posterior fossa anomalies. There are two reports of autosomal dominant syndromes with overlapping features that have digital anomalies not seen in Noonan syndrome — camptodactyly/postminimus and proximally placed small thumbs.

MANIFESTATIONS AND MANAGEMENT

Growth and Feeding

Birth weight usually is normal, although edema may cause a transient increase (Allanson, 1987; Patton, 1994). Almost a quarter of infants with Noonan syndrome have no feeding difficulties; however, poor suck with prolonged feeding time (15%), very poor suck and slow feeding with recurrent vomiting (38%), and severe feeding problems that require tube feeding for 2 weeks or more (24%) are described (Sharland et al., 1992a). Typically, this period of failure to thrive is self-limited, although poor weight gain may persist for up to 18 months (personal experience).

Length at birth is usually normal. Mean height follows the third centile until puberty, when below-average growth velocity and attenuated adolescent growth spurt tend to occur. Bone age (Greulich-Pyle method) is usually 2 years delayed, leading to prolonged growth potential into the 20s (Allanson, 1987; Sharland et al., 1992a). Final adult height approached the lower limit of normal (162.5 cm in men and 151 cm in women) at the end of the second decade of life in one mixed cross-sectional and longitudinal study (Witt et al., 1986). Growth curves have been developed from these cross-sectional retrospective data (Witt et al., 1986).

Early studies of the etiology of short stature in Noonan syndrome demonstrated normal resting and stimulated levels of growth hormone with mild elevation in somatomedin levels. Two large studies of growth hormone treatment in Noonan syndrome have been completed. The National Cooperative Growth Study (U.S.A) has a large data set and long duration with 150 patients enrolled, 97 of them male (Romano

et al., 1996). Participation was 3 years on average. Mean height at enrollment was -3.5 SD (-1.35 SD when standardized to the Noonan syndrome data of Ranke et al., (1988)). Stimulated peak growth hormone levels were $<10\mu g/L$ in 45%. Growth rates for years 1, 2, 3, and 4 of therapy were significantly greater than baseline. Height gain over 4 years was approximately 1 SD and was sustained. Six boys reached heights considered their final adult status, despite a mean age at enrollment of 13.6 years. Three of the six exceeded their Bayley-Pinneau-predicted heights. In some individuals, bone age appeared to advance disproportionately in comparison to gain in height age. This initial advance in bone age is not unique to Noonan syndrome and may reflect a greater baseline bone age deficit.

Thirty subjects were enrolled in a British study of growth hormone treatment (4 IU/m^2/day); (Cotterill et al., 1996): all were prepubertal, with growth 2 SD or more below the mean for average British children, normal left ventricular wall thickness, and no chronic illness. Low responses to glucagon provocation were noted in one third. Growth was monitored for 12 months before and at 3-month intervals during therapy. Twenty-seven patients completed 12 months of therapy with height SD score and height velocity increasing significantly. The comparison group with untreated Noonan syndrome showed no such changes. Insulin-like growth factor (IGF)-1 and IGF-binding protein 3 (IGFBP-3) increased, which, together with low responses to provocation, suggest impaired growth hormone release in some patients. Significant reduction in body fat, reflected in lowered skinfold thickness and body mass index score, was observed. In children who have continued growth hormone therapy, there is a suggestion that growth velocity gradually begins to fall after 3 years (Kelnar and Patton, personal communication). As a result, a new British study is planned, in which some children will be randomized to 2 years of growth hormone, followed by discontinuation of treatment until puberty, at which time further randomization will allow some children to restart growth hormone. Such intermittent treatment may prevent the waning efficacy over time (Kelnar and Patton, personal communication).

A small number of insignificant adverse events were documented in these studies, including joint swelling of hand and knee (1), transient hand and face edema (1), a raspy voice (1), and recurrence of a previously diagnosed maxillary giant cell tumor (1). No abnormal anabolic effects of growth hormone on the left ventricular wall were seen. No changes in glycosylated hemoglobin, triglycerides, or cholesterol were noted (Cotterill et al., 1996; Romano et al., 1996).

Evaluation

- There are significant differences in the utilization of growth hormone studies and in the approach to treatment between countries. In Canada, growth hormone deficiency must be documented before growth hormone treatment is sanctioned. In the United States and Britain, some endocrinologists may choose to treat any small individual with growth hormone, irrespective of growth hormone testing results, beginning at age 7–8 years (Romano, personal experience).
- Growth velocity should be monitored for 6–12 months, using regular, not syndrome specific, growth charts. If growth velocity is normal, height should be measured every 6 months.
- If deficiency is noted, nutritional status should be evaluated and chronic illness ruled out.
- Initial testing for growth deficiency should include thyroid function tests, bone age, complete blood count, blood chemistries, sedimentation rate, and IGF-1 and usually IGFBP-3.

- Provocation testing should be performed using standard methods.
- If growth hormone deficiency is found, panhypopituitarism should be assessed by specific hormone testing and magnetic imaging of the brain.
- Cardiac status must be evaluated in the child on growth hormone treatment. Cardiomyopathy is not a complete contraindication to treatment, but close monitoring with echocardiography must be put in place.
- The child on growth hormone should have periodic assessment of growth velocity (every 6 months), bone age (every 12 months), and thyroid function tests and blood chemistries (annually).

Treatment

- Initiation of treatment with growth hormone should be considered once deficiency is proven. Some clinicians would institute treatment in any child with Noonan syndrome who is small, irrespective of results, beginning at 7 or 8 years (Romano, personal experience). Treatment is currently a daily injection or application to the skin surface using a gunlike device. Alternate vehicles are under development.

Development and Behavior

Early developmental milestones may be delayed, with mean age of sitting at 10 months, first unsupported walking at 21 months, and simple two-word sentences at 31 months. Motor milestone delay, in part, is likely to be influenced by hyperextensibility and hypotonia. Most school-age children perform well in a normal educational setting but 10–15% require special education (Sharland et al., 1992a; Lee et al., unpublished data). Mild mental retardation is seen in up to one-third of individuals (Mendez and Opitz, 1985; Allanson, 1987). In general, IQ falls within the normal range, but more children fall into the low average range than one would expect (Lee et al., unpublished data). Verbal performance is frequently lower than nonverbal performance (Lee et al., unpublished data). There are reports of individuals with very superior IQ, good organizational skills, concentration, and persistence, relative strengths in mental computation, social awareness, and judgment, and an intact visual-perceptual-motor system (Finegan and Hughes, 1998). Even when full-scale IQ is low, it does not necessarily signify straightforward mental retardation but rather a specific cognitive disability, either in verbal or praxic reasoning, requiring a special academic strategy and school placement.

Good peer and social interactions and self-esteem are generally evident, with no particular syndrome of behavioral disability or psychopathology, although there may be an increased likelihood of clumsy, fidgety, stubborn, and irritable behavior (Lee et al., unpublished data). One recent survey of families suggests that children with Noonan syndrome are less likely to be socially competent and may have more behavioral problems than their age-matched peers; however, the problems appear to be relatively mild and do not reach a level of clinical significance (Witt and Stoltzfus, 1999). Notably few children are reported with autistic features, sleep difficulties, severe aggression, or anxiety.

Articulation deficiency is common (72%) but should respond well to intervention therapy. Language delay may be related to hearing loss, perceptual motor disabilities, or articulation deficiencies (Allanson, 1987).

Evaluation

- A screening developmental assessment, with such tools as the Denver Developmental Screening Test, should be done at diagnosis and at least annually on all patients with Noonan syndrome.
- A full developmental assessment should be done if delays are ascertained.
- School difficulties deserve formal psychological assessment to determine whether a specific cognitive disability is

present that might respond to an alternate teaching method.
- Any delay in speech acquisition should prompt an assessment by speech pathology.

Treatment

- Hypotonia will respond to physical and occupational therapies over time.
- An infant stimulation program should be initiated if delays are noted early.
- Special individualized education strategies are needed if indicated by detailed testing.
- Speech therapy is suggested where delays or articulation deficiencies are identified.

Ears and Hearing

Hearing loss is reported in more than one-third of children and generally is secondary to serous otitis media. Sensorineural deafness is unusual (3%) (Sharland et al., 1992a), and congenital ossicular chain anomaly is rare. Articulation problems may result.

Evaluation

- Hearing testing should begin in infancy and continue annually through early childhood.

Treatment

- Aggressive treatment of otitis media with antibiotics is recommended.
- Sensorineural hearing loss may require hearing aids.

Cardiovascular

It is important to recognize the possibility of bias when estimating the frequency of congenital heart disease, because many clinicians require the presence of cardiac anomalies for diagnosis of Noonan syndrome (Sharland et al., 1992a) and frequently the reports in the literature come from tertiary and quaternary medical centers, where the most serious manifestations of a condition are likely to be present–the so-called "worst case scenario." The frequency of congenital heart disease in Noonan syndrome is estimated to be between 50% and 80% (Allanson, 1987; Patton, 1994). The frequency of Noonan syndrome in children with congenital heart disease is 1.4%.

A stenotic and often dysplastic pulmonary valve is the most common cardiac anomaly in Noonan syndrome, found in 20–50% of affected individuals (Allanson, 1987; Sharland et al., 1992a; Ishizawa et al., 1996); it may be isolated or associated with other defects. The frequency of Noonan syndrome in children with pulmonary stenosis is 7%. The sequelae of severe valve dysfunction are similar to those in nonsyndromic pulmonary valve stenosis, with right ventricular hypertrophy, dysfunction, and fibrosis resulting if it is left untreated.

Hypertrophic cardiomyopathy is found in 20–30% of affected individuals (Allanson, 1987; Sharland et al., 1992a; Patton, 1994; Ishizawa et al., 1996). It may present at birth, in infancy or childhood. Nonobstructive and obstructive hypertrophic cardiomyopathy are likely extensions of the same clinical spectrum. Both may be associated with poor ventricular compliance, leading to diastolic dysfunction that may mimic a restrictive cardiomyopathy. The clinical, echocardiographic, and histopathological phenotype (myocardial hypertrophy with pathological myofibrillar disarray) is indistinguishable from nonsyndromic hypertrophic cardiomyopathy, although arrhythmia and sudden death are more common in nonsyndromic cases (Patton, 1994). Newborn mortality secondary to hypertrophic cardiomyopathy is 20%.

Other structural defects frequently seen in Noonan syndrome include atrial septal defect (10–20%), ventricular septal defect (5–15%), branch pulmonary artery stenosis, and tetralogy of Fallot (Allanson, 1987; Ishizawa et al., 1996). Coarctation of the aorta was thought to be unusual and found more frequently in Turner syndrome. It would appear to be more common than

realized previously (9%) (Digilio et al., 1998). Rare anomalies include aortic stenosis, Ebstein anomaly, coronary artery fistulae, and anomalous pulmonary venous return.

An electrocardiographic abnormality is documented in 87% of individuals with Noonan syndrome (Sharland et al., 1992a). Extreme right axis deviation with superior counterclockwise frontal QRS loop (40%) is likely to be related to asymmetric septal hypertrophy. Superior or left axis deviation may be secondary to a conduction abnormality; there may also be left anterior hemiblock or an RSR' pattern in lead V1.

Echocardiographic predictors of poor prognosis include greater left ventricular posterior wall thickness (>2SD), with consequent lower ventricular septum:left ventricular posterior wall ratio (<2); progression of hypertrophy with reduction in asymmetry; and congestive cardiac failure. Alteration of left ventricular function with reduced ejection fraction may predict poor outcome but cannot be used alone.

Children generally do very well after valvotomy. In adults, prognosis is excellent when pulmonary stenosis is trivial, but results may not be uniformly good because of persistent right ventricular dysfunction. Favorable prognostic features include absence of symptoms, normal resting cardiac output, peak right ventricular pressure less than 100 mm Hg, and normal pulmonary artery pressure.

Evaluation

- Clinical assessment, electrocardiogram (with particular attention to the QRS axis), and echocardiogram are recommended at the initial assessment.

- Subsequent management and follow-up are dictated by these investigations and the clinical course.

- A malformed pulmonary valve should be evident at initial assessment but may become more stenotic with time. Cardiac hypertrophy may progress without changes in clinical status. Therefore, echocardiographic follow-up, at least every 2 years, is important regardless of the finding of a normal myocardium at presentation.

Treatment

- β-Blockade or calcium channel blockers have been used most frequently in the treatment of obstructive cardiomyopathy, although attempts to improve diastolic function with both classes of drug are often contemplated (Ishizawa et al., 1996).

- If there is no response to drug therapy, surgery is indicated for left ventricular outflow obstruction. Both surgical myomectomy and transplantation are reported (Sharland et al., 1992a).

- Intervention for pulmonary outflow tract obstruction caused by valvular dysplasia is recommended at any age if right ventricular pressure exceeds 80 mmHg. Results are good. The initial palliative surgery of choice (Ishizawa et al., 1996) is balloon valvuloplasty, although it is widely accepted that results in the presence of a dysplastic valve may not be as good as in nonsyndromic pulmonary valve stenosis. Frequently, open pulmonary valvotomy, with annulus enlargement, is needed. Severe cases may require pulmonary valve debridement or replacement, typically with a bioprosthesis (Ishizawa et al., 1996). Recurrent stenosis rarely occurs, although a mild decease in gradient may occur in the late postoperative period.

- Subacute bacterial endocarditis prophylaxis is required for dental work, surgery, catheterization, and other circumstances likely to promote a bacteremia.

Neurologic

Joint hyperextensibility and hypotonia are very common features of Noonan syndrome. Recurrent seizures are less frequently described (13%) (Sharland et al., 1992a). Rare neurological structural anomalies include schwannoma, multiple cutaneous granular cell schwannoma (myoblastoma), peripheral neuropathy, syringomyelia with Chiari type I malformation, hydrocephalus, Dandy-Walker malformation, cerebral (basal) arteriovenous malformation (1 case), hypoplastic posterior cerebral blood vessels (1 case), and lateral meningoceles.

The association between Noonan syndrome and malignant hyperthermia is poorly understood; creatine kinase usually is normal in Noonan syndrome (Sharland et al., 1992a), although in King syndrome, which may have a Noonan syndrome phenotype and muscle fibers of variable diameter, creatine kinase is elevated (King and Denborough, 1973). Malignant hyperthermia is of greater concern when there is a subclinical myopathy or elevated creatine kinase (Mendez and Opitz, 1985).

Evaluation

- Neurological investigation should be prompted by signs and symptoms and may include thorough neurological examination, electroencephalogram, electromyogram, and/or nerve conduction velocities.

- Creatine kinase analysis is recommended before anesthesia or dental work.

Treatment

- Anticonvulsant therapy is indicated for a seizure disorder, and treatment does not differ from that in the general population.

- Dantrolene prophylaxis should be used during anesthesia when creatine kinase levels are increased or if there is a clinical suspicion of malignant hyperthermia or myopathy.

- Surgery may be required for a rare brain structural anomaly such as hydrocephalus.

Ophthalmologic

Differences in shape and size of the eyes and periorbital structures are hallmark features of Noonan syndrome. The iris frequently is an attractive and striking pale blue or green with sparseness of the usual trabeculae, crypts, and furrows. Ocular findings are among the most common features of Noonan syndrome, seen in up to 95%. They include strabismus (48–63%), refractive errors (60–70%) (36% astigmatism, 13% myopia, 35% hypermetropia), amblyopia (33%), and nystagmus (9%). Anterior segment changes (63%) include prominent corneal nerves (46%), anterior stromal dystrophy (94%), cataracts (8%), and panuveitis (2%). Fundal changes are less frequent, occurring in 20%, and include optic head drusen, optic disk hypoplasia, colobomas, and myelinated nerves (Sharland et al., 1992a; Lee et al., 1992).

Retinitis pigmentosa was described in one patient with Noonan syndrome but also in several individuals reported with cardio-facio-cutaneous syndrome. Cardio-facio-cutaneous syndrome also is associated with optic disk anomalies, cataracts, refractive errors, strabismus, nystagmus, hypertelorism, ptosis, and epicanthic folds.

Evaluation

- A detailed visual assessment in infancy is indicated.
- Continuing periodic ophthalmologic evaluation should be done if anomalies are found (Lee et al., 1992).

Treatment

- Most ocular defects require nonsurgical treatment, such as glasses and occlusion for amblyopia and correction of refractive errors.
- Surgery may be required for cataracts and ptosis (in 10%).

Hematologic-Oncologic

Several different coagulation defects may occur in Noonan syndrome, either singly or in combination. They affect about one-third of all individuals (Witt et al., 1987). However, two-thirds of individuals with Noonan syndrome will give a history of abnormal bleeding or mild to severe bruising (Sharland et al., 1992b). The coagulopathy may manifest as severe surgical hemorrhage, clinically mild but detectable bruising, or laboratory abnormalities with no clinical sequelae. There is a poor correlation between history and the actual coagulation factor deficit. Although the factor deficiencies are generally stable, there may be clinical amelioration with age. There is no apparent relationship between age, sex, type or severity of bleeding, and cardiac abnormality present. No evidence of hepatic dysfunction, vitamin K-dependent coagulation factor deficiency, or disseminated intravascular coagulation is reported in Noonan syndrome (Sharland et al., 1992b).

Laboratory findings include von Willebrand disease, prolonged partial thromboplastin time (40%) and bleeding time, thrombocytopenia, varied coagulation factor defects (factors V, VIII, XI, XII, protein C), alone or in combination (50%), and platelet dysfunction (abnormal platelet aggregation studies with epinephrine, ADP, and collagen). Noonan syndrome may be accompanied less often by abnormalities of regulation of the intrinsic system (contact activation), platelet dysfunction associated with trimethylaminuria, or defective thromboplastin regeneration (a pattern of platelet aggregation defects mimicking aspirin-induced effects, pointing to an abnormality of prostaglandin synthesis or action) (Witt et al., 1987; Sharland et al., 1992b).

Hepatosplenomegaly is evident clinically (25%) and ultrasonographically (51%) (Sharland et al., 1992a). Splenomegaly is present in one-half, with concomitant hepatomegaly in one-quarter of these cases. No associated changes in spleen echogenicity are noted, and there is no apparent reason for enlargement.

Acute myelogenous or lymphatic leukemia, congenital hypoplastic anemia, decreased erythroid and myeloid precursors, neuroblastoma, and vaginal rhabdomyosarcoma are all reported rarely.

Evaluation

- Inquiries should be made about a history of easy bruising or prolonged bleeding after venipuncture.
- Clinical evidence of abnormal bleeding should be sought.
- Routine screening tests at diagnosis should include prothrombin time, activated partial thromboplastin time, bleeding time, and platelet count. Recent aspirin exposure must be excluded.
- Additional specific testing of coagulation factors, von Willebrand factor antigen, and functional epitope and platelet function is advised if indicated by the screening results (Witt et al., 1987; Sharland et al., 1992b).

Treatment

- Aspirin and aspirin-containing medications should be avoided.
- Individualized hemostatic support may be required, depending on the specific hemorrhagic diathesis identified.

Lymphatic

Fewer than 20% of individuals with Noonan syndrome have a lymphatic abnormality; however, many varied differences are described (Mendez and Opitz, 1985; Witt et al., 1987). The lymphatic abnormality may be manifest in several ways: it may be localized or widespread, prenatal and/or postnatal. It is most commonly obvious at birth, although onset may be delayed until adulthood. Dorsal limb lymphedema is most common. It may contribute to increased birth weight (mean birth weight

is 3450 g) (Sharland et al., 1992a), and it usually resolves in childhood. Less common findings include intestinal, pulmonary, or testicular lymphangiectasia, chylous effusions of pleural space and peritoneum, and localized lymphedema of scrotum or vulva. Rare lymphatic abnormalities include single cases of lip lymphatic dysplasia, neck lymphangioma, orbital edema, and facial lymphangioma. The most common underlying pathological finding is lymphatic hyperplasia with or without thoracic duct anomaly. Lymphatic aplasia or hypoplasia and megalymphatics are reported (Witt et al., 1987).

A common prenatal indicator of lymphatic dysfunction or abnormality, seen on ultrasound, is a cystic hygroma, which is often accompanied by scalp edema, polyhydramnios, pleural and pericardial effusions, ascites, and/or frank hydrops. The presence of these findings, particularly in the absence of a chromosome abnormality, should prompt a search for cardiac and other malformations. Cystic hygroma is usually caused by delayed connection of the jugular lymph sac and the left internal jugular vein. It may regress, leaving redundant neck skin at birth (Witt et al., 1987; Benacerraf et al., 1989). However, not all cystic hygromas resolve, and some progress to hydrops. Timing of regression may be a useful factor in determining survival. Regression before the mid-second trimester appears to be associated with a more favorable prognosis (Benacerraf et al., 1989). Chorioangiomas also are described, and these vascular lesions may play a role in edema formation through loss of α-fetoprotein into amniotic fluid with resultant decrease in fetal oncotic pressure.

Severe lymphatic dysplasia with chylous effusions can lead to protein loss, malnutrition, and lymphopenia, especially of the T-helper cells.

Evaluation

- Prenatal: In the presence of a cystic hygroma or thickened nuchal fold, maternal serum screening or invasive testing with chromosome analysis should be pursued. A detailed sonographic search for other anomalies should be carried out.

- Postnatal: The objectives of evaluation of lymphedema are twofold—to discover the cause of the lymphatic problem and to define the type. Radionuclide scanning is advocated by many as a first step. Intradermal injection in the first interdigital web space of the lower limb is followed by serial scintiscans of the ilioinguinal region. Direct lymphangiography can then be used to define the type of anomaly.

- The majority of individuals with intestinal lymphangiectasia manifest diarrhea, with or without steatorrhea, and diagnosis often begins, as a consequence, with studies to detect and quantify protein loss. Barium meal appearance is characteristic, and peroral jejunal biopsy and lymphography provide definitive diagnosis.

- Chylous complications often are related to lymph vessel hyperplasia with abnormalities of the thoracic duct or presence of megalymphatics. Diagnosis of chylothorax depends on accurate assessment of clinical features, chest radiographs, and demonstration of chyle in pleural fluid obtained by thoracocentesis. Computerized tomographic scanning and lymphoscintigraphy are useful adjuncts that may delineate obstruction to the cisterna chyli with chylous reflux in both chylothorax and chylous ascites.

Treatment

- Chronic lymphedema of the lower extremities, albeit rare, is frequently associated with infection. Foot hygiene is extremely important. Carefully fitting shoes and support stockings are useful, along with antibacterial cleaning solutions. Daily examination for web-space fissures, paronychias, impetigo, and folliculitis should be instituted, with prompt use of systemic antibiotics where indicated to decrease the incidence of severe infection. Prophylactic penicillin may be warranted when hygiene measures alone are inadequate (White, 1984).

- Treatment options for chylothorax include drainage by repeated thoracentesis, chest tube, or pleuroperitoneal shunt; reduction of chyle production by low-fat diet or parenteral nutrition; and, if conservative measures fail, surgical modification of lymph flow by thoracic duct ligation, chemical pleurodesis, or pleurectomy. Most chylothoraces resolve with drainage and dietary modification. Long periods of drainage are complicated by weight loss, hypoalbuminemia, lymphopenia, and infection, which can be fatal. Successful prednisone therapy has been reported. The effect of steroids may be to increase plasma oncotic pressure through increased rate of breakdown of extrahepatic proteins, freeing amino acids and facilitating liver synthesis of more plasma proteins.

Genitourinary

Renal abnormalities, generally mild, are found on ultrasound in 11% of individuals with Noonan syndrome although prior studies in smaller groups of patients suggested an anomaly rate up to 60% (Noonan, 1994). The most commonly reported finding is dilatation of the renal pelvis resembling pelviureteric junction obstruction. Duplex systems, minor rotational anomalies, distal ureteric stenosis, renal hypoplasia, unilateral renal agenesis, unilateral renal ectopia, and bilateral cysts with scarring are reported less commonly (George et al., 1993).

Male pubertal development and subsequent fertility may be normal, delayed, or inadequate with associated deficient spermatogenesis (Mendez and Opitz, 1985; Sharland et al., 1992a). The latter may be related to cryptorchidism, which is noted in 60–80% of males (Patton, 1994; personal experience). Such males may have primary hypogonadism with high FSH levels. Cryptorchidism and consequent impaired spermatogenesis are also likely to be associated with reduced paternal transmission of Noonan syndrome (personal observation). Sexual function is not affected, but onset of sexual activity may be later in those males with delayed puberty.

Puberty may be delayed in females, with mean age at menarche being 14.6 ± 1.17 years (Sharland et al., 1992a). Normal fertility is the rule.

Evaluation

- Renal ultrasound is recommended in newborns to assess for malformations and disruptions.
- Serial reevaluation may be suggested, depending on the findings.
- Periodic urinalysis is warranted if the genitourinary tract is abnormal, because of increased frequency of urinary tract infection in these circumstances.
- Evaluation of the pituitary-gonadal axis before puberty is suggested to assess the need for hormone replacement therapy.

Treatment

- The presence of cryptorchidism at birth should lead to a referral to an appropriate surgeon for consideration of a trial of hCG injection and/or surgery before school entry. The approach to treatment is the same as in the general population.
- Urinary tract infection should be treated with appropriate antibiotics.
- Testosterone replacement should be considered in males with primary hypogonadism.

Musculoskeletal

The classical pectus deformity, with carinatum superiorly and excavatum inferiorly, is seen in 90–95% of individuals with Noonan syndrome. It is often evident by early childhood. Wide-spaced and apparently low-set nipples and rounded shoulders are common (Allanson, 1987). Scoliosis is reported in 10–15%. Other spinal anomalies include kyphosis, spina bifida, vertebral and rib anomalies, and genu valgum. Talipes equinovarus is described in 10–15%, other joint contractures in 4%, radio-ulnar synostosis in 2%, and cervical spine fusion in 2%. The range of forearm carrying angle generally is 14–15 degrees in girls and 10–11 degrees in boys. Abnormal angles (cubitus valgus) are found in more than half the males and females with Noonan syndrome (Sharland et al., 1992a).

A high-arched palate is common, with a high incidence of class II, division I malocclusion of the teeth. The association of Noonan syndrome and cherubism, a giant cell lesion of the jaws with rare extragnathic skeletal involvement, has been reported several times, likely a coincidental association because both are relatively common autosomal dominant disorders.

Hyperextensibility is common.

Evaluation

- Annual assessment of chest cage and spine, both clinical and radiological, is recommended.
- Dental evaluation and monitoring should begin in early childhood, so that appropriate referral to orthodontics can be facilitated.

Treatment

- Scoliosis may require bracing or surgery, as in the general population.
- Malocclusion may need orthodontic intervention, as in the general population.

Dermatologic

There is a considerable range of changes in skin, one of the most common being follicular keratosis, predominantly over extensor surfaces and face (14%) (Pierini and Pierini, 1979; Sharland et al., 1992a). Keratosis pilaris atrophicans faciei (ulerythema ophryogenes) is characterized by horny, whitish, hemispherical or acuminate papules at the opening of the pilosebaceous follicles and is caused by disturbances in the keratinization process of hair follicles. It involves the face, manifesting itself a few months after birth, in the external third of the eyebrows and may extend over the preauricular area, cheeks, and scalp. Generally, progression occurs until puberty, when it becomes quiescent. It may leave pitted scars and atrophic skin and interfere with beard and eyebrow growth (Pierini and Pierini, 1979).

Abnormalities of scalp and body hair are often described. Scalp hair may be curly, thick, and wooly or sparse and poor growing with easy breakage. Microscopically, there is variation in hair shaft diameter.

Café-au-lait spots (10%) and lentigines (2%) are described in Noonan syndrome (Allanson, 1987; Sharland et al., 1992a). Several individuals with both neurofibromatosis type 1 and Noonan syndrome are reported (Allanson et al., 1985b). The Noonan syndrome phenotype is also described in some of the members of published families with neurofibromatosis 1. This so-called neurofibromatosis/Noonan syndrome is likely to be a chance association of the two phenotypes (Colley et al., 1996). This conclusion is supported by the lack of linkage between Noonan syndrome and the *NF1* locus on chromosome 17 (Sharland et al., 1992c).

Prominent fetal finger pads are common (67%) (Sharland et al., 1992a). Rare skin anomalies reported in Noonan syndrome include xanthomas of skin and tongue, redundant, molluscoid skin over the scalp, which demonstrates hyperplasia with radiating adipocyte proliferation histologically, leukokeratosis of the lip and gingiva, and vulvar angiokeratoma.

Evaluation

- Dermatological problems should be referred to a specialist and management planned as in the general population.

Treatment

- Local medication for keratosis pilaris atrophicans faciei is usually unsuccessful.

Miscellaneous

Hypothyroidism is described in 5% of individuals with Noonan syndrome, although antimicrosomal thyroid antibodies are more frequently found (38%) (M. Patton, personal communication). Other autoantibodies are found at a higher frequency than one would expect (M. Patton, personal communication). Further evidence for autoimmune dysfunction includes vasculitis, vitiligo, anterior uveitis (all single cases) (Sharland et al., 1992a).

RESOURCES

Brochures and Newsletters

USA support group (Noonan Syndrome, Inc): contact Wanda Robinson, PO Box 145, Upperco, MD 21155; 410-239-6926, or through the internet (see below).

UK brochure available through the Birth Defects Foundation, Martindale, Hawks Green, Cannock, Staffs. WS11 2XN, UK. Helpline: 08700 70 70 20, or through the Internet (see below).

Internet

USA support group (TNSSG, Inc): *wandar@bellatlantic.net*

UK support group is part of *www.birthdefects.co.uk*

REFERENCES

Allanson JE (1987) Noonan syndrome. *J Med Genet* 24:9–13.

Allanson JE, Hall JG, Hughes HE, Preus M, Witt RD (1985a) Noonan syndrome: The changing phenotype. *Am J Med Genet* 21:507–514.

Allanson JE, Hall JG, Van Allen MI (1985b) Noonan phenotype associated with neurofibromatosis. *Am J Med Genet* 21:457–462.

Allanson JE, Upadhyaya M, Watson GH, Partington MW, Mackenzie A, Lahey D, MacLeod H, Sarfarazi M, Broadhead W, Harper PS, Huson SM (1991) Watson syndrome: Is it a subtype of type 1 neurofibromatosis? *J Med Genet* 28:752–756.

Benacerraf BR, Greene MF, Holmes LB (1989) The prenatal sonographic features of Noonan's syndrome. *J Ultrasound Med* 8:59–63.

Brady AF, Patton MA (1996) Web-neck anomaly and its association with congenital heart disease. *Am J Med Genet* 64:605.

Colley A, Donnai D, Evans DGR (1996) Neurofibromatosis/Noonan phenotype: A variable feature of type 1 neurofibromatosis. *Clin Genet* 49:59–64.

Cotterill AM, McKenna WJ, Brady AF, Sharland M, Elsawi M, Yamada M, Camacho-Hubner C, Kelnar CJ, Dunger DB, Patton MA, Savage MO (1996) The short-term effects of growth hormone therapy on height velocity and cardiac ventricular wall thickness in children with Noonan's syndrome. *J Clin Endocrinol Metab* 81:2291–2297.

Digilio MC, Marino B, Picchio F, Prandstraller D, Toscana A, Giannotti A, Dallapiccola B (1998) Noonan syndrome and aortic coarctation. *Am J Med Genet* 80:160–162.

Finegan JK, Hughes HE (1988) Very superior intelligence in a child with Noonan syndrome. *Am J Med Genet* 31:385-389.

Fryer AE, Holt PJ, Hughes HE (1991) The cardio-facio-cutaneous syndrome and Noonan syndrome: Are they the same? *Am J Med Genet* 38:548–551.

George CD, Patton MA, El Sawi M, Sharland M, Adam EJ (1993) Abdominal ultrasound in Noonan syndrome: A study of 44 patients. *Pediatr Radiol* 23:316–318.

Ishizawa A, Oho S-I, Dodo H, Katori T, Homma S-I (1996) Cardiovascular abnormalities in Noonan syndrome: The clinical findings and treatment. *Acta Paediatr Jpn* 38:84–90.

Jamieson RC, van der Burgt I, Brady AF, van Reen M, Elsawi MM, Hol F, Jeffery S, Patton M, Mariman E (1994) Mapping a gene for Noonan syndrome to the long arm of chromosome 12. *Nat Genet* 8:357–360.

King JO, Denborough MA (1973) Anaesthetic-induced malignant hyperpyrexia in children. *J Pediatr* 83:37–40.

Lee D, Portnoy S, Hill P, Patton MA Psychological aspects of children with Noonan Syndrome (unpublished).

Lee NB, Kelly L, Sharland M (1992) Ocular manifestations of Noonan syndrome. *Eye* 6: 328–334.

Legius E, Schollen E, Matthijs G, Fryns J-P (1998) Fine mapping of the Noonan/cardio-facio-cutaneous syndrome in a large family. *Eur J Hum Genet* 6:32–37.

Mendez HMM, Opitz JM (1985) Noonan syndrome: A review. *Am J Med Genet* 21:493–506.

Neri G, Zollino M, Reynolds JF (1991) The Noonan-CFC controversy. *Am J Med Genet* 39:367–370.

Noonan JA (1994) Noonan syndrome: Update and review for the primary pediatrician. *Clin Pediatr* 33:548–555.

Noonan JA, Ehmke DA (1963) Associated non-cardiac malformations in children with congenital heart disease. *J Pediatr* 63:468–470.

Patton MA (1994) Noonan syndrome: A review. *Growth, Genetics and Hormones* 33:10:1–3.

Pierini DO, Pierini AM (1979) Keratosis pilaris atrophicans faciei (ulerythema ophryogenes): A cutaneous marker in the Noonan syndrome. *Br J Dermatol* 100:409–416.

Ranke MB, Heidemann P, Knupfer C, Enders H, Schmaltz AA, Bierich JR (1988) Noonan syndrome: Growth and clinical manifestations in 144 cases. *Eur J Pediatr* 148:220–227.

Romano AA, Blethen SL, Dana K, Noto RA (1996) Growth hormone treatment in Noonan syndrome: The National Cooperative Growth Study experience. *J Pediatr* 128:S18–S21.

Sharland M, Burch M, McKenna WM, Patton MA (1992a) A clinical study of Noonan syndrome. *Arch Dis Child* 67:178–183.

Sharland M, Patton MA, Talbot S, Chitolie A, Bevan DH (1992b) Coagulation-factor deficiencies and abnormal bleeding in Noonan's syndrome. *Lancet* 339:19–21.

Sharland M, Taylor R, Patton MA, Jeffrey S (1992c) Absence of linkage of Noonan syndrome to the neurofibromatosis type 1 locus. *J Med Genet* 29:188–190.

van der Burgt I, Berends E, Lommen E, van Beersum S, Hamel B, Mariman E (1994). Clinical and molecular studies in a large Dutch family with Noonan syndrome. *Am J Med Genet* 53:187–191.

White SW (1984) Lymphedema in Noonan's syndrome. *Int J Dermatol* 23:656–7.

Witt DR, Keena BA, Hall JG, Allanson JE (1986) Growth curves for height in Noonan syndrome. *Clin Genet* 30:150–153.

Witt DR, Hoyme HE, Zonana J, Manchester DK, Fryns JP, Stevenson JG, Curry CJR, Hall JG (1987) Lymphedema in Noonan syndrome: Clues to pathogenesis and prenatal diagnosis and review of the literature. *Am J Med Genet* 27:841–856.

Witt DR, Stoltzfus C (1999) Behavioral phenotype in Noonan syndrome. *Proc Greenwood Genet Ctr* 18:149–150.

CHAPTER 16

OCULO-AURICULO-VERTEBRAL SPECTRUM

ROBERT J. GORLIN

INTRODUCTION

Incidence

Oculo-auriculo-vertebral spectrum was probably first described by Canton in 1861 and von Arlt in 1881. Many good reviews are available (Harvold et al., 1983; Rollnick et al., 1987; Cohen et al., 1989; Gorlin et al., 1995).

Oculo-auriculo-vertebral spectrum has been variously called hemifacial microsomia, craniofacial microsomia, Goldenhar syndrome, Goldenhar-Gorlin syndrome, first and second branchial arch syndrome, first arch syndrome, facio-auriculo-vertebral syndrome, and lateral facial dysplasia. Oculo-auriculo-vertebral spectrum occurs with a frequency of approximately 1 in 5,600 births. The male-to-female ratio is at least 3:2. Because of markedly variable expression, the exact frequency of the disorder is not known, many mild cases not having been categorized as such.

Diagnostic Criteria

Craniofacial findings usually bring the patient to the clinician's attention (Figs. 16.1 and 16.2). Facial asymmetry, frequently but not always obvious in infancy, may become more evident with age. The ear on the involved side is often dysmorphic, microtic, and displaced. One or more ear tags may be present from the tragus to the angle of the mouth. The mouth may be larger on the affected side, the mastoid bone may be small, and there may be facial paralysis on the same side. Rarely, there is bilateral involvement. There may be epibulbar dermoids on one or both sides and occasionally colobomas of the upper eyelids. Some vertebral bodies may be malformed, and various forms of congenital heart disease may be found.

Despite the name Oculo-auriculo-vertebral spectrum, involvement is often remarkably catholic. It has been estimated that about 50% of patients have involvement of other than the craniofacial area. One of the cardinal features of the syndrome is facial asymmetry. However, not all patients exhibit facial asymmetry.

There have been many attempts to classify the Oculo-auriculo-vertebral spectrum. Many systems have been limited because they have focused on one or two anatomic variables (Lauritzen et al., 1985, David et al., 1987).

Using the mandible and temporomandibular joint as reference centers, Kaban et al., (1988) modified Pruzansky's earlier system of classification, separating the mandibular form in Oculo-auriculo-vertebral spectrum into three basic types: type I, miniature mandible with normal morphology; type IIA,

Management of Genetic Syndromes, Edited by Suzanne B. Cassidy and Judith E. Allanson
ISBN 0-471-31286-X   Copyright © 2001 by Wiley-Liss, Inc.

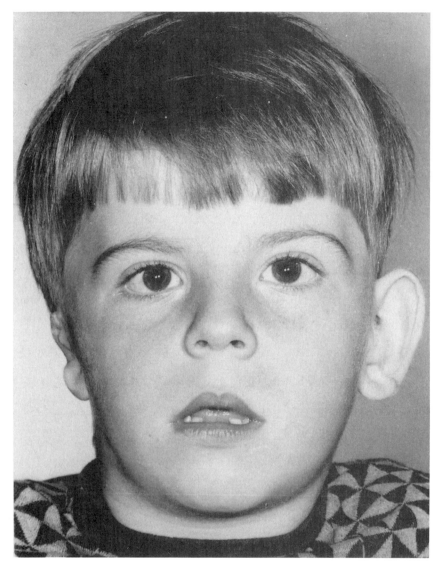

FIGURE 16.1. This young boy has right hemifacial microsomia with right microtia.

mandibular ramus abnormal in size and shape; type IIB, mandibular ramus abnormal in size, shape, and location requiring costo-chondral graft construction; type III, absent ramus, condyle, and temporomandibular joint. In all three types, the temporal bone, orbit, zygoma, nasal bones, and maxilla may be distorted. The temporal bone and glenoid fossa are often displaced anteriorly. The zygomatic arch may also be small or absent in all three types. The orbit may be hypoplastic and inferiorly displaced, partic-ularly in types IIB and III. Patients with type III have the greatest potential growth deficiency. Obliquity of the occlusal plane develops at an earlier age than in types I and IIA.

A more comprehensive attempt is that of Vento et al., (1991), which the authors chose to name OMENS classification (O = orbital distortion, M = mandibular hypopla-sia, E = ear anomaly, N = nerve, S = soft

(a) 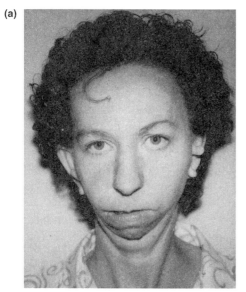   (b)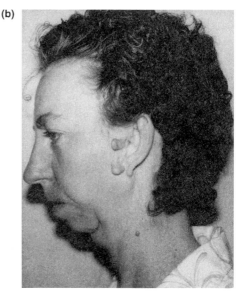

FIGURE 16.2. This adult woman demonstrates mild facial asymmetry, marked micrognathia, a right lateral cleft of the mouth, and multiple preauricular tags.

tissue deficiency). This classification easily adapts to data storage, retrieval, and analysis for craniofacial evaluation, surgical and other treatment modalities, and orthodontic therapy (Cousley, 1993). However, it undervalues anomalies of other systems (cardiac, CNS, skeletal, renal, etc.). Rollnick et al., (1987) provided a system for inclusion of systemic abnormalities.

Etiology, Pathogenesis, and Genetics

The constellation of anomalies in Oculo-auriculo-vertebral spectrum suggests an origin at about 30–45 days of gestation. This has been confirmed in humans by demonstration of disruption of vascular supply. Poswillo (1973), using an animal model, showed that early vascular disruption with expanding hematoma formation in utero resulted in destruction of differentiating tissues in the region of the ear and jaw. The severity appeared to be related to the degree of local destruction (Poswillo, 1973; Robinson et al., 1987). Another possible mechanism is that disturbances in the branchial arches or various populations of neural crest

cells may impede development of adjacent medial or frontonasal processes. First and second branchial arch anomalies are often seen in association with facial palsy in infants born to women exposed to thalidomide, primidone, and retinoic acid in utero. The Oculo-auriculo-vertebral spectrum phenotype has also been noted in infants born to diabetic mothers.

Although most cases of Oculo-auriculo-vertebral spectrum are isolated, several large families have been observed. Expression varies within these families. There are reports of ear and mandibular involvement in first-degree relatives and reports of isolated microtia or preauricular tags in first-degree relatives of patients with ear and mandibular involvement. Whether isolated microtia or preauricular tags represent the mildest expression of the disorder has never been established. It should be pointed out that preauricular skin tags or nodules occur in about 1% of the normal population.

Against the possibility of single-gene inheritance, as in most cases, is discordance in monozygotic twins, which has been reported frequently. Only rarely has concordance been documented in monozygotic twins. There have been an ample number of affected individuals in two generations and a few affected sibs with normal parents. A recurrence risk of 2–3% has been estimated. It should also be mentioned that a few families (possibly representing 1–2%) have autosomal dominant inheritance.

Oculo-auriculo-vertebral spectrum is caused by several factors. There is a remarkable collection of reports in which some aspects of the spectrum have been seen in a wide variety of chromosomal aneuploidies, including del(5p), del(6q), trisomy 7 mosaicism, del(8q), trisomy 9 mosaicism, trisomy 18, del(18q), del(21q), del(22q), and several variants of Klinefelter syndrome (Gorlin et al., 1995). These chromosomal anomalies may indicate multiple causative or contributory genes, may be coincidental, or may represent misdiagnosis.

Diagnostic Testing

There is no test for the Oculo-auriculo-vertebral spectrum. Diagnosis is made on clinical judgement. A chromosome analysis is appropriate in most cases, given the number of anomalies found in affected patients.

Differential Diagnosis

The Oculo-auriculo-vertebral spectrum, as indicated above, is remarkably variable and undoubtedly causally heterogeneous. One must exclude various chromosome disorders. In addition, several syndromes have overlapping features. Townes-Brocks syndrome consists of dysplastic ears, ear tags, and hearing loss in addition to thumb anomalies (most commonly triphalangeal thumb), anal defects, and renal anomalies. It has autosomal dominant inheritance. The branchio-oto-renal (BOR) syndrome has mixed hearing loss, preauricular pits, branchial cysts or fistulas, anomalous pinnae, malformations of the middle or inner ear, lacrimal duct stenosis, and/or renal dysplasia. It also has autosomal dominant inheritance with variable expression. Families have been reported in which first-degree relatives have varying features of hemifacial microsomia and/or branchio-oto-renal syndrome. However, the gene for brachio-oto-renal syndrome has been located at 8q13. The characteristic features of the Oculo-auriculo-vertebral spectrum should be distinguishable from mandibulofacial dysostosis (Treacher Collins syndrome), maxillofacial dysostosis, Nager acrofacial dysostosis, and postaxial acrofacial dysostosis, all of which tend to have bilateral, reasonably symmetrical involvement. As noted above, facial involvement in the Oculo-auriculo-vertebral spectrum is usually asymmetric. Partial to total absence of the lower eyelashes has not been reported in the Oculo-auriculo-vertebral spectrum, whereas colobomas of the upper eyelids are not infrequent. Characteristics of the VATER association (see Chapter 28), the CHARGE association (see Chapter 5), and the MURCS association (müllerian duct aplasia, renal aplasia, and cervical thoracic vertebral dysplasia) overlap with the Oculo-auriculo-vertebral spectrum.

MANIFESTATIONS AND MANAGEMENT

Because the Oculo-auriculo-vertebral spectrum is so complex, a team approach is necessary (Harvold et al., 1983; Munro, 1987; Kaban et al., 1988; Chibbaro, 1999). Treatment is long-term, and although some surgical procedures are carried out early, others may extend into adulthood.

Growth and Feeding

Affected infants are often small for dates (Avon and Shively, 1988). However, later growth abnormalities have not been documented in Oculo-auriculo-vertebral spectrum.

Development and Behavior

Estimates of the frequency of cognitive deficits have ranged from 5–15%; however, this has not been adequately investigated. There is some evidence to suggest that children with Oculo-auriculo-vertebral spectrum are at risk for psychosocial problems and that measures of self-concept are low (Padwa et al., 1991). These children are also at risk for speech problems. D'Antonia et al., (1998) found a higher than expected occurrence of pharyngeal and laryngeal abnormalities affecting speech production. They found asymmetric soft palate elevation and lack of sufficient velopharyngeal closure resulting in excessive nasality in several patients with Oculo-auriculo-vertebral spectrum, increased articulation errors likely related to velopharyngeal issues and/or malocclusions, and reduced overall speech intelligibility. Small laryngeal structures, asymmetric function, and narrowing of the airway at the laryngeal level were also described, resulting in voice deviation and concern about apnea for some.

Evaluation

- It is important that people with Oculo-auriculo-vertebral spectrum be followed periodically by an interdisciplinary craniofacial team for evaluation by psychologists and speech-language pathologists to identify problems and to intervene when appropriate. The value of comprehensive interdisciplinary evaluation addressing the range of structural manifestations of the disorder and potential effects in psychosocial and speech behavior cannot be overemphasized.

Treatment

- Psychological counseling is indicated for those patients where problems have been identified.
- Speech treatment is frequently needed, focusing on articulation, resources, or voice concerns.

- Not infrequently, consideration may need to be given to surgical or prosthodontic improvement of velopharyngeal closure. Surgical techniques are the same as those used in the general population.

Craniofacial

Skull defects include cranium bifidum, microcephaly, dolichocephaly, and plagiocephaly. Mild facial asymmetry is evident in about 65%, with marked asymmetry noted in roughly 20% (Fig. 16.1). The facial asymmetry is a function of age and is related to unusual bone growth. The temporal, maxillary, and malar bones on the more severely involved side are often reduced in dimension and flattened. Although this is generally considered to be a unilateral disorder, about 10–30% have bilateral involvement. For unknown reasons, the right side is generally more severely involved than the left. The mandibular ramus and condyle may be aplastic or hypoplastic (Fig. 16.2). The hypoplasia is often found in association with macrostomia of mild degree and, as noted above, is more common on the right side (R : L = 3 : 2). Unilateral or bilateral cleft lip and/or cleft palate occur in 7–15%, and macrostomia (lateral facial cleft) is present in at least 30% to some degree. Because the parotid glands have their embryonic origin at the corners of the mouth, it is not unusual for parotid duct development to have been disturbed in the general process. In some cases, there is unilateral parotid gland agenesis. Malocclusion is extremely frequent.

Longitudinal studies have established that hemifacial microsomia is a progressive condition. Until relatively recent times, treatment was delayed until the deformity reached "end-state." Good evidence has accumulated to indicate that this is not always wise. In the case of mild examples, delay probably does not cause serious facial skeletal changes or psychological impairment. However, with severe forms of Oculo-auriculo-vertebral spectrum that have not been corrected in childhood, extensive surgical procedures carried out on both the upper and lower jaw and occasional orbital osteotomies are required. As the normal side grows, the shortened and deformed hypoplastic mandible results in secondary deformation of the orbit, nose, and maxilla. Decreased mandibular growth prevents vertical elongation of the ipsilateral face. This, in turn, results in canting of the maxilla and the occlusal plane. Failure of downward growth of the maxilla also results in secondary orbital displacement.

Evaluation

- Before CT scans and MRI, the degree of hypoplasia and distortion of the mandible was examined in three standard X-ray planes, the frontal plane being seen in anteroposterior (AP) cephalometric radiographs, which allowed estimation of discrepancy in ramus height, tilting of maxilla, pyriform apertures, and orbits, and the extent of mandibular rotation toward the affected side. Lateral cephalograms and panorex studies allowed examination of the sagittal plane. The temporomandibular joint was examined, and discrepancy in height of mandibular rami in relationship to the upper jaws and to the base of the skull was assessed. The transverse plane was examined by a submental vertex radiograph to demonstrate shape and width of the mandibular body, the degree of asymmetry of zygomatic arches, and, if possible, displacement of the temporomandibular joint.
- In most major medical centers these three radiographic views have become auxiliary, having been largely replaced by three-dimensional CT reconstruction.

Treatment

- Correction of macrostomia should begin in the first 6 months.

- In the mildest form of hemifacial microsomia, and if the individual is less than 6 years of age, a functional orthodontic appliance is used to guide the mandibular remnant into a better, more normal position for bringing the affected side of the jaw downward, forward, and toward the midline. The appliance also stimulates skeletal growth by placing tension on the affected muscles. This can first be done when the child is 3–4 years of age.
- If the appliance is not effective, the hypoplastic mandible is surgically advanced, elongated, and rotated into correct position. This creates a posterior open bite on the affected side. In some cases, a compensatory osteotomy may be required on the contralateral side to allow rotation without disturbing the joint. The posterior open bite is progressively reduced by an orthodontic appliance.
- In more severe cases (types IIB and III), during the deciduous dentition stage, construction of the zygoma, glenoid fossa, temporomandibular joint, condyle, and ramus should be carried out so that symmetry with the opposite joint is achieved. The zygomatic arch is usually made from rib grafts or even cranial bone grafts. The glenoid fossa is lined with perichondrium. In construction of the temporomandibular joint, a bone graft is placed medial to the newly constructed zygomatic arch and hollowed to receive the condylar graft. The ramus is constructed from full-thickness rib graft, iliac graft, or calvarial material (Lindquist et al., 1986).
- The various surgical procedures used for treatment of Oculo-auriculo-vertebral spectrum, such as mandibular osteotomies, costochondral grafts, and maxillary osteotomies done at an early age or after permanent dentition has been completed, often affect the vitality of tooth

buds and often are followed by relapses. This requires several operations.

- It is likely that many of the surgical procedures that have been used for correction of the Oculo-auriculo-vertebral spectrum will be replaced within the next few years by bone distraction, the technique originally used by Ilizarov et al. in the early 1950s to align fractured segments of long bones and later to elongate the bones without a bone graft (Molina and Ortiz-Monasterio, 1995). The technique employed is roughly as follows. An oblique corticotomy is made in the external cortex of the mandible at the level of the gonial angle. Stainless steel points are inserted and joined by a softer distraction screw. Cuts are made in the mandible either unilaterally or bilaterally. Extraoral devices were used initially but are being replaced by intraoral devices. New bone is deposited in the space created by the cut at the rate of approximately 1–2 mm per day. This technique obviates the need for blood transfusion, harvesting of bone grafts, tracheotomy, and even, in some cases, intramaxillary fixation. The potential for bone regeneration is highest in younger individuals.

Ears and Hearing

Abnormalities of the external ear range from anotia (absence) to an ill-defined mass of tissue displaced anteriorly and inferiorly to a mildly dysmorphic ear (Figs. 16.1 and 16.2). Rarely, there is bilateral involvement. Preauricular tags of skin and cartilage are extremely common and may be unilateral or bilateral (Fig. 16.2). These ear tags are located anywhere from the tragus to the angle of the mouth. They are most commonly seen in patients with macrostomia and/or aplasia of the parotid gland and epibulbar dermoids. Preauricular sinuses may be noted. In milder cases, the external auditory canals

are narrow, with severe pinnal anomalies being associated with atretic canals. Rarely, small pinnae with normal architecture are seen, and, as noted above, isolated microtia is considered by some to be a microform of the spectrum.

Both conductive (75%) and, less frequently, sensorineural (10%) hearing loss have been reported in about 75% of patients with Oculo-auriculo-vertebral spectrum. Mixed hearing loss is noted in many patients (10%). Despite unilateral external ear involvement, it is not unusual for conductive hearing loss to be present on the contralateral side (Carvalho et al., 1999). The etiology of hearing loss is diverse and includes anomalies of the middle and external ears, hypoplasia or agenesis of ossicles, aberrant facial nerves, patulous eustachian tubes, and abnormalities of the skull base (Kaye et al., 1989; Bassila and Goldberg, 1989). Persons with unilateral hearing loss are at higher risk for educational problems and grade failure. It has been suggested that 25% of children with unilateral hearing loss repeat one or more grades, especially if the loss is severe to profound and/or is in the right ear (Bess and Humes, 1990).

Evaluation

- Otoscopy should be part of the routine physical examination.
- It is imperative that hearing be evaluated bilaterally to determine the nature and extent of the hearing loss. Educational audiologists serving school districts or clinical audiologists associated with otolaryngology practice or interdisciplinary craniofacial teams should evaluate hearing (air and bone conduction) and middle ear functions via tympanometry (when possible) at least on a 6-month basis.
- In very young children where behavioral audiometric procedures are not possible, auditory brain stem response (ABR) or otoacoustic emission assessments should be done.

Treatment

- Surgical treatment during the first 6 months involves removal of skin tags under local anesthesia.
- A hypoplastic, badly positioned ear can be moved into the correct location in frontal and sagittal planes.
- Very often, early ear construction results in misplaced auricular framework, the malaligned ear usually being located anterior and inferior. It is best to wait until adolescence to achieve ultimate symmetry. Early correction, not uncommonly, leaves residual soft tissue defects, and dermal fat grafts or de-epithelialized free vascularized scapular flaps may be required.
- Depending on the nature and extent of the hearing loss, children need to be evaluated for potential benefits of personal and/or classroom amplifications (FM systems).
- Preferential classroom seating is mandated with the better ear toward the source of auditory information and away from extraneous noises such as vents and fans.
- Surgical improvement of hearing on the affected side should be considered and is dependent on anatomical status, position, and, of course, the facial nerve, and choice of the patient and family. Again, interdisciplinary craniofacial treatment planning is important. Ear procedures may be done in conjunction with other surgical and/or dental procedures.
- Antibiotic treatment for middle ear disease in the better or normal ear is recommended.
- If middle ear effusion persists, myringotomy and ventilation tube insertion must be considered.

Neurologic

A wide range of neurologic defects has been found. Lower facial nerve weakness, seen in about 20% (Bassila and Goldberg, 1989; Carvalho et al., 1999), is probably related to bony involvement in the region of the facial canal. Nearly all cranial nerves have been reported to be affected on occasion. In the so-called expanded Oculo-auriculo-vertebral spectrum, brain malformations including encephalocele, hydrocephaly, lipoma, dermoid cysts, teratoma, Arnold-Chiari malformation, lissencephaly, arachnoid cyst, holoprosencephaly, unilateral arhinencephaly, and hypoplasia of the corpus callosum have been described. Lower facial nerve weakness correlates with severity of ear involvement but not with the degree of mandibular hypoplasia. It is not unusual for the soft palate to deviate to the contralateral side. Asymmetric velar elevation may affect adequacy of velopharyngeal closure for speech.

Evaluation

- Patients need to be evaluated to determine the effect of neurologic involvement on specific oral-pharyngeal functions such as speech, feeding, and swallowing. All may be involved in some patients. Ideally, these evaluations are carried out periodically by speech-language pathologists in an interdisciplinary setting.

Treatment

- Patients frequently benefit from speech treatment focusing on compensatory strategies to optimize speech intelligibility and articulation.
- Depending on the status of velopharyngeal closure, speech therapy and surgical and prosthodontic treatment may be required.
- Temporalis muscle transfer can improve facial animation on the affected side.

Ophthalmologic

Eye anomalies are extremely common. They include epibulbar dermoids (35%), blepharoptosis or narrowing of the palpebral fissure on the involved side (10%), and clinical anophthalmia or microphthalmia (rare). The latter may be correlated with the presence of mental retardation (personal observation). Coloboma of the upper lid has been noted unilaterally in about 20% and bilaterally in possibly 3%.

Evaluation

- Complete eye evaluation should be carried out at diagnosis.
- Periodic ophthalmologic evaluation in the interdisciplinary craniofacial clinic is also desirable.

Treatment

- Frequently, surgical management of epibulbar dermoids, ptosis, and colobomas can be coordinated with other procedures in the same surgical setting.

Cardiovascular

Various forms of heart anomalies have been recorded. These are probably present in about 35% (range 5–60%). Ventriculoseptal defect and tetralogy of Fallot account for about 50% of structural defects, although no single cardiac lesion is characteristic. A wide variety of other lesions have been documented, including transposition of great vessels, hypoplasia of the aortic arch, isolation of the left innominate artery with bilateral patent ductus arteriosus, pulmonary stenosis, and dextrocardia (Pierpont et al., 1982; Morrison et al., 1992; Kumar et al., 1993).

Evaluation

- If a heart murmur is detected by the physician in the neonatal period, the infant should be referred to a pediatric cardiologist for evaluation.

Treatment

- Depending on the anomaly present, cardiac surgery may be required.

- The infant should be in good cardiac status before any surgical procedure is considered.

Musculoskeletal

Cervical vertebral fusions have been demonstrated in about 20–35%, whereas platybasia and occipitalization of the atlas have been found with about the same frequency. However, a wide variety of spinal anomalies have been reported: spina bifida, hemivertebrae, butterfly vertebrae, fused and hypoplastic vertebrae, Klippel-Feil anomaly, scoliosis, and anomalous ribs. Collectively, these are present in about 30% (Gibson et al., 1996).

Talipes equinovarus (club feet) has been noted in about 20%, with radial limb anomalies in about 10%. These usually take the form of hypoplasia or aplasia of the radius and/or thumb and bifid or digitalized thumb (Figueroa and Friede, 1985).

Evaluation

- The primary care physician should conduct a careful musculoskeletal evaluation.
- Consultation with an orthopedic surgeon for several of the anomalies (scoliosis, talipes equinovarus) is mandated.

Treatment

- Scoliosis and talipes equinovarus should be treated in the standard fashion by the orthopedic surgeon.
- Cervical vertebral fusions do not usually produce symptoms, and no therapy is required.

Respiratory

Lung anomalies range from incomplete lobulation to hypoplasia to agenesis. These findings have been rare, probably on the order of 5%. They can be unilateral or bilateral. Pulmonary agenesis usually occurs on the same side as the facial anomalies. Tracheoesophageal fistula has also been documented. Obstructive sleep apnea has been reported.

Evaluation

- Tracheoesophageal fistula may be suspected in the newborn period if it is difficult to pass a suction tube to clear tracheal secretions.
- If obstructive sleep apnea is suspected, a full sleep study should be arranged.

Treatment

- Surgical correction of tracheoesophageal fistula is performed using standard techniques.
- Treatment of apnea will depend on the cause.

Genitourinary

Renal anomalies, which are rare, have included renal agenesis, double ureter, crossed renal ectopia, renovascular anomalies, hydronephrosis, and hydroureter.

Evaluation

- If a child has recurrent urinary tract infections, a search should be made for an underlying structural anomaly.

Treatment

- The associated renal anomalies are rarely severe and seldom need surgical correction unless there is obstruction or reflux.

Gastrointestinal

Rarely reported is imperforate anus with or without rectovaginal fistula.

Evaluation

- At birth, patency of the anus should be established.

Treatment

- Surgical treatment of anal anomalies, when present, is standard.

RESOURCES

AboutFace USA
  1002 Liberty Lane
  Warrington, PA 18976
  800-225-FACE

Children's Craniofacial Association
  PO Box 280297
  Dallas, TX 75243-4522
  972-994-9902

FACES — National Association for the Craniofacially Handicapped
  PO Box 11082
  Chattanooga, TN 37401
  800-332-2373 (Contact: Priscilla Caine)

Let's Face It, Inc.
  PO Box 29972
  Bellingham, WA 98228-1972
  Contact: Betsy Wilson, Director
  360-676-7325
  Website: *http://www.nas.com/~letsfaceit/*

Ear Anomalies Reconstructed (EAR)
  Atresia-Microtia Support Group
  72 Durand Rd.
  Maplewood, NJ 07040
  201-761-5438 (Contact: Jack Gross or Betsy Olds)

NORD: National Organization for Rare Disorders, Inc.
  100 Rt. 37, PO Box 8923
  New Fairfield
  CT 06812-8923
  Ph: 203-746-6518
  Email: *orphan@nord-rdb.com*
  Internet:
  http://www.nord-rdb.com/~orphan

About Face
  99 Crowns Lane
  Toronto M59 3P4
  Ontario, Canada
  800-665-FACE
  Email: *abtface@interlog.com* (attention: Laura)

Changing Faces (UK)
0171-706-4232
Email: *info@faces.demon.co.uk*

REFERENCES

Avon SW, Shively JL (1988) Orthopaedic manifestations of Goldenhar syndrome. *J Pediatr Orthop* 8:683–686.

Bassila MK, Goldberg R (1989) The association of facial palsy and/or sensorineural hearing loss in patients with hemifacial microsomia. *Cleft Palate J* 26:287–291.

Bess FH, Humes LE (1990) *Audiology: The Fundamentals.* Baltimore, MD: Williams and Wilkins.

Carvalho GJ, Song CS, Vargervik K, Lalwani AK (1999) Auditory and facial nerve dysfunction in patients with hemifacial microsomia. *Arch Otolaryngol Head Neck Surg* 125:209–212.

Chibbaro PD (1999) Living with craniofacial microsomia: Support for the patient and family. *Cleft Palate Craniofac J* 36:40–42.

Cohen MM Jr, Rollnick BR, Kaye CI (1989) Oculo-auriculo-vertebral spectrum: An updated critique. *Cleft Palate J* 26:276–286.

Cousley RRJ (1993) A comparison of two classification systems for hemifacial microsomia. *Br J Oral Maxillofac Surg* 31:78–82.

David DJ, Mahatumarat C, Cooter RD (1987) Hemifacial microsomia: A multisystem classification. *Plast Reconstr Surg* 80:525–533.

D'Antonia LL, Rice RD, Fink SC (1998) Evaluation of pharyngeal and laryngeal structure and function in patients with oculo-auriculo-vertebral spectrum. *Cleft Palate Craniofac J* 35:333–341.

Figueroa AA, Friede H (1985) Costovertebral malformation in hemifacial microsomia. *J Craniofac Genet Dev Biol Suppl* 1:167–178.

Gibson JNA, Sillence DO, Taylor TKF (1996) Abnormalities of the spine in Goldenhar's syndrome. *J Pediatr Orthopaed* 16:344–349.

Gorlin RJ, Toriello HV, Cohen MM Jr (1995) *Hereditary Hearing Loss and Its Syndromes.* New York: Oxford University Press.

Harvold EP, Vargevik K, Chierici G, eds. (1983) *Treatment of hemifacial microsomia.* New York: Liss.

Kaban LB, Moses MH, Mulliken JB (1988) Surgical correction of hemifacial microsomia. *Plast Reconstr Surg* 82:9–19.

Kaye CI, Rollnick BR, Hauck WW, Martin AO, Richtsmeyer JT, Nagatoshi K (1989) Microtia and associated anomalies. *Am J Med Genet* 34:574–578.

Kumar A, Friedman JM, Taylor GP, Patterson MWH (1993) Pattern of cardiac malformation in oculo-auriculo-vertebral spectrum. *Am J Med Genet* 46:423–426.

Lauritzen C, Munro IF, Ross RB (1985) Classification and treatment of hemifacial microsomia. *Scand J Plast Reconstr Surg* 19:33–39.

Lindquist C, Pihakari A, Tasanen A, Hampf G (1986) Autogenous costochondral grafts in temporomandibular joint arthroplasty. *J Maxillofac Surg* 14:143–149.

Molina F, Ortiz-Monasterio F (1995) Mandibular elongation and remodeling by distraction: A farewell to major osteotomies. *Plast Reconstr Surg* 96:825–45.

Morrison PJ, Mulholland HC, Craig BG, Nevin NC (1992) Cardiovascular abnormalities in the oculo-auriculo-vertebral spectrum (Goldenhar syndrome). *Am J Med Genet* 44:425–428.

Munro IR (1987) Treatment of craniofacial microsomia. *Clin Plast Surg* 14:177–186.

Padwa BL, Evans CA, Pillemer FC (1991) Psychosocial adjustments in children with hemifacial microsomia and other craniofacial deformities. *Cleft Palate Craniofac J* 28:354–359.

Pierpont MEM, Moller JH, Gorlin RJ, Edwards JE (1982) Congenital cardiac, pulmonary and vascular malformations in oculo-auriculo-vertebral dysplasia. *Ped Cardiol* 2:297–302.

Poswillo D (1973) The pathogenesis of the first and second branchial arch syndrome. *Oral Surg* 35:302–329.

Robinson L, Hoyme HE, Edwards DK, Jones KL (1987) The vascular pathogenesis of unilateral craniofacial defects. *J Pediatr* 111:236–239.

Rollnick BR, Kaye CE, Nagatoski K (1987) Oculo-auriculo-vertebral dysplasia and variants: Phenotypic characteristics of 194 patients. *Am J Med Genet* 26:361–375.

Vento AR, LaBrie RA, Mulliken JB (1991) The O.M.E.N.S. classification of hemifacial microsomia. *Cleft Palate J* 28:68–76.

CHAPTER 17

OSTEOGENESIS IMPERFECTA

JOAN C. MARINI AND EDITH J. CHERNOFF

INTRODUCTION

Osteogenesis imperfecta is an autosomal dominant disorder of type I collagen, more commonly known as "brittle bone disease." The occurrence of osteogenesis imperfecta can be traced to early human history. The earliest case with good skeletal documentation is that of an Egyptian mummy dating from about 1000 B.C. The first description of osteogenesis imperfecta in the medical literature was published in 1788 by Ekman, in which he described "osteomalacia congenita" (Ekman, 1788). Vrolik coined the term osteogenesis imperfecta in 1849 (Vrolik, 1849) and Looser divided the disorder into "congenita" and "tarda" forms in 1906 (Looser, 1906). However, it was not until 1918 that Van der Hoeve and de Kleyn (1918) described the triad of fragile bones, blue sclerae, and early-onset deafness as a distinct syndrome. The terms "congenita" and "tarda" have since fallen into disuse, because they fail to adequately describe the variability in osteogenesis imperfecta.

Incidence

The overall frequency of osteogenesis imperfecta identifiable at birth is estimated to be between 1 in 20,000 and 1 in 30,000. In the United States, the incidence is 1 in 20,000 if all children diagnosed within 1 year of birth are included. A survey of Victoria, Australia yielded a type II osteogenesis imperfecta frequency of 1 in 62,000 births and a type III osteogenesis imperfecta frequency of 1 in 68,000 births (Sillence et al., 1986). The minimum frequency of type I osteogenesis imperfecta in Victoria, Australia was estimated to be approximately 1 in 30,000. There is no preferential distribution of osteogenesis imperfecta by gender, race, or ethnic group (McKusick, 1972).

Diagnostic Criteria

Osteogenesis imperfecta is characterized by bone fragility such that affected individuals sustain fractures after very mild trauma. In fact, the trauma is sometimes so insignificant that patients cannot identify when or how a fracture occurred. In addition, the disorder often includes other skeletal features, such as short stature, relative macrocephaly, scoliosis, and bowing of the long bones. Because osteogenesis imperfecta is a generalized connective tissue disorder, other typical features include blue sclerae, dentinogenesis imperfecta, hearing loss, cardiopulmonary abnormalities, easy bruisability, excessive sweating, and loose joints.

Management of Genetic Syndromes, Edited by Suzanne B. Cassidy and Judith E. Allanson
ISBN 0-471-31286-X   Copyright © 2001 by Wiley-Liss, Inc.

Phenotypic diversity has prompted multiple attempts at classification of osteogenesis imperfecta. The system currently accepted was devised in 1979 by Sillence (Sillence et al., 1979). Affected individuals are separated into four types based on clinical, radiographic, and genetic findings. Given the variability of the disease, it should not be surprising that many affected individuals do not fit exactly into these rigid categories; however, the typing allows a common groundwork for discussion and research.

Osteogenesis imperfecta type I is the mildest form of the disorder. This phenotype includes postnatal onset of fractures, generally without ultimate bony deformity, hyperextensible joints, blue sclerae, early hearing loss, and easy bruisability. This category may be subdivided into types IA and IB based on the absence or presence of dentinogenesis imperfecta (Levin et al., 1978).

The most severe form of osteogenesis imperfecta is type II, which is almost uniformly lethal. This form of the disorder is characterized by extreme bone fragility, leading to fetal demise or death in the perinatal period (Sillence, 1981). Infants are often delivered prematurely or stillborn, and some are hydropic. Both weight and length are small for gestational age. Prenatal long bone fractures, shortening, and poor mineralization are detectable; fetal head size is large for body size, with radiographs revealing multiple wormian bones. On physical examination the "caput membranaceum" is soft to palpation, and the infants have flat triangular facies with a small, beaked nose. Scleral color is usually blue-gray. The thorax is narrow and small, and palpation of the ribs may feel similar to a rachitic rosary due to callus formation associated with multiple healing fractures sustained *in utero*. In addition, there is striking micromelia (small hands and feet) and bowing of the extremities. Legs are usually held in the frog leg position, with hips abducted and knees flexed.

Infants with type II osteogenesis imperfecta are extremely fragile, and delivery via cesarean section is recommended to avoid avulsion of body parts or intracranial hemorrhage. Affected newborns show markedly reduced ossification, especially of the skull, ribs, and tubular bones. Infants who survive the perinatal period generally die from pneumonia or respiratory insufficiency secondary to inadequate pulmonary volume. With optimum delivery and neonatal care, some infants with osteogenesis imperfecta type II have survived for months to years. On pathologic examination, the bones of these infants are severely porotic with no evidence of haversian canals or lamellar bone.

Type III osteogenesis imperfecta is known as the progressive deforming form (Fig. 17.1*A* and *B*) (Sillence et al., 1986). The presentation at birth is similar phenotypically to the milder end of the spectrum of type II disease. Although this form of the disorder is compatible with a long life, many children die in infancy of respiratory difficulties, whereas others die in childhood of pneumonia, cor pulmonale, or trauma. For those who survive, there is gradual deformity of the long bones (Fig. 17.2) and spine (Fig. 17.3), even in the absence of fractures, which, in combination with compression of vertebrae, contributes to marked short stature. Clinically, these patients have triangular facies and relative macrocephaly. Initially blue sclerae whiten with age. If dentinogenesis imperfecta is present, it is usually of the transparent, grayish variety. Affected individuals are intellectually normal barring significant birth trauma. Radiographically, one sees generalized osteoporosis, wormian bones, "codfish" vertebrae, and multiple deformities (Fig. 17.2). As childhood progresses, a cystic "popcorn" appearance of flared long bone metaphyses develops and the long bones may appear thin and twisted or cylindrical and crumpled (Fig. 17.4) (Sillence et al., 1984). Most of these patients are severely physically handicapped and have traditionally required multiple orthopedic rodding procedures and wheelchairs

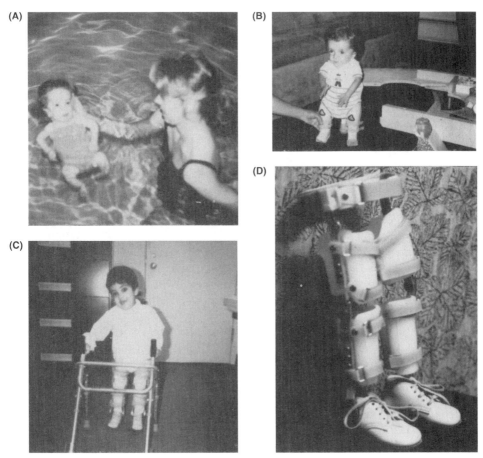

FIGURE 17.1. Rehabilitation of children with osteogenesis imperfecta. A: 1-year-old infant with severe osteogenesis imperfecta swimming with her mother. B: 3-year-old child in a standing frame. Note play table made by patient's family. C: 5-year-old boy walking with braces and a walker. D: Example of braces used for ambulation.

for mobility. Aggressive early intervention for rehabilitation and ambulation has been demonstrated to improve the prognosis for these children, especially in terms of their potential for self-care.

Finally, osteogenesis imperfecta type IV represents the moderately severe spectrum of this bone disease. The diagnosis may be recognized at birth because of prenatal fractures, although diagnosis may be delayed until the child begins to ambulate. During childhood, these children often have several fractures per year and moderate bowing of their long bones (Fig. 17.5). Fracture rate decreases at puberty. Most affected individuals have moderately short stature. In addition to moderate osteoporosis and modeling abnormalities of the long bones, radiographs demonstrate platyspondyly and mild scoliosis (Fig. 17.6). Division into types IVA or IVB is again based on the absence or presence of dentinogenesis imperfecta (Levin et al., 1978). Although the Sillence criteria emphasize scleral hue as a distinction between osteogenesis imperfecta types I and IV, patients have been described with bone disease consistent with osteogenesis imperfecta type IV and blue sclerae. It is unclear how this distinction will hold up as molecular diagnosis improves.

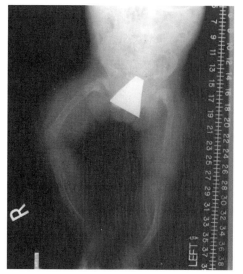

FIGURE 17.2. Lower extremity X rays of a 6-month-old child with osteogenesis imperfecta type III. Note bowing of limbs and thinning of cortices.

Etiology, Pathogenesis, and Genetics

Osteogenesis imperfecta is an autosomal dominant disorder caused by defects in type I collagen (Kuivaniemi et al., 1997). The collagens are a family of extracellular matrix proteins that are closely related but distinct. There are approximately 19 collagen types, each of which is composed of three α chains in a triple helical formation (Fig. 17.7). Type I collagen is the most abundant of the collagens and is the major constituent of most connective tissues, including bone, tendon, skin, dentin, ligament, fascia, and many blood vessels. It is composed of three α chains, two copies of the $\alpha 1$ chain and one copy of the $\alpha 2$ chain, which coil around each other to form a triple helix. Both chains are composed of uninterrupted repetitions of the amino acid sequence Gly-X-Y, in which a glycine residue holds every third position, X is frequently proline, and Y is frequently hydroxyproline. All collagen molecules form fibrils, which are supramolecular aggregates that are stabilized by interactions between the triple helix domains (Kivirikko, 1993) (Fig. 17.7).

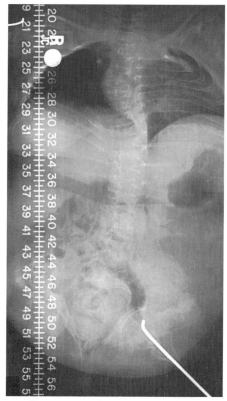

FIGURE 17.3. Chest film of an 11-year-old child with osteogenesis imperfecta type III showing scoliosis, collapse of multiple vertebrae, and thin, misshapen ribs.

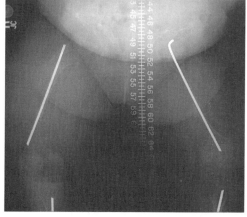

FIGURE 17.4. Lower extremity X rays of an 11-year-old child with osteogenesis imperfecta type III showing misshapen limbs and popcorning at the joints.

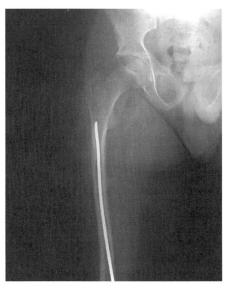

FIGURE 17.5. Lower extremity X ray of an 11-year-old child with osteogenesis imperfecta type IV. Note thicker cortex than in the child with osteogenesis imperfecta type III (Fig. 17.4) and rod in place.

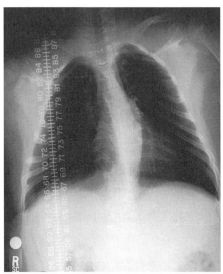

FIGURE 17.6. Chest film of an 11-year-old child with osteogenesis imperfecta type IV showing slight scoliosis and vertebrae thicker than in the child with osteogenesis imperfecta type III (Fig. 17.3).

Osteogenesis imperfecta is caused by mutations in the genes *COL1A1* and *COL1A2*, which reside on chromosomes 7 and 17, respectively, and which encode the $\alpha1$ and $\alpha2$ chains. Biosynthesis of type I collagen requires a large number of post-translational modifications that can be divided into two groups. The intracellular stage results in the formation of the triple helix procollagen molecules and requires at least 8 specific enzymes, whereas the extracellular stage leads to conversion of the procollagen molecule into collagen and incorporation of the collagen into stable, cross-linked fibrils.

The protein α chains of collagen are synthesized in procollagen forms, with globular extensions at both the amino and carboxyl terminal ends. Helix formation then occurs spontaneously in the carboxyl-to-amino direction, opposite to that of protein synthesis. Concomitant with helix formation, proline and lysine residues are hydroxylated. Some lysine residues that have been hydroxylated are also glycosylated. Biochemically, structural collagen defects are usually detected as collagen overmodification. Procollagen overmodification frequently decreases helix secretion from the cell, resulting in increased intracellular degradation. In contrast, mutations causing null $\alpha1$ alleles (i.e., no protein synthesis) are detected indirectly at the biochemical level. In these cases, the decreased type I collagen results in an increase in the type III:type I collagen ratio. Once secreted into the pericellular space, the procollagen terminal extensions are cleaved by specific amino-terminal and carboxyl-terminal peptidases. The resulting collagen molecules undergo self-assembly into fibrils that are stabilized by cross-links formed by lysyl oxidase.

Over 200 mutations have been recognized to cause osteogenesis imperfecta. Most are unique to an individual family. Initial descriptions of type II osteogenesis imperfecta attributed it to both autosomal recessive and autosomal dominant inheritance. The basis of proposing an autosomal recessive form was the occurrence of consanguinity in some families in the original series and the absence of clinical findings in parents

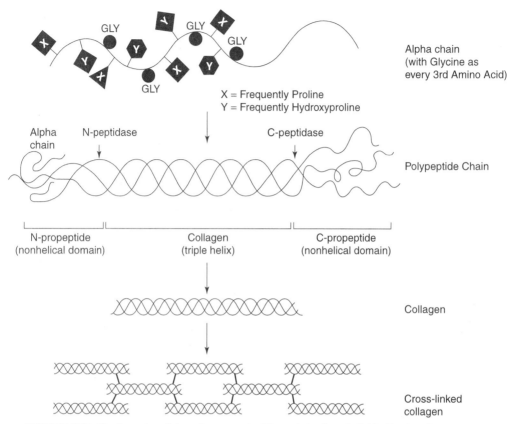

FIGURE 17.7. The formation of the collagen matrix. The α chains form individually; they then aggregate into triple helices with propeptide chains on either end. The propeptide chains are cleaved, and the fully formed triple helix is incorporated into the collagen matrix by crosslinking with other collagen triple helices. It is the regularity of the helices and their placement with crosslinking into the matrix that gives the tissues their strength.

with more than one affected child. More recent data have demonstrated that osteogenesis imperfecta type II, like the other forms of the disorder, is inherited in a dominant fashion and is most commonly caused by new dominant mutations.

The recurrence risk for osteogenesis imperfecta depends on the individual family's situation. Most cases of osteogenesis imperfecta, especially type II, are caused by a new mutation in the affected individual. Risk of recurrence in a subsequent child is due to mosaic carrier status in one parent, recurrence being caused by parental gonadal mosaicism. In families with unaffected parents and one affected child, the empiric risk for recurrence is 6–7%. The empiric recurrence risk increases to 28% if more than one affected child has been born to unaffected parents. Mosaicism is a mechanism by which a proportion of the cells and/or tissues of the body are normal whereas others carry the mutation. Thus an unaffected or minimally affected parent can have a severely affected child (Pepin et al., 1997). Examination of some of these parents reveals mild manifestations of the disorder, including osteoporosis. Findings depend on the developmental stage at which the mutation arose, the amount of abnormal collagen present in the various tissues, and how effective these tissues are at suppressing the mutation by negative selection. Eighteen cases of mosaicism have been documented in the literature, twelve paternal and six maternal; approximately one-third of these parents were mildly affected, as defined by their fracture history and/or scleral hue. When the mutation was known in the proband, all carrier parents had evidence of mosaicism in their leukocytes; however, not all had a detectable collagen abnormality in cultured fibroblasts. To date, no pure germ line carrier has been described. Once the mutation has been identified, the parent on whose collagen allele the mutation occurred can be assessed for proportion of the mutant allele and tissue distribution. By identifying the mutation in tissues, including sperm, the percent mosaicism can be quantified and a more accurate recurrence risk can be given. In mosaic fathers, investigation of the proportion of mutation in sperm provides the most accurate recurrence risk. When individuals with osteogenesis imperfecta become parents, the risk to their offspring rises to 50%, consistent with an autosomal dominant mutation.

There is great variability in the presentation of osteogenesis imperfecta. The correlation of phenotype with genotype is still not completely understood and is an active area of investigation. It has been noted that, even within families, affected individuals may display considerable phenotypic heterogeneity. Unrelated individuals with identical mutations may have similar or distinct phenotypes. Furthermore, individuals with almost identical phenotypes often have different molecular defects. Lethal and nonlethal mutations are both represented approximately equally on α1 and α2 chains.

Phenotype appears to be determined by the nature of the specific mutation, the chain in which it occurs, and its location in the chain. Recently, a regional model was proposed suggesting that phenotype could be predicted on the basis of the location of the mutation within a series of alternating lethal and nonlethal regions along the α chain. This model accounts for approximately 86% of mutations on the α2 chain but does not account for α1 mutations (Marini et al., 1993).

There exist two broad categories of molecular genetic mutations that generally correlate with the Sillence classification of osteogenesis imperfecta, null mutations and structural mutations. Null mutations dramatically decrease the amount of functional α chain made from the collagen allele containing the mutation. The null mutations described in α1 cause premature chain termination. These patients make half the normal amount of α1 chain, but all the type I collagen they make is structurally normal. These mutations correlate with the mild type I osteogenesis imperfecta phenotype (Willing et al., 1993).

The more severe forms of osteogenesis imperfecta, types II, III, and IV, are caused by structural mutations. The majority (85%) cause substitution of a glycine residue with a bulkier amino acid. Single exon splicing defects cause 10% of osteogenesis imperfecta mutations, and the remainder are a variety of insertions, duplications, and large deletions. These mutations cause varying degrees of collagen overmodification, intracellular protein suicide, and abnormal fibril formation (Prockop, 1997).

To better understand the pathophysiology of osteogenesis imperfecta, it is important to understand the function of osteoblasts and fibroblasts and the formation of collagen matrix. Research into collagen matrix formation may be helpful in correlating mutation to phenotype, as well as illuminating disease pathophysiology.

Normal bone formation involves the deposition of a collagen fibrillar network composed primarily of type I collagen with a minor proportion of type V collagen. Noncollagenous proteins are incorporated into the extracellular matrix. Hydroxyapetite crystals are then deposited along the fibrils. The proportions of all components of the matrix are crucial for bone mineralization and functional strength (Fedarko et al., 1992).

In vitro studies of fibroblasts derived from patients with osteogenesis imperfecta reveal a decrease in the amount of secreted collagen, resulting in poor matrix deposition. Mutant collagen tends to be selectively degraded after incorporation into the matrix (Bateman and Golub, 1994). Tissue-specific differences in the metabolism of mutant type I collagen may explain why osteogenesis imperfecta manifests primarily as a disease of brittle bones despite type I collagen being secreted by multiple tissues (Sarafova et al., 1998).

The bony matrix of patients with osteogenesis imperfecta contains relatively increased type III and V collagen and decreased type I collagen. In addition, there are decreased levels of osteonectin, large chondroitin sulfate, biglycan and decorin, and increased levels of fibronectin, thrombospondin and hyaluronate (Prockop, 1997). Because decorin and biglycan have a role in binding transforming growth factor β, which is a stimulant of bone cell proliferation and matrix synthesis, it has been hypothesized that a decrease in these two proteoglycans may contribute to the growth retardation seen in patients with osteogenesis imperfecta through alteration in local transforming growth factor β concentration (Prockop, 1997).

Diagnostic Testing

Clinical diagnosis is primarily based on family history, physical, and radiographic findings, as delineated in **Diagnostic Criteria**. Analysis of defects in collagen synthesis or secretion is available. Although osteogenesis imperfecta remains a clinical diagnosis, testing confirms the diagnosis and identification of a mutation allows one to test the parents; this is important with respect to prenatal diagnosis and counseling of recurrence risk.

Prenatal diagnosis for osteogenesis imperfecta can be accomplished by noninvasive testing or invasive methods. The main mode of noninvasive prenatal diagnosis is ultrasound. Ultrasonography is the only option for prenatal diagnosis when the collagen defect and the mutation are both unknown. It is useful for the diagnosis of severe cases, but milder forms are often missed and detection may only occur late in the second trimester. If there is a known risk of osteogenesis imperfecta type II, detection may be possible as early as 15 weeks gestation. In cases of osteogenesis imperfecta type III or type IV, diagnosis cannot be made reliably until after 20 weeks, as limb shortness may not become apparent until then.

Ultrasound findings that suggest a diagnosis of osteogenesis imperfecta include low echogenicity of all bones due to their poor mineralization and abnormalities in long bones, especially in the femora, such as shortening, angulation, bowing, and fractures. Rib cage deformity is also common, with the chest appearing narrow at the apices and the ribs flared. The skull may be thinner than normal, and light compression by the ultrasound receiver may result in deformation of the cranial outline (Thompson, 1993).

If the mutation is known, molecular analysis performed on a chorionic villus sample is highly accurate and has the advantage of being available in early gestation. Even when the mutation in the first affected child has not been identified, biochemical studies of collagen synthesis, performed directly on the chorionic villi or after sample culture, may detect abnormal collagen in a subsequent pregnancy (Pepin et al., 1997). As discussed previously in this chapter, structural collagen defects can be detected as overmodification of the protein; thus these studies will be most accurate for cases in which there is a substantial overmodification of type I collagen caused by mutations located in the carboxyl half of the collagen helix.

Amniocentesis is useful only if the mutation is known and if linkage studies or restriction enzyme analysis can be performed on cultured amniocytes. It is not suitable for biochemical testing in osteogenesis imperfecta because of false positive overmodification. In other words, analysis may be carried out on DNA but not on protein; thus the mutation must be known in advance. There are currently two groups in the United States that do clinical testing for osteogenesis imperfecta. One group does biochemical testing on all cases received and mutation identification on selected cases. The other group offers DNA analysis (mutational identification) but not biochemical testing. Mutational identification is also available on a research basis. Information as to the location of these laboratories is available through GeneTests.

Differential Diagnosis

Because the four types of osteogenesis imperfecta vary widely in clinical appearance and in the timing of onset of symptoms, the differential diagnosis depends on the age of the patient in question. Prenatally, osteogenesis imperfecta type II can be difficult to distinguish from some of the chondrodystrophies, especially thanatophoric dysplasia, campomelic dwarfism, and achondrogenesis type I. Neonatally, there may be some difficulty in distinguishing between osteogenesis imperfecta type III and infantile hypophosphatasia, and in older children with type I osteogenesis imperfecta there may be confusion with juvenile osteoporosis. The major differential diagnosis with type I and IV osteogenesis imperfecta is child abuse. It is often difficult to distinguish clinically between child abuse and osteogenesis imperfecta types I and IV. Although the children with osteogenesis imperfecta may have blue sclerae, unaffected infants may also have this finding. Finding decreased bone mineral density, wormian bones, or evidence of osteoporosis on X ray may be helpful in differentiating between abuse and osteogenesis imperfecta. In addition, children with osteogenesis imperfecta should not have other evidence of abuse or neglect. They should not have excessive bruising,

burns, or cuts that may be seen in children who have been abused. Obviously, a molecular diagnosis consistent with osteogenesis imperfecta would be the definitive distinction.

Thanatophoric dysplasia is a lethal chondrodystrophy caused by mutations in fibroblast growth factor receptor 3. It occurs with a frequency of 1 in 20,000 and is inherited as an autosomal dominant mutation. Affected fetuses are characterized by markedly shortened extremities, relatively large cranium, and narrow thorax. Diagnosis can be made using ultrasound between 20 and 24 weeks, which reveals an increased biparietal diameter and very short limbs without polydactyly (Camera et al., 1983; Elejalde and de Elejalde, 1985).

Campomelic dysplasia is a syndrome that includes a large dolichocephalic head, disproportionate limb shortness, hypoplastic scapulae, pelvic and spine changes, and small thorax with 11 pairs of ribs. The lower extremities are often bowed with pretibial dimples, congenital hip dislocation, and talipes equinovarus. It is an autosomal dominant disorder caused by mutation of the *SOX9* gene. Death due to respiratory insufficiency usually occurs within the first months of life. Prenatal ultrasound evaluation reveals a large skull, often with hydrocephaly and poorly ossified tubular bones. Hydrocephaly can be seen as early as 16 weeks gestation and may be important in differentiating this syndrome from other short-limbed entities like osteogenesis imperfecta (Fryns et al., 1981).

Achondrogenesis type I is another lethal chondrodystophy. Radiographically, the disorder presents with micromelia, large cranium due to soft tissue swelling, deficient ossification in lumbar vertebrae, and absent ossification in sacral, pubic, and ischial bones. Type I achondrogenesis can be further subdivided into type IA and type IB based on histologic examination of chondro-osseous morphology. Inheritance is likely autosomal recessive, but this has not been proven (Borochowitz et al., 1988).

Hypophosphatasia is an autosomal recessive genetic disorder that can be divided into three types, infantile, childhood, and adult onset. The infantile form has its onset prenatally or early in postnatal life and is usually fatal in infancy. Prenatally, "spurs" of the limbs, small thornlike structures that extend from the sides of the knee and elbow joints, are diagnostic. These can be seen only by X-ray, however, and not on ultrasound (Whyte, 1995). Infants present with craniostenosis, hypercalcemia, and bony abnormalities including severe osteoporosis and micromelia, with severe epiphyseal and metaphyseal disturbances in the long bones, vertebrae, and ribs. Diagnosis can be made by determination of serum alkaline phosphatase (low), phosphoethanolamine (increased), and inorganic pyrophosphate (increased). In osteogenesis imperfecta, alkaline phosphatase is normal or elevated.

Osteoporosis occurs rarely in childhood. The differential diagnosis for primary osteoporosis in childhood includes juvenile and idiopathic osteoporosis. Children affected by juvenile osteoporosis are usually brought to light by the development of long bone fractures or the complaint of back pain. X-rays reveal generalized osteoporosis with compression fractures of the vertebrae and metaphyses of long bones. Bone histology shows an excess of osteocytes associated with woven bone and normal collagen. Routine biochemical studies tend to be normal for age. The mean age of onset is 7 years, and most affected children improve at puberty. Idiopathic osteoporosis is more variable, it has no obvious cause, and it may represent a state of either high or low bone turnover. Its course may be transient and self-limited or progressive and disabling and is difficult to predict at the onset. Other causes of osteoporosis in children are secondary osteoporoses such as glucocorticoid-induced osteoporosis, osteoporosis due to hypogonadism, or osteoporosis secondary to malignancy (Williams, 1998)

MANIFESTATIONS AND MANAGEMENT

Growth and Feeding

Growth deficiency and short stature are common features in all patients with osteogenesis imperfecta regardless of type. Patients with mild (type I) osteogenesis imperfecta are of average size at birth. They may fall below the growth curve by school age and grow parallel to the normal curve to achieve a final height slightly below normal adult range. Alternatively, they may grow in the normal range and have a final height several inches shorter than unaffected siblings of the same gender. The growth of those with moderate (type IV) osteogenesis imperfecta includes a plateau phase between the ages of 1 and 3–4 years during which there is minimal growth. After this period, children with type IV osteogenesis imperfecta grow parallel to the growth curve, achieving a final height comparable to an unaffected individual in midadolescence. Finally, the patients with severe (type III) osteogenesis imperfecta are small-to normal-sized infants who rapidly fall below the growth curve and have growth rates far below normal for age throughout life. They achieve a final adult height in the prepubertal range (Marini, Bordenick et al., 1993a). The cause of growth deficiency is not clear and is likely multifactorial. Short stature can not be explained wholly by vertebral compression fractures, and the role of the skeletal matrix in growth deficiency is an area of active investigation.

Examination of causes of growth deficiency in patients with osteogenesis imperfecta has included evaluation of response to growth hormone-releasing hormone, growth hormone provocative tests, somatomedin generation tests, and 24-hour unstimulated growth hormone secretion. Test results do not correlate with type of osteogenesis imperfecta or degree of growth deficiency. All children with osteogenesis imperfecta synthesize and release growth hormone in response to provocative testing with results similar to children with idiopathic short stature. There are two groups of children with respect to response to growth hormone-releasing hormone: a group whose responses are similar to children with growth hormone deficiency and another group whose mean response is within normal limits for age. In addition, most children with osteogenesis imperfecta have a lower area under the 24-hour curve of unstimulated growth hormone and a blunted response to somatomedin generation, suggesting that some patients with osteogenesis imperfecta have a hypoactive growth hormone axis at the hypothalamic-pituitary level or at the tissue response level (Marini, Bordenick et al., 1993a,b).

Administration of exogenous growth hormone to children with type III and IV osteogenesis imperfecta significantly increases the linear growth rate of about half of them, and withdrawal results in a return to pretreatment growth rate. Children with type IV osteogenesis imperfecta compose the majority of the responder group. Although the use of growth hormone in children with osteogenesis imperfecta is still under investigation, currently available data suggest that children with osteogenesis imperfecta types I and IV are responsive to its administration, at times attaining heights within the normal growth curves (Marini, Bordenick et al., 1993a,b).

Evaluation

- Consideration should be given to testing patients with all types of osteogenesis imperfecta with standard growth hormone stimulation.
- Aberration in thyroid function is not associated with osteogenesis imperfecta.
- Children with osteogenesis imperfecta should be carefully measured at all visits, including head circumference, weight, sitting height, and length taking into account any contractures of the limbs.
- Excess caloric intake tends to be a problem in children who are immobile; the subsequent development of

obesity further decreases their activity, because they cannot support their own weight and therefore cannot move themselves from wheelchair to walker or wheelchair to seat or bed.

Treatment

- Although most of these children do not have documented growth hormone deficiency, therapy is effective in most children with type I and in approximately half of children with type IV osteogenesis imperfecta. There is value to a 6-month empiric treatment trial for children with osteogenesis imperfecta type IV to determine whether they will respond (personal experience), but this approach cannot yet be considered standard of care.
- Exogenous growth hormone treatment seems to improve bone density without advancing bone age and without worsening skeletal deformity. There is an increase in blood levels of all components of bone turnover due to an increased rate of whole body remodeling associated with rapid bone gain.
- Growth hormone treatment has the additional effect of increasing muscle mass and strength, which may lead to increased activity benefiting skeletal integrity (Antoniazzi et al., 1995).

Development and Behavior

Children with osteogenesis imperfecta tend to have minimal delay in fine motor development but significant delays in their gross motor skills (Marini and Gerber, 1997). Intelligence and language development are unaffected by this disorder.

Evaluation

- The presence of a delay in development should prompt a complete developmental assessment.

Treatment

- Infant stimulation and physical therapy can be extremely valuable.
- Programs must be highly individualized to the specific disabilities of the child.
- Rodding procedures on the lower extremities before the age of $3\frac{1}{2}$ years may improve motor development (Engelbert et al., 1995).

Musculoskeletal

Although many physicians place importance on the number of fractures sustained by children with osteogenesis imperfecta, it is important to keep in mind that the least active children, those with osteogenesis imperfecta type III, may have bones that are so soft that they tend to deform rather than fracture. In these cases, fracture number becomes a less useful index for measuring the severity of the disease. Fracture number may not be as important as the degree of trauma needed to create a fracture. In general, children with osteogenesis imperfecta type III sustain more fractures with trivial trauma and in areas that are more difficult to break (arms and ribs) than those with type IV, who in turn sustain more fractures than those with type I.

Repeated fractures can lead to progressive muscle weakness and decreased progress toward ambulation and other activities of daily living (Marini and Gerber, 1997).

Many children with moderate to severe osteogenesis imperfecta develop significant spinal scoliosis (Figs. 17.3 and 17.6) and kyphosis, and the resultant deformities of the thorax can lead to pulmonary compromise. This is more often the case in type III osteogenesis imperfecta than in type IV. Development of scoliosis does not correlate directly with the number of collapsed vertebrae. In addition, patients with type III osteogenesis imperfecta with multiple severe compression fractures may not progress to severe scoliosis, whereas others with type IV osteogenesis imperfecta and only a few wedge-shaped vertebrae may progress to significant deformity.

Compression fractures generally begin in the thoracolumbar region.

Infants with moderate to severe osteogenesis imperfecta tend to develop positional torticollis and hip abduction contractures caused by being kept supine on a soft surface. This will interfere with the development of sitting and standing if left uncorrected (Binder et al., 1993). Infants who can tolerate the prone position will later be able to roll and sit (Binder et al., 1993).

Evaluation

- Fractures should be evaluated with standard X-rays. Bone scans to discover clinical fractures that are not apparent on plain film are not useful because the bones of children with osteogenesis imperfecta have a high turnover rate and will "light up" in multiple locations.
- Scoliosis progresses in fits and starts, making annual chest films in PA and lateral position warranted in patients with types III and IV to monitor the progression of curvature (Engelbert et al., 1998).

Treatment

- Management of children with osteogenesis imperfecta should include the close involvement of an orthopedic surgeon who has some experience in the treatment of this disorder.
- Early intervention should include lessons for caregivers in infant handling and positioning, head support to avoid torticollis, and neutral alignment of the femora (Gerber et al., 1990).
- Use of a regular mattress covered with a sheepskin mat or liner will allow the child greater movement.
- Turning the infant from side to side and into a prone position is useful for strengthening neck extensors and upper extremities and also allows the hip abductors to stretch.

- Use of custom-molded seats or sand-bags will help to assure lower extremity alignment as well as improve positioning of head and spine in severely affected infants (Gerber et al., 1990).
- Exercise programs must be based on functional level and current ability. In general, programs should ensure that children have at least 3+/5 muscle grade strength (the ability to lift a limb against gravity) in their deltoid and biceps in the upper extremities and in the gluteus maximus and medius and trunk extensors of the lower extremities. This will allow at least independent transferring. The children should be able to supinate their hands, and to touch the top and back of their head with their hands, and their hips and knees should reach full extension or have no greater than $-20°$ contracture while in extension (Marini and Gerber, 1997).
- The goal of rehabilitation therapy for the child with osteogenesis imperfecta is to promote and maintain optimal function in all aspects of the child's life. To accomplish this, a program combining early intervention, muscle strengthening and aerobic conditioning, and, if possible, protected ambulation should be initiated early in life.
- Strength and mobility can be accomplished using isotonic strengthening and aerobic conditioning. Swimming should be encouraged, because many exercises are more easily performed in water (Fig. 17.1). Strengthening exercises should be done daily for a few minutes at a time.
- Individuals with osteogenesis imperfecta who have the potential for ambulation, even if only for short distances (household ambulators), should be encouraged to do so. This often requires a combination of bracing (Fig. 17.1), surgical intervention, and physical therapy to strengthen muscles and improve stamina.

- Use of braces and orthopedic intervention can help to maximize function while minimizing the risk of fracture (Gerber et al., 1990).
- Long leg bracing is recommended to provide support for weak muscles, control joint alignment, and decrease motion and pain. Braces improve upright balance but do not unload the limb. Ultralightweight plastic clamshell braces (Fig. 17.1) are designed to provide a more natural alignment, to unweight the limb, and to supply $360°$ compression using the anterior clamshell contoured supports. Their use promotes independent activity by providing stability to the pelvic girdle, controlling knee recurvatum and severe hindfoot valgus, as well as decreasing tibial bowing. Braces are not protective or are minimally protective against fractures. In fact, they promote increased activity, which may even put these children at increased risk for fractures. However, the advantage of increased function and independence is often judged to outweigh this disadvantage.
- Fractures should not be allowed to heal without reduction and realignment to prevent loss of function.
- In general, fractures should be managed with traction and casts as would a similar fracture in an unaffected child, except that the period of immobilization should be kept to a minimum to avoid worsening osteoporosis and muscular atrophy.
- The goal of surgery is to improve ambulation, strengthen long bones and prevent a cycle of fracturing, deformity, osteoporosis, and refracturing, as well as to allow long limb bracing. The classic surgical procedure is the Sofield and Millar procedure of multiple osteotomies, realignment, and intramedullary rod fixation (Fig. 17.5).
- Decisions about when to intervene surgically must be highly individualized.

In deciding when to schedule osteotomy procedures, it is appropriate to take into account the child's developmental as well as functional status. If a patient is making progress, it is often prudent to postpone surgery and allow the child to achieve maximal presurgical function. In addition, it is a matter for debate as to whether the results of osteotomy are improved if the procedure is done electively as opposed to after fracture.

- It has been shown that most affected children have improved neuromuscular development and meet their motor milestones at a more normal rate if they have rodding procedures on their lower extremities before the age of $3\frac{1}{2}$ years (Engelbert et al., 1995).

- Indications for surgical intervention include long bone angulation of greater than 40°, because the risk of fracture increases at greater than 40°, functional valgus or varus deformity which interferes with gait, or more than two fractures in the same bone within a 6-month period.

- With respect to the classic Sofield and Millar procedure, a number of rods are currently being used, the main choices being elongating (Bailey-Dubow) or non-elongating (Rush) rods. Each has its advantages and disadvantages and is highly lauded by its proponents. Most patients with osteogenesis imperfecta will not have achieved skeletal maturity at the time of rod placement and so will continue to grow beyond the rod tip, leaving a segment of bone unsupported and at risk for fracture. Rush rods need revision every $2-2\frac{1}{2}$ years, although children with moderate to severe osteogenesis imperfecta whose growth rate is slow may not need revisions that frequently. The Bailey-Dubow extensible rod device passively elongates with growth. These rods need

to be revised less often, with an average revision interval of 5 ± 1 years (Luhmann et al., 1998). They achieve the same stabilization as non-elongating rods and have no advantage in the prevention of fractures or the recovery of walking. Because they have a wider diameter than the nonextending rods, they often cannot be placed into the limb of a child less than 4 years old. More complications are associated with the placement of elongating rods (Zionts et al., 1998; Porat et al., 1991), including migration of the implant outside the bony cortex, internal migration with or without fracture and bending of the nail after trauma. These complications are more likely to occur in children less than 5 years of age. One-third of children in whom Bailey-Dubow rods are placed will need surgical revision because of migration or other mechanical problems (Zionts et al., 1998), making this revision rate about the same as the revision rate for nonelongating rods (Porat et al., 1991). Our preference is to use non-elongating rods (personal experience).

- The major disadvantage of intramedullary stabilization is that children develop significant cortical atrophy and osteoporosis, especially in the diaphysis, because of unloading of mechanical weight.

- Historically, other procedures used to treat bone deformity in osteogenesis imperfecta include the use of plates and screws, and percutaneous rodding. A series of plates and screws spanning from metaphysis to metaphysis has been used to correct deformity of the limb; however, this leads to softening of the underlying cortex and loosening of the screws. In addition, once the screws are removed, the holes serve as weak points for new fractures. This procedure is best used in mild osteogenesis imperfecta for rapid correction of alignment.

- For children who are too fragile to undergo an open procedure, percutaneous intramedullary fixation of long bone has been done in children less than 3 years of age and as young as 8 months of age. This procedure has fallen into disfavor because it did not achieve the desired long-term results.

- The progressive scoliosis of osteogenesis imperfecta does not respond to conservative management with Milwaukee bracing; spinal fusion with Harrington rod placement is often necessary. This procedure has a high complication rate, but stabilization of the fused spine is generally good. The best surgical results are achieved when correction is done at less than a 60° curvature.

- There is currently no curative treatment for osteogenesis imperfecta. In the past, several potentially reasonable pharmacologic therapies have been tried unsuccessfully. The compounds most studied are calcitonin and fluoride. Neither is currently believed to have positive long-term effects.

- Recently, there has been some excitement over the use of bisphosphonates in the treatment of patients with osteogenesis imperfecta. These compounds are synthetic analogs of inorganic pyrophosphate that have been used successfully in the treatment of postmenopausal osteoporosis and hypercalcemia of malignancy. They act by inhibiting osteoclast resorption of bone, but they would presumably not affect the deposition of abnormal collagen into bone matrix in osteogenesis imperfecta. An uncontrolled study of administration of pamidronate, an intravenous form of the compound, in 30 children with osteogenesis imperfecta types III and IV reported an increase in bone mineral density and vertebral body height, decreased fractures, improved ambulation, and decreased bone pain (Glorieux et al., 1998). Further investigation into this therapy is currently under way.

Neurologic

It has become evident that there are two patterns of cranial growth in children with osteogenesis imperfecta. One group demonstrates a normal rate of head growth, whereas another crosses percentile lines between ages 2 and 3 years. Prominence of the sulci and ventriculomegaly are common findings in children with osteogenesis imperfecta, even in those without absolute macrocephaly. These imaging findings are sometimes interpreted as cortical atrophy. However, this diagnosis is not consistent with psychometric testing, which shows these children to have normal to above average intelligence. More likely, a distinction should be made between true atrophy and ventriculomegaly (Charnas and Marini, 1993).

Basilar invagination occurs with high frequency in patients with severe osteogenesis imperfecta. Patients with larger head circumferences appear to be at greater risk (Charnas and Marini, 1993). It has been hypothesized that larger cranial mass, combined with upright posture, increases the risk. Some authors have proposed that there is a connection between basilar invagination and the benign communicating hydrocephalus seen in some individuals with osteogenesis imperfecta.

The earliest signs of basilar invagination include nystagmus, followed by long tract signs, whereas the earliest symptom and most common complaint is headache that is worse with movement, cough, sneezing, or straining. Basilar invagination generally progresses slowly in childhood, and neurological signs may be present for years before symptoms. Most patients are asymptomatic into the second decade of life despite radiographic evidence of basilar invagination from as early as 5 years. A good outcome is obtained by delaying surgical intervention until symptoms develop (personal experience).

Evaluation

- Screening for basilar invagination with a CT scan and complete neurologic exam at an early age is recommended.
- Follow-up should occur every 3–5 years, provided findings are normal.
- If there is radiographic evidence of basilar invagination, annual follow-up with MRI is appropriate.

Treatment

- Surgical suboccipital craniectomy with occipitocervical fusion is performed for symptomatic basilar invagination. Only a few centers have experience with this procedure in osteogenesis imperfecta at the time of this writing.
- Postoperatively, prolonged external orthotic immobilization is recommended to prevent progression of basilar invagination (Sawin and Menezes, 1997).

Ears and Hearing

Hearing loss is a characteristic finding in a sizable proportion of patients with type I osteogenesis imperfecta; it also occurs in types III and IV. Although there may be high-frequency loss in prepubertal years, it is unusual to see clinically significant loss before young adulthood. Combined sensorineural and conductive hearing deficits are responsible for this loss (Garretsen et al., 1997). Clinically, the deficits in osteogenesis imperfecta are very similar to those in otosclerosis. However, the hearing loss in osteogenesis imperfecta tends to occur at an earlier age and has more severe middle ear involvement.

Evaluation

- Assessment using tympanometry and acoustic reflexes are recommended. Abnormalities are suggestive of stapedial fixation.

Treatment

- Surgical intervention with a stapedectomy gives satisfactory long-term results in osteogenesis imperfecta with severe hearing loss but should not be undertaken routinely, because conductive hearing loss may be relieved by surgery but the sensorineural component progresses despite intervention (Pedersen, 1984).
- Hearing aids help with conductive hearing loss more than sensorineural loss and should be considered when hearing loss is clinically significant.
- Referral to a center with experience with osteogenesis imperfecta should be made when a hearing aid is no longer ample intervention.

Dental

Dentinogenesis imperfecta is a heritable dental dysplasia of variable phenotype. The majority of patients with osteogenesis imperfecta have some degree of dentinogenesis imperfecta. Dentinogenesis imperfecta varies in severity between individuals and is almost always more severe in deciduous teeth than in permanent teeth. Affected teeth vary in color from blue-gray to yellow-brown opalescence. Consistent features include early obliteration of pulpal tissues, severe microscopic disturbances in dentin, constriction of the cemento-enamel junctions, and short, narrow roots (Lund et al., 1998). The enamel, although itself unaffected, cracks at the defective dentinogenesis imperfecta junction, and the exposed dentin wears down rapidly (Ranta et al., 1993).

Histologically, there appears to be normal mantle dentin and lamellated, disorganized circumpulpal dentin with a decreased number of scattered dentinal tubules. Similar to collagen analysis of bone and skin, the dentinal matrix reveals an increase in collagen types

III and V, abnormal fibronectin concentration, and abnormal collagen type I.

Patients with osteogenesis imperfecta have been noted to have significant dental malocclusion. It has been hypothesized that this is caused by increased growth in the anterior direction of the mandible, creating a profile of midface hypoplasia. This tends to occur during adolescence, and some patients have found their appearance so displeasing that they have sought surgical correction. In addition, this group of patients has a high incidence of anterior and posterior crossbites and opened bites in both primary and permanent dentition.

Evaluation

- Ability to chew solids without discomfort should be a major consideration when evaluating whether intervention is needed for primary dentition, and esthetic considerations should not be undervalued.
- A standard dental panorex will most commonly reveal obliteration of the pulp chambers, even in patients with apparently normal teeth (Lund et al., 1998).
- Referral to orthodontics is recommended once permanent teeth erupt for assessment of malocclusion and intervention.

Treatment

- The aim of treatment should be to ensure favorable conditions for the eruption of permanent teeth and for normal growth of the facial bone and temporomandibular joint.
- In areas that are occlusally nonstressed, glass ionomers such as fluoride-releasing and chemical-attacking materials are recommended.
- New composites combined with dental bonding agents are recommended over occlusal areas (Ranta et al., 1993).
- Management decisions can be aided by assessment of the color of the teeth.

Yellow-brown teeth are seen with a higher frequency, occupy more of the total dental surface area, and have a tendency toward increased attrition and enamel fracture; therefore, more patients with teeth of this color need placement of crowns on their primary dentition to maintain vertical dimension (O'Connell et al., 1999).

- The presence of anterior open bite correlates highly with the use of a pacifier in infancy, so parents should be counseled against this practice. (O'Connell et al., 1999)

Cardiovascular

Osteogenesis imperfecta can be complicated by aortic root dilatation (12% of all individuals with osteogenesis imperfecta, 28% of persons with type III osteogenesis imperfecta) (Vetter et al., 1989). Both aortic and mitral regurgitation are noted occasionally. However, these phenomena are not as commonly associated with this disorder as they are with other connective tissue disorders such as Marfan syndrome. The development of aortic root dilatation is generally proportional to body growth, and, although it may be worsened by hypertension, it does not appear to be progressive and rarely needs surgical intervention (Hortop et al., 1986). Abnormalities in the aortic root and mitral valve may lead to aortic insufficiency and mitral regurgitation, respectively. In both situations, the valves have been described histopathologically as having myxoid degeneration. Mitral valve prolapse has been described in patients with osteogenesis imperfecta; however, it does not appear to be more prevalent than in the general population (5–7%).

Evaluation

- No standard regimen of cardiac evaluation has been delineated; therefore, echocardiography should be prompted by clinical signs and symptoms.

Treatment

- The need for antibiotic prophylaxis should be addressed in all patients with mitral valve prolapse, as in the general population.

Respiratory

The cardiopulmonary aspect of osteogenesis imperfecta is a significant cause of morbidity and mortality in affected adults. Because of the development of kyphoscoliosis and vertebral collapse, many individuals with osteogenesis imperfecta have restrictive lung disease. Although this is not well studied, it is well recognized that this may progress to cor pulmonale.

Evaluation

- Evaluation by and follow-up with a cardiologist and/or pulmonologist is a necessity for children with severe chest deformities or scoliosis. Pulmonary function should be evaluated initially at a young age (between 4 and 6 years of age) and reassessed every 2–3 years if normal.

Treatment

- Restrictive lung disease is managed with conventional therapies including chronic oxygen administration.
- The need for chronic oxygen may arise as early as adolescence.

Ophthalmologic

There is a well-known association between osteogenesis imperfecta and blue sclerae, especially in types I and III. The blueness is often less intense near the limbus and has been noted to decrease in intensity with age. This blue color has been attributed to differential scattering of light of different wavelengths through abnormal connective tissue (Sillence et al., 1993). Whether it is the abnormal collagen itself or other factors such as water or mucopolysaccharide content that affect the scattering coefficient is unclear. In addition, blue sclerae have been associated with decreased ocular rigidity not related to myopic refractive error. Blue sclerae are not exclusive to osteogenesis imperfecta and may be seen in association with other connective tissue disorders or in the normal population, particularly in infancy. Additional ocular findings noted in osteogenesis imperfecta patients are rare and apparently not associated with the disorder itself.

RESOURCES

Osteogenesis Imperfecta Foundation

804 West Diamond Ave., Suite 210
  Gaithersburg, MD 20878
  E-mail: *bonelink@oif.org*
  Homepage : *www.oif.org*

REFERENCES

Antoniazzi F, Bertoldo F, Mottes M, Valli M, Sirpresi S, Zamboni G, Valentini R, Tato L (1995) Growth hormone treatment in osteogenesis imperfecta with quantitative defect of type I collagen synthesis. *J Pediatr* 129:432–439.

Bateman JF, Golub SR (1994) Deposition and selective degradation of structurally abnormal type I collagen in a collagen matrix produced by osteogenesis imperfecta fibroblasts in vitro. *Matrix Biol* 14:251–262.

Binder HB, Conway A, Hason S, Gerber LH, Marini JC, Berry R, Weintrob J (1993) Comprehensive rehabilitation of the child with osteogenesis imperfecta. *Am J Med Genet* 45:265–269.

Borochowitz Z, Lachman R, Adomian GE, Spear G, Jones K, Rimoin DL (1988) Achondrogenesis type I: Delineation of further heterogeneity and identification of two distinct subgroups. *J Pediatr* 112:23–31.

Camera G, Dodero D, De Pascale S (1983) *Prenatal Diagnosis of Thanatophoric Dysplasia at 24 Weeks*. New York: Liss, p. 39–43.

Charnas LR, Marini JC (1993) Communicating hydrocephalus, basilar invagination and other neurologic features in osteogenesis imperfecta. *Neurology* 43:2603–2608.

Ekman O (1788) *Dissertatio medica descriptionem et casus aliquot ostoemalaciae sistens.* Uppsala.

Elejalde BR, de Elejalde MM (1985) Thanatophoric dysplasia: Fetal manifestations and prenatal diagnosis. *Am J Med Genet* 22:669–683.

Engelbert RHH, Helders PJM, Keessen W, Pruijs HE, Gooskens RHJM (1995) Intramedullary rodding in type III osteogenesis imperfecta: Effects on neuromotor development in 10 children. *Acta Orthop Scand* 66:361–364.

Engelbert RH, Gerver WJ, Breslau-Siderius LJ (1998) Spinal complications in osteogenesis imperfecta: 47 patients 1–16 years of age. *Acta Orthop Scand* 69:283–286.

Fedarko NS, Moerike M, Brenner R, Robey PG, Vetter U (1992) Extracellular matrix formation by osteoblasts from patients with osteogenesis imperfecta. *J Bone Min Res* 7:921–929.

Fryns JP, van den Berghe K, van Assche A, van den Berghe H (1981) Prenatal diagnosis of campomelic dwarfism. *Clin Genet* 19:199–201.

Garretsen AJ, Cremers CW, Huygen PL (1997) Hearing loss (in nonoperated ears) in relation to age in osteogenesis imperfecta type I. *Ann Otol Rhinol Laryngol* 106:575–582.

Gerber LH, Binder H, Weintrob J, Grange DK, Shapiro J, Fromherz WF, Berry R, Conway A, Nason S, Marini JC (1990) Rehabilitation of children and infants with osteogenesis imperfecta. A program for ambulation. *Clin Ortho Rel Res* 251:254–262.

Glorieux FH, Bishop NJ, Plotkin H, Chabot G, Lanoue G, Travers R (1998) Cyclical administration of pamidronate therapy in children with severe osteogenesis imperfecta. *N Engl J Med* 339:947–952.

Gruber HE, Baylink DJ (1991) The effects of fluoride on bone. *Clin Ortho Rel Res* 267:264–277.

Hortop J, Tsipouras P, Hanley J, Maron B, Shapiro J (1986) Cardiovascular involvement in osteogenesis imperfecta. *Circulation* 73:54–61.

Kivirikko KI (1993) Collagens and their abnormalities in a wide spectrum of diseases. *Ann Med* 25:113–126.

Kuivaniemi H, Tromp G, Prockop DJ (1997) Mutations in fibrillar collagens (types I, II, III and XI), fibril-associated collagen (type IX), and network-forming collagen (type X) cause a spectrum of diseases of bone, cartilage and blood vessels. *Hum Mut* 9: 300–315.

Levin LS, Salinas CF, Jorenson RJ (1978) Classification of osteogenesis imperfecta by dental characteristics. *Lancet* 1:332.

Looser, E (1906) Zur kenntnis der osteogenesis imperfecta congenita et tarda. *Mitt Girenzgeb Med Chir* 15:161.

Luhmann SJ, Sheridan JJ, Capelli AM, Schoenecker PL (1998) Management of lower extremity deformities in osteogenesis imperfecta with extensible intramedullary rod technique: A twenty year experience. *J Pediatr Orthop* 18:88–94.

Lund AM, Jensen BL, Nielson LA, Skovby F (1998) Dental manifestations of osteogenesis imperfecta and abnormalities of collagen metabolism. *J Craniofac Genet Dev Biol* 18:30–37.

Marini JC, Lewis MB, Wang Q, Chen KJ, Orrison BM (1993) Serine for glycine substitutions in type I collagen in two cases of type IV osteogenesis imperfecta. *J Biol Chem* 268:2667–2673.

Marini JC and Gerber NL (1997) Osteogenesis imperfecta: Rehabilitation and prospects for gene therapy. *JAMA* 277:746–750.

Marini JC, Bordenick S, Heavner G, Rose S, Chrousos GP (1993a) Evaluation of growth hormone axis and responsiveness to growth stimulation of short children with osteogenesis imperfecta. *Am J Med Genet* 45:261–264.

Marini JC, Bordenick S, Heavner G, Rose S, Hintz R, Rosenfeld R, Chrousos GP (1993b) The growth hormone and somatomedin axis in short children with osteogenesis imperfecta. *J Clin Endocrin Metab* 76:251–256.

McKusick VA (1972) Osteogenesis imperfecta. In *Heritable Disorders of Connective Tissue*, 4th ed. St Louis, MO: Mosby.

O 'Connell AC, Dent, B, Marini JC. (1999) Evaluation of oral problems in an osteogenesis imperfecta population. *Oral Surg Oral Med Oral Path* 87:189–196.

Pedersen U (1984) Hearing loss in patients with osteogenesis imperfecta. A clinical and audiological study of 201 patients. *Scand Audiol* 13:67–74.

Pepin M, Atkinson M, Starman BJ, Byers PH (1997) Strategies and outcomes of prenatal diagnosis for osteogenesis imperfecta: A review of biochemical and molecular studies completed in 129 pregnancies. *Prenat Diagn* 17:559–570.

Porat S, Heller E, Seidman DS, Meyer S (1991) Functional results of operation in osteogenesis imperfecta: Elongating and nonelongating rods. *J Pediatr Orthop* 11:200–203

Prockop DJ (1997) What holds us together? Why do some of us fall apart? What can we do about it? *Matrix Biol* 16:519–528.

Ranta H, Lukinmaas P, Waltimo J (1993) Heritable dentin defects: Nosology, pathology and treatment. *Am J Med Genet* 45:193–200.

Rebelo I, da Silva P, Blanco JC, Monteiro MES, Ferreira NC (1989) Effects of synthetic salmon calcitonin therapy in children with osteogenesis imperfecta. *J Intern Med Res* 17:401–405.

Sarafova AP, Choi H, Forlino A, Gajko A, Cabral WA, Tosi L, Reing CM, Marini JC (1998) Three novel type I collagen mutations in osteogenesis imperfecta type IV probands are associated with discrepancies between electrophoretic migration of osteoblast and fibroblast collagen. *Hum Mut* 11:395–403.

Sawin PD, Menezes AH (1997) Basilar invagination in osteogenesis imperfecta and related osteochondrodysplasias: Medical and surgical management. *J Neurosurg* 86:950–960.

Sillence DO, Senn A, Danks DM (1979) Genetic heterogeneity in osteogenesis imperfecta. *J Med Genet* 16:101–116.

Sillence DO (1981) Osteogenesis imperfecta: An expanding panorama of variants. *Clin Ortho Rel Res* 159:11–25.

Sillence DO, Barlow KK, Garber AP, Hall JG, Rimoin DL (1984) Osteogenesis imperfecta type II: Delineation of the phenotype with reference to genetic heterogeneity. *Am J Med Genet* 17:407.

Sillence DO, Barlow KK, Cole WG, Dietrich S, Garber AP, Rimoin DL (1986) Osteogenesis type III: Delineation of phenotype with reference to genetic heterogeneity. *Am J Med Genet* 23:821.

Sillence D, Butler B, Latham M, Barlow K (1993) Natural history of blue sclerae in osteogenesis imperfecta. *Am J Med Genet* 45:183–186.

Talbot JR, Fischer MM, Farley SM, Libanati C, Farley J, Tabuenca A, Baylink DJ (1996) The increase in spinal bone density that occurs in response to fluoride therapy for osteoporosis is not maintained after the therapy is discontinued. *Osteop Int* 6:442–447.

Thompson EM (1993) Non-invasive prenatal diagnosis of osteogenesis imperfecta. *Am J Med Genet* 45:201–206.

Van der Hoeve J, de Kleyn A (1918) Blaue sclerae, knochenbruchigkeit und schwerhorigkeit. *Arch Ophthal* 95:81.

Vetter U, Maierhofer B, Muller M, Teller W, Brenner R, Frohneberg D, Wordsdorfer O (1989) Osteogenesis imperfecta in childhood: Cardiac and renal manifestations. *Eur J Pediatr* 149:184–187.

Vrolik W (1849) *Tabulae ad illustrandam embryogenesium hominis et mammalium tam naturalem quam abnormen.* Amsterdam.

Whyte, MP (1995) Hypophosphatasia. In *The Metabolic Basis of Inherited Diseases*, Scriver CR, Beaudet AL, Sly WS, Valle D, eds. McGraw Hill, Inc. New York. Chapter 136; p. 4095–4111.

Williams, JD (1998) *Textbook of Endocrinology*, 9th ed. Pages 1221–1228. Wilson, Foster DW, Kronenberg HK, Larsen PR eds. Saunders, Philadelphia, PA: 1221–1228.

Willing MC, Pruchno CJ, Byers PH (1993) Molecular heterogeneity in osteogenesis imperfecta type I. *Am J Med Genet* 45:223–227.

Zionts LE, Edward A, Stott NS (1998) Complications in the use of the Bailey-Dubow extensible nail. *Clin Ortho Rel Res* 348:186–195.

CHAPTER 18

PRADER-WILLI SYNDROME

SUZANNE B. CASSIDY

INTRODUCTION

Prader-Willi syndrome is a complex, multi-system mental retardation disorder that was first described in 1956 (Prader et al., 1956). For many years, its cause was unknown, and it was believed that affected individuals were doomed to die young of complications of the associated obesity. Twenty-five years later, Prader-Willi syndrome captured the interest of geneticists because it was the first recognized microdeletion syndrome identified when high-resolution chromosome analysis was introduced (Ledbetter et al., 1981). Prader-Willi syndrome is now known to be one of the most common microdeletion syndromes, one of the most frequent disorders seen in genetics clinics, and the most common recognized genetic form of obesity. It is also the first recognized human genomic imprinting disorder and the first recognized as resulting from uniparental disomy (Nicholls et al., 1989). Prader-Willi syndrome thus occupies an important place in the contemporary history of human genetic disorders. It is, in addition, distinguished by being a syndrome caused by several different genetic alterations of proximal chromosome 15q (genetic heterogeneity), and it is typified by a distinctive behavioral phenotype (Dykens et al., 1992; Holm et al., 1993; Dykens et al., 1996).

Incidence

Approximately 1 in 10,000–15,000 individuals is diagnosed with Prader-Willi syndrome, and it occurs in both sexes and all races. The vast majority of affected individuals are the only affected individuals in their family. Despite the availability of clinical diagnostic criteria (Holm et al., 1993), diagnosis is still delayed or missed in many cases. The consequence is often delay in intervention. Appropriate management can have a significant positive impact on health and quality of life, but controlling the characteristic obesity and difficult behavior constitutes a major challenge, requiring cooperative input from geneticists, primary care physicians, endocrinologists, nutritionists, psychologists, psychiatrists, educators, as well as families and other caregivers.

Diagnostic Criteria

Clinical diagnostic criteria were developed by consensus before the availability of complete sensitive and specific laboratory testing

Management of Genetic Syndromes, Edited by Suzanne B. Cassidy and Judith E. Allanson
ISBN 0-471-31286-X   Copyright © 2001 by Wiley-Liss, Inc.

(Holm et al., 1993). These are still extremely valuable in suggesting the diagnosis and indicating the need for diagnostic testing (see Table 18.1). The cardinal features of Prader-Willi syndrome are neonatal hypotonia and failure to thrive, developmental delay and mild cognitive impairment, characteristic facial appearance, early-childhood-onset obesity, hypogonadism with genital hypoplasia, mild short stature, and a characteristic behavior disorder. These and the more minor but often more distinctive features have been well described in a number of reviews (Cassidy, 1984; Butler, 1990; Cassidy, 1997).

The central hypotonia that predominates the infancy period in Prader-Willi syndrome is prenatal in onset and is nearly uniformly present. It causes decreased fetal movement, frequent abnormal fetal position, and difficulty at the time of delivery, often necessitating cesarean section. Reflexes may be decreased or absent. The neonatal central hypotonia and a state of hypoarousal are almost invariably associated with poor suck and lack of awakening to feed, with consequent failure to thrive and the necessity for gavage or other special feeding techniques. Infantile lethargy, with decreased arousal and weak cry, are also prominent findings. Neuromuscular electrophysiological and biopsy studies are normal or nonspecific, and the hypotonia gradually improves. Motor milestones are delayed, and average age of sitting is 12 months and of walking is 24 months. Adults remain mildly hypotonic with decreased muscle bulk and tone. This hypotonia is such a significant finding that it is recommended that all newborns with persistent hypotonia be tested for Prader-Willi syndrome (Miller et al., 1999).

Language development is also delayed. Verbal skills are an ultimate strength in most patients, although speech is often poorly articulated, having a nasal and/or slurred character. Cognitive abnormalities are evident, and most patients are mildly retarded (mean IQ 60s–low 70s) (Dykens et al., 1992; Curfs, 1992; Curfs and Fryns, 1992).

TABLE 18.1. Diagnostic Criteria for Prader-Willi Syndrome

Major Criteria (1 point each)

Infantile central hypotonia
Infantile feeding problems/failure to thrive
Rapid weight gain between 1 and 6 years
Characteristic facial features
Hypogonadism: genital hypoplasia, pubertal deficiency
Developmental delay/mental retardation

Minor Criteria (1/2 point each)

Decreased fetal movement and infantile lethargy
Typical behavior problems
Sleep disturbance/sleep apnea
Short stature for the family by age 15 years
Hypopigmentation
Small hands and feet for height age
Narrow hands with straight ulnar border
Esotropia, myopia
Thick, viscous saliva
Speech articulation defects
Skin picking

Supportive Criteria (no points)

High pain threshold
Decreased vomiting
Temperature control problems
Scoliosis and/or kyphosis
Early adrenarche
Osteoporosis
Unusual skill with jigsaw puzzles
Normal neuromuscular studies

In children under 3 years of age with 5 points (3 from major criteria) or those above 3 years with 8 points (4 from major criteria), diagnosis should be suspected. The original diagnostic criteria, developed before the availability of sensitive and specific genetic testing, included a major criteria of chromosome 15 deletion or other chromosome 15 anomaly. Adapted from Holm et al. (1993).

Approximately 40% have borderline retardation or low normal intelligence, and about 20% have moderate retardation. Academic performance is poor for cognitive ability. Specific patterns of cognitive strength and weakness have begun to emerge, frequently with relative strength in reading, visual-spatial skills and long-term memory and weakness in arithmetic, sequential processing, and short-term memory (Dykens and Cassidy, 1996). Coming to clinic with a book of word-find puzzles can almost be considered a diagnostic sign for Prader-Willi syndrome (personal observation), and unusual skill with jigsaw puzzles is common.

Hypogonadism is prenatal in onset and persists throughout life. At birth it is evident as genital hypoplasia. Hypogonadism is also evident in abnormal pubertal development. In both males and females, sexual activity is uncommon and fertility is rare.

Although the proportion of fat mass to lean body mass is high even in thin infants with Prader-Willi syndrome (Butler, 1990), significant obesity is not found in young infants. Rather, it generally begins after hyperphagia has its onset, generally between ages 1 and 6 years, and usually between 2 and 4 years (Fig. 18.1). Hyperphagia is due to a hypothalamic abnormality resulting in lack of satiety (Zipf and Bernston, 1987; Holland et al., 1993). In addition, there is a decreased caloric requirement (Holm and Pipes, 1976), likely related to hypotonia and decreased activity. Food-seeking behavior, with hoarding or foraging for food, eating of unappealing substances such as garbage, pet food, and frozen food, and stealing food or money to buy food are common. A high threshold for vomiting may complicate bingeing on spoiled food from the garbage or such items as boxes of sugar or frozen uncooked meat, and toxicity from ineffective emetics used to induce vomiting has occurred. The obesity is central in distribution, with relative sparing of the distal extremities, and even individuals who are not overweight tend to deposit fat on the abdomen, buttocks, and thighs (Figs. 18.1 and 18.2). Obesity is the major cause of morbidity and mortality in Prader-Willi syndrome, and longevity may be nearly normal

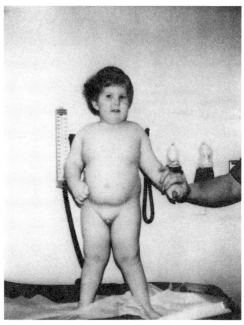

FIGURE 18.1. Four year old boy with Prader-Willi syndrome. Note typical facial appearance, emerging obesity, and characteristic body habitus with genu valgus and straight leg borders.

if it is avoided (Greenswag, 1987; Cassidy et al., 1994). Cardiopulmonary compromise (pickwickian syndrome) results from excessive obesity, as can type II diabetes mellitus, hypertension, thrombophlebitis, and chronic leg edema. Sleep apnea occurs at increased frequency, but the other sleep disturbances seen in Prader-Willi syndrome appear to be unrelated to obesity (Hertz et al., 1995).

Characteristic facial features, including narrow bifrontal diameter, almond-shaped palpebral fissures, narrow nasal bridge, and downturned mouth with a thin upper lip, are either present from birth or evolve over time in most patients (Figs. 18.1, 18.2 and 18.3). Small, narrow hands with a straight ulnar border and sometimes tapering fingers and short, often broad feet are usually present by age 10. African-Americans are less likely to have small hands and feet (Hudgins et al., 1998). A characteristic body habitus, including sloping shoulders, heavy midsection, and genu valgus with straight

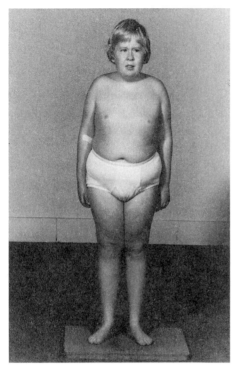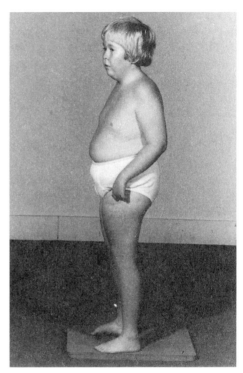

FIGURE 18.2. Fifteen-year-old with Prader-Willi syndrome. Note facial appearance, fat distribution, small distal extremities, and small genitalia.

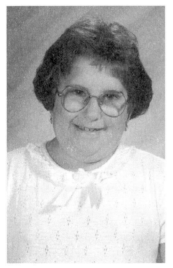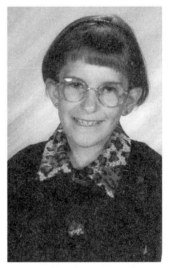

FIGURE 18.3. Girl with Prader-Willi syndrome at 7 (*left*) and 8 (*right*) years of age. The diagnosis of this condition was made at 7 years, and diet, exercise and restriction of access to food resulted in significant weight loss over a 1-year period. The difficulty of making a diagnosis in a thin individual with Prader-Willi syndrome can be appreciated in the figure on the *right*, despite typical facial appearance when obese (*left*).

lower leg borders, is usually present from toddlerhood (Figs. 18.1 and 18.2). Hypopigmentation for the family, manifested as fairer skin, hair, and eye color, occurs in about one-third of affected individuals. Strabismus is often present. Scoliosis and/or kyphosis are common, the former occurring at any age and the latter developing in early adulthood.

Birth weight and length are usually within normal limits, but the early period of failure to thrive may result in both weight and length being below the third centile. Short stature, if not apparent in childhood, is almost always present by the second half of the second decade, associated with lack of a pubertal growth spurt. Average height is 155 cm for males and 148 cm for females. African-Americans tend to be taller (Hudgins et al., 1998).

A characteristic behavior profile becomes evident in early childhood, with temper tantrums, stubbornness, controlling and manipulative behavior, obsessive-compulsive characteristics, and difficulty with change in routine (Dykens et al., 1992; Dykens and Cassidy, 1996). Lying, stealing and aggressive behavior are common. True psychosis is evident in young adulthood in approximately 5–10% of patients. Behavioral and psychiatric problems interfere the most with quality of life in adulthood.

A variety of less well-understood findings are somewhat unique to this condition, including thick, viscous saliva that may predispose to dental caries and contribute to articulation abnormalities; high pain threshold; skin picking; and high threshold for vomiting. Sleep disturbances, especially excessive daytime sleepiness and oxygen desaturation in REM sleep, are common even in the absence of obesity (Hertz et al., 1995). Osteoporosis is frequent but as yet poorly studied.

Etiology, Pathogenesis, and Genetics

Many of the manifestations of Prader-Willi syndrome are referable to insufficient functioning of the hypothalamus. However, no structural defect of the hypothalamus has been documented on postmortem examination. Therefore, the deficiency must be functional, but its nature has not yet been identified. On the other hand, the genetic basis for Prader-Willi syndrome has been intensely investigated.

Prader-Willi syndrome is caused by the lack of expression of normally active paternally inherited genes at chromosome 15q11–q13; the maternally inherited genes are normally inactive because of a phenomenon called genetic imprinting by which some genes are modified in different ways depending on the gender of the parent from whom they were inherited. As a result, there are three ways in which Prader-Willi syndrome can be caused. In approximately 75% of patients with Prader-Willi syndrome, there is a small deletion in the paternally contributed chromosome 15 between bands 15q11 and 15q13. In the vast majority of cases, the same breakpoints on the chromosome have resulted in a 4-Mb deletion, although a small number of patients has a smaller deletion. Most of the remaining patients with Prader-Willi syndrome have inherited two maternal chromosomes 15 but no paternal chromosome 15, a situation known as uniparental disomy 15. Of these two groups, approximately 2–5% of patients with Prader-Willi syndrome have either their deletion or their maternal uniparental disomy for the critical region as a result of a translocation or other structural abnormality involving chromosome 15. The third cause of Prader-Willi syndrome, which occurs in approximately 1% of patients, is neither deletion nor uniparental disomy but rather a defect in the imprinting process. In the latter group, a proportion of affected individuals have been shown to have a very small deletion or other abnormality in the center that controls imprinting within 15q11–q13, the imprinting center. Others have not had a detectable mutation or deletion in the imprinting center but nonetheless have biparental inheritance and a maternal-only pattern. All studied families in which there has been a recurrence of Prader-Willi syndrome have had an imprinting mutation.

The actual genes whose deficiency that cause the phenotypic effects in Prader-Willi syndrome have not been identified as yet. A number of imprinted and nonimprinted genes have been found to exist within the usual deletion region [the PWS/AS critical region; see also Angelman syndrome (AS), Chapter 3] (Nicholls, 1993, Buiting et al., 1994, Glenn et al., 1997). For most of these it is unclear how underexpression of the gene is involved in the pathogenesis. The major exception is the nonimprinted *P* gene, which codes for tyrosinase-positive albinism; its deletion is associated with the hypopigmentation seen in about one-third of patients with Prader-Willi syndrome. *SNRPN* is the best-described gene that is likely to cause some of the features of Prader-Willi syndrome (Ozcelik et al., 1992). This gene codes for a small nuclear ribonucleoprotein, which is a ribosome-associated protein that functions in controlling gene splicing and therefore may be pivotally involved in the control of synthesis of some proteins. *SNRPN* is known to be imprinted in the brain, the focus of most of the abnormalities seen in Prader-Willi syndrome. It is the most frequently used gene for clinical testing purposes. Upstream of the *SNRPN* gene, in a region called *SNURF* (*SNRPN* upstream reading frame), is a putative imprinting control element for the region. Very small deletions within it have been identified in a few patients with Prader-Willi syndrome who have maternal-specific methylation patterns but who do not have either the usual large paternally derived deletion of the PWS/AS region or maternal uniparental disomy (Saitoh et al., 1997).

GABRB3, *GABRA5*, and *GABRG3*, are all nonimprinted receptor subunit genes for the neurotransmitter GABA (γ-aminobutyric acid). *UBE3A*, the gene for Angelman syndrome, is also present in the PWS/AS critical region (see Chapter 3). It codes for a ubiquitin protein ligase (E6AP) that is involved in degradation of proteins and thus in control of protein turnover in the cell. There are also several identified imprinted genes and transcripts whose functions are unknown. *ZNF127* is an imprinted zinc finger gene of unknown function. *NDN* (Necdin) is an imprinted gene that encodes a DNA-binding protein. *IPW* is another imprinted gene, and it is thought to be an RNA transcript only, because it does not encode a protein. Two imprinted anonymous transcripts (DNA segments without identified genes), PAR1 and PAR5, have also been identified. *PW71* is another imprinted gene of unknown function; it has been used as a methylation probe for some clinical and research studies. A number of other genes and transcripts in this region have been identified more recently, but no pathogenetic relationship to the phenotype of Prader-Willi syndrome has yet been found.

Prader-Willi syndrome caused by either the common large deletion in the absence of a structural chromosome abnormality or by uniparental disomy has not been reported to recur. However, a paternal balanced insertion or gonadal mosaicism is possible, and therefore a recurrence risk of approximately 1% or less is appropriate for genetic counseling purposes. Uniparental disomy is caused by nondisjunction, as evidenced by advanced maternal age in this group, and by documentation of trisomy 15 on chorionic villus sampling with resultant maternal uniparental disomy at birth (Robinson et al., 1991). Because nondisjunction can recur, a recurrence risk of 1% or less is appropriate for genetic counseling purposes (Ledbetter and Engel, 1995; Kennerknecht, 1992). In those families with a detected imprinting mutation (small deletion in *SNURF*), and with a presumed imprinting defect based on maternal-only methylation pattern when other testing fails to demonstrate deletion or uniparental disomy, a recurrence risk of up to 50% pertains, because this is likely to be an imprinted dominant mutation that occured in the paternal grandmother's germ line. Prenatal diagnosis by detection of a methylation defect (see below) is possible.

Diagnostic Testing

This topic has been the focus of much literature and a statement from the American Society of Human Genetics Joint Test and Technology Transfer Committee (American Society of Human Genetics/American College of Medical Genetics, 1996). To understand diagnostic testing, it is necessary to appreciate the complexity of the genetic basis for this disorder.

Because there are three different causes of Prader-Willi syndrome, there are a number of different tests that can be used to confirm the diagnosis. Inactivation of the maternal genes causing Prader-Willi syndrome is known to be caused by methylation of cytosine residues in the DNA. Methylation is the best known mechanism for genomic imprinting in general, and methylation has been demonstrated for several genes identified within the Prader-Willi syndrome chromosome region. Unfortunately, little is known about the function of these genes or how their absence leads to the manifestations of Prader-Willi syndrome. Nevertheless, the fact that methylation of the genes in this area is associated with their being unexpressed, and, conversely, that lack of methylation allows expression of the genes in chromosome 15q11–q13, has led to the most efficient test to confirm the diagnosis. So-called methylation analysis, originally accomplished by Southern blotting and now done by PCR, can detect all three causes of Prader-Willi syndrome, because all three causes result in the genes for Prader-Willi syndrome being methylated. This test can be done because methylated DNA is cut differently by some restriction enzymes than unmethylated DNA, and the differences in the size of DNA fragments can be detected. Methylation analysis has been validated for prenatal as well as postnatal use.

However, there are also other methods of detecting the genetic causes of Prader-Willi syndrome, and these all have a use in certain circumstances. In addition, determining the exact cause of Prader-Willi syndrome is important for genetic counseling purposes. Deletion in 15q11–q13 can most accurately be identified by doing a chromosome analysis and using the FISH probe for *SNRPN*, a candidate gene within the deletion. High-resolution chromosome analysis alone is insufficient, because false positives and false negatives have occurred using this method without FISH. Uniparental disomy can be identified by using so-called microsatellite repeat sequences on chromosome 15 in the patient and both parents; if none of the variants of these repeats that are present in the father is seen in the child, then all the genetic information on chromosome 15 has been derived from the mother and uniparental disomy is confirmed. This test requires DNA from the parents as well as the child. The presence of a defect in the imprinting center is not a clinically available test but is implied from an abnormal methylation analysis in the presence of normal FISH and uniparental disomy studies. Mutations in the imprinting center can be detected, and this is accomplished in one of a few laboratories on a research basis.

Differential Diagnosis

The differential diagnosis for Prader-Willi syndrome in infancy includes many causes of neonatal hypotonia, particularly neuromuscular disorders. Later in childhood and adulthood, a number of conditions in which mental retardation/developmental delay is associated with obesity are in the differential, including Bardet-Biedl syndrome, Albright hereditary osteodystrophy, and Cohen syndrome (Gunay-Aygun et al., 1997). Mental retardation disorders in which obesity is an occasional finding, such as fragile X syndrome, Down syndrome, and Angelman syndrome, may also be confused with Prader-Willi syndrome. Acquired hypothalamic injury from accidents, tumors, or surgical complications can closely mimic Prader-Willi syndrome. Most people with developmental disability and childhood-onset obesity have them on the basis of an unknown cause. Familial obesity should be sought in the family history.

MANIFESTATIONS AND MANAGEMENT

Intervention and management of Prader-Willi syndrome can significantly impact the health, functional abilities, and longevity of affected individuals. Despite the relatively mild mental impairment in Prader-Willi syndrome, most patients require sheltered living and working environments and considerable medical monitoring because of their disorder, with 24-hour supervision to control the consequences of their hyperphagia and behavioral outbursts.

The reader should be aware that most of the recommendations for management of Prader-Willi syndrome are based on the experience of experts rather than on controlled studies, with the exception of those relating to growth hormone replacement. However, there is considerable communication among the experts on Prader-Willi syndrome, with annual national scientific meetings in the United States, and an international scientific meeting every 3 years. Many of the suggestions for management described here are based on personal experience with 18 years of Prader-Willi syndrome clinics, in conjunction with review of published experience and the input of other experienced physicians. Recently, the PWSA(USA) (United States Prader-Willi Syndrome Association) has developed health care guidelines for Prader-Willi syndrome, which can be obtained by contacting them.

Growth and Feeding

Infantile Failure to Thrive. Infantile hypotonia (see below) causes great difficulty with sucking. Breast feeding is rarely possible, and special feeding techniques, including special nipples or gavage feeding, may be necessary for weeks to months to assure adequate nutrition and avoid failure to thrive. Eventually, with improving muscle tone comes improved sucking, and a period of relatively normal eating behavior usually occurs.

Short Stature. Approximately 90–95% of people with Prader-Willi syndrome have short stature, although the frequency is somewhat lower in African-Americans (Hudgins et al., 1998). Growth pattern is abnormal in Prader-Willi syndrome, and growth charts representing typical growth patterns have been published (Bray et al., 1983; Butler and Meaney, 1991). In infants, length is below the 50th percentile in most and below the 3rd percentile in some, despite adequate nutrition. With the end of the severe neonatal hypotonia phase, a normal growth rate is usually found until early in the second decade of life, although height may be below the 5th percentile. Small hands and feet are typical, although they may be normal in the first decade (Hudgins et al., 1991) and are more normal in African-Americans (Hudgins et al., 1998).

Short stature in comparison with the family is the rule, likely related at least in part to growth hormone deficiency and lack of an adolescent growth spurt. Without intervention, average height is 155 cm for males and 148 cm for females, although it is a little higher in African-Americans (Hudgins et al., 1998). Until recently, this was attributed exclusively to hypogonadism, but in recent years a number of anecdotal (Angulo et al., 1996) and controlled (Lindgren et al., 1997, 1998; Eiholzer et al., 1998; Carrel et al., 1999) studies have demonstrated decreased growth hormone secretion with low IGF-1 (insulin-like growth factor-1) in most individuals and an excellent response to growth hormone in nearly all in whom it is used. Those who are treated can obtain an adolescent growth spurt and enter the normal height range. Longer-term studies, studies of treatment in infancy, studies of the use of lower than usual dosage of growth hormone, and studies of growth hormone use in adults are currently in progress.

Obesity. This major problem is discussed in a separate section.

Evaluation

- Both height and weight should be monitored frequently by the physician and plotted on growth charts, with frequent assessment of the adequacy of caloric intake.
- All patients should have height measured regularly and plotted along either standard growth charts or growth charts for Prader-Willi syndrome.
- Patients who have growth deficiency even after infancy should be assessed for possible hypothyroidism. Even though there is no reported increase in frequency of hypothyroidism, some patients with poor growth and prolonged hypotonia have hypothyroidism as a cause (personal observation). TSH, T4, and T3 uptake should be assessed in these patients.
- Standard growth hormone stimulation testing (i.e., growth hormone response to L-DOPA or clonidine) remains the standard of assessment in patients with growth deficiency. Many patients with Prader-Willi syndrome who are not growth deficient also have blunted growth hormone response to stimulation, and these patients also benefit from growth hormone treatment. This is true even of individuals who are not obese. There is still controversy as to whether the diagnosis of Prader-Willi syndrome alone (without demonstration of growth hormone deficiency by standard stimulation tests) should be adequate indication to begin replacement therapy. Recently, one growth hormone preparation has been FDA approved for the indication Prader-Willi syndrome,

and stimulation studies are no longer required.

- During growth hormone treatment, it is vital to closely monitor the patient for scoliosis, because acceleration of scoliosis has been identified in a number of patients on treatment. This can be done through clinical examinations at quarterly visits or can be augmented with annual scoliosis X-ray series.

Treatment

- The child must usually be awakened to feed for at least the first several weeks of life. High-calorie formula with or without supplemental oil or other calorie source may be needed. Attention should be paid to the length of time to feed, because the work of feeding may exceed the caloric benefit if prolonged feeding times are allowed. A gastrostomy tube is rarely necessary because the severity of the hypotonia improves with time and poor feeding is transient.
- In early infancy, it is inappropriate to be concerned about avoiding fats, because they are needed for nervous system development and growth.
- Supportive counseling for parents is an important function of the care provider during this difficult time for families, and assurance that the child will overcome this phase of the disorder is beneficial.
- Thyroid hormone should be replaced if it is deficient. Standard doses are appropriate.
- If the child is growth hormone deficient, growth hormone replacement therapy, should be started using standard protocols. It may be that people with Prader-Willi syndrome require lower doses of growth hormone because they are often only partially deficient, but studies using lower doses have not yet been completed. The age for starting growth hormone replacement is still

controversial. Studies have largely been conducted on patients at least 6 years of age (Lindgren et al., 1997, 1998; Carrel et al., 1999). However, there is considerable experience among endocrinologists in treating patients between 2 and 6 years and even below 2 years. These individuals grow extremely well on treatment, improve their body composition, and become more normal in facial appearance and hand and foot length (personal observation).

- If scoliosis is accelerated in conjunction with growth hormone therapy, the decision as to whether to stop the replacement therapy should be made through consensus of the endocrinologist, the orthopedist and the family.

Development and Behavior

Delayed motor milestones are evident, and average age of sitting is 12 months and of walking is 24 months. Poor coordination is common, particularly in those who are not physically active starting early in life (personal observation). Eventually, the majority of patients learn to pedal a tricycle or bicycle. Adults remain mildly hypotonic with decreased muscle bulk and tone. Upper body strength is particularly deficient.

Language development is also delayed. Verbal skills are an ultimate strength in most affected individuals, although speech is often poorly articulated, having a nasal and/or slurred character. A minority of affected individuals have persistence of very immature speech.

Cognitive abnormalities are evident, and most patients are mildly retarded (mean IQ 60s–low 70s) (Curfs, 1992; Curfs and Fryns, 1992; Dykens et al., 1992). Approximately 40% have borderline retardation or low normal intelligence, and about 20% have moderate retardation. Academic performance is often below what is expected for the individual's cognitive ability. Specific patterns of cognitive strength and weakness have begun to emerge, frequently with relative strength in reading, visual-spatial skills, and long-term memory and weakness in arithmetic, sequential processing, and short-term memory (Curfs and Fryns, 1992; Dykens et al., 1992). However, this pattern is not seen consistently. Coming to clinic with a book of word-find puzzles can almost be considered a diagnostic sign for Prader-Willi syndrome (personal observation), and unusual skill with jigsaw puzzles is common. Most individuals can read, write, and do simple mathematics.

A characteristic behavior profile becomes evident in early childhood, with temper tantrums, stubbornness, controlling and manipulative behavior, obsessive-compulsive characteristics, and difficulty with change in routine (Curfs, 1992; Dykens et al., 1992; Dykens and Cassidy, 1996). Lying, stealing, and aggressive behavior are common. Several studies have documented a high prevalence of obsessive-compulsive symptoms (Dykens and Cassidy, 1996; Dykens et al., 1996; State et al., 1999). Although these problems are not unique to Prader-Willi syndrome, they do occur with greater severity and frequency in people with Prader-Willi syndrome relative to some other groups with mild to moderate mental retardation. About 70% of affected individuals show a mixture of compulsive behaviors such as hoarding, ordering and arranging, redoing, and needing to tell or ask (Dykens et al., 1996). Parents often complain about repetitive question asking and getting stuck on ideas (personal observation). Many people with Prader-Willi syndrome are also described as quite clever and manipulative, particularly in regard to obtaining food. Behavioral issues not infrequently jeopardize home life, group home placements, and school and employment situations (personal experience). Skin picking and rectal picking may also be considered behavioral findings, and are discussed under **Dermatologic**.

True psychosis occurs in approximately 5–10% of patients, although some report a higher prevalence (Clarke, 1998; Beardsmore et al., 1998). Onset is often in young adulthood. Cycloid psychosis, a specific type of psychosis, has been noted in a significant proportion of those with psychosis (Verhoeven et al., 1998). These findings may guide treatment.

There is preliminary evidence that patients who have Prader-Willi syndrome on the basis of a 15q deletion have more numerous and more severe behavioral disturbances, although both genotypes are associated with significant problems in this area (Dykens et al., 1999). Although autism spectrum problems are not common in conjunction with Prader-Willi syndrome, there have been a few reported cases of this dual diagnosis, and all cases have had uniparental disomy as the etiology of the Prader-Willi syndrome. Because autism is known to be associated with duplication of the same region of chromosome 15 as is deleted in patients with deletion-based Prader-Willi syndrome (Schroer et al., 1998; see Gillberg, 1999 for review), it is presumed that overexpression of a gene in this region is responsible for autism.

Behavioral and psychiatric problems interfere the most with quality of life in adults with Prader-Willi syndrome. Behavior and its management are reviewed in Dykens and Cassidy (1999).

Evaluation

- Developmental skills attainment should be closely evaluated in infancy and toddlerhood.
- A careful educational, behavioral, and psychological assessment should be conducted for any affected individual. This should include an evaluation of cognitive strengths and weaknesses.
- Assessment should be made for evidence of obsessive-compulsive disorder, impulse control problems, and depressive disorders. Determination of whether compulsive tendencies lead to getting stuck on thoughts should be

made, and extra support should be provided with transitions. Intervention can be directed at these problems, if they are identified.
- Assessment of family support and psychosocial/emotional needs will assist in designing family interventions.

Treatment

- The child should be involved in early intervention services beginning as early as possible.
- Educational intervention throughout the school years (at a minimum) should include addressing individual strengths and weaknesses and taking into account the behavior disorder. Most children with Prader-Willi syndrome require either placement in a special educational classroom or special assistance in a regular classroom. Both inclusion and self-contained classroom settings have been effective, depending on the level of skills and the extent of behavior disorder (personal experience). Individual aides in the classroom can be invaluable in assuring that the child attends to task, and the use of aides has been particularly effective when the child is in an inclusion program or a regular classroom.
- Speech therapy and physical/occupational therapies, increased physical activity, and supervision during lunches are all important for most individuals with Prader-Willi syndrome during school.
- Provision of clear behavioral expectations and limits, beginning at an early age, is an extremely important part of behavior management. Applying consistent limits at home and school and/or work is critical. Preparing parents very early in the life of the affected individual to be able to set and enforce limits consistently appears to be a good predictor of fewer behavior problems in the future (personal experience).

- Formal social skills training is invaluable, because most individuals with Prader-Willi syndrome have difficulty reading social cues and maintaining friendships with peers.

- Before graduation from school, planning for vocational placement is essential. Most people require sheltered work or work with a job coach. Optimal work settings involve physical activity and absence of exposure to available food. Some of the occupations that have been excellent for affected individuals are landscaping, mail or flyer delivery, working at a florist shop, maintenance work, child or pet care, and other active employment. Inactive piecework at a sheltered workshop is far less desirable than many other jobs. If given responsibility and respect, most affected individuals will rise to the occasion.

- It is important for care providers to maintain consistency in daily routines. The individual should be prepared in advance for changes in routine or in planned activities.

- Appreciation of the impact of tantrums and other maladaptive behaviors on family stress can be very helpful.

- Many people with Prader-Willi syndrome and severe behavior problems respond to individual psychotherapy or, in some cases, group therapy with other developmentally disabled individuals. Selecting a behavior therapist interested in working with the disabled is not always easy, but such people exist and can be extremely helpful.

- Pharmaceutical treatment of behavior and psychiatric problems in people with Prader-Willi syndrome is often needed and is frequently helpful. Sometimes, this treatment is required in childhood, although use is much more frequent in adults. In particular, specific serotonin reuptake inhibitors have been beneficial. Affected individuals appear to be more sensitive to all medications than the average individual, so starting with a low dose is recommended. For those with evidence of psychosis, risperidone has been valuable.

- For adults who leave their family home, careful consideration must be given to living situation. Although a variety of options have been successful in individual situations, the most successful setting for the largest number of individuals has been in group homes specifically designed for Prader-Willi syndrome. These homes have only low-calorie foods, everyone is on a special diet, and food is inaccessible. Behavioral limits can be more strictly enforced. Studies have shown that dedicated group homes are the most effective in reducing and maintaining weight over time and in managing behavioral difficulties (Greenswag, 1987; Cassidy et al., 1994; Greenswag and Alexander, 1995).

Obesity

Obesity is nearly always present in Prader-Willi syndrome after 6 years of age, if it is not actively avoided. Avoidance of obesity is one of the most difficult problems of Prader-Willi syndrome, and obesity is the major cause of morbidity and mortality in this disorder. One consequence of hypotonia in Prader-Willi syndrome is a decrease in lean body mass (Schoeller et al., 1988). This results in a relatively high ratio of fat to lean body mass even in children whose weight-to-height ratio is normal (Butler et al., 1988). It also is the suspected cause of the decreased caloric requirement (Holland et al., 1993). The ratio of fat to lean body mass is also helpful in recognizing the early signs of hyperphagia and resultant obesity, which have their onset soon after the neonatal hypotonia seems to improve, usually between ages 1 and 6 years, with an average age range of 2–4 years. At the point of increasing weight-to-height ratio, a plan should be developed to avoid increasing obesity.

The obesity is central in distribution, with relative sparing of the distal extremities (Figs. 18.1 and 18.2). Even individuals who are not overweight tend to deposit fat on the abdomen, buttocks, and thighs.

Cardiopulmonary compromise (pickwickian syndrome) results from excessive obesity, as can type II diabetes mellitus, hypertension, thrombophlebitis, and chronic leg edema. Sleep apnea occurs at increased frequency, but the other sleep disturbances seen in Prader-Willi syndrome appear to be unrelated to obesity (Hertz et al., 1995). Breakdown of skin in the intertriginous skin folds is common in those with significant obesity (personal experience).

The major contributor to obesity is likely to be the excessive eating, or hyperphagia, that characterizes the majority of affected patients. This appears to be the consequence of a hypothalamic defect that results in lack of satiety (Holland et al., 1993). Although there is variation in the severity of hyperphagia, it is almost always present and causes the individual to constantly seek food, forage for food, and eat food that most people would consider inedible (e.g., a bag of sugar, garbage, or rotten or frozen food). A high threshold for vomiting may complicate bingeing on spoiled food from the garbage or such items as boxes of sugar or frozen uncooked meat, and toxicity from ineffective emetics used to induce vomiting has occurred. However, with proper management, the obesity can be controlled (Fig. 18.3).

Attempting to reach an "ideal" body weight is usually impractical in this disorder. Aiming for 2 standard deviations above the weight that is average for height age is reasonable (personal experience).

Hyperphagia and the potential for obesity are long-term problems in Prader-Willi syndrome. It is unreasonable to expect that individuals with Prader-Willi syndrome will eventually learn to control their own food intake. Until a medication or other treatment for hyperphagia can be found, a supportive living environment sensitive to this problem is essential.

Evaluation

- Close monitoring of weight percentiles and height-to-weight ratio, including plotting on growth charts to identify crossed percentiles, is critical throughout life. This is particularly true in the first few years, to recognize when obesity has its onset.

- Assessment of glycosylated hemoglobin levels in those who are significantly obese and in those who have experienced a rapid weight gain in a short period of time is helpful in early identification of diabetes.

Treatment

- Unfortunately, no medication or surgical procedure available at the time of writing has had long-term effectiveness in controlling appetite. Therefore, a low-calorie, well-balanced diet combined with a regular exercise program and close supervision to minimize food stealing should be instituted early, but no later than when excessive weight gain is first noted through crossing of weight percentiles.

- Decreased caloric requirement should be kept in mind in planning diets (Holm and Pipes, 1976). Intake should rarely be above 1000–1200 Kcal/day. There is considerable variability in dietary recommendations among those who conduct specialized programs for management of Prader-Willi syndrome. Approximately 800–900 Kcal/day is a good level at which to start in toddlers and very young children, working slowly up by increments of 100 Kcal as judged by the growth chart (personal experience). The extent of activity and the patient's height have a small influence on allowable caloric intake. For those who have already become obese, intake of approximately 1000 Kcal/day in individuals over age 6 years will result in slow but steady weight loss and is adequate for healthy nutrition (personal experience). For such individuals, some people have recommended diets as low as 600 Kcal/day (Mullins and Maier, 1987), deciding on caloric intake based on height (Holm and Pipes, 1976), or using a ketogenic diet (Bistrian et al., 1977).

- Regardless of diet type, supplemental vitamins and intake of the recommended daily allowance of calcium should be assured, the latter because of preliminary evidence for osteoporosis.

- Access to food should be as limited as possible, because in many cases the prescribed diet is only part of food intake if additional food is obtainable. Keeping temptation out of reach allows the individual to turn his or her attention to other matters (personal experience). In most cases, this entails locking the kitchen or locking the refrigerator and pantry. It is important to help families determine how best to respect the rights of other members of the household while still reducing temptation to take extra food away by the affected individual. One family used an elaborate system of motion detection alarms in their kitchen.

- Encouraging families to keep only healthy, low-calorie food in the house is appropriate. Arranging for supervision of school children during lunch time to prevent them from finishing other children's lunches has been effective, as has allowing no pocket money to buy food at school or work in older children and adults. Schools can provide low-calorie lunches, if requested.

- Teachers and employers of people with Prader-Willi syndrome should be educated about the importance of decreased food intake to health, and other students or co-workers should also be informed. Family or other home care providers and those responsible for day programs should be encouraged to communicate regarding "treats" and food sneaking, and dinner intake can be adjusted to compensate for excesses earlier in the day.

- Behavioral management programs, including firm limit setting and enforcement, should be instituted simultaneously with diet and as early as possible. People with Prader-Willi syndrome can be very convincing and can develop elaborate tales of having missed meals, and many have been found to be getting two breakfasts or two lunches this way. Consistency over time and communication among all care providers is essential.

- Many families have difficulty denying their child food, particularly among ethnic groups that associate feeding the child with loving him or her. Supportive counseling is critical. A behavioral psychologist or other behavior specialist is an important part of the management team (personal experience).

- Regular exercise is also an extremely important part of weight management, and most affected individuals have a strong tendency to inactivity. Exercise can build muscle mass as well as burn calories, thus increasing metabolic rate. At least 30 minutes of some type of physical activity daily, with rewards or other behavior modification techniques to encourage exercise, is appropriate (personal experience). Initiating a daily exercise program as young as possible, and making it part of the daily routine, has been the most effective. Some adults who do 45–60 minutes of exercise biking or similar activity daily have been able to eat essentially a normal diet (i.e., 1,800–2,000 Kcal/day) once they have reached a healthy weight (personal experience).

- Treatment of severe obesity accompanied by cardiopulmonary compromise or other major medical problems is complicated. Despite difficulties with resistance to hospital admission for treatment of obesity, and problems convincing insurance companies that this is not just an esthetic issue, experience has indicated that it can be arranged, and is usually necessary if there is significant morbidity (personal experience). On occasion, this can be accomplished as an outpatient by removing the individual from his or her current living situation and placing him or her in a more restrictive environment in which firmer limit setting takes place. If hospitalization is needed, care should be taken to alter the environment that allowed the individual to become morbidly obese, and education of parents and/or care providers about avoidance of morbidity is critical.

- A significant benefit has been noted in individuals with Prader-Willi syndrome who have been treated with growth hormone in that there is a trend to normalize the body composition through decreased fat mass and increased muscle and bone mass (Lindgren et al., 1997; 1998; Carrel et al., 1999). Some studies have indicated that many of those treated actually lose weight (Angulo et al., 1996), although others have not (Davies et al., 1998), but most improve their body mass index and can eat more without gaining weight. Treated individuals have also been preliminarily shown to be more active and more agile (Eiholzer et al., 1998; Carrel et al., 1999). These effects appear to revert to pre-treatment status with cessation of growth hormone administration.

- Treatment of the complications of obesity does not differ significantly from that in the general population. However, in treating diabetes, the possibility of poor compliance with diet should be kept in mind, and frequent monitoring of fasting blood glucose and/or glycosylated hemoglobin should be used to assess compliance.

Neurologic

Hypotonia is a medically and developmentally significant finding in infants and children, although it is less so in adults. However, adults do have generalized mild hypotonia. In virtually all cases, the neonatal period is dominated by hypotonia, lethargy, and weak suck leading to feeding difficulties. Deep tendon reflexes may be absent. Muscle electrophysiological and biopsy studies, often done early in life, are normal or nonspecifically abnormal. These manifestations usually lead to prolonged hospital stay to assure adequate feeding and growth. A small proportion of infants with Prader-Willi syndrome has severe hypotonia lasting more than 2 years. This is uncommon and necessitates evaluation for other causes of hypotonia. In particular, hypothyroidism may occur at slightly increased frequency in Prader-Willi syndrome (personal experience). Hypotonia also likely contributes to strabismus.

The hypotonia at all ages is reflected in decreased muscle bulk and tone as well as poor coordination and, often, decreased strength. One consequence of hypotonia in Prader-Willi syndrome is a decrease in the proportion of lean body mass (Schoeller et al., 1988). The hypotonia likely contributes to a lower metabolic rate (Holland et al., 1993) and results in an inclination to inactivity. Both of these complicate the management of obesity.

A number of findings suggest a variety of other neurologic symptoms. Abnormalities of the autonomic nervous system have been reported (DiMario et al., 1994;

1996), and these may be responsible for the decreased salivary flow (Hart, 1998) and the high threshold for vomiting. A high threshold for pain is also described by parents and care providers, and it contributes to morbidity and mortality in that affected individuals often will not complain very much when they have broken bones (personal experience) or have severe abdominal problems (Wharton et al., 1997). Impaired peripheral somatosensory function has been demonstrated in one study of Prader-Willi syndrome, possibly reflecting a low density of peripheral nerve fibers (Brandt and Rosen, 1998). The latter has led to ruptured internal viscera before care providers were aware of significant problems.

Evaluation

- Physical therapy evaluation is appropriate for all infants and children with Prader-Willi syndrome, to assess the necessity for ongoing therapy.
- Infants and young children with prolonged symptomatic hypotonia leading to prolonged failure to thrive and lethargy or severe developmental lag compared with the average for Prader-Willi syndrome should be evaluated for other causes, including hypothyroidism.

Treatment

- Early intervention, particularly physical therapy, is recommended from early infancy to avert muscle atrophy from inactivity. It may be of value in improving muscle strength and encouraging achievement of developmental milestones. For the most part, long-term physical therapy is of benefit to compensate for persistent hypotonia and poor coordination through improved muscle strength, agility, and activity.
- Growth hormone has been used (though not systematically studied) at this early age to improve muscle mass and should

be considered early in cases with prolonged severe and symptomatic hypotonia (e.g., more than 1 year).

Endocrine

In addition to the growth hormone deficiency (discussed in the **Growth and Feeding** section) and diabetes (discussed under **Obesity**), hypogonadism is present in the majority but not in all individuals with Prader-Willi syndrome and is of prenatal onset. It is hypothalamic in origin, and gonadotropins, estrogen, and testosterone generally are usually deficient. Because the pituitary gland and gonads are normal but understimulated, treatment with pituitary or gonadal hormones can improve secondary sex characteristics.

Hypogonadism is evident at birth as genital hypoplasia. It is manifested by cryptorchidism, scrotal hypoplasia (small, hypopigmented, and poorly rugated), and sometimes a small penis in males and by hypoplasia of the labia minora and clitoris in females. It may be difficult to appreciate in prepubertal girls. The genital hypoplasia persists throughout life, although in males spontaneous descent of testes has been reported up to adolescence.

Hypogonadism is also evident in abnormal pubertal development in both sexes with Prader-Willi syndrome. Although pubic and axillary hair may develop early or normally, the remainder of pubertal development is usually delayed and incomplete. Adult males only occasionally have voice change, male body habitus, or substantial facial or body hair. In females, breast development generally begins at a normal age, but there is usually amenorrhea or oligomenorrhea. Menarche may occur as late as the 30s, particularly in association with significant weight loss. In both males and females, sexual activity is uncommon. Only one adult with molecularly confirmed Prader-Willi syndrome, a female, has been documented to be fertile (Akefeldt et al., 1999).

Evaluation

- The possibility of cryptorchidism should be assessed in every affected male, and the position of the testes should continue to be monitored, because retractile testes, and the need for repeat orchiopexy have been noted repeatedly (personal experience).
- Measurement of testosterone in males or estradiol in females in the early pubertal years is necessary before consideration of replacement therapy.

Treatment

- Administration of human chorionic gonadotropin (hCG) occasionally may stimulate testicular descent, but frequently it enlarges the scrotum, improving the success of orchiopexy. In addition, it improves muscle bulk and therefore accelerates early motor milestones, activity, and feeding in infancy.
- In the general population, orchiopexy is done in the early months to preserve full fertility, to avoid neoplasia, and for psychological and cosmetic reasons. There are no published guidelines for when to do orchiopexy in males with Prader-Willi syndrome. However, it is relevant that fertility is not an issue, and testicular neoplasia has only been reported on one occasion in Prader-Willi syndrome (although there are a few additional anecdotal cases). It is probably appropriate to leave the issue of timing of testicular surgery up to the surgeon and the family until data are published that suggest otherwise.
- Improvement in secondary sex characteristics can be accomplished by the administration of testosterone in males or estrogen in females, although there is considerable controversy among physicians experienced with Prader-Willi syndrome as to whether to use them and on whom.

- In males, not only can voice change and body hair, beard growth, and genital size be improved, but a more masculine body habitus and increased muscle bulk and strength usually occur with testosterone treatment. One approach is to begin testosterone replacement at age 13–14 years with a relatively low dose (50–75 mg IM. depotestosterone every 3–4 weeks, or a single testosterone patch daily), working up slowly in dose to about 150 mg every 3–4 weeks (personal experience). Although this is a relatively low dose, blood levels should be monitored during mid-month and the dose can be titrated against behavior problems. In males, an increase in aggressive behavior is the greatest concern, because these individuals usually already have behavioral disturbance. Some parents have objected to the increase in body hair. With the recent introduction of testosterone by daily skin patch, a more consistent level of testosterone may be achieved, thus avoiding the usual increase in aggression in the week or so after an injection is given. Care must be taken, as always, to avoid abnormal acceleration of bone growth with ultimate shorter stature, so bone age should be monitored in treated growing individuals.
- Simultaneous treatment with growth hormone and testosterone should probably be monitored by an endocrinologist.
- In females, estrogen treatment or, preferably, cycling hormones or birth control pills can increase breast size if desired and also results in menstrual periods. A surprising number of women with Prader-Willi syndrome want to have their periods like other women, at least for a while. The benefits of hormone replacement therapy to the cardiovascular system and to prevention of osteoporosis have not been studied but are documented in other conditions with low estrogen levels such as

Turner syndrome and postmenopausal women. The risk of thrombosis is of concern but, again, has not been studied.

- Sex education is as important in Prader-Willi syndrome as in the general population.

Opthalmologic

Strabismus is frequent, likely caused by muscular hypotonia, although a contribution from albinoidism has also been documented in individuals with fair coloring (Wiesner et al., 1987). Myopia and hyperopia are common.

Evaluation

- All infants and young children should be screened for stabismus during routine well child visits, including use of the cover/uncover test for detecting esophoria.
- A formal ophthalmologic evaluation between ages 1 and 3 years is appropriate.

Treatment

- Strabismus should be managed as for any infant, keeping in mind muscular hypotonia and the possibility of hypopigmentation and its consequences.
- Visual acuity problems should be treated as in the geneal population.

Dental

Dental anomalies have been frequently reported and include dental crowding, carious teeth, and decreased saliva flow. Thick, sticky, and ropy saliva often leaves dried material on the lips and, anecdotally, makes articulation more difficult. One study documented that affected individuals have approximately 20% of the salivary flow of unaffected individuals (Hertz et al., 1995). This may be related to decreased autonomic stimulation of the saliva glands, which can be stimulated to increase flow by autonomic stimulants.

Evaluation

- Regular, routine semiannual dental examination and prophylaxis, starting no later than age 3, is important. Some dentists who have seen a large number of affected patients recommend that they be performed four times per year.
- The quality and quantity of saliva should be evaluated through a search for crusted matter on the lips, ropes or strings of saliva in the mouth, or very dry mouth.

Treatment

- Emphasis should be placed on good dental hygiene.
- Products that increase saliva flow have appeared on the market in the past decade. These include toothpaste, mouthwash, and sugarless gums. Biotene has been effective in increasing saliva flow and consistency (personal experience). These should be used in patients with decreased saliva flow.

Musculoskeletal

The major musculoskeletal problems relate to the increased incidence of scoliosis and/or kyphosis and to osteoporosis, for which there is preliminary evidence of an increase in Prader-Willi syndrome.

Scoliosis is presumed to be related to muscular hypotonia, because there are no underlying structural anomalies. Scoliosis can occur at any age during childhood, including early infancy. When it occurs in infancy, it is often quite severe (personal experience). Kyphosis occurs commonly in adolescents and adults with Prader-Willi syndrome but is rarely a cause of morbidity.

Osteoporosis has been anecdotally reported (Rubin and Cassidy, 1988), but there are no controlled studies or treatment trials. There are a number of contributory factors, including hypogonadism, hypotonia, inactivity, and, often, low-dairy diets resulting in decreased calcium intake. An increased fracture rate may be present.

Evaluation

- Clinical screening for scoliosis should be done at all routine health care visits by assessing the symmetry of the back in the "diving" position.
- Any suspicion of scoliosis should prompt a scoliosis X-ray series.
- The criteria used for referral to an orthopedist for scoliosis should be the same as those in the general population.
- Bone densitometry is appropriate in adulthood or in any child with frequent fractures or fractures with apparently inadequate trauma.

Treatment

- Scoliosis in Prader-Willi syndrome should be treated as in the general population. The prolonged period of growth caused by pubertal deficiency should be kept in mind. Bracing and surgical procedures are sometimes necessary.
- Calcium and vitamin D intake at least to RDA-recommended levels should be assured. Calcium and vitamin D supplementation is appropriate in all patients. Taking Tums to accomplish this has been well tolerated (personal experience), although other supplements may also be used.
- Weight-bearing exercise should be encouraged throughout life.
- The use of sex hormone supplementation and, potentially, growth hormone may prevent or limit osteoporosis, although this has not been studied.
- The use of bisphosphonates has not yet been studied in Prader-Willi syndrome.

Dermatologic

One of the more difficult problems in Prader-Willi syndrome is picking at the skin or mucosal areas such as the nose, rectum, or vagina, which occurs in over half of affected individuals. Difficulties with sores kept open for months or years and subsequent scarring and pigmentary changes are not uncommon among those who do skin picking. Anxiety and stress seem to increase the severity of picking behavior.

Peripheral edema, later leading to chronic skin changes of the legs, is not uncommon in Prader-Willi syndrome.

Evaluation

- Examination of the skin and exposed mucosal areas for evidence of complications of picking should occur at routine medical visits.
- A history of frequent nose bleeds or rectal bleeds should prompt examination of these areas for sores resulting from picking.

Treatment

- Treatment of picking is very resistant to most therapies and rarely responds to medications such as specific serotonin reuptake inhibitors.
- Keeping lesions moist and covered, keeping the fingernails short, and using behavior modification techniques may be beneficial in controlling picking behavior.
- Individuals who spend long periods of time in the bathroom are frequently the ones doing rectal picking. Limiting the amount of time that can be spent in the bathroom may be helpful.
- Peripheral edema and chronic skin changes should be treated as for the general population. Weight loss is often very helpful as well.

RESOURCES

Prader-Willi Syndrome Association (USA)

5700 Midnight Pass Road, Suite 6
Sarasota, FL 34242

Phone: 1-800-926-4797
Web: *http://www.pwsausa.org*

Prader-Willi Syndrome Association of the United Kingdom 33 Leopold Street

Derby DE1 2HF
England
Phone: (01332) 365676
Web: *http://www.pwsa-uk.demon.co.uk*

International Prader-Willi Syndrome Organisation

http://www.ipwso.org
(an organization of country chapters)

The Prader-Willi Foundation

223 Main Street
Port Washington, N.Y. 11050
(800) 253-7993
(516) 944-3173 - fax
E-mail: *PWSAUSA@aol.com*

Written Resources

Greenswag LR, Alexander RC, eds. (1995) *Management of Prader-Willi Syndrome*, 2nd ed. New York: Springer.

Multiple written resources are available from the support groups

REFERENCES

Åkefeldt A, Törnhage CJ, Gillberg C (1999) A woman with Prader-Willi syndrome gives birth to a healthy baby girl. *Dev Med Child Neurol* 41:789–790.

American Society of Human Genetics/American College of Medical Genetics (1996) Diagnostic testing for Prader-Willi and Angelman syndromes: Report of the ASHG/ACMG Joint Test and Technology Transfer Committee. *Am J Hum Genet* 58:1085–1088.

Angulo M, Castro-Magana M, Mazur B, Canas JA, Vitollo PM, Sarrantonio M (1996) Growth hormone secretion and effects of growth hormone therapy on growth velocity and weight gain in children with Prader-Willi syndrome. *J Pediatr Endocrinol Metab* 9:393–400.

Beardsmore A, Dorman T, Cooper SA, Webb T (1998) Affective psychosis and Prader-Willi syndrome. *J Intellect Disabil Res* 42:463–471.

Bistrian BR, Blackburn GL, Stanbury JB (1977) Metabolic aspects of a protein-sparing modified fast in the dietary management of Prader-Willi obesity. *N Engl J Med* 296:774–779 .

Brandt BR, Rosen I (1998) Impaired peripheral somatosensory function in children with Prader-Willi syndrome. *Neuropediatrics* 29: 124–126.

Bray G, Dahms W, Swerdloff R, Fiser R, Atkinson R, Carrell R (1983) The Prader-Willi syndrome: A study of 40 patients and a review of the literature. *Medicine* 62:59–80.

Buiting K, Saitoh S, Gross S, Dittrich B, Schwartz S, Nicholls RD, Horsthemke B (1994) Inherited microdeletions in the Angelman and Prader-Willi syndromes define an imprinting centre on human chromosome 15. *Nat Genet* 9:395–400.

Butler MG (1990) Prader-Willi syndrome: Current understanding of cause and diagnosis. *Am J Med Genet* 35:319–332.

Butler MG, Butler RI, Meaney FJ (1988) The use of skinfold measurements to judge obesity during the early phase of Prader-Labhart-Willi syndrome. *Int J Obesity* 12:417–422.

Butler MG, Meaney FJ (1991) Standards for selected anthropometric measurements in Prader-Willi syndrome. *Pediatrics* 88:853–860.

Carrel AL, Myers SE, Whitman BY, Allen DB (1999) Growth hormone improves body composition, fat utilization, physical strength and agility, and growth in Prader-Willi syndrome: A controlled study. *J Pediatr* 134:215–221.

Cassidy SB (1984) Prader-Willi syndrome *Curr Probl Pediatr* 14:1–55.

Cassidy SB (1997): Prader-Willi syndrome *J Med Genet* 34:917–923.

Cassidy SB, Devi A, Mukaida C (1994) Aging in Prader-Willi syndrome: 22 patients over age 30 years. *Proc Greenwood Genet Ctr* 13:102–103.

Clarke D (1998) Prader-Willi syndrome and psychotic symptoms 2. A preliminary study of prevalence using the Psychopathology Assessment Schedule for Adults with Developmental Disability checklist. *J Intellect Disabil Res* 42:451–454.

Curfs LG (1992) Psychological profile and behavioral characteristics in Prader-Willi syndrome. In: *Prader-Willi Syndrome and Other 15q Deletion Disorders*, Cassidy SB, ed. Berlin: Springer, p. 211–222.

Curfs LM, Fryns JP (1992) Prader-Willi syndrome: A review with special attention to the cognitive and behavioral profile. *Birth Defects Orig Artic Ser* 28:99–104.

Curfs LM, Wiegers AM, Sommers JR, Borghgraef M, Fryns JP (1991) Strengths and weaknesses in the cognitive profile of youngsters with Prader-Willi syndrome. *Clin Genet* 40:430–434.

Davies PS, Evans S, Broomhead S, Clough H, Day JM, Laidlaw A, Barnes ND (1998) Effect of growth hormone on height, weight, and body composition in Prader-Willi syndrome. *Arch Dis Child* 78:474–476.

DiMario FJ Jr, Bauer L, Volpe J, Cassidy SB (1996) Respiratory sinus arrhythmia in patients with Prader-Willi syndrome. *Child Neurol* 11:121–125.

DiMario FJ Jr, Dunham B, Burleson JA, Moskovitz J, Cassidy SB (1994) An evaluation of autonomic nervous system function in patients with Prader-Willi syndrome. *Pediatrics* 93:76–81.

Dykens EM, Hodapp RM, Walsh K, Nash L (1992) Profiles, correlates and trajectories of intelligence in individuals with Prader-Willi syndrome. *J Am Acad Child Adolesc Psychiatry* 31:1125–1130.

Dykens EM, Cassidy SB (1996) Prader-Willi syndrome: Genetic, behavioral and treatment issues. *Child Adolesc Clin N Am* 5:913–927.

Dykens EM, Cassidy SB (1999) Prader-Willi syndrome. In *Neurodevelopmental and Genetic Disorders in Children*, Goldstein S and Reynolds C, eds. New York: Guilford, p. 525–554.

Dykens EM, Cassidy SB, King BH (1999) Maladaptive behavior differences in Prader-Willi syndrome due to paternal deletion versus maternal uniparental disomy. *Am J Ment Retard* 104:67–77.

Dykens EM, Leckman JF, Cassidy SB (1996) Obsessions and compulsions in Prader-Willi syndrome. *J Child Psychol Psychiatry* 37:995–1002.

Eiholzer U, Gisin R, Weinmann C, Kriemler S, Steinert H, Torresani T, Zachmann M, Prader A (1998) Treatment with human growth hormone in patients with Prader-Labhart-Willi syndrome reduces body fat and increases muscle mass and physical performance. *Eur J Pediatr* 157:368–377.

Gillberg C (1999) Chromosomal disorders and autism. *J Autism Dev Disord* 28:415–425.

Glenn CC, Driscoll DJ, Yang TP, Nicholls RD (1997) Genetic imprinting: Potential function and mechanisms revealed by the Prader-Willi and Angelman syndromes. *Mol Hum Reprod* 3:321–332.

Greenswag LR (1987) Adults with Prader-Willi syndrome. A survey of 22 cases. *Dev Med Child Neurol* 29:145–152.

Greenswag LR, Alexander RC, eds. (1995) *Management of Prader-Willi syndrome*, 2nd ed. New York: Springer.

Gunay-Aygun M, Cassidy SB, Nicholls RD (1997) Prader-Willi and other syndromes associated with obesity and mental retardation. *Behav Gene* 27:307–324.

Hart PS (1998) Salivary abnormalities in Prader-Willi syndrome. *Ann NY Acad Sci* 842:125–131.

Hertz G, Cataletto M, Feinsilver SH, Angulo M (1995) Developmental trends of sleep-disordered breathing in Prader-Willi syndrome: The role of obesity. *Am J Med Genet* 56:188–190.

Holland AJ, Treasure J, Coskeran P, Dallow J, Milton N, Hillhouse E (1993) Measurement of excessive appetite and metabolic changes in Prader-Willi syndrome. *Int J Obes* 17:526–532.

Holm VA, Cassidy SB, Butler MG, Hanchett JM, Greenswag LR, Whitman BY, Greenberg F (1993) Prader-Willi syndrome: Consensus diagnostic criteria. *Pediatrics* 91:398–402.

Holm VA, Pipes PL (1976) Food and children with Prader-Willi syndrome *Am J Dis Child* 130:1063–1067.

Hudgins LH, McKillop JA, Cassidy SB (1991) Hand and foot lengths in Prader-Willi syndrome. *Am J Med Genet* 41:5–9.

Hudgins L, Geer JS, Cassidy SB (1998) Phenotypic differences in African-Americans with Prader-Willi syndrome. *Genet Med* 1:49–51.

Kennerknecht I (1992) Differentiated recurrence risk estimations in the Prader-Willi syndrome. *Clin Genet* 41:303–308.

Ledbetter DH, Engel E (1995) Uniparental disomy in humans. Development of an imprinting map and its implications for prenatal diagnosis. *Hum Mol Genet* 4:1757–1764.

Ledbetter DH, Riccardi VM, Airhart SD, Strobel RJ, Keenen SB, Crawford JD (1981) Deletions of chromosome 15 as a cause of the Prader-Willi syndrome. *N Engl J Med* 304: 325–329.

Lindgren AC, Hagenäs L, Müller J, Blichfeldt S, Rosenborg M, Brismar T, Ritzen EM (1997) Effects of growth hormone on growth and body composition in Prader-Willi syndrome: A preliminary report. *Acta Paediatr Suppl* 423:60–62.

Lindgren AC, Hagenäs L, Müller J, Blichfeldt S, Rosenborg M, Brismar T, Ritzen EM (1998) Growth hormone treatment of children with Prader-Willi syndrome affects linear growth and body composition favourably. *Acta Paediatr* 87:28–31.

Miller SP, Riley P, Shevell MI (1999) The neonatal presentation of Prader-Willi syndrome revisited. *Pediatrics* 134:226–228 .

Mullins J, Maier B (1987) Weight management of youth with Prader-Willi syndrome. *Int J Eating Disord* 6:419–427.

Nicholls RD, Knoll JHM, Butler MG, Karam S, Lalande M (1989) Genetic imprinting suggested by maternal heterodisomy in nondeletion Prader-Willi syndrome. *Nature* 342: 281–285.

Nicholls RD (1993) Genomic imprinting and uniparental disomy in Angelman and Prader-Willi syndrome: A review. *Am J Med Genet* 46:16–25.

Ozcelik T, Leff S, Robinson W, Donlon T, Lalande H, Sanjines E, Schinzel A, Francke U (1992) Small nuclear ribonucleoprotein polypeptide N (*SNRPN*), an expressed gene in the Prader-Willi syndrome critical region. *Nat Genet* 2:265–269.

Prader A, Labhart A, Willi H (1956) Ein Syndrom von Adipositas, Kleinwuchs, Kryptorchismus und Oligophrenie nach myotoniertigem Zustand im Neugeborenalter. *Schweiz Med Wochenschr* 86:1260–1261.

Robinson WP, Bottani A, Yagang X, Balakrishman J, Binkert F, Machler M, Prader A, Schinzel A (1991) Molecular, cytogenetic and clinical investigations of Prader-Willi syndrome patients. *Am J Hum Genet* 49:1219–1234.

Rubin KG, Cassidy SB (1988) Endocrine abnormalities and osteoporosis. In: *Management of Prader-Willi Syndrome*, Greenswag LR and Alexander R, eds. New York: Springer, Chapter 3, p. 23–33.

Saitoh S, Buiting K, Cassidy SB, Conroy JM, Driscoll DJ, Gabriel JM, Gillessen–Kaesbach G, Glenn CC, Greenswag LR, Horsthemke B, Kondo I, Kuwajima K, Niikawa N, Rogan PK, Schwartz S, Seip J, Williams CA, Wiznitzer M, Nicholls RD (1997) Clinical spectrum and molecular diagnosis of Angelman and Prader-Willi syndrome imprinting mutation patients. *Am J Med Genet* 68:195–206.

Schoeller DA, Levitsky LL, Bandini LG, Dretz WW, Walczak A (1988) Energy expenditure and body composition in Prader-Willi syndrome. *Metabolism* 39:115–120.

Schroer RJ, Phelan MC, Michaelis RC, Crawford EC, Skinner SA, Cuccaro M, Simensen RJ, Bishop J, Skinner C, Fender D, Stevenson RE (1998) Autism and maternally derived aberrations of chromosome 15q. *Am J Med Genet* 76:327–336.

State MW, Dykens EM, Rosner B, Martin A, King BH (1999) Obsessive-compulsive symptoms in Prader-Willi and "Prader-Willi-like" patients. *J Am Acad Child Adolesc Psychiatry* 38:329–334.

Verhoeven WM, Curfs LM, Tuinier SJ (1998) Prader-Willi syndrome and cycloid psychoses. *J Intellect Disabil Res* 42:455–462.

Wharton RH, Wang T, Graeme-Cook F, Briggs S, Cole RE (1997) Acute idiopathic gastric dilation with gastric necrosis in individuals with Prader-Willi syndrome. *Am J Med Genet* 73: 437–441.

Wiesner GL, Bendel CM, Olds DP, White JG, Arthur DC, Ball DW, King RA (1987) Hypopigmentation in the Prader-Willi syndrome. *Am J Med Genet* 40:431–442.

Zipf WB, Bernston GG (1987) Characteristics of abnormal food-intake patterns in children with Prader-Willi syndrome and study of effects of naloxone. *Am J Clin Nutr* 46:277–281.

CHAPTER 19

ROBIN SEQUENCE

ROBERT J. SHPRINTZEN

INTRODUCTION

Incidence

Robin sequence was named after the French stomatologist Pierre Robin (Robin, 1923) and has typically been regarded as the association of micrognathia, a wide, U-shaped cleft palate, and upper airway obstruction (Randall et al., 1965; Shprintzen, 1988; Shprintzen and Singer, 1992). In 1934, Robin mentioned cleft palate as an aggravating factor leading to airway obstruction in infants, although that feature was not part of his original description (Robin, 1934). Now recognized as an etiologically heterogeneous disorder that most often occurs as a sequence of other syndromes (Cohen, 1976; Shprintzen, 1988; Shprintzen and Singer, 1992, Shprintzen, 1992), its incidence has been estimated to be approximately 1 in 2,000 births. This figure is based on the prevalence of Robin sequence in a large sample of cases with cleft palate (Shprintzen et al; 1985), and on a survey of a single hospital system with approximately 9,000 births per year over a 4-year period (personal data). Some babies with Robin sequence die shortly after birth because of severe airway obstruction or a variety of underlying syndromes incompatible with life (such as trisomy 13, velocardiofacial syndrome with severe heart anomalies, or X-linked arthrogryposis, type I). Therefore, population prevalence is slightly lower than birth incidence.

Diagnostic Criteria

It has been demonstrated that the large majority of cases of Robin sequence are associated with other multiple-anomaly syndromes (Shprintzen, 1988; Shprintzen and Singer, 1992; Shprintzen, 1992). In one large series of cases meeting the criteria for Robin sequence in a single center, only 17% were isolated. In the remainder, Robin sequence was part of a multiple-anomaly syndrome (Shprintzen, 1988; Shprintzen and Singer, 1992; Shprintzen, 1992). Two syndromes constituted over 40% of all cases of Robin sequence. Stickler syndrome was the most common associated diagnosis (34%), and velocardiofacial syndrome was second most common (11%) (Shprintzen and Singer, 1992; Shprintzen, 1992). Therefore, an initial diagnosis of Robin sequence must be regarded as a starting point in the diagnostic search, not an ending point. In addition, Robin sequence may be associated with mandibular anomalies other

Management of Genetic Syndromes, Edited by Suzanne B. Cassidy and Judith E. Allanson
ISBN 0-471-31286-X   Copyright © 2001 by Wiley-Liss, Inc.

than micrognathia, including retrognathia and mandibular asymmetry.

Micrognathia may best be described as hypoplasia of the ramus, mandibular body, or both (Fig. 19.1). Retrognathia is a retruded mandible. The mandible is typically of normal size and morphology but is retruded (positioned posteriorly) because the skull base is flat (platybasia) and the temporomandibular joint is more posterior than normal, for example in velocardiofacial syndrome (Arvystas and Shprintzen, 1984). Although micrognathia and retrognathia are not mutually exclusive, there are only a few syndromes in which both may occur together. Robin sequence may also be caused by macroglossia and severe muscle weakness, as will be described in the next section.

Although the majority of clinicians cite the triad of clinical findings of micrognathia, U-shaped cleft palate, and upper airway obstruction as the criteria for Robin sequence, many clinicians stretch the boundaries of the diagnosis so that only two of the features of the triad may prompt the label of Robin sequence (Sadewitz and Shprintzen, 1986), as in micrognathia with cleft palate without airway obstruction, or micrognathia with airway obstruction without a U-shaped cleft. Because Robin sequence is most often secondary to another syndromic diagnosis, many other anomalies may coexist with the Robin triad. For example, many patients with Treacher Collins syndrome have the Robin triad. Micrognathia occurs in nearly all cases of Treacher Collins syndrome, airway obstruction is also very common, and a wide U-shaped cleft palate is seen in at least 10% of cases (personal experience). However, because the facial features associated with Treacher Collins syndromes (when severe) are so striking, clinicians may not consider the diagnosis of Robin sequence to be applicable even though accurate.

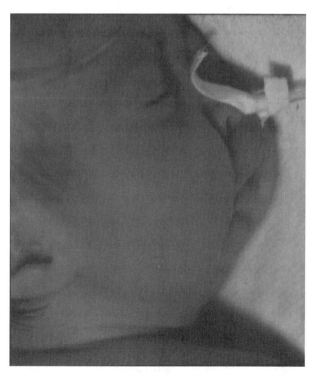

FIGURE 19.1. Infant with Robin sequence and severe micrognathia.

Etiology, Pathogenesis, and Genetics

To discuss the pathogenesis of Robin sequence, it is first important to recall the difference between a syndrome and a sequence (see **Introduction**), especially because many clinicians still refer to "Pierre Robin syndrome." The term syndrome is used when multiple anomalies in a single individual are caused by a single etiology. The term sequence is used when an individual has multiple anomalies caused secondarily by a single known or presumed structural anomaly or error in morphogenesis; that is, it is a cascade of events. However, the single primary structural defect that causes the other anomalies may itself have multiple possible causes.

Robin is a sequence, not a syndrome. In the case of Robin sequence, the primary anomaly, which interrupts the normal developmental process, is micrognathia or occasionally retrognathia. Palate fusion, which occurs between 9 and 11 weeks of embryonic development, is a precisely choreographed interaction between increasing size of the oral cavity, medial growth of the maxillary processes, and increasing growth of the head. At approximately 8 weeks after fertilization, the mandible is very short, with little height in the portion that will develop into the ramus. As a result, the vertical dimension of the oral cavity is very small and the tongue rests against the skull base. The embryonic palatal shelves, which are portions of the bilateral maxillary processes, are oriented vertically alongside the tongue. Because there is an increase in neural crest migration to the mandible and maxillary processes, there is a spurt in vertical growth of the mandible that allows the mandible to descend in the oral cavity, moving the tongue out of the space between the vertical palatal shelves. This process is enhanced by the normal mandibular movements being made by the fetus at this time. The palatal shelves are thus impulsed into a horizontal position, where they are aligned for continued medial growth and eventual fusion. At the same time, the head is growing wider, thus requiring the rate of medial growth of the palate to exceed the rate of lateral growth of the cranium. If for any reason the medial growth of the palatal shelves is temporally delayed, the head will be too wide for the palate's growth potential and fusion may fail to occur, resulting in a palatal cleft.

In the case of Robin sequence, micrognathia or retrognathia is present at the time that palate fusion is genetically programmed to begin. Because of the mandibular anomaly, the tongue is not free to descend from between the vertical palatal shelves. The tongue's presence between the palatal shelves physically prevents them from orienting horizontally and growing medially toward fusion. Although the tongue may eventually descend in the oral cavity and away from the cranial base, it may do so after lateral head growth is too great for the remaining palatal growth to overcome or the period of programmed growth may be over. After birth, micrognathia persists. Newborns are reflexively obligate nose breathers. With the mouth closed and a small or retruded mandible present, the tongue is retrodisplaced in the pharynx (glossoptosis), which causes airway obstruction and failure to thrive. Thus micrognathia leads to the third feature of the triad, airway obstruction and failure to thrive.

Malformations of either the ramus or the body of the mandible may result in Robin sequence. Syndromes with anomalies of the ramus are far more common than syndromes in which only the mandibular body is small. Lack of vertical development of the ramus would be expected in syndromes in which the cell populations that constitute the ramus are either deficient in number or abnormally organized (dysplasia). For example, there are a number of syndromes that have been linked to mutations in genes that regulate the formation of collagen, which is a component of the early matrix for bone deposition in the ramus. Stickler syndrome and spondyloepiphyseal dysplasia congenita are caused by different mutations in type II collagen. Stickler syndrome, one of the most common genetic forms of connective tissue dysplasia in humans (see Chapter 24) accounts for over a third of all cases of Robin sequence (Herrmann and Opitz, 1975; Shprintzen, 1988; Shprintzen and Singer, 1992). The ramus is also short in Freeman-Sheldon syndrome, femoral hypoplasia-unusual facies syndrome, FG syndrome, multiple pterygium syndrome, fetal alcohol syndrome (see Chapter 9), and otopalatodigital syndrome (both type I and type II).

An important component of care of the individual who has Robin sequence is understanding its etiologic heterogeneity and recognizing that the sequence may be instigated by either a malformation process (i.e., an intrinsic anomaly of the mandible) or a deformation process (i.e., an extrinsic mechanical force). A short mandibular body in the presence of a normal ramus is a more unusual finding in Robin sequence.

The most common occurrence of a short mandibular body is in positional mandibular deformation, an extrinsic mechanical force. This may occur as a result of fetal crowding caused, for example, by the presence of multiple fetuses, abnormal fetal position, uterine anomalies including tumors or malformations, or decreased amniotic fluid levels as in oligohydramnios. Associated deformations may include clubfoot, crumpled ear, or limb contractures. Positional deformations represent the only category of isolated Robin sequence in which the etiology is purely mechanical, and one would not expect to find other anomalies that were not related to mechanical constriction. Therefore, the association of other malformations such as congenital heart anomalies, internal organ anomalies, or dysplasias would indicate that the Robin sequence is not an isolated abnormality secondary to mechanical forces. In cases of positional deformation, once the mechanical force has been removed, it would be expected that mandibular growth would

proceed normally because the problem is not one of hypoplasia at the cellular level.

In some syndromes, malformation of both the mandibular body and ramus may occur simultaneously. Treacher Collins syndrome, Nager syndrome, and Stickler syndrome (see Chapter 24) all have anomalies of both the ramus and the body of the mandible. In these three syndromes, the ramus is short (far more hypoplastic in Treacher Collins and Nager syndromes) and the body of the mandible is smaller than normal with antegonial notching, bowing that is easily palpable on clinical examination and that is a good sign of a primary mandibular malformation with possible syndromic association. Antegonial notching of the mandible is common in Treacher Collins syndrome, Nager syndrome, Stickler syndrome, spondyloepiphyseal dysplasia, Freeman-Sheldon syndrome, Steinert syndrome, oculo-auriculo-vertebral spectrum (usually unilateral (see Chapter 16)), Wildervanck syndrome, cerebrocostomandibular syndrome, Christian syndrome, cornelia de Lange syndrome (see Chapter 6), Escobar syndrome, femoral hypoplasia-unusual facies syndrome, FG syndrome, Miller syndrome, multiple pterygium syndrome, otopalatodigital syndrome types I and II, and retinoic acid embryopathy. All of these syndromes may result in Robin sequence secondarily. There are a number of chromosomal syndromes that also have similar mandibular anomalies and result in Robin sequence, including trisomy 13 and 18 (see Chapter 25), 6q deletion syndrome, deletion 2p, and Turner syndrome (see Chapter 27).

The most common cause of retrognathia is platybasia, which draws the glenoid fossa and the temporomandibular joint backward away from the maxilla. Platybasia has been observed in a number of craniofacial syndromes (Shprintzen, 1982). The most common association of Robin sequence with platybasia is in velocardiofacial syndrome (see Chapter 29) (Arvystas and Shprintzen, 1984; Shprintzen et al., 1985; Shprintzen, 1988; Shprintzen and Singer, 1992).

Robin sequence may also be caused by macroglossia or severe facial hypotonia. Robin sequence has been reported in association with Beckwith-Wiedemann syndrome (see Chapter 4), presumably secondary to the large tongue interfering with palatal fusion (Cohen, 1976). Robin sequence has also been reported in association with Steinert syndrome (myotonic dystrophy) presumably secondary to a lack of embryonic mandibular exercise, thus preventing the tongue from descending from between the developing palatal shelves (Cohen, 1976).

The majority of the syndromes that result in Robin sequence are single-gene disorders, often inherited in an autosomal dominant manner, although there are several X-linked recessive disorders (such as otopalatodigital syndrome, type I) and recessive disorders (such as Nager syndrome). Among teratogenic disorders, the most common cause of Robin sequence is probably fetal alcohol syndrome (Shprintzen and Singer, 1992) (see Chapter 9), although other teratogens have also been implicated, including phenytoin and retinoic acid.

Diagnostic Testing

There is no specific testing for Robin sequence other than the observation of the clinical features either prenatally or postnatally. Both micrognathia and cleft palate can be detected with sonography in the fetus. All the chromosomal and many of the single-gene syndromes that can lead to Robin sequence may be detected individually by chromosomal or molecular procedures. Because two syndromes, specifically Stickler syndrome (34%) (see Chapter 24) and velocardiofacial syndrome (11%) (see Chapter 29), account for nearly half of all cases of Robin sequence, it is appropriate to screen all newborns with Robin sequence for these disorders before searching for other disorders, which are far less common. The vast majority of cases of velocardiofacial syndrome will be accurately detected by FISH for deletion 22q. Although

Stickler syndrome is known to be caused by *COL2A1* mutations in many cases, there are also mutations in other collagen genes that can cause the disorder. *COL11A1* and *COL11A2* genes have also been implicated in Stickler syndrome. Testing for any of these is not routinely clinically available at the time of this writing. There are, however, a few laboratories that perform these tests for clinical purposes.

Differential Diagnosis

Once micrognathia, cleft palate, and airway obstruction are recognized, this should initiate the process of seeking a syndromic diagnosis. The clinician should evaluate the child for any associated anomalies before concluding that the Robin sequence is an isolated event presumed to be caused by positional deformation. Shprintzen and Singer (1992) listed a series of 15 multiple-anomaly syndromes constituting 100 consecutive cases of Robin sequence seen within a single institution. Only 17 cases were found to be isolated, meaning that they were not associated with other syndromes. Thus the search for differential diagnosis should focus on anomalies other than the obvious presentation of micrognathia and cleft palate. The challenge for the clinician is that many anomalies commonly associated with syndromes that cause Robin sequence may not necessarily be evident at birth. For example, in children with velocardiofacial syndrome (Chapter 29) who lack a cardiac malformation, no obvious manifestation of the syndrome may be present until later in childhood when language impairment or learning disabilities become obvious. Stickler syndrome (Chapter 24) may also be difficult to diagnose in infancy if the clinician does not specifically assess for myopia. Furthermore, myopia is not present in all cases. Epiphyseal dysplasia will not be evident until the epiphyses are sufficiently formed for radiographic assessment. Table 19.1 provides an extensive list of syndromes associated with Robin sequence.

TABLE 19.1. A Partial List of Some of the More Common Syndromes Associated with Robin Sequence.

Syndrome	Associated Findings
Campomelic dysplasia	Small stature, hypertelorism, curved limbs, clubfoot, mental retardation, male sex reversal (deletion 17q24.3–q25.1/mutation of SOX9)
Catel-Manzke syndrome	Clubfoot, ventriculoseptal defect, anomalous index finger (unknown)
Cerebrocostomandibular syndrome	Costovertebral gaps, small stature, mental retardation (unknown)
Christian syndrome	CNS demyelination, mental retardation, small stature, clubfoot, imperforate anus, glucose intolerance, joint limitation, adducted thumbs, scoliosis, cervical spine fusions, absent sacrum, hemivertebrae, hirsutism, metopic ridging (X-linked recessive)
Cri-du-chat syndrome	High-pitched cry, mental retardation, early hypotonia followed by hypertonia and hyperreflexia, bowel malrotation, megacolon, joint contractures, short stature (deletion 5p15.2)
Diastrophic dysplasia	Short stature, short limbs, skeletal dysplasia, cartilage calcification, kyphoscoliosis, cervical spine subluxation (autosomal recessive)
Distal arthrogryposis	Multiple joint contractures, clubfoot (autosomal dominant)
Dubowitz syndrome	Small stature, mental retardation, ptosis, short palpebral fissures, anal anomalies, eczema, sparse hair, immune deficiency, increased frequency of malignancy (autosomal recessive)
Femoral hypoplasia-unusual facies syndrome	Absent or hypoplastic femurs, polysyndactyly, absent labia majora in females, spine anomalies, rib anomalies (autosomal dominant)
Fetal alcohol syndrome	Low birth weight, small stature, mental retardation, heart anomalies, microcephaly, small eyes, minor limb anomalies
Freeman-Sheldon syndrome	Joint contractures, ulnar deviation of the fingers, "puckered" appearance of mouth, keel-shaped forehead, short stature (autosomal dominant)
Kniest syndrome	Myopia, macrocephaly, platyspondyly, joint enlargement and limitation, lordosis, atlantooccipital instability (autosomal dominant)
Lenz syndrome	Microphthalmia, strabismus, nystagmus, microcornea, microcephaly, mental retardation, hypoplastic clavicles, lordosis, kyphosis, narrow, sloping shoulders, genital anomalies, anal anomalies, renal anomalies (X-linked recessive)
Marden-Walker syndrome	Hypertelorism, facial paresis or hypotonia, mental retardation, cerebellar hypoplasia, kyphoscoliosis, ptosis, small eyes, microcystic kidneys (autosomal recessive)
Marshall syndrome	Hypertelorism, cutis aplasia, myopia (autosomal dominant)
Myotonic dystrophy (congenital)	Myotonia, progressive muscle wasting, clubfoot, thin ribs, cognitive impairment, eyelid ptosis, facial diplegia, cataracts, lens opacities, hypogonadism, megacolon, constipation, malignant hyperthermia in reponse to anesthesia (autosomal dominant)
Nager syndrome	Hypoplasia or absence of thumbs, radial-ulnar fusion, radial hypoplasia/aplasia, conductive hearing loss, ossicular anomalies, microtia, zygomatic hypoplasia/aplasia (most sporadic, some dominant and recessive families)
Otopalatodigital syndrome, type 1	Conductive hearing loss, short halluces, thickened finger and toe pads, radial head dislocation, mental retardation, hypodontia, small stature (X-linked recessive)

TABLE 19.1. (*continued.*)

Syndrome	Associated Findings
Otopalatodigital syndrome, type 2	Anomalous fingers and toes (probably x-linked)
Pena-Shokeir syndrome	Multiple joint contractures, adrenal hypoplasia, Meckel diverticulum, cryptorchidism, hypospadias, rocker-bottom feet, primary motor neuropathy, pulmonary hypoplasia, heart anomalies (etiologically heterogenous)
Smith-Lemli-Opitz syndrome	Mental retardation, severe hypotonia, infantile irritability, cortical hypoplasia, cerebellar hypoplasia, absence of the corpus callosum, hydrocephalus, small stature, microglossia, microcephaly, square, high forehead, short nose with anteverted nostrils, micropenis, ambiguous genitalia, cryptorchidism, kidney anomalies, hydronephrosis, heart anomalies, including tetralogy of Fallot or ventriculoseptal defect, pulmonary hypoplasia, pyloric stenosis, polydactyly, finger contractures, hip dislocation, decreased serum cholesterol (autosomal recessive)
Spondyloepiphyseal dysplasia congenita	Short stature (short trunk variety), micrognathia, cleft palate, flat midface, myopia, retinal detachment, flattened vertebrae, short neck, cervical spine subluxation, odontoid hypoplasia, kyphoscoliosis, lumbar lordosis, pectus excavatum or carinatum (autosomal dominant)
Stickler syndrome	Myopia, retinal detachment, epiphyseal dysplasia, joint laxity, flat midface, depressed nasal root (autosomal dominant)
Treacher Collins syndrome	Severe micrognathia, conductive hearing loss secondary to ossicular anomalies, microtia, zygomatic cleft or aplasia, skeletal malar clefts, airway obstruction, absent eyelashes on the inner third of the lower lid, projection of hair onto the cheeks (autosomal dominant)
Turner syndrome	Short stature, gonadal aplasia, kidney anomalies, low-set posteriorly rotated ears, prominent ears, low posterior hairline, broad chest resulting in wide-spaced nipples, scoliosis, skeletal dysplasia, cubitus valgus, spoon-shaped nails, short fourth metatarsal and metacarpal, multiple pigmented nevi, tendency to form keloid scars, webbing of the neck (pterygium coli), aortic valve anomalies, coarctation of the aorta, absence of secondary sexual characteristics, diabetes mellitus, thyroid disorders, strabismus, ptosis (X chromosome monosomy)
Velocardiofacial syndrome	Conotruncal heart anomalies, immune disorders, developmental delay, hypotonia, kidney anomalies, hernias, minor auricular anomalies, prominent nose, seizures, vascular anomalies, hypospadias, learning disabilities, attention deficit/hyperactivity, eventual psychiatric disorders, hypocalcemia (deletion 22q11.2)

Syndromes that have Robin sequence as a frequent secondary manifestation are listed in italics. Potentially, any syndrome that has micrognathia or retrognathia as a clinical feature, or even macroglossia [as in Beckwith-Wiedemann syndrome (Chapter 4)], may yield a number of cases of Robin sequence, but this list of syndromes accounts for the majority of syndromic associations.

MANIFESTATIONS AND MANAGEMENT

Growth and Feeding

Evidence of respiratory difficulty may not necessarily be present immediately, and often the first manifestations that cause concern relate to feeding. Babies with Robin sequence may have marginal airways that permit sufficient respiration to sustain life, but there is difficulty maintaining the airway while feeding. Failure to thrive becomes evident in the neonatal period and is marked by struggling during feeding, inability to nurse, long feeding periods with irritability, and exhaustion during and after feeding. Aspiration during feeding is not common but may be a concern in children who are persistently creating negative pressure in the upper airway during feeding.

Failure to thrive and long-term feeding problems occur in well over 50% of babies with Robin sequence (personal experience). Many clinicians recommend observing respiration and color as an indicator of early difficulty. However, because the respiratory problems in infants with Robin sequence are obstructive in nature, it may appear that respiration is normal because the baby is making effort to breathe even if he or she is not exchanging air. In my experience, cyanosis is not particularly common in babies with Robin sequence, and using a change in color as an indicator of difficulty is not definitive.

Evaluation

- Respiratory sounds should be assessed at the nose, mouth, neck, and chest by stethoscope during feeding and at rest. Noises consistent with obstruction or constriction should be noted along with the pattern of respiration during feeding. The association of obstructive respiratory sounds in association with feeding is often a clear indication of the primary reason for failure to thrive and increased effort on the part of the baby to maintain an airway during feeding.

- Fiber optic endoscopic examination of swallowing (FEES) is a relatively new procedure that can be very helpful in assessing pharyngeal, palatal, lingual, and laryngeal movements during feeding and swallowing. Patterns of airway obstruction can be observed (Sher et al., 1986), as well as evidence of aspiration or penetration of fluids or foods into the glottis.

- Clinical examination during nursing should also include assessment of the movement of the chest, neck, and back for evidence of substernal, suprasternal, or intercostal retractions.

Treatment

- Failure to thrive is often misinterpreted as being caused by a swallowing or feeding problem; in some institutions it is routinely treated by gastrostomy. This is rarely necessary in Robin sequence, unless the primary cause of the sequence (i.e., an underlying syndrome) has neurological or structural problems that contribute to feeding disorders, such as a tracheoesophageal fistula or severe neurologic impairment.

- In the overwhelming majority of cases, resolution of the airway problem (see also below) results in resolution of the feeding problem.

Development and Behavior

Cognitive and motor development are normal in isolated Robin sequence but may be abnormal depending on the underlying syndromic diagnosis. Chronic hypoxia may also cause developmental abnormalities.

Evaluation

- Because impairment of developmental skills will depend on the underlying disorder and on acquired hypoxic damage, developmental milestone achievement should be closely monitored by the physician at regular office visits.

- Significant developmental delay should result in detailed developmental assessment.
- Other evaluation depends on the underlying cause.

Treatment

- Treatment depends on the underlying cause and is generally no different than would be expected in a child with developmental delay of other cause.

Respiratory

Robin sequence is typically evident at birth or shortly after because of the potentially life-threatening effects of upper airway obstruction. A deep pectus excavatum is commonly seen with each inspiration and may be accompanied by suprasternal and intercostal retractions. The apneic events that are frequent in neonates with Robin sequence are typically silent because the neonatal lung capacity cannot create the high negative pressures that would prompt loud noises or snoring. However, stridor and stertor are often detected during feeding. Cyanosis is not common but may occur, especially if Robin sequence is a secondary manifestation of a syndrome with associated heart anomalies, such as velocardiofacial syndrome or fetal alcohol syndrome. Initially, babies with Robin sequence who are struggling to breathe actually appear pink, if not brighter red, even though their oxygen saturation is falling. The struggle to breathe usually induces tachypnea and tachycardia, which cause the baby to appear a brighter red than normal.

Although glossoptosis associated with micrognathia is typically suspected to be the cause of airway obstruction and apnea, there are other types of upper airway obstruction that occur in Robin sequence (Sher et al., 1986). In cases in which the pharynx is hypotonic, as in velocardiofacial syndrome, upper airway collapse may be related to the absence of adequate muscle tone to maintain a patent airway when any degree of negative pressure is induced. Laryngeal anomalies such as laryngomalacia, laryngeal cleft, or laryngeal web may be features of syndromes associated with Robin sequence. Tracheomalacia may be found on occasion in Stickler syndrome and other connective tissue dysplasias. In some syndromes associated with Robin sequence, there is also choanal stenosis or atresia, although choanal atresia would be unusual in cases in which the cleft extends to the hard palate.

The prognosis for the resolution of breathing disorders, as for feeding problems, is excellent unless the underlying syndromic diagnosis involves anomalies that would predict a negative outcome. In isolated deformational Robin sequence, the prognosis is far better because there is no intrinsic anomaly of the mandible, and normal growth after birth would be expected.

Complications of continuing obstructive airway disorders include sudden death, failure to thrive, a persistent deformation of the sternum resulting in a permanent pectus excavatum, decreased pulmonary function, and the potential for the long-term cognitive effects of chronic hypoxia. In a retrospective study, it was reported that a number of children diagnosed with Robin sequence at a major medical center succumbed to sudden death, sometimes later in childhood, presumably from airway obstruction or an acute apneic episode (Sadewitz and Shprintzen, 1986). Thus the early management of the airway problem is critical. Sudden death is probably unusual in Robin sequence (personal experience).

Evaluation

- Monitoring by pulse oximetry is important initially to document drops in oxygen saturation. The use of "apnea monitors," meaning thoraco-abdominal devices that monitor breath effort (i.e., chest movements) and heart rate will not adequately detect the type of respiratory problem experienced by most children with Robin sequence, because they are designed to detect lack of effort. Pulse oximetry responds more rapidly to the primary effect of obstructive apnea.

- Flexible fiber optic nasopharyngoscopy can be used to identify the exact mechanism of upper airway obstruction (Sher et al., 1986; Shprintzen and Singer, 1992).

- The tongue must be examined to determine whether the sublingual frenulum is too short. Micrognathia is often accompanied by a short attachment of the genioglossus muscle that does not allow the tongue to move forward (Argamaso, 1992). Because the tongue is limited from moving forward, it is more likely to drop posteriorly, obstructing the airway.

- If the baby with Robin sequence survives the neonatal period without treatment, then the clinician should be concerned about chronic storage of carbon dioxide, which may not be adequately assessed by standard blood gas workups or pulse oximetry. It is therefore recommended that serum bicarbonate be assessed to rule out chronic elevation of bicarbonate. Elevated serum bicarbonate can be found in the presence of normal oxygen levels and therefore must be assessed separately.

Treatment

- Treatment is primarily dependent on the severity of airway obstruction, which can be quite variable in Robin sequence. The more severe the airway obstruction, the more urgent the treatment must be, although severity does not necessarily predict the type of treatment.

- Clinicians often initially rely on positioning to relieve upper airway obstruction, frequently placing babies on their bellies in an attempt to allow gravity to draw the mandible forward. This mechanism of treatment fails frequently, and

it presents some danger relative to detecting the extent of the problem. When the baby is in a prone position, the chest cannot be easily seen during respiration and substernal retractions cannot be easily visualized. Because babies with airway obstruction are typically silent, the clinician may be misled into believing that respiration is proceeding comfortably. Monitoring with pulse oximetry may help to avoid this type of circumstance.

- In rare cases of marginal obstruction, positioning may assist the neonate during quiet respiration. With age and growth, the infant may learn to protect the airway adequately, but this approach should be utilized with caution and should be accompanied by frequent checks for acidosis.

- Placement of a nasogastric tube for early feeding is often sufficient to stent the tongue forward and the airway open, thus allowing the baby to breathe and gain weight by gavage feeding for several days or a week. In some cases, the gavage tube can be withdrawn and the baby nippled if the obstruction is not too severe. However, if airway obstruction persists, some other form of management is necessary.

- Another temporary treatment that has been shown to be effective is the placement of a nasopharyngeal tube (Sher et al., 1986; Shprintzen and Singer, 1992). An endotracheal tube can be cut short and gradually passed through the nostril until breath sounds are heard through the tube or misting is seen in the tube. The tube can then be taped securely, which allows the baby to breathe comfortably through the nose while stenting the tongue forward. In these circumstances, feeding is best accomplished by gavage. The tube may be left in place for a week or two, allowing additional growth and maturation of the infant, and then can be withdrawn to see whether the baby can protect the airway.

- Surgical management of upper airway obstruction falls into three categories: tracheotomy, glossopexy, and mandibular distraction.

- Glossopexy is a procedure designed to draw the tongue forward and attach it to an anterior structure so that it will not drop posteriorly in the airway. Many different types of glossopexy procedures have been suggested, but it is generally agreed that the original lip-tongue fusions first described over 40 years ago (often referred to as a Beverly Douglas procedure) are not effective because attachment of the tongue is to the lower lip only. This cannot anchor the tongue forward sufficiently because the lip itself is mobile. These procedures often dehisce because of the constant movement of the lip and tongue. In addition, it has been found that the genioglossus attachment of the tongue in the floor of the mandible is often short, preventing sufficient advancement of the tongue to open the airway. Therefore, the recommended procedure for glossopexy is that described by Argamaso (1992). This procedure involves undermining the base of the tongue to free up the genioglossus attachment, which advances the tongue. The tongue is then attached to the anterior mandible with a buried circum-mandibular suture as well as to the lower lip. The success rate with this procedure has been shown to be excellent in cases in which glossoptosis could be documented endoscopically. However, this procedure would not be expected to have a positive outcome if the mechanism of airway obstruction is not related to glossoptosis (Sher et al., 1986).

- Mandibular distraction is a new approach to airway problems that has a great deal of hypothetical appeal, but there are not sufficient objective data to demonstrate its effectiveness. Mandibular distraction involves a surgical incision in the mandible followed by the application of traction to the bone, which stimulates new bone growth in the areas of bone incised, so that the advancement of the mandible and resolution of micrognathia is based on intrinsic development of new bone tissue. Until recently, the devices used to apply traction were external to the face and involved indwelling pins in the mandible. New devices are being developed that will perform the same function internally (surgically implanted on the mandible), but there is little experience with the technique as yet, and there is no scientific study of the effects on airway development.

- Tracheotomy should not be necessary in the majority of Robin sequence cases unless more conservative treatments have not proven successful or unless there is good endoscopic evidence that the airway cannot be protected by any other means. In some syndromes associated with Robin sequence, the airway is so small that there is no other option, as in some cases of Treacher Collins syndrome, Nager syndrome, or cerebrocostomandibular syndrome. Assessment using flexible fiber optic endoscopy is critical in making this decision.

- Tracheotomy should be used as a last resort because, when implemented in the neonatal period, it is difficult to decanulate the child early. Presence of a tracheotomy is a major obstacle to early speech development depending on the ability to use prostheses and valves (such as the Blom-Singer valve).

Craniofacial

When the ramus is short, the body of the mandible often undergoes secondary growth changes with age. A vertical mandibular growth pattern is a common secondary effect of ramus hypoplasia and results in a facial configuration known as "long face syndrome" because of the increased length of the lower third of the face. This pattern of growth becomes evident in childhood as more teeth erupt, and the mandibular growth pattern becomes pronounced with the 6-year growth spurt. An anterior skeletal open bite is often the long-term outcome.

Normal mandibular growth, often referred to as "catch-up growth," is not typical for Robin sequence unless it is secondary to mechanical constraint (deformation sequence). Once the mechanical constraint is removed (at birth), the mandible should achieve normal size and shape within the first 2 years of life. In syndromes that have intrinsic mandibular anomalies at the root of the

sequence, mandibular growth will remain deficient. However, in some syndromes, such as Stickler syndrome, the maxilla is also hypoplastic so that with time, the mandible and maxilla become proportionate.

The cleft palate typically associated with Robin sequence is a wide, U-shaped cleft (Fig. 19.2). However, many clinicians apply the diagnosis of Robin sequence if the cleft is of the more typical V shape or even when only micrognathia and airway obstruction are present (Sadewitz and Shprintzen, 1986). This stretching of diagnostic criteria is actually inconsequential in most instances because the diagnosis of Robin sequence is etiologically nonspecific. Clefts in Stickler syndrome may be overt, submucous, wide U-shaped, or narrow V-shaped. The only instances in which the shape of the cleft may

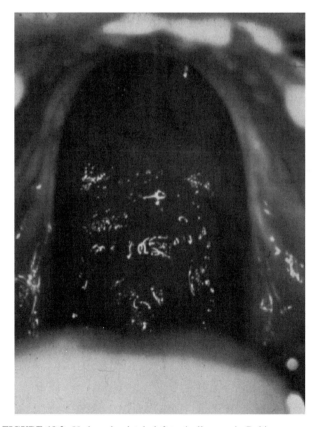

FIGURE 19.2. U-shaped palatal cleft typically seen in Robin sequence.

be of some importance is in cases of isolated Robin sequence that are suspected to be related to positional deformation. In such cases, the presence of the U-shaped cleft does not imply a genetic contribution to clefting and the recurrence risk for cleft palate would be extremely low.

Evaluation

- Identification of the underlying cause of the micrognathia is invaluable in deciding whether or not to intervene, and if so, how.
- Cephalometric radiographs are indicated because the mandibular measurements can be compared to well-established norms for height of the ramus, length of the body, and angulation of growth. Cranial base angle also becomes evident in a cephalogram. Abnormal cranial base angles have been noted in Stickler syndrome, Treacher Collins syndrome, and velocardiofacial syndrome (Shprintzen, 1982).
- Nasopharyngoscopy should be performed to assess pharyngeal morphology, function (including during speech), and the potential for airway obstruction.
- Orthodontic assessment should be initiated early in life (4 years of age or sooner) to obtain baseline records related to mandibular and facial growth.

Treatment

- Treatment options include mandibular distraction, which is discussed above (see **Respiratory**).
- Orthognathic surgery to align the jaws is an option in teen years. Early costochondral grafts may be indicated in cases of severe micrognathia if distraction is not possible.
- Orthodontic treatment is not typically initiated until the early mixed dentition stage (7 or 8 years of age).

Ears and Hearing

Because cleft palate is one of the triad of findings in Robin sequence, middle ear disease is likely to be more common among those with Robin sequence than in the general population. However, chronic middle ear disease is also a component of many of the syndromes that result in the Robin triad, including velocardiofacial syndrome, fetal alcohol syndrome, Smith-Lemli-Opitz syndrome, and others. Middle ear malformations giving rise to conductive hearing loss are common in Treacher Collins syndrome, Nager syndrome, and otopalatodigital syndrome, types 1 and 2. Sensorineural hearing loss is commonly found in Stickler syndrome and velocardiofacial syndrome, among others. Therefore, the presence of hearing loss caused by anything other than middle ear effusion should raise the question of the presence of an associated syndrome.

Evaluation

- In the presence of cleft palate, hearing should be assessed at diagnosis and at least annually thereafter, depending on the frequency of otitis media.
- Tympanic membranes should be examined at each physician encounter and at least twice annually in the first 3 years.

Treatment

- Otitis media should aggressively treated be with antibiotics.
- Hearing aids may be of benefit in some cases.

RESOURCES

Pierre Robin Network *http://www.pierre robin.org/*. This web site also has links to other internet listings.

American Cleft Palate-Craniofacial Association (ACPA). *http://www.cleft.com/*.

REFERENCES

Argamaso RV (1992) Glossopexy for upper airway obstruction in Robin sequence. *Cleft Palate-Craniofac J* 29:232–238.

Arvystas M, Shprintzen RJ (1984) Craniofacial morphology in the velo-cardio-facial syndrome. *J Craniofac Genet Dev Biol* 4:39–45.

Cohen MM Jr (1976) The Robin anomalad: Its nonspecificity and associated syndromes. *J Oral Surg* 34:587–598.

Gorlin RJ, Cohen MM Jr, Levin LS (1990) *Syndromes of the Head and Neck.* New York: Oxford University Press, p. 700–7075.

Herrmann J, Opitz JM (1975) The Stickler syndrome (hereditary arthroophthalmopathy). *Birth Defects Orig Artic Ser* 11:76–103.

Randall P, Krogman WM, Jahina S (1965) Pierre Robin and the syndrome that bears his name. *Cleft Palate J* 2:237–244.

Robin P (1923) La chute de la base de la langue considérée comme une nouvelle cause de gene dans la respiration naso-pharyngienne. *Bull Acad Natl Med (Paris)* 89:37–41.

Robin P (1934) Glossoptosis due to atresia and hypotrophy of the mandible. *Am J Dis Child* 48:541–547.

Sadewitz VL, Shprintzen RJ (1986) *Pierre Robin: A new look at an old disorder.* White Plains, NY: March of Dimes Birth Defects Foundation (Videotape).

Sher AE, Shprintzen RJ, Thorpy MJ (1986) Endoscopic observations of obstructive sleep apnea in children with anomalous upper airways: Predictive and therapeutic value. *Int J Pediatr Otorhinolaryngol* 11: 135–146.

Shprintzen RJ (1982) Palatal and pharyngeal anomalies in craniofacial syndromes. *Birth Defects Orig Artic Ser* 18:53–78.

Shprintzen RJ (1988) Pierre Robin, micrognathia, and airway obstruction: The dependency of treatment on accurate diagnosis. *Int Anesthesiol Clin* 26:64–71.

Shprintzen RJ (1992) The implications of the diagnosis of Robin sequence. *Cleft Palate-Craniofac J* 29:205–209.

Shprintzen RJ, Siegel-Sadewitz VL, Amato J, Goldberg RB (1985) Anomalies associated with cleft lip, cleft palate, or both. *Am J Med Genet* 20:585–596.

Shprintzen RJ, Singer L (1992) Upper airway obstruction and the Robin sequence. *Int Anesthesiol Clin* 30:109–114.

CHAPTER 20

RUSSELL-SILVER SYNDROME

HOWARD M. SAAL

INTRODUCTION

Russell-Silver syndrome is a genetically heterogeneous condition characterized by primordial growth failure, normal head circumference, triangular face, variable degrees of body asymmetry, fifth finger clinodactyly, and normal intelligence (Saal et al., 1985). This condition was independently described by Silver et al. (1953), who reported two patients, and Russell (1954), who reported five individuals with the disorder. It is important to note that of Russell's five patients, only two had body asymmetry and all had disproportionate shortening of the upper limbs, reinforcing the variable nature of this condition.

Incidence

This diagnosis has been made in children with intrauterine growth retardation caused by various etiologies, and therefore, the number of described clinical features found in the literature has been greatly expanded. This adds to confusion with regard to the true incidence and natural history of the Russell-Silver syndrome as well as to how this information may be used in counseling individual families regarding anticipatory management and recurrence risk. It is probably of greatest benefit to identify this condition as a phenotype, reserving the diagnosis of Russell-Silver syndrome for patients with all classical features. Because of the genetic heterogeneity of Russell-Silver syndrome, the true prevalence of this condition is not known.

Diagnostic Criteria

Minimal diagnostic criteria should include intrauterine growth retardation (birth weight <3 standard deviations below the mean), postnatal growth retardation, normal head circumference, triangular face, fifth finger clinodactyly, and normal psychomotor development (Saal et al., 1985) (Figs. 20.1 and 20.2). Many other features can also be identified but are not diagnostic (Table 20.1). These include limb length asymmetry (involving upper extremities, lower extremities, or both), arm span less than height (in the presence of a normal upper-to-lower segment ratio), hypogenitalism or cryptorchidism in males, and hypotonia. Because the head circumference is normal but the face may be small, there is a triangular appearance to the face with a broad-appearing forehead and a small, pointed chin. The mouth tends to be wide with downturned corners.

Micrognathia can occur, rarely causing Pierre Robin sequence (Escobar et al., 1978)

Management of Genetic Syndromes, Edited by Suzanne B. Cassidy and Judith E. Allanson
ISBN 0-471-31286-X   Copyright © 2001 by Wiley-Liss, Inc.

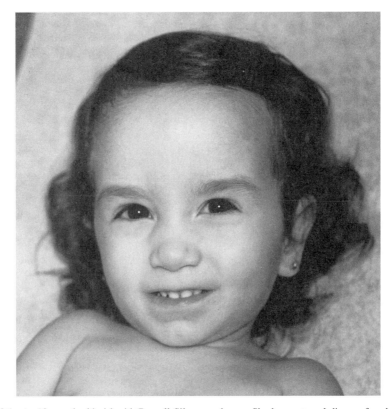

FIGURE 20.1. An 18-month-old girl with Russell-Silver syndrome. She has maternal disomy for chromosome 7.

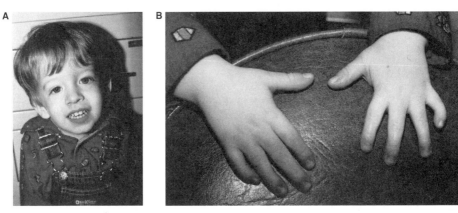

FIGURE 20.2. A: A $2\frac{1}{2}$-year-old boy with Russell-Silver syndrome. B: Fifth finger clinodactyly in this boy with Russell-Silver syndrome.

(see Chapter 19).Therefore, respiratory status, especially with respect to upper airway obstruction, should be evaluated carefully in all children with Russell-Silver syndrome.

Limb asymmetry is very common and can be variable (Tanner et al., 1975).

Approximately 60% of patients with Russell-Silver syndrome will have limb length asymmetry (Patton, 1988).There appears to be no asymmetry of other body parts.The limb length asymmetry may be progressive, but in most patients the asymmetry remains

TABLE 20.1. Clinical Signs and Symptoms of Russell-Silver Syndrome

---

Major (Diagnostic) Signs

Intrauterine growth retardation
Proportionate short stature
Normal head circumference
Triangular face
Fifth finger clinodactyly

Minor (Supportive) Criteria

Short arm span
Limb length asymmetry
Cryptorchidism
Hypotonia
Normal intelligence

---

proportionate with growth. One other significant finding pertinent to limb length is that of short upper extremities. This finding was reported by Silver et al. (1953) in his original five cases. This appears to be a frequently overlooked clinical feature and may be a valuable clue to the diagnosis of Russell-Silver syndrome. There is no similar shortening of lower extremities. Fifth finger clinodactyly is a constant feature of Russell-Silver syndrome (Fig. 20.2*B*). This is a minor anomaly and not specific to or diagnostic of this disorder. Brachydactyly of the fifth finger is also commonly seen. Other significant digital anomalies are not encountered.

Etiology, Pathogenesis, and Genetics

Russell-Silver syndrome is a genetically heterogeneous condition, as evidenced by the numerous reports of familial cases and associated chromosome aberrations. Most cases are sporadic, and the cause of the Russell-Silver syndrome is usually not known in these individuals. Many may represent new mutations for what is possibly an autosomal dominant gene. Some families with apparent autosomal dominant inheritance have been reported (Escobar et al., 1978; Duncan et al.,

1990). Several affected sib pairs with normal parents have been described in the literature, suggesting autosomal recessive inheritance (Escobar et al., 1978; Teebi, 1992).

There have been reported cases of monozygotic twins discordant for Russell-Silver syndrome, although it is difficult to explain the mechanism of discordance unless postzygotic somatic mutation is identified. (Bailey et al., 1995; Sagot et al., 1996). Russell-Silver syndrome, however, may be a reasonable explanation for discordant size in some cases of dizygotic twins (Leppig, 1991).

Numerous reports of individuals with the Russell-Silver phenotype associated with chromosome anomalies are found throughout the literature (Saal et al., 1985). Early cases include deletion of the short arm of chromosome 18, mosaic Turner syndrome, and trisomy 18 mosaicism (Tulinius et al., 1972; Chauvel et al., 1975; Christensen and Nielsen, 1978). It is arguable whether these patients actually had Russell-Silver syndrome. A case of Russell-Silver syndrome associated with an interstitial deletion of the Y chromosome in a male twin raises the issue of whether Yq deletions actually can cause Russell-Silver syndrome, especially because many affected males have hypogonadism (Leppig et al., 1991).

Recent discoveries have led to greater understanding of the heterogeneity of the causes of Russell-Silver syndrome. The initial breakthrough case was that of a girl with Russell-Silver syndrome who had a paternally derived balanced chromosome translocation between the long arms of chromosomes 17 and 20, 46,XX,t(17;20)(q25;q13) pat (Ramirez-Duenas et al., 1992). A second case involving a balanced chromosome translocation between chromosomes 1 and 17 with a breakpoint at 17q25.3 was a boy with Russell-Silver syndrome reported by Midro et al., (1993). These two cases support the possibility that a gene for autosomal dominant Russell-Silver syndrome may map to the long arm of chromosome 17 at band 17q25.

More intriguing are the cases of Russell-Silver syndrome associated with maternal disomy for chromosome 7; that is, both members of the pair of chromosomes 7 are of maternal origin with no chromosome 7 contribution from the father. The remaining 22 chromosome pairs reflect equal maternal and paternal contributions. Uniparental disomy can only be identified by testing for microsatellite chromosome markers, which are very heterogeneous variations of the DNA (see **Introduction**). Maternal disomy was first identified in two patients who were homozygous for a cystic fibrosis mutation for which their mother was heterozygous, but their father was normal. Three relatively large studies of Russell-Silver syndrome, looking for uniparental disomy, identified 11 of 114 patients with this chromosome finding, suggesting that this mechanism accounts for approximately 10% of all cases of Russell-Silver syndrome (Kotzot et al., 1995; Eggermann et al., 1997; Price et al., 1999). The presence of uniparental disomy suggests that a mechanism called genetic imprinting may play a role in the pathogenesis of Russell-Silver syndrome in some patients. Imprinting refers to the differential expression of a gene or genes depending on whether the gene was inherited from the mother or the father. If such a gene can be found on chromosome 7, for which paternal contribution is necessary for normal growth, then it may be possible to develop a simple molecular test to evaluate all patients with suspected Russell-Silver syndrome. A great deal of research is directed at finding candidate gene(s) on chromosome 7 that may play major roles in the pathogenesis of Russell-Silver syndrome.

Although numerous other chromosome anomalies have been reported as being associated with Russell-Silver syndrome, it must be emphasized that most of the individuals with these chromosome anomalies do not have Russell-Silver syndrome but rather have a chromosome disorder with clinical

TABLE 20.2. Diagnostic Evaluation of Russell-Silver Syndrome

Thorough pregnancy history
    Teratogenic exposures
    Intrauterine infections
    History of maternal hypertension
Family history
    Parental and sibling heights
    Parental and sibling birth weights
Placental pathology
Examination of parents and siblings (with
   growth parameters)
Chromosome studies
Special studies for maternal disomy of
   chromosome 7
Skeletal radiograph survey
Growth hormone studies

features that overlap those of Russell-Silver syndrome.

Diagnostic Testing

Because the specific cause of Russell-Silver syndrome is unknown, the diagnosis rests on finding the characteristic pattern of clinical findings. However, it is appropriate to conduct molecular studies of microsatellite markers on chromosome 7 to seek uniparental disomy 7. This test is available in some clinical laboratories. Other diagnostic studies are performed to exclude other genetic conditions with overlapping features (Table 20.2).

Differential Diagnosis

The differential diagnosis of Russell-Silver syndrome should include any condition that can cause intrauterine growth retardation and short stature.This includes many chromosome disorders. This is especially true of patients with a deletion of distal chromosome 15 (15q26.1–qter), which results in deletion of the insulin-like growth factor I receptor gene. The clinical features of patients with deletions of chromosome 15 generally differ from those of Russell-Silver syndrome by the presence of microcephaly, the lack of a triangular face, and the presence of mental retardation. Asymmetry is rarely seen. Studies seeking a deletion of the insulin-like growth factor receptor gene in patients diagnosed with Russell-Silver syndrome found none to be deleted for this gene (Rogan et al., 1996; Abu-Amero et al., 1997). The chromosome breakage syndromes, including Bloom syndrome, Fanconi anemia, and Nijmegen immunodeficiency syndrome, share physical features with Russell-Silver syndrome. Although these patients may have normal psychomotor development, they tend to have microcephaly, which should lead to the exclusion of Russell-Silver syndrome. Additionally, efforts should be made to rule out chromosomal mosaicism, because diploid/triploid mixoploidy and 45,X/46,XX Turner syndrome mosaicism can be confused with Russell-Silver syndrome, especially because asymmetry may be seen in patients with chromosome mosaicism (Graham et al., 1981).

Children with fetal alcohol syndrome (see Chapter 9) generally present with intrauterine growth deficiency. They often have a somewhat similar appearance with triangular face, small chin, and fifth finger clinodactyly. What distinguishes fetal alcohol syndrome from Russell-Silver syndrome is the frequent presence of microcephaly, developmental disabilities, and other additional minor anomalies, including short palpebral fissures, long hypoplastic philtrum, thin upper lip, and nail hypoplasia.

There is an entity called X-linked short stature with skin pigmentation. These patients have many features in common with Russell-Silver syndrome, and this condition may be difficult to distinguish from Russell-Silver syndrome in the absence of a positive family history of affected males (Partington, 1986).

The 3-M syndrome may be confused with the Russell-Silver syndrome. Individuals with this autosomal recessive condition have intrauterine growth retardation but lack the triangular face of Russell-Silver syndrome. patients with the 3-M syndrome also have numerous skeletal changes on radiograph, and tend to be shorter than those with Russell-Silver syndrome (Feldmann et al., 1989). Patients with short upper and lower limbs should be evaluated for a skeletal dysplasia.

Some patients with pituitary disorders will present with a Russell-Silver phenotype, but these patients generally do not have the minor anomalies of classical Russell-Silver syndrome and frequently have normal birth size.

It may also be important to compare the child's growth to that of parents and siblings, to rule out familial short stature.

MANIFESTATIONS AND MANAGEMENT

Growth and Feeding

Intrauterine growth retardation is an essential feature for the diagnosis. Growth retardation is often not evident until the third trimester. In most cases, the birth weight is more than 3 standard deviations below the mean for gestational age. The diagnosis becomes more challenging in the face of premature birth, because not all features can be readily identified. Most cases of Russell-Silver syndrome, however, are delivered at term. The birth length is also proportionally diminished but may not exactly parallel the low birth weight, because most infants with Russell-Silver syndrome appear to have diminished subcutaneous fat. The head circumference is normal at birth. Some infants have demonstrated feeding difficulties, but most feed normally.

Although, by definition, all individuals with this disorder are small at birth and remain small up to adulthood, most patients with Russell-Silver syndrome will demonstrate a normal growth velocity. If growth is followed over a long period of time, the growth curve of a child with Russell-Silver syndrome should parallel the normal growth curve (Tanner et al., 1975). There have been rare instances of growth hormone deficiency in Russell-Silver syndrome, but these cases are exceptions rather than the rule (Cassidy et al., 1986).

Catch-up growth is not expected to occur in Russell-Silver syndrome; however, some patients suspected of having this disorder have been observed to demonstrate catch-up growth. This may indicate difficulties with the diagnostic criteria for Russell-Silver syndrome, given the "soft" features for diagnosis. In one study, 5 of 15 patients with Russell-Silver syndrome and intrauterine growth retardation showed catch-up growth between 4 and 8 years of age, with heights ranging from the 5th to the 40th centile. None of the patients had received any growth-enhancing medications (Saal et al., 1985). No clinical signs were helpful to determine which patients were most likely to demonstrate catch-up growth. In the same study, 10 of the 15 patients had heights 3 or more standard deviations below the mean.

Because the head is of normal size, it appears disproportionately large compared with the rest of the body. This appearance has been termed "pseudohydrocephaly" (Szalay, 1973). However, the head growth is normal in children with Russell-Silver syndrome, and true hydrocephalus is an exceptional event and probably indicates a disorder other than Russell-Silver syndrome.

Evaluation

- Gestational causes of growth interference, especially placental insufficiency, should be excluded by careful pathological examination. The prenatal history should also be directed at identifying maternal factors that contribute to intrauterine growth retardation, including maternal hypertension, insulin-dependent diabetes, maternal infections, and teratogen exposure, especially cigarettes and alcohol.
- It is essential to obtain a family history, and this should include growth data of parents, siblings, and other pertinent relatives. If available, birth weights of parents and siblings should be recorded.
- The physical examination should emphasize documentation of weight, length, and head circumference. Skeletal examination should include documentation of span, limb lengths, upper-to-lower segment ratio, and presence of fifth finger clinodactyly. It may be necessary to examine parents and siblings for signs of Russell-Silver syndrome or other possible causes of short stature.
- Laboratory evaluation should be directed at exclusion of other causes of intrauterine growth retardation and short stature. This should include routine chromosome studies and evaluation for maternal disomy of chromosome 7 (available at selected genetics centers). Chromosome breakage studies may be warranted to rule out a chromosome breakage syndrome associated with short stature such as Bloom syndrome, Fanconi anemia, or Nijmegen chromosome breakage syndrome.
- Abnormal growth velocity deserves further testing for all possible causes of growth failure, including renal disease, growth hormone deficiency, hypothyroidism, and skeletal dysplasia.

Treatment

- Those few patients with documented growth hormone deficiency require growth hormone to achieve normal growth velocities.
- The studies of growth hormone supplementation for children with Russell-Silver syndrome without growth hormone deficiency have yielded conflicting results. A positive short-term response to growth hormone is seen for most patients with Russell-Silver syndrome. However, one European study of a limited number of patients has shown that growth hormone treatment

can induce sustained catch-up growth in children with intrauterine growth retardation, including those with Russell-Silver syndrome (Albanese and Stanhope, 1997). A larger collaborative study done in the United States showed that there may be little increase in predicted adult height despite treatment with growth hormone in children with intrauterine growth retardation (Chernausek et al., 1996). At this time, the use of growth hormone to treat short stature in Russell-Silver syndrome remains controversial, especially in the presence of normal growth velocity and normal growth hormone levels. Additional long-term studies must be completed before the role of growth hormone in treatment of short stature in Russell-Silver syndrome is ultimately defined.

Development and Behavior

The IQ is normal in most individuals with Russell-Silver syndrome. If a child does have mental retardation, other causes should be explored, especially chromosome anomalies. There is frequent early gross motor delay, most likely related to the small birth size, mild hypotonia, and relatively large head seen in infants. Although no systematic study of psychomotor development exists, anecdotal data indicate a higher incidence of learning disabilities in older children. One study of 20 children with Russell-Silver syndrome between the ages of 6 and 12 years showed that most had some degree of developmental delay. The average IQ in this group was 86. Additionally, 32% of these patients scored within the learning disability range, with 36% of subjects requiring special education and 48% speech therapy (Lai et al., 1994).

Evaluation

- The child with Russell-Silver syndrome should be evaluated for gross motor, fine motor, and speech and language abilities using standard developmental screening tools.
- Older children may need comprehensive educational evaluations for learning disabilities, especially those related to speech and language difficulties.

Treatment

- Early developmental problems related to hypotonia should be managed with early intervention and physical therapy. Seldom will long-term intervention be necessary.
- When learning disabilites are encountered, appropriate educational evaluations with appropriate delivery of therapeutic services are indicated.
- Occasionally, psychological counseling is necessary for the child with Russell-Silver syndrome to help deal with peer relationships and body self-image issues.

Craniofacial

Dental anomalies are relatively common and include microdontia (Cullen and Wesley, 1987).

Micrognathia is common and can cause cleft palate secondary to the Robin sequence (see Chapter 19). These patients must be closely monitored for feeding difficulties and upper airway obstruction. In addition to micrognathia, most patients have narrow, arched palates, which are likely to cause dental crowding and increased overjet.

Evaluation

- Affected individuals should begin evaluation relatively early in childhood with a pediatric dentist.
- Evaluation and management by an orthodontist is needed in many patients who have significant dental crowding and micrognathia.
- Some patients will need evaluation by a multidisciplinary craniofacial team.

Treatment

- Occasionally, dental extraction will be necessary if crowding cannot be otherwise managed.
- The narrow palate often requires orthodontic expansion of the dental arch.

Musculoskeletal

Orthopedic complications, with the exception of limb length asymmetry, are rare. Two males have been reported with aseptic necrosis of the hip that responded to conservative management, and one patient had slipped capital femoral epiphysis (Limbird, 1989; Hotokebuchi et al., 1994).

Evaluation

- Patients should be carefully measured for possible limb length discrepancies of greater than 1 cm.
- Those individuals with limb length asymmetry should be evaluated by a pediatric orthopedist.
- Full skeletal X-ray studies should be performed for patients with suspected skeletal dysplasia.
- Bone age X rays (left hand and wrist) should be performed as indicated to follow skeletal maturity.

Treatment

- The management of asymmetry and growth deficiency is complicated and depends on severity and interference with normal function. If asymmetry is recognized in childhood, evaluation by an orthopedist is indicated. Asymmetry of the lower extremities requires active intervention generally when the difference in leg length is greater than 4 cm.
- During growth in childhood, leg length discrepancy is best managed by placing a lift in the shoe of the shorter extremity.

- When growth has ceased, equality of limb length can be achieved surgically, with a bone-lengthening procedure called bone distraction. This is a generally safe and effective approach to limb length discrepancy.
- Another approach to managing limb length discrepancy is to interrupt the growth of the longer limb by ablating the growth plate during adolescence, a procedure known as epiphysiodesis.

Genitourinary

Genitourinary anomalies can be seen in males with Russell-Silver syndrome. Cryptorchidism and hypospadias are most common (Weiss and Garnick, 1981; Patton, 1988).

Occasional renal anomalies have been reported including hydronephrosis, renal tubular acidosis, posterior urethral valves, and a single case of horseshoe kidney (Arai et al., 1988; Ortiz et al., 1991).

Most individuals with Russell-Silver syndrome will have normal secondary sexual development and puberty.

Evaluation

- Genitourinary examination should document testicular descent and penile size.
- When hypogonadism or micropenis are seen, an evaluation for other conditions, such as chromosome anomalies or hypopituitarism, should be pursued.
- Renal function studies, including a renal ultrasound, should be performed as part of the evaluation of short stature if other causes of growth disturbance are considered.

Treatment

- Treatment of cryptorchidism is straightforward. If the testis has not descended into the scrotum by age 1 year, orchiopexy is indicated. Untreated cryptorchidism increases the risk for gonadoblastoma, as would be the case for any child with an intra-abdominal testis.

- The occasional renal anomalies should be treated as in any other individual.

Neoplasia

Malignancies are rare in Russell-Silver syndrome and are probably not related to the primary condition. There has been a single report of a child with Russell-Silver syndrome and hepatocellular carcinoma (Chitayat et al., 1988). There is another report of a patient with a craniopharyngioma (Draznin et al., 1980). Testicular cancer can occur if cryptorchidism remains untreated. This complication is not specific for Russell-Silver syndrome.

Despite the limb length asymmetry in many patients, there does not appear to be an increased risk for developing intra-abdominal or retroperitoneal tumors, as is the case in overgrowth syndromes and hemi-hyperplasia, because the pathophysiology of overgrowth and asymmetry appears to be different in these syndromes. Therefore, it is not necessary to screen patients with Russell-Silver syndrome for these tumors.

Evaluation

- No specific routine evaluation for tumors is indicated.

Treatment

- Treatment for tumors should be targeted to the specific tumor type. There is no specific treatment regimen for patients with Russell-Silver syndrome.

RESOURCES

Association for Children with Russell-Silver Syndrome, Inc.
22 Hoyt St.
Madison, NJ 07940
Phone: (201) 377-4531

Fax: (201) 822-2715
This is a comprehensive support organization.

Russell-Silver Support Group (MAGIC Foundation)
1327 N. Harlem Ave.
Oak Park, IL 60302
Phone: (313) 586-8038
(800) 3-MAGIC-3
E-mail: *slantana@awol.com*
Web site: *http://www.nettap.com/~magic/*

National Organization for Rare Disorders, Inc. (NORD)
P.O. Box 8923
New Fairfield, CT 06812-8923
Phone: (203) 746-6518
(800) 999-6673
Fax: (203) 746-6481
TDD: (203) 746-6927
E-mail: *orphan@nord-rdb.com*

Little People of America, Inc.
P.O. Box 745
Lubbock, TX 79408

REFERENCES

Abu-Amero S, Price S, Wakeling E, Stanier P, Trembath R, Preece MA, Moore GE (1997) Lack of hemizygosity for the insulin-like growth factor 1 receptor gene in a quantitative study of 33 Silver-Russell syndrome probands and their families. *Eur J Hum Genet* 5:235–241.

Albanese A, Stanhope R (1997) GH treatment induces sustained catch-up growth in children with intrauterine growth retardation: 7-year results. *Horm Res* 48:173–177.

Arai Y, Wakabayashi Y, Pak K, Tomoyoshi T (1998) Horseshoe kidney in Russell-Silver syndrome. *Urology* 31:321–323.

Bailey W, Popovich B, Jones KL (1995) Monozygotic twins discordant for the Russell-Silver syndrome. *Am J Med Genet* 58:101–105.

Cassidy SB, Blonder O, Courtney VW, Ratzan SK, Carey DE (1986) Russell-Silver syndrome and hypopituitarism. Patient report and literature review. *Am J Dis Child* 140:155–159.

Chauvel PJ, Moore CM, Haslam RHA (1975) Trisomy-18 mosaicism with features of Russell-Silver syndrome. *Dev Med Child Neurol* 17:220–224.

Chernausek SD, Breen TJ, Frank GR (1996) Linear growth in response to growth hormone treatment in children with short stature associated with intrauterine growth retardation: The National Cooperative Growth Study experience. *J Pediatr* 128:S22–S27.

Chitayat D, Friedman JM, Anderson L, Dimmick JE (1988) Hepatocellular carcinoma in a child with familial Russell-Silver syndrome. *Am J Med Genet* 31:909–914.

Christensen MF, Nielsen J (1978) Deletion short arm 18 and Silver-Russell syndrome. *Acta Paediatr Scand* 67:101–103.

Cullen CL, Wesley RK (1987) Russell-Silver syndrome: Microdontia and other pertinent oral findings. *ASDC J Dent Child* 54:201–204.

Draznin MB, Stelling MN, Johnson AJ (1980) Silver-Russell syndrome and craniopharyngioma. *J Pediatr* 96:887–889.

Duncan PA, Hall JG, Shapiro LR, Vibert BK (1990) Three-generation dominant transmission of the Silver-Russell syndrome. *Am J Med Genet* 35:245–250.

Eggermann T, Wollmann HA, Kuner R, Eggermann K, Enders H, Kaiser P, Ranke MB (1997) 37 Silver-Russell syndrome patients: Frequency and etiology of uniparental disomy. *Hum Genet* 100:415–419.

Escobar V, Gleiser S, Weaver DD (1978) Phenotypic and genetic analysis of the Silver-Russell syndrome. *Clin Genet* 13:278–288.

Feldmann M, Gilgenkrantz S, Parisot S, Zarini G, Marchal C (1989) 3M dwarfism: A study of two further sibs. *J Med Genet* 26:583–585.

Graham JM, Hoehn H, Lin MS, Smith DW (1981) Diploid-triploid mixoploidy: Clinical and cytogenetic aspects. *Pediatrics* 68:23–28.

Hotokebuchi T, Miyahara T, Sugioka Y (1994) Legg-Calve-Perthes' disease in the Russell-Silver syndrome. A report of two cases and a review of the literature. *Int Orthopaed* 18:32–37.

Kotzot D, Schmitt S, Bernasconi F, Robinson WP, Lurie IW, Ilyina H, Mehes K, Hamel BC, Ottern BJ, Hergersberg M (1995) Uniparental disomy 7 in Silver-Russell syndrome and primordial growth retardation. *Hum Mol Genet* 4:583–587.

Lai KY, Skuse D, Stanhope R, Hindmarsh P (1994) Cognitive abilities associated with the Silver-Russell syndrome. *Arch Dis Child* 71:490–496.

Leppig KA, Saal HM, Simpson E, Disteche CM (1991) Distal deletion of Yq in a patient with phenotype of Russell-Silver syndrome. *Am J Med Genet* 49:301.

Limbird TJ (1989) Slipped capital femoral epiphysis associated with Russell-Silver syndrome. *Southern Med J* 82:902–904.

Midro AT, Devek K, Sawicka A, Marcinkiewicz D, Rogowska M (1993) Second observation of Silver-Russell syndrome in a carrier of a reciprocal translocation with one breakpoint at site 17q25. *Clin Genet* 44:53–55.

Ortiz C, Cleveland RH, Jaramillo D, Blickman JG, Crawfore J (1991) Urethral valves in Russell-Silver syndrome. *J Pediatr* 119:776–778.

Partington MW (1986) X-linked short stature with skin pigmentation: Evidence for heterogeneity of the Russell-Silver syndrome. *Clin Genet* 29:151–156.

Patton MA (1988) Russell-Silver syndrome. *J Med Genet* 25:557–560.

Price SM, Stanhope R, Garrett C, Preece MA, Trembath RC (1999) The spectrum of Silver-Russell syndrome: A clinical and molecular genetic study and new diagnostic criteria. *J Med Genet* 36:837–842.

Ramirez-Duenas ML, Medina C, Ocampo-Campos R, Rivera H (1992) Severe Silver-Russell syndrome and translocation (17;20)(q25;q13). *Clin Genet* 41:51–53.

Rogan PK, Seip JR, Driscoll DJ, Papenhausen P, Johnson P, Raskin S, Woodward AL, Butler MG (1996) Distinct 15q genotypes in Russell-Silver and ring 15 syndromes. *Am J Med Genet* 62:10–15.

Russell A (1954) Syndrome of "intra-uterine" dwarfism recognizable at birth with craniofacial dysostosis, disproportionately short arms, and other anomalies. *Proc R Soc Med* 47:1040–1044.

Saal HM, Pagon RA, Pepin MG (1985) Reevaluation of Russell-Silver syndrome. *J Pediatr* 107:733–737.

Sagot P, David A, Talmant C, Pascal O, Winer N, Boog G (1996) Russell-Silver syndrome: An explanation for discordant growth in monozygotic twins. *Fetal Diagn Ther* 11: 72–78.

Silver HK, Kiyasu W, George J, Deamer WC (1953) Syndrome of congenital hemihypertrophy, shortness of stature, and elevated urinary gonadotrophins. *Pediatrics* 12:368–375.

Szalay GC (1973) Definition of the Russell-Silver syndrome. *Pediatrics* 52:309–310.

Tanner JM, Lejarrage H, Cameron N (1975) The natural history of the Silver-Russell syndrome: A longitudinal study of thirty-nine cases. *Pediatr Res* 9:611–623.

Teebi AS (1992) Autosomal recessive Silver-Russell syndrome. *Clin Dysmorphol* 1:151–156.

Tulinius H, Tryggvason K, Hauksdottir H (1972) 45,X-46,XY chromosome mosaic with features of the Russell-Silver syndrome: A case report with a review of the literature. *Dev Med Child Neurol* 14:161–172.

Weiss GR, Garnick MB (1981) Testicular cancer in a Russell-Silver dwarf. *J Urology* 126:836–837.

CHAPTER 21

SMITH-LEMLI-OPITZ SYNDROME

CHRISTOPHER CUNNIFF

INTRODUCTION

Incidence

Smith-Lemli-Opitz syndrome was first described in 3 boys with a characteristic pattern of malformation including growth deficiency, developmental delay, ptosis, downslanting palpebral fissures, and hypospadias (Smith et al., 1964). Since that time over 250 cases have been described, and the phenotypic spectrum of the disorder has become well delineated. For almost 30 years after the initial patients were described, the cause of Smith-Lemli-Opitz syndrome was unknown. However, in 1993 Irons et al. found low cholesterol and elevated 7-dehydrocholesterol (7DHC) levels in their patients with Smith-Lemli-Opitz syndrome. Subsequent studies have shown conclusively that Smith-Lemli-Opitz syndrome is caused by deficiency of the enzyme 7-dehydrocholesterol reductase (7DHCR), the final step of the cholesterol biogenesis pathway.

From birth defects surveillance data in British Columbia, Lowry and Yong (1980) estimated an incidence of 1 in 40,000 (Lowry and Yong, 1980). Ryan et al., (1998) used data from biochemically confirmed cases in the United Kingdom to derive a minimum incidence of 1 in 60,000 and a carrier frequency of 1 in 122 (0.8%). Smith-Lemli-Opitz syndrome appears to be more common in people of European background and has been seen rarely in those of African or Asian descent. There is an excess of males diagnosed with Smith-Lemli-Opitz syndrome. The skewed sex distribution represents a bias of ascertainment as a result of the hypogenitalism seen in boys.

Although the phenotype is highly variable, there is generally concordance within a sibship. Although there are a number of good clinical reviews of the spectrum of phenotypic findings, the most reliable information can be found in recent publications of biochemically confirmed cases (Tint et al., 1995; Cunniff et al., 1997; Ryan et al., 1998).

Diagnostic Criteria

No standard diagnostic criteria have been formulated for Smith-Lemli-Opitz syndrome. The diagnosis is usually made based on the recognition of a constellation of characteristic clinical features, with diagnostic confirmation by measurement of elevated 7DHC in plasma or other tissues. The cardinal features of Smith-Lemli-Opitz syndrome are prenatal-onset growth deficiency, developmental delay, characteristic facial features, cleft palate,

Management of Genetic Syndromes, Edited by Suzanne B. Cassidy and Judith E. Allanson
ISBN 0-471-31286-X   Copyright © 2001 by Wiley-Liss, Inc.

cardiac defects, hypospadias, polydactyly, and 2-3 toe syndactyly. Almost all affected individuals have developmental delay or mental retardation. Cutaneous syndactyly of the second and third toes appears to be the most consistent structural anomaly, present in over 90% of biochemically confirmed cases (Fig. 21.1).

The facial appearance is characterized by narrow bifrontal diameter, ptosis, down-slanting palpebral fissures, and a short nose with depressed nasal bridge with anteverted nares (Fig. 21.2). The ears are frequently low set and posteriorly rotated. There is often retrognathia. These features change with age and are often difficult to discern in adulthood (Ryan et al., 1998). Early photographs may be helpful diagnostically. In the evaluation of adults it is necessary to have a high index of suspicion and initiate laboratory evaluation.

Etiology, Pathogenesis, and Genetics

Smith-Lemli-Opitz syndrome is inherited as an autosomal recessive trait with widely variable expression. Because it is an autosomal recessive condition, the recurrence risk for parents who have one affected child is 25%.

The etiology of Smith-Lemli-Opitz syndrome is deficiency of the enzyme 7DHCR, the final enzymatic step in the Kandutsch-Russell pathway of cholesterol biogenesis. It is now known that the gene encoding 7DHCR is located at chromosome position 11q12-13 and is named *DHCR7*. Mutations in *DHCR7* have recently been reported in 19 patients (Fitzky et al., 1998; Wassif et al., 1998; Waterham et al., 1998). Nineteen different mutations have been characterized, including 13 missense mutations, 5 frame-shift mutations, and 1 nonsense mutation. Two individuals with a severe presentation were found to be homozygous for a 134-base pair insertion that is believed to result in a completely nonfunctional enzyme. Milder presentations have been seen in individuals with mutations that result in some residual enzymatic activity. Most mutations have been located in or near one of the 9 putative transmembrane segments of the protein.

The pathogenetic mechanism leading to the manifestations in affected individuals appears to be a deficiency of cholesterol (Cunniff et al., 1997), although some data suggest that excess 7DHC may also play a role (Ryan et al., 1998). It is unclear what the relative contributions of these two abnormalities are in producing all the phenotypic features encountered in patients with

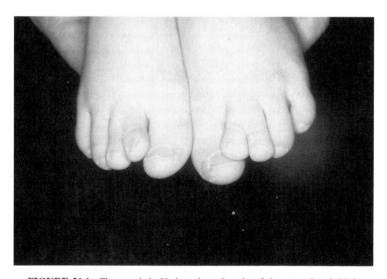

FIGURE 21.1. Characteristic Y-shaped syndactyly of the second and third.

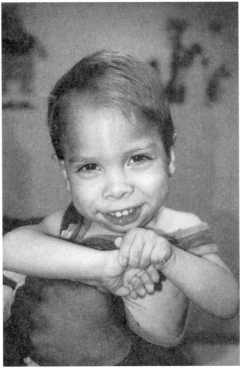

FIGURE 21.2. Two year-old boy with frontal hair upsweep, telecanthus, anteverted nares, smooth-appearing philtrum, and a postaxial scar on the left hand from removal of a supernumerary digit.

Smith-Lemli-Opitz syndrome. Some studies have suggested an inverse correlation between cholesterol level and severity (Tint et al., 1995; Cunniff et al., 1997), especially among patients under age 2 years. However, Ryan et al., (1998) found a weak correlation between severity and 7DHC level and no correlation between cholesterol and severity for 19 patients from the United Kingdom.

Whether the primary pathogenetic mechanism is a decrease in cholesterol or an increase in 7DHC, it is clear that derangements of sterol quantity and/or type are the major factors responsible for the clinical abnormalities in individuals with Smith-Lemli-Opitz syndrome. Because cholesterol and related compounds such as 7DHC are critical components of myelin and other central nervous system proteins, the altered sterol profile in Smith-Lemli-Opitz syndrome is associated with abnormal intellectual and motor function. The identification of patients with Smith-Lemli-Opitz syndrome and holoprosencephaly has led to the implication of Sonic hedgehog, a signaling protein, and Patched, a putative Sonic hedgehog receptor, in the co-occurrence of these two abnormalities (Kelley, 1998). Sonic hedgehog (*shh*) is known to cause holoprosencephaly in humans, and the Sonic hedgehog protein product undergoes autoproteolysis to form a cholesterol-modified active product. Because cholesterol is an important precursor of the sex steroids testosterone and estrogen, hypocholesterolemia results in deficiency of these hormones. Both prenatal and postnatal testosterone levels are decreased, leading to undervirilization of genotypic males, and underproduction of estrogen results in low maternal serum estriol levels detected prenatally in some pregnancies (Rossiter et al., 1995). The pathogenesis of other features such as polydactyly and cleft palate is less obvious but may be the result of abnormal cell-to-cell interactions that result from derangement of sterol composition in the cell membranes of the developing embryo. The positive growth response seen in children treated with dietary cholesterol suggests that growth deficiency is at least partly a result of hypocholesterolemia.

Diagnostic Testing

Definitive diagnosis of Smith-Lemli-Opitz syndrome is by the detection of increased 7DHC levels in blood or other tissues. Although cholesterol is usually decreased, about 10% of patients have levels in the normal range, especially those with mild disease (Cunniff et al., 1997). Prenatal diagnosis is by measurement of elevated 7DHC in amniotic fluid or chorionic villi (Abuelo et al., 1995). Reliable heterozygote detection by measurement of 7DHC or cholesterol is not feasible because the population distribution of cholesterol and 7DHC levels does not allow for a clear distinction between heterozygotes and homozygous normal individuals in the general population. Although heterozygotes have higher mean 7DHC levels than normal controls, the range of values between heterozygotes and controls overlaps considerably, making measurement of 7DHC an unsuitable test for heterozygote detection. With the discovery of *DHCR7*, it is hoped that mutation analysis will assist in heterozygote identification, especially for relatives of affected individuals.

Differential Diagnosis

Because the cardinal features of Smith-Lemli-Opitz syndrome include developmental delay, growth deficiency, cleft palate, polydactyly, and hypogenitalism, it must be distinguished from other disorders with one or more of these features. There are a number of chromosome anomaly syndromes with features that overlap those seen in Smith-Lemli-Opitz syndrome. Growth deficiency, cleft palate, and developmental delay occur frequently in individuals with trisomy 18; and growth deficiency, polydactyly, and developmental delay are seen in those with trisomy 13. Severe hypogenitalism has been described in children with deletion of chromosomal material from the long arm of chromosome 10 (Wulfsberg et al., 1989). Chromosome analysis will readily distinguish between Smith-Lemli-Opitz syndrome and these chromosome anomaly syndromes.

The differential diagnosis of Smith-Lemli-Opitz syndrome should include a number of single-gene disorders. Children with Noonan syndrome, an autosomal dominant condition, frequently have short stature, developmental disabilities, cardiac defects, and cryptorchidism (see Chapter 15). The differences in facial appearance, the pattern of cardiac defects and the presence or absence of polydactyly and toe syndactyly will usually allow the clinician to make a distinction between individuals with Noonan syndrome and those with Smith-Lemli-Opitz syndrome. Polydactyly is a feature of many malformation syndromes such as Simpson-Golabi-Behmel syndrome, Pallister-Hall syndrome, and Meckel syndrome. Individuals with Simpson-Golabi-Behmel syndrome, an X-linked recessive condition, have macrosomia, macroglossia, accessory nipples, and other features not encountered in children with Smith-Lemli-Opitz syndrome. Pallister-Hall syndrome is a variable autosomal dominant disorder with hypothalamic hamartoblastoma in addition to polydactyly. Abnormal facial features, syndactyly, and genital abnormalities are usually not present. Meckel syndrome is an almost uniformly lethal autosomal recessive disorder associated with encephalocele and cystic renal disease in addition to polydactyly and sometimes hypogenitalism.

Before to the availability of biochemical testing for Smith-Lemli-Opitz syndrome, a group of patients with a severe phenotype including XY sex reversal and early lethality was described (Curry et al., 1987). It is now known that these children, who were considered to have Smith-Lemli-Opitz syndrome syndrome type II, actually represent the severely affected end of the biochemical and phenotypic spectrum of children with Smith-Lemli-Opitz syndrome (Cunniff et al., 1997).

MANIFESTATIONS AND MANAGEMENT

Growth and Feeding

As described in the original patients reported by Smith, Lemli, and Opitz, most individuals with Smith-Lemli-Opitz syndrome have height and weight below the 3rd centile. Neonates with Smith-Lemli-Opitz syndrome usually have normal length and weight but gradually decelerate in their linear growth and weight gain so that they are below the 3rd centile by age 6 months. In the report of Ryan et al., (1998), 21 of 24 (88%) of their living patients were considered to have failure to thrive. Although weight gain may improve in infancy and childhood, final adult stature is usually below the 3rd centile.

Most patients have feeding difficulty in infancy (Ryan et al., 1998). At least part of this difficulty may relate to hypotonia, with a poor suck, listlessness, and disinterest in feeding. Nasogastric or orogastric feedings are frequently necessary. Vomiting and gastroesophageal reflux are also prominent features, and the reflux is often refractory to medical management. The feeding problems tend to improve with age. However, fundoplication was required in 8 of 24 patients discussed by Ryan et al., (1998). In assessing children with Smith-Lemli-Opitz syndrome and poor feeding, it should be recognized that some patients will have gastrointestinal complications that should be considered in any plan for dietary treatment and monitoring. Pyloric stenosis, Hirschsprung disease, malrotation, and cholestatic liver disease have all

been seen with some frequency and should be evaluated and treated when signs and symptoms point to one of these conditions.

Because Smith-Lemli-Opitz syndrome results from defective cholesterol synthesis, the focus of treatment has been dietary (Elias et al., 1997; Irons et al., 1997; Nwokoro and Mulvihill, 1997), with the goal of providing supplementary cholesterol to improve, or even normalize, plasma cholesterol levels. A total of 20 patients have been reported on to date, with the length of dietary treatment ranging between 8 and 27 months (Irons et al., 1997; Nwokoro and Mulvihill, 1997). Cholesterol supplementation in most patients consisted of a commercial preparation of pure cholesterol dissolved in soybean oil, with a concentration of 200 mg/ml. The cholesterol dose varied between 40 and 120 mg/kg/day, with most patients taking about 100–125 mg/kg/day by the end of the study period. Initially, these patients also received chenodeoxycholic and ursodeoxycholic acid therapy to replace the abnormal bile acids produced as a result of deranged sterol metabolism and to aid in cholesterol absorption. However, because plasma cholesterol levels and the percent of total sterols present as cholesterol were not appreciably different between patients who were and were not receiving bile acid replacement, it was discontinued. All patients are now maintained on cholesterol supplements alone. Although there was initially concern that altered bile acid metabolism would lead to malabsorption of vitamins and minerals, it appears that patients with Smith-Lemli-Opitz syndrome do not have a deficiency of fat-soluble vitamins. Improvement in weight gain, an increase in plasma cholesterol levels, and an increase in cholesterol as a percentage of total sterols have been seen in almost all patients on this regimen. However, other clinical benefits have been more difficult to quantitate. There is evidence from parental report and unblinded investigator observation that the number of infectious illnesses is decreased, feeding tolerance is enhanced, behavior is improved, rashes and photosensitivity are diminished, and patients are less irritable and more manageable. It should be emphasized that these latter findings are very difficult to document in an objective manner and will require randomization to determine conclusively. There is a suggestion that neurodevelopmental progress is enhanced in the treatment group, but there are few data to determine conclusively that there is a developmental benefit of cholesterol supplementation. Alternatively, it should also be noted that no untoward side effects of dietary treatment have been seen by any investigators.

In addition to postnatal treatment with dietary cholesterol, prenatal treatment has also been attempted in at least one case (Abuelo et al., 1995). During a pregnancy with an affected fetus, increased maternal consumption of cholesterol was encouraged. Cholesterol levels remained below the lower limit of the 95% confidence interval for normal controls throughout the pregnancy. There was no discernible advantage detected in the neonate at birth. It is unclear to what degree cholesterol crosses the placenta during gestation, especially during the critical first trimester when organogenesis occurs. It is therefore difficult to judge whether prenatal treatment from conception might decrease the number or severity of malformations seen. The degree to which cholesterol, especially maternally ingested cholesterol, crosses the blood-brain barrier is also not known, further complicating the assessment of prenatal treatment of Smith-Lemli-Opitz syndrome to prevent related developmental disabilities.

Although it is expected that most individuals with Smith-Lemli-Opitz syndrome will have short stature, it may be possible to achieve normal weight for height with appropriate caloric intake, either orally or through gavage feedings. The feeding difficulty, poor suck, and irritability that are seen in infants gradually improve with age. Cholesterol supplementation appears to improve growth but has not been shown conclusively to affect other parameters such as irritability and poor suck.

Gastroesophageal reflux may not respond to medical management and may require surgical intervention in the form of fundoplication. Because reflux tends to improve with age, a course of aggressive medical management should precede the decision to intervene surgically.

Evaluation

- Height, weight, and head circumference should be measured at initial evaluation and during health supervision visits. Because most individuals with Smith-Lemli-Opitz syndrome will have linear growth deficiency, it is important to consider weight for height in addition to charting absolute centile measurements for these parameters.

- For children who are unable to take adequate calories orally, a feeding evaluation should be undertaken. This should include an assessment of parent abilities and responses, oral motor skills of the infant, the number of calories being consumed, and any signs of gastroesophageal reflux

- When gastroesophageal reflux is suspected, consideration should be given to a full diagnostic evaluation. There are no recommendations that evaluation of gastroesophageal reflux in individuals with Smith-Lemli-Opitz syndrome should be conducted differently than such reflux evaluation in other children, especially those with developmental disabilities.

Treatment

- Adequate caloric intake should be ensured.

- Consideration should be given to cholesterol supplementation to improve weight gain. Provision of 40–120 mg/kg/day of cholesterol has been shown to improve weight gain in treated patients.

- Oral-motor training with an occupational therapist or feeding specialist may assist the patient in taking all feedings orally.
- For those who are unable to consume adequate calories orally, nasogastric, orogastric, or gastrostomy tube feedings should be considered.
- Appropriate positioning, low-volume and frequent feedings, and antireflux medications should be considered in treating gastroesophageal reflux.
- For patients who are refractory to medical management, fundoplication may be the only viable treatment alternative.

Development and Behavior

Almost all children with Smith-Lemli-Opitz syndrome are mentally retarded, most commonly in the moderately to severely retarded range of functioning. The range of intellectual outcomes is great, however, with some patients functioning in the normal or near-normal range, especially in infancy and early childhood. In general, children with more severe malformations have a more severe intellectual prognosis, but strict correlation is not possible.

There is only one systematic evaluation of the behavioral phenotype in Smith-Lemli-Opitz syndrome (Ryan et al., 1998). Questionnaires were completed by the parents of 23 living children and adults aged 6 months and older. Sleep disturbance was particularly common (70%). Although children were often sleepy and hypotonic in early infancy, they had long periods of wakefulness in early childhood, sometimes requiring no more than 2-3 hours of sleep per 24-hour period. Most were difficult to settle and had frequent and early awakening that was refractory to treatment with sedatives. Sleep patterns tended to normalize by school age.

Other commonly reported behavioral characteristics were aggressive (52%) and self-injurious (35%) behavior. Ritualistic or obsessive behaviors were seen in 52% of patients. Many children were reported to be inappropriately affectionate with strangers.

Evaluation

- Developmental screening should be performed at health supervision visits. A variety of methods might be adopted for screening, including such tools as the Parent Development Questionnaire, the Denver Developmental Screening Test, or other objective measures as appropriate.
- Because of the frequency of behavioral abnormalities, it is suggested that these be inquired about specifically. Particular attention may be given to the behavioral disturbances discussed above, especially in regard to sleep and aggressive or self-injurious behavior.

Treatment

- Children and adults with Smith-Lemli-Opitz syndrome should have the opportunity to enroll in early intervention programs, special education programs, and other systems of care that enhance their developmental potential. Specific developmental or educational strategies have not been examined systematically for patients with Smith-Lemli-Opitz syndrome. It is presumed that programs geared to the developmental and behavioral concerns of the individual are most likely to be beneficial. Instruction in a special education classroom setting is common.
- Adults will usually require some type of supervised care setting such as a group home.
- As noted in the section on **Growth and Feeding**, there are reports of improved development and behavior in children and adults receiving cholesterol supplementation. Because the number of patients studied is few and the subjectivity of most of the measures is high, these reports should be viewed with cautious optimism.

- Behavioral strategies for treatment of persons with Smith-Lemli-Opitz syndrome have not been examined systematically. For treatment of abnormal sleep patterns, general strategies such as scheduled bedtimes, positive routines, and good sleep hygiene can be recommended. Cautious medication trials may be warranted for particularly refractory cases.

- For aggressive or self-injurious individuals, behavioral strategies such as redirection, time-out, and positive rewards may be helpful, but again it should be noted that there are no specific studies of these strategies in children with Smith-Lemli-Opitz syndrome.

Neurologic

A variety of develomental abnormalities of the brain have been seen in individuals with Smith-Lemli-Opitz syndrome. Six of 28 patients (21%) who had neuroimaging studies in the series of Ryan et al., (1998) had some type of brain malformation. These included 2 patients with delayed myelination and one patient each with lissencephaly and agenesis of the corpus callosum, hypoplasia of the corpus callosum, choroidal cyst, and cerebellar hypoplasia. One of the most striking central nervous system findings in individuals with Smith-Lemli-Opitz syndrome is holoprosencephaly, which has now been observed in 7 patients (Kelley, 1998). The pathogenesis of holoprosencephaly in Smith-Lemli-Opitz syndrome is unknown. An embryonic signaling protein known as Sonic hedgehog (Shh), which causes autosomal dominant holoprosencephaly, has been implicated, as has its putative receptor, Patched. Other studies have suggested a role for cholesterol deficiency in the neural plate ectoderm, the precursor tissue for the fetal brain (Kelley, 1998).

The primary disabilities resulting from central nervous system dysfunction in Smith-Lemli-Opitz syndrome are mental retardation and behavioral abnormalities. Seizures are generally not observed.

Evaluation

- Careful neurological evaluation is recommended for all newly diagnosed patients.

- Neuroimaging studies can be reserved for individuals with signs of holoprosencephaly such as hypotelorism or agenesis of the premaxilla or for children with evidence of hypopituitarism such as diabetes insipidus.

Treatment

- The brain abnormalities seen in Smith-Lemli-Opitz syndrome rarely require specific treatment.

- Children with endocrine disturbances resulting from hypopituitarism will need hormonal treatment directed to the specific deficiencies observed.

Craniofacial

Most children with Smith-Lemli-Opitz syndrome are born with microcephaly that persists throughout life. Cleft palate is seen in 37–52% (Cunniff et al., 1997; Ryan et al., 1998) and most commonly affects the soft palate, although there can be cleft of the hard palate, soft palate, or both. The gingivae may be hyperplastic and rugated, and the alveolar ridge is often broad. Tongue hamartomata have been observed in some patients with severe phenotypic features.

Evaluation

- All patients should have a careful physical examination of the palate and other mouth structures for abnormalities.

- Children with cleft palate will need surgical evaluation.

- Attention should also be directed to the infant's ability to take oral feedings, because feeding problems are encountered frequently in patients with

Smith-Lemli-Opitz syndrome, particularly those with cleft palate. Evaluation by a feeding specialist such as an occupational therapist is indicated for children with feeding difficulties.

Treatment

- Cleft palate repair is usually performed at age 12–18 months. The timing, method, or approach to repair has not been addressed specifically in children with Smith-Lemli-Opitz syndrome. The approach to surgical treatment is generally not altered on the basis of the diagnosis of Smith-Lemli-Opitz syndrome.
- As with other at-risk newborns, children with Smith-Lemli-Opitz syndrome and feeding difficulties may benefit from oral-motor training.
- If adequate calories cannot be taken orally, consideration should be given to orogastric, nasogastric, or gastrostomy feedings.

Ophthalmologic

Ptosis is seen in about half of reported patients (Ryan et al., 1998), and cataracts are present in 12–18% (Cunniff et al., 1997; Ryan et al., 1998). Additional ophthalmologic findings include strabismus, retinal hemangiomata, demyelination of the optic nerves, sclerosis of the lateral geniculate bodies, and the lack of a visual following response (Fierro et al., 1977).

There are no outcome studies of visual function in children with Smith-Lemli-Opitz syndrome.

Evaluation

- The ocular examination of children with Smith-Lemli-Opitz syndrome should receive special attention, including assessment as to whether ptosis is obstructing the visual axis.
- Because congenital cataracts may be found, it is important that the red reflex

be elicited in newborns and that there be a clear view of the fundus in older individuals.
- If there is a suggestion of visual compromise from ptosis, congenital cataracts, ocular motility abnormalities, or any other abnormal ophthalmologic signs, referral to an ophthalmologist is recommended.

Treatment

- There is no systematic study of cataract treatment in individuals with Smith-Lemli-Opitz syndrome. Clinical criteria for medical and surgical management should generally be the same as for other children.
- For children with ocular motility abnormalities or ptosis that may impair vision, the treatment plan should be formulated based on a full visual assessment.

Cardiovascular

Congenital heart disease is present in 36–38% of patients with Smith-Lemli-Opitz syndrome (Cunniff et al., 1997; Lin et al., 1997; Ryan et al., 1998). Lin et al., (1997) reported on 215 patients with Smith-Lemli-Opitz syndrome (59 biochemically confirmed cases and 156 from the medical literature). They found a disproportionate number of patients with atrioventricular canal defects and total anomalous pulmonary venous return when compared with an unselected population of children with congenital heart defects. Complex conotruncal anomalies were very uncommon; complex single-ventricle malformations and heterotaxies were not reported. These findings suggest that two of the important pathogenetic mechanisms that produce cardiac malformations in Smith-Lemli-Opitz syndrome are altered extracellular matrix and abnormal targeted cell growth.

Evaluation

- Cardiac evaluation is recommended at the time of diagnosis, with follow-up determined by the severity of any abnormalities identified.
- Evaluation should include ECG with assessment of axis and an echocardiogram with special attention to the atrial and ventricular septa and the pulmonary veins.

Treatment

- Treatment of the cardiovascular malformations in Smith-Lemli-Opitz syndrome is specific to the malformation identified.
- Careful consideration should be given to surgical or other invasive treatment in those children with a poor prognosis in whom medical or other palliative treatment might provide a good short-term outcome.

Gastrointestinal

Gastrointestinal abnormalities have been described in 25% (Cunniff et al., 1997) to 29% (Ryan et al., 1998) of biochemically confirmed cases. A variety of both specific and nonspecific features have been seen. Chronic constipation or diarrhea has also been noted. Pyloric stenosis, malrotation, and Hirschsprung disease have all been described. Of particular note are 5 patients with cholestatic liver disease (Cunniff et al., 1997; Ryan et al., 1998), 2 of whom died. This abnormality is presumed to be the result of abnormal bile acids, although the exact pathogenetic mechanism is unknown. Perhaps cholesterol supplementation could be beneficial by providing appropriate amounts of cholesterol substrate to produce normal bile acids, although results of treatment with this modality have not been reported.

Generally, poor feeding and vomiting without an underlying structural abnormality improve as children become older.

Evaluation

- Liver enzymes and total and direct bilirubin levels should be performed at the time of diagnosis.
- Young infants with persistent projectile vomiting and failure to thrive should be evaluated for pyloric stenosis. In addition to careful physical examination, an ultrasound examination of the pylorus is recommended. Electrolyte analysis may show evidence of hypochloremic alkalosis.
- Individuals with chronic constipation or alternating constipation and diarrhea, especially if associated with other signs of Hirschsprung disease, should have a barium enema and/or small bowel biopsy. Surgical evaluation is also recommended if Hirschsprung disease is suspected.
- Children with evidence of bowel obstruction should have surgical evaluation.

Treatment

- Surgical referral and standard treatment are recommended for infants with evidence of pyloric stenosis, malrotation, or Hirschsprung disease.
- Although there are no data on treatment of cholestasis in Smith-Lemli-Opitz syndrome, a trial of cholesterol supplementation is warranted for children with evidence of cholestatic liver disease (personal experience). This is based on the presumptive pathogenetic mechanism of altered bile acid profile in Smith-Lemli-Opitz syndrome and the potential beneficial effects of increasing plasma cholesterol and increasing the percentage of sterols that are present as cholesterol.
- Long-term gastrostomy placement, with or without fundoplication, is necessary for some with persistent inability to feed orally.

Genitourinary

Joseph et al. (1987) reported on 29 males and 15 females ascertained before the advent of biochemical testing. Evaluation of the upper urinary tract in 21 of their 44 cases and in 31 cases from the literature revealed abnormalities in 31 of these 52 children (60%). There was no difference in the incidence between boys and girls, and there was no correlation between upper tract anomalies and abnormal external genitalia. Reported abnormalities included cystic renal dysplasia (29%), renal positional abnormalities (19%), hydronephrosis (16%), ureteropelvic junction obstruction (13%), renal duplication (13%), and renal agenesis (6%).

Renal defects were reported in 13% (Cunniff et al., 1997) and 29% (Ryan et al., 1998) of biochemically confirmed cases. Abnormalities ranged from lack of fetal lobulation to bilateral renal agenesis. These figures probably represent a minimal estimate because all patients did not undergo renal imaging studies. Long-term studies of renal function are not available for children with Smith-Lemli-Opitz syndrome. Case reports have not generally identified any serious sequelae such as recurrent infections or renal insufficiency.

Genital abnormalities are present in 91% (Ryan et al., 1998) to 100% (Joseph et al., 1987) of affected males. Most commonly there is hypospadias, cryptorchidism, or a combination of the two. However, there is a spectrum of undervirilization seen in boys with Smith-Lemli-Opitz syndrome. Of the 35 males reported in the series of Ryan et al., 8 (23%) had sex reversal and 11 (31%) had what were described as ambiguous genitalia. Genital abnormalities are generally not seen in affected girls, although 2 of 12 girls reported by Joseph et al., (1987) had clitoral enlargement.

The prognosis for boys with genital abnormalities is related to the severity of abnormalities encountered. Repair of hypospadias generally produces a good functional and cosmetic result. Because of the related developmental disabilities in Smith-Lemli-Opitz syndrome, affected individuals have not been known to have sexual relationships, although it is presumed that many have the physical capability, especially affected women.

Evaluation

- Ultrasonography of the urinary tract is recommended at the time of diagnosis.
- On the basis of findings detected on ultrasonography, additional studies may be recommended. For example, children with hydronephrosis identified by ultrasound examination should have a voiding cystourethrogram to assess for vesicoureteral reflux that will require antibiotic prophylaxis and possibly surgical intervention.
- For individuals with an unambiguous female genital appearance, no additional evaluations are suggested.
- For patients who have any degree of genital ambiguity, chromosome analysis is warranted.
- If the karyotype is 46,XY, it is important to evaluate for signs of appropriate virilization: Is the penis of normal size? Are the testes palpable? Is hypospadias present? These will be important factors to consider in decisions about sex of rearing. Careful palpation for testes in the scrotum and in the inguinal areas should be carried out during the initial physical examination. The patient should be in a warm room, and the examiner's hands should also be warmed to facilitate palpation in boys with retractile testes. If the testes are not palpable on initial examination, additional attempts should be made at subsequent health supervision visits.
- Referral to a urologist is recommended for all boys with hypospadias, cryptorchidism, or other genital abnormalities such as micropenis.

Treatment

- Treatment of upper urinary tract anomalies is dependent on the nature of the abnormality identified. Although renal malposition will rarely require any kind of treatment, almost all children with renal duplication will require surgical treatment by a urologist.

- With modern surgical techniques, satisfactory repair of hypospadias can usually be accomplished easily.

- Boys with cryptorchidism should be observed over the first year of life to see whether spontaneous testicular descent will occur. Orchiopexy is recommended for boys with persistent cryptorchidism.

- If penile size is in the normal range, usually defined as a stretched length of 2.5 cm or greater in the newborn, male sex of rearing is appropriate. If the penis is hypoplastic, female sex of rearing may be more appropriate. Boys with micropenis or any significant degree of genital ambiguity should evaluated carefully to determine appropriate sex of rearing. This may best be accomplished by a team approach including a urologist, an endocrinologist, and a geneticist. Strong consideration should be given to female sex of rearing when penile reconstruction is unlikely to produce a functionally adequate penis. Several factors should be considered in decisions regarding sex assignment. First, there is a positive correlation between general clinical severity and the severity of genital abnormalities in boys (Bialer et al., 1987). This means that boys with the most severe genital abnormalities tend to have the poorest prognosis. The benefits of genital surgery should be weighed carefully against the psychological anguish and disruption that parents undergo around the process of gender reassignment. Decisions about genital surgery and gender reassignment should be made in the context of the functional status of the child and the prognosis for long-term survival, developmental outcome, and social awareness.

- Orchidectomy and scrotoplasty are performed for 46,XY individuals who will undergo gender reassignment.

Musculoskeletal

The most commonly reported musculoskeletal abnormality is syndactyly of the second and third toes, present in more than 95% of biochemically confirmed cases (Tint et al., 1995; Cunniff et al., 1997; Ryan et al., 1998). In most cases this syndactyly is distinctive, with what has been termed a "Y shape." The stem of the "Y" is produced by tight cutaneous syndactyly of the toes to the level of the distal interphalangeal joint, and the fork of the "Y" is produced by the distal phalanges. This appearance is not an obligate feature and may not be present in mildly affected patients. It causes no functional abnormalities.

Postaxial polydactyly is present in about half of the patients reported. It appears more commonly on the hands than on the feet and usually is present in the form of a pedunculated postminimus. Abnormally short or proximally placed thumbs are also seen in about half of patients, more commonly in those who are more severely affected. Additional skeletal abnormalities reported include dislocated hips (18%), limb shortening (12%), brachydactyly (20%), ulnar deviation of the fingers (14%), and positional foot deformities (31%) (Ryan et al., 1998).

There are no clinical data regarding the functional outcomes of procedures to correct these abnormalities, and the prognosis must be considered in light of the overall status of the child.

Evaluation

- Routine physical examination should be sufficient to detect musculoskeletal abnormalities in all patients.

- For those with polydactyly, surgical evaluation is recommended.
- Particular attention should be given to examination of the hips. Those with abnormal hip position, limitation of abduction, or a positive Ortolani sign or Barlow test may have hip dysplasia and should be referred for orthopedic evaluation.
- Patients with positional foot abnormalities such as talipes equinovarus or calcaneovalgus should also be referred for orthopedic evaluation.

Treatment

- Simple excision of supernumerary digits can usually be performed easily as a day procedure, although some children with polydactyly of the feet may have a more fully developed extra digit that requires a more complex surgical approach.
- It is presumed that treatment of hip dysplasia will produce a stable hip joint and that treatment of foot deformities will provide appropriate foot positioning.
- There are no data to suggest that treatment of musculoskeletal problems in children with Smith-Lemli-Opitz syndrome should differ from treatment of unaffected children.

Skin

It has been recognized recently that individuals with Smith-Lemli-Opitz syndrome can have a variety of skin manifestations. Most have fair complexion and light hair coloration when compared with their unaffected first-degree relatives (Ryan et al., 1998). Almost all report erythematous reactions to sunlight, so that parents frequently keep their children indoors or otherwise restrict their sun exposure. Eczema is reported in up to 10% of patients. The skin manifestations of Smith-Lemli-Opitz syndrome are generally not serious and can be treated with preventive measures.

Evaluation

- Inspection of the skin should identify any abnormalities requiring treatment.

Treatment

- Dietary cholesterol treatment has been reported to cause a decrease in photosensitivity and skin rashes (Elias et al., 1997; Nwokoro and Mulvihill, 1997). It should be remembered, however, that documentation of this benefit is solely by parent and investigator report.
- Sun photosensitivity reactions can be minimized by limiting the length of exposure, wearing protective clothing, and using sunscreen.
- Exacerbations of eczema may benefit from treatment with topical steroids.

RESOURCES

Smith-Lemli-Opitz Syndrome Advocacy and Exchange

32 Ivy Lane
Glen Mills PA 19342
(610) 361-9663
Contact person: Barbara Hook
email: *bhook@erols.com*
Internet address:
http://members.aol.com/slo97/index.html

REFERENCES

Abuelo DN, Tint GS, Kelley R, Batta AK, Shefer S, Salen G (1995) Prenatal detection of the cholesterol biosynthetic defect in the Smith-Lemli-Opitz syndrome by the analysis of amniotic fluid sterols. *Am J Med Genet* 56:281–285.

Bialer MG, Penchaszadeh VB, Kahn E, Libes R, Krigsman G, Lesser ML (1987) Female external genitalia and müllerian duct derivatives in a 46,XY infant with the Smith-Lemli-Opitz syndrome. *Am J Med Genet* 28:23–31.

Cunniff C, Kratz LE, Moser A, Natowicz MR, Kelley RI (1997) Clinical and biochemical spectrum of patients with RSH/Smith-Lemli-Opitz syndrome and abnormal cholesterol metabolism. *Am J Med Genet* 68:328–337.

Curry CJ, Carey JC, Holland JS, Chopra D, Fineman R, Golabi M, Sherman S, Pagon RA, Allanson J, Shulman S, Barr M, McGravey V, Dabiri C, Schimke N, Ives E, Hall BD (1987) Smith-Lemli-Opitz syndrome-type II: Multiple congenital anomalies with male pseudohermaphroditism and frequent early lethality. *Am J Med Genet* 26:45–57

Elias ER, Irons MB, Hurley AD, Tint GS, Salen G (1997) Clinical effects of cholesterol supplementation in six patients with the Smith-Lemli-Opitz syndrome. *Am J Med Genet* 68:305–310.

Fierro M, Martinez AJ, Harbison JW, Hay SH (1997) Smith-Lemli-Opitz syndrome: Neuropathological and ophthalmological observations. *Dev Med Child Neurol* 19:57–62.

Fitzky BU, Witsch-Baumgartner M, Erdel M, Lee JN, Paik YK, Glossman H, Utermann G, Moebius FF (1998) Mutations in the Δ7-sterol reductase gene in patients with the Smith-Lemli-Opitz syndrome. *Proc Natl Acad Sci USA* 95:8181–8186.

Irons M, Elias ER, Salen G, Tint GS, Batta AK (1993) Defective cholesterol biosynthesis in Smith-Lemli-Opitz syndrome. *Lancet* 341:1414.

Irons M, Elias ER, Abuelo D Bull MJ, Greene CL, Johnson VP, Keppen L, Schanen C, Tint GS, Salen G (1997) Treatment of Smith-Lemli-Opitz syndrome: Results of a multicenter trial. *Am J Med Genet* 68:311–314.

Joseph DB, Uehling DT, Gilbert E, Laxova R (1987) Genitourinary abnormalities associated with the Smith-Lemli-Opitz syndrome. *J Urol* 137:719–721.

Kelley RI (1998) RSH/Smith-Lemli-Opitz syndrome: mutations and metabolic morphogenesis. *Am J Hum Genet* 63:322–326.

Lin AE, Ardinger HH, Ardinger RH Jr, Cunniff C, Kelley RI (1997) Cardiovascular malformations in Smith-Lemli-Opitz syndrome. *Am J Med Genet* 68:270–278.

Lowry RB, Yong SL (1980) Borderline normal intelligence in the Smith-Lemli-Opitz (RSH) syndrome. *Am J Med Genet* 5:137–143.

Nwokoro NA, Mulvihill JJ (1997) Cholesterol and bile acid replacement in children and adults with Smith-Lemli-Opitz (RSH/Smith-Lemli-Opitz syndrome) syndrome. *Am J Med Genet* 68:315–321.

Rossiter JP, Hofman KJ, Kelley RI (1995) Smith-Lemli-Opitz syndrome: Prenatal diagnosis by quantification of cholesterol precursors in amniotic fluid. *Am J Med Genet* 56:272–275.

Ryan AK, Bartlett K, Clayton P, Eaton S, Mills L, Donnai D, Winter RM, Burn J (1998) Smith-Lemli-Opitz syndrome: A variable clinical and biochemical phenotype. *J Med Genet* 35:558–565.

Smith DW, Lemli L, Opitz JM (1964) A newly recognized syndrome of multiple congenital anomalies. *J Pediatr* 64:210–217.

Tint GS, Salen G, Batta AK, Shefer S, Irons M, Elias ER, Abuelo DN, Johnson VP, Lambert M, Lutz R, Schanen C, Morris CA, Hoganson G, Hughes-Benzie R (1995) Correlation of severity and outcome with plasma sterol levels in variants of the Smith-Lemli-Opitz syndrome. *J Pediatr* 127:82–87.

Wassif CA, Maslen C, Kachilele-Linjewile S, Lin D, Linck LM, Connor WE, Steiner RD, Porter FD (1998) Mutations in the human sterol Δ7-reductase gene at 11q12-13 cause Smith-Lemli-Opitz syndrome. *Am J Hum Genet* 63:55–62.

Waterham HR, Wijburg FA, Hennekam RCM, Vreken P, Poll-The BT, Dorland L, Duran M, Jira PE, Smeitink JAM, Wevers RA, Wanders RJA (1998) Smith-Lemli-Opitz syndrome is caused by mutations in the 7-dehydrocholesterol reductase gene. *Am J Hum Genet* 63:329–338.

Wulfsberg EA, Weaver RP, Cunniff CM, Jones MC, Jones KL (1989) Chromosome 10qter deletion syndrome: A review and report of three new cases. *Am J Med Genet* 32:364–367.

CHAPTER 22

SMITH-MAGENIS SYNDROME

ANN C. M. SMITH AND ANDREA GROPMAN

INTRODUCTION

Incidence

Smith-Magenis syndrome, a contiguous gene syndrome caused by an interstitial deletion of chromosome 17p11.2, is a multisystem multiple congenital anomaly/mental retardation syndrome. The deletion was first reported in 1982 (Smith et al., 1982) and the phenotypic spectrum was subsequently more fully delineated in 1986, through tandem articles describing a series of 15 patients with del(17)(p11.2) (Smith et al., 1986; Stratton et al, 1986). More than 150 cases, ranging from 1 month to 72 years of age, have been identified worldwide from a diversity of ethnic groups. In all cases, the 17p11.2 deletion has been associated with a distinct and clinically recognizable complex phenotype now referred to as the Smith-Magenis syndrome. Comprehensive reviews are available delineating the clinical (Greenberg et al., 1991, 1996; Finucane, 1993b; Chen KS et al., 1996; Chen RM et al., 1996, Allanson et al., 1999; Hagerman, 1999) and neurobehavioral (Smith et al., 1998a,b; Dykens et al., 1997; Dykens and Smith, 1998) aspects of Smith-Magenis syndrome.

Smith-Magenis syndrome is probably more common than previously recognized. Greenberg et al. (1991) report a minimum prevalence of Smith-Magenis syndrome of 1 in 25,000 births in Harris County, Texas, over a 2-year period. However, the vast majority of cases have been identified in the last 5 years as a result of improved cytogenetic techniques, suggesting that this is a probable underestimation. The availability of fluorescence *in situ* hybridization (FISH) probes specific for Smith-Magenis syndrome proves beneficial in equivocal cases (Elsea et al., 1997; Juyal et al., 1995a,b). Delayed diagnosis with reportedly normal standard chromosome analysis is not uncommon, especially among older individuals.

Smith-Magenis syndrome does not appear to be associated with reduced lifespan, and reported patient ages range from birth to over 70 years of age (Smith et al., 1986). Deaths have not been reported, with the exception of two reported cases of early demise: one died at 6 months of postcardiogenic shock (Smith et al., 1986), and the other died unexpectedly at 11 months of adrenal aplasia-hypoplasia after perioperative stress following palatoplasty (Denny et al., 1992).

Diagnostic Criteria

The diagnosis of Smith-Magenis syndrome is based on the clinical recognition of a unique and complex phenotypic pattern of physical, developmental, and behavioral features,

Management of Genetic Syndromes, Edited by Suzanne B. Cassidy and Judith E. Allanson
ISBN 0-471-31286-X   Copyright © 2001 by Wiley-Liss, Inc.

with diagnostic confirmation of an interstitial deletion of 17p11.2 cytogenetically and/or by FISH. Many of the features are subtle in early childhood, becoming more distinctive with advancing age. Common features seen in over two-thirds of individuals with Smith-Magenis syndrome include a characteristic craniofacial appearance (Fig. 22.1), ocular abnormalities (85%), speech delay with or without associated hearing loss (96%), short stature with failure to thrive (78%), brachy-dactyly (81%), signs of peripheral neuropathy (pes planus or cavus, depressed deep tendon reflexes, insensitivity to pain) (75%), scoliosis (65%), variable levels of mental retardation (100%); and neurobehavioral problems including sleep disturbance and self-injurious behaviors (Greenberg et al., 1996; Smith et al., 1998a,b; Gropman et al., 1998a). The voice is hoarse and low pitched (82%) and serves as a diagnostic marker of the syndrome. Functional impairment of voice and speech have also been reported (Sonies et al., 1997).

Several distinctive features characterize the infantile phenotype of Smith-Magenis syndrome, including hypotonia (100%), hyporeflexia (84%), generalized lethargy (100%), complacency (100%) with increased sleepiness and napping, oromotor dysfunction (100%), feeding difficulties with failure to thrive, and delayed gross motor and expressive language skills in the presence of relatively appropriate social skills (80%) (Gropman et al., 1998b; Gropman et al., 1999). Although failure to thrive does occur, some infants actually appear "chubby," with redundant fat folds similar to a "Michelin man" (Smith et al., 1998a). Crying is infrequent (95%), and babbling and vocalizations are markedly decreased for age in virtually all infants. Sleep disturbances are evident in infancy, marked by hypersomnolence and lethargy, which is replaced by the frequent nocturnal awakenings and fragmented sleep seen later in childhood. The infant with Smith-Magenis syndrome shares many features with Down syndrome, including

hypotonia, brachycephaly, round face with upslanting eyes, and midface hypoplasia. Chromosome analysis may be initiated for this reason, fortuitously leading to the correct diagnosis.

The facial appearance in Smith-Magenis syndrome is distinctive and changes over time (Fig. 22.1). These changes are described in detail in the **Craniofacial** section below. Briefly, the face is square and broad with mild brachycephaly. The face is "cherubic" with full cheeks, upslanting and deep-set eyes, marked midfacial hypoplasia with depressed broad nasal root, and micrognathia (Smith et al., 1998a). The distinctive shape of the mouth includes a fleshy upper lip and a cupid's bow or tented appearance due to bulky philtral pillars (Allanson et al., 1999). Over time, heavy brows and prognathism develop.

Developmental delay and/or mental retardation are found in all patients and are highly variable. The majority of affected individuals are moderately retarded (Greenberg et al., 1996). A distinct and complex behavioral phenotype is seen in Smith-Magenis syndrome, with several neurobehavioral aspects appearing unique to the syndrome. Unusual maladaptive, self-injurious, and stereotypic behaviors occur in 40–100% of both children and adults with Smith-Magenis syndrome (Smith et al., 1986; Stratton et al., 1986; Colley et al., 1990, de Rijk-van Andel et al., 1991; Greenberg et al., 1991 and 1996; Finucane et al., 1994; Dykens et al., 1997; Dykens and Smith, 1998 Smith et al., 1998a,b). Two behaviors possibly unique to Smith-Magenis syndrome are onychotillomania, or nail yanking, and polyembolokoilamania, or bodily insertions (Greenberg et al., 1991). Two stereotypic behaviors have also been described, the spasmodic upper body squeeze, or "self-hug" (Finucane et al., 1994), and a hand-licking and page flipping, or "lick and flip" behavior (Dykens et al., 1997; Dykens and Smith, 1998), providing other effective diagnostic markers for the syndrome.

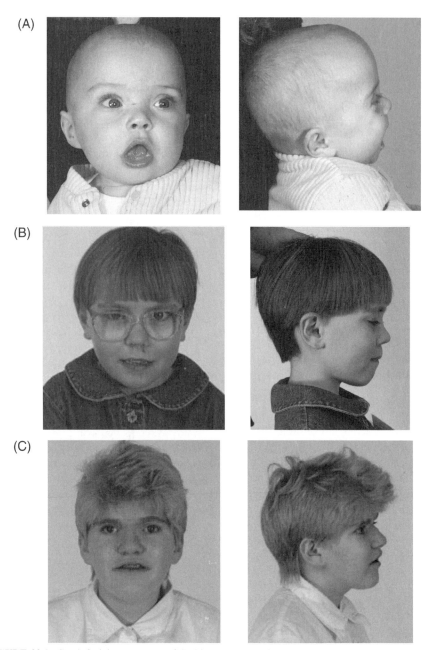

FIGURE 22.1. Craniofacial appearance of Smith-Magenis syndrome in three unrelated children at ages 9 months (A) 7 years, 4 months (B) and 16.5 years (C) In infant (*A*), note mild brachycephaly with square-shaped face, "cherubic" appearance due to prominent "pudgy" cheeks with a flushed ("rosy") appearance, upslanting palpebral fissures with deep-set and close-set eyes, marked midfacial hypoplasia with depressed broad nasal root, and micrognathia. The mouth is characteristic, with cupid's bow or tented appearance and open-mouth posture. In the older child, the facial appearance is more distinct (*B* and *C*) with broad, square shape, marked broadening of the jaw, increasing midface hypoplasia and relative prognathism. Brows appear heavy, almost pugilistic, often extending laterally, and eyes appear deep set. The downturned mouth and characteristic cupid bow upper lip remain apparent. The nasal bridge becomes almost "ski jump" in shape with age.

Several clinical features of Smith-Magenis syndrome appear to be age dependent, including the prominent forehead, midface hypoplasia, prognathism, brachycephaly, hoarse voice, and ophthalmologic findings, specifically high myopia with and without retinal detachment (Smith et al., 1998a). Although sleep disturbance is present from early infancy, the stereotypies and self-injurious behaviors generally do not begin until after the first 18 months of life. Many believe that the early behavioral problems, including head banging, self-biting, and self-hitting, are in part related to the general frustrations experienced with poor expressive language skills (Greenberg et al., 1996; Smith et al., 1998a). The sleep disturbance and self-abusive behaviors also appear to escalate with age, often at expected stages of the life cycle, specifically, at 18–24 months, at school age, and with pubertal onset.

Etiology, Pathogenesis, and Genetics

Smith-Magenis syndrome is considered to be a contiguous gene syndrome (Greenberg et al., 1991), which by definition suggests that haploinsufficiency of multiple, functionally unrelated genes located in close proximity is responsible for the phenotype (Schmickel, 1986). The vast majority of patients with Smith-Magenis syndrome have been identified in the last 5 years as a result of improved cytogenetic techniques, including FISH. With few exceptions, (Howard-Peeples et al., 1985; Zori et al., 1993), all cases of Smith-Magenis syndrome occur *de novo*, suggesting a low recurrence risk. However, parental cytogenetic analyses are recommended for all newly diagnosed cases. To date, there is no evidence to suggest an obvious parental age contribution for the deletion or unusual sex distribution of cases (Lockwood et al., 1988). Random parental origin of the 17p deletion has been documented, suggesting that imprinting does not play a role in the expression of the Smith-Magenis syndrome phenotype (Greenberg et al, 1991).

The underlying pathogenetic mechanism leading to the features of Smith-Magenis syndrome has yet to be identified. Molecular studies demonstrate that the majority of patients have a common deletion interval spanning 4–5 megabases (Juyal et al., 1996). However, deletions have ranged from <2 to >9 megabases (Trask et al., 1996). Potentially, this region may contain more than 100 genes (Elsea et al., 1997). With the use of somatic cell hybrid panels, a bin map of 17p11.2 was constructed to determine the shortest region of overlap, further refining the Smith-Magenis syndrome critical interval (Elsea et al., 1997; Liang et al., 1998). Gene(s) responsible for behavior are hypothesized to be located in the proximal part of the critical interval, whereas gene(s) affecting physical and mental development may fall in the distal part of the critical region (Elsea et al., 1997). Further genotype/phenotype correlations are needed to confirm this hypothesis.

In 1993, Moncla et al. (1993) suggested that an unstable region, located between Smith-Magenis syndrome and CMT1A (Charcot-Marie-Tooth disease type1A), might be a hot spot for rearrangements, leading distally to *CMT1A* duplications and proximally to Smith-Magenis syndrome microdeletions. On the basis of the presence of a low-copy repeated gene cluster, Chen et al. (1997) showed that homologous recombination of a flanking repeat gene cluster is the mechanism leading to the Smith-Magenis syndrome deletion. Such low-copy repeats have been identified for several other contiguous gene syndromes, including Williams syndrome (see Chapter 30), Prader-Willi syndrome/Angelman syndrome (see Chapters 3 and 18), and DiGeorge/velocardiofacial syndrome (see Chapter 29) (Lupski, 1998).

Over the past five years, multiple genes have been mapped to the 17p11.2 Smith-Magenis syndrome critical region (http.//www.ncbi.nlm.nih.gov). However, only a few of these have been found to be consistently deleted in patients with Smith-Magenis syndrome. The role of each of these is not yet known. Because the deletion occurs on only one chromosome, haploinsuffiency for several genes is likely to account for the phenotype.

Several genes mapped to the Smith-Magenis syndrome critical region are worthy of mention. Chen et al. (1995; 1996) suggested that the human homolog of the *Drosophila melangaster flightless-I* gene (human = *FLII*), which is involved in protein-protein interactions, might interact with proteins such as collagen and elastin, thereby offering a possible explanation for the ocular, cardiovascular, and skeletal abnormalities in Smith-Magenis syndrome. Another gene mapped to 17p11.2 is the human microfibril-associated protein gene (*MFAP4*), which encodes a calcium-dependent adhesive protein associated with elastin microfibrils and integrin (Zhao et al., 1995). *MFAP4* may also play a role in the connective tissue aspects of Smith-Magenis syndrome.

Haploinsufficiency for the gene for cytosolic serine hydroxymethyltransferase (*cSHMT*) was demonstrated among all 26 patients with Smith-Magenis syndrome in one study (Elsea et al., 1995). This enzyme was decreased by 50% in lymphoblasts from all three patients tested and may result in neurotoxicity (Elsea et al., 1995).

Another gene, *COP9*, recently mapped to the Smith-Magenis syndrome critical region (Potocki et al., 1999) is intriguing, because it is a conserved protein that is ubiquitously expressed and appears to act as a developmental switch. Found to be 45% conserved from plants to humans, *COP9* is a multi-subunit complex protein shown to be a nuclear regulator in humans; in plants, it responds to environmental light signals and regulates development (Potocki et al., 1999). Given the recent confirmation of a circadian rhythm disturbance in Smith-Magenis syndrome (De Leersnyder et al., 1999 Potocki et al., 2000), this gene may play a role in this aspect of the phenotype. Further studies are required to answer this question.

Recent studies have demonstrated hypercholesterolemia in patients with Smith-Magenis syndrome (Finucane et al., 1996; Smith et al., 1998). The common Smith-Magenis syndrome deletion interval contains the gene for sterol regulatory element-binding protein (*SREBF1*), a transcription factor involved in cholesterol homeostasis. Among 20 children with Smith-Magenis syndrome deleted for *SREBF1*, 8 (40%) had a mean total cholesterol of >90%, 11 (55%) had LDL cholesterol >90%, and 13 (65%) had elevated triglycerides. Functional studies are needed to determine the role of haploinsufficiency for *SREBF1* in altered cholesterol homeostasis and its potential contribution to the pathogenesis of Smith-Magenis syndrome.

The increased frequency of sensorineural hearing loss seen in Smith-Magenis syndrome may be secondary to loss of heterozygosity at the locus with a mutation of *MYO15*, a gene for nonsyndromic recessive hearing loss (Friedman et al., 1995).

Diagnostic Testing

Definitive diagnosis of Smith-Magenis syndrome is based on diagnostic confirmation of the deletion of 17p11.2 cytogenetically and/or by FISH. Virtually all cases (95%) have cytogenetically detectable deletions of 17p11.2. Moderate quality and 450- to 550-band resolution is generally adequate for detection of the deletion (Behjati et al. 1997). The availability of a FISH probe specific for Smith-Magenis syndrome has proven beneficial in confirming equivocal cases (Elsea et al., 1996; Juyal et al., 1995a,b). Previously "normal" karyotypes in patients subsequently documented to have Smith-Magenis syndrome by repeat cytogenetic study are not uncommon, confirming the importance of clinical diagnostic criteria. Although at least one FISH probe, D17S258, is deleted in all patients examined to date (Elsea et al., 1997), another commercial FISH probe (D17S29) is present in all Smith-Magenis syndrome patients (Juyal et al., 1996; Elsea et al., 1997). Hence, repeat cytogenetic analysis accompanied by FISH should be considered for those patients in whom a prior cytogenetic study was interpreted as "normal," especially in cases where a subtle deletion may have been missed or for whom an early suspected diagnosis of Down syndrome was not confirmed.

Recently, a few individuals with clinically suspected Smith-Magenis syndrome phenotype have been identified who fail to demonstrate the cytogenetic deletion on high-resolution analysis and/or with commercial Smith-Magenis syndrome FISH probes, thereby eluding customary diagnostic confirmation. Whether such cases represent smaller molecular deletions, point mutations, or genetic phenocopies has yet to be determined; however, they become valuable in narrowing the Smith-Magenis syndrome critical region.

Differential Diagnosis

Delayed diagnosis in Smith-Magenis syndrome is common. In infancy, children with Smith-Magenis syndrome are often thought to have Down syndrome because of infantile hypotonia and several facial stigmata suggestive of this diagnosis, including a flat midface and upslanting palpebral fissures (Gropman et al., 1998; Allanson et al., 1999) (see Chapter 7). Among a cohort of 19 patients with Smith-Magenis syndrome evaluated by the authors, over one-third underwent an initial chromosome analysis to rule out Down syndrome. Fortuitous diagnosis of del 17p11.2 and Smith-Magenis syndrome was confirmed in a few of these infants; however, the majority remained undiagnosed until repeat chromosome analysis at school age. Other diagnoses considered before confirmation of Smith-Magenis syndrome include the following: Prader-Willi syndrome, because of infantile hypotonia,

lethargy, and feeding and sleep disorders (see Chapter 18); velocardiofacial syndrome, because of marked speech delay and cardiac anomalies (see Chapter 29); and fragile X syndrome (see Chapter 10). Clinically, many of the children have been given the diagnosis of autism/pervasive developmental disorder because of abnormalities of language and stereotypic behaviors (Gropman et al., 1998).

MANIFESTATIONS AND MANAGEMENT

Growth and Feeding

Since the early delineation of the syndrome by Smith et al. (1986), short stature and/or failure to thrive remain consistent findings, seen in 78% of individuals with Smith-Magenis syndrome (Smith et al., 1998a). Prenatal histories are notable for decreased fetal movement in 50% of cases (Gropman et al., 1998b). Although weight, length, and head circumference are generally within the normal range at birth (Smith et al., 1986), height and weight gradually decelerate in early infancy. Head circumference usually plots within the normal range, although about 20% have head circumference less than the 3rd centile for age (Stratton et al., 1986; personal observation).

Short stature is characterized by heights generally 2–3 SD below the mean for age during infancy and childhood (Greenberg et al., 1991); however, adult heights generally fall in the low range of normal (<10%). Several patients with Smith-Magenis syndrome have been reported who are notably short and obese. In some cases, this has led to an initial suspected diagnosis of Prader-Willi syndrome, especially in the presence of a history of infantile hypotonia and feeding problems, food foraging and/or evidence of behavioral dysfunction (Stratton et al., 1986; Del Vecchio et al., 1998; personal experience).

Feeding difficulties during infancy occur in the majority of cases, caused in part by infantile hypotonia, general lethargy, and major oral-motor dysfunction and poor suck and swallowing abilities. Oral sensorimotor dysfunction is seen in virtually all cases examined, characterized by lingual findings (weakness, asymmetry, and/or limited motion) in 100% and at least one laryngeal finding (Sonies et al., 1997). Nasogastric or gastrostomy tube feedings are sometimes necessary, and gastroesophageal reflux has been observed (Sonies et al., 1997). Additional findings that can impact feeding include weak bilabial seal (64%), palatal anomalies including velopharyngeal insufficiency (75%), and open mouth posture with tongue protrusion (<30%). Tracheobronchial signs are reported in over half of cases. Oral-motor dysfunction may result in refusal of highly textured foods and contribute to failure to thrive.

Evaluation

- Height, weight, and head circumference (with percentile plots) should be measured at initial evaluation and during subsequent health maintenance visits. It is important to consider comparison of weight to height in addition to charting absolute percentile measurements for these parameters.
- Oral feeding and swallowing evaluations to include assessment of caloric intake, swallowing abilities, oral-motor skills, gastroesophageal reflux signs and symptoms, along with assessment of parental feeding concerns are highly recommended for all affected infants. Suspected gastroesophageal reflux warrants consideration of full diagnostic evaluation.
- Occupational and speech evaluations are indicated to assess oral-motor dysfunction because it interferes with feeding.

Treatment

- Oral-motor therapy with a speech pathologist, clinical feeding specialist, or occupational therapist is suggested. Emphasis on increasing labial and lingual movements for swallowing and transitioning to varying food textures is also beneficial for a child's oral-motor and swallowing maturation.
- Neurodevelopmental training has been used in several cases and has proven beneficial for enhancing feeding and swallowing skills (personal experience).
- Gastrostomy or nasogastric tube feedings may be required.

Development and Behavior

In contrast to the extensive clinical and molecular reviews of Smith-Magenis syndrome, systematic study of the cognitive and behavioral phenotype of Smith-Magenis syndrome has been more limited (Finucane et al., 1994; Dykens et al., 1997; Smith et al., 1998a,b; Dykens and Smith, 1998). Yet it is the complex neurobehavioral phenotype associated with Smith-Magenis syndrome that represents the major management problem for both parents and professionals working with this syndrome. Moreover, the behavioral phenotype proves useful to clinical diagnosis of Smith-Magenis syndrome.

Developmental delay or mental retardation is found to some degree in all patients, ranging from profound to borderline functioning. Greenberg et al. (1996) found IQ scores ranging from 20 to 78 in a series of 27 patients, with the majority falling in the moderate range of mental retardation at 40–54. However, 6 of 25 patients evaluated had IQ scores in the mild and one in the borderline range. As infants, subtle motor delays may be evident, with gross motor delays of 2–24 months; however, social-emotional function can be within the normal range, further confirming the need for diagnostic work up (Gropman et al., 1998; Gropman et al, 1999). In general, expressive language delays are out of proportion to receptive language skills, especially during early childhood (Greenberg et al., 1996; Smith et al.,

1998a; Gropman et al., 1998). Studies by Sonies et al. (1997) suggest that the severe oral-motor dysfunction and apraxia may be caused in part by bilateral dysfunction of structures subserving the muscles needed for swallowing and speech (palate, pharyngeal, buccal, etc.).

Dykens et al. (1997) described specific cognitive profiles in 10 subjects with Smith-Magenis syndrome with relative weaknesses observed in sequential processing and short-term memory; relative strengths were found in long-term memory and perceptual closure. Relative strengths in receptive language skills and attention span were found compared with relative weaknesses in expressive language and fine motor skills. (Gropman et al., 1999).

Significant speech/language delay, with or without associated hearing loss, occurs in over 90% of individuals with Smith-Magenis syndrome. Infants and toddlers make limited vocalizations and exhibit poor vocal sound production because of underlying oral sensorimotor anomalies. Expressive language skills remain delayed in early childhood. With aggressive speech/language therapy accompanied by sign language and a total communication program, fairly understandable expressive language is usually present by school age. Some parents report that the onset of language, specifically, speaking in full sentences, occurs when their child begins to read (personal observation). Speech parameters include hypernasality with a harsh, hoarse vocal quality. Speech intensity may be mildly elevated with a rapid rate and moderate explosiveness (Sonies et al., 1997). Once verbal, children with Smith-Magenis syndrome are incessant talkers, asking constant, often repetitive questions. Verbal teens and adults with Smith-Magenis syndrome often demonstrate a good sense of humor, with a unique propensity for "one-liners," and excellent long-term memory.

Behavioral problems, including maladaptive behaviors and stereotypic behaviors, are frequent in Smith-Magenis syndrome

(60–80%) and represent the major management problem for both parents and professionals working with this syndrome (Finucane et al., 1994; Greenberg et al., 1991; Dykens et al., 1997; Smith et al., 1998a,b). Dykens and Smith (1998) examined the distinctiveness and correlates of maladaptive behavior as well as prevalence of self-injurious and stereotypical behaviors further delineating the behavioral phenotype of Smith-Magenis syndrome. With the use of the Child Behavior Check List score, 35 children with Smith-Magenis syndrome were compared to age- and gender-matched subjects with Prader-Willi syndrome or mixed mental retardation. All but four subjects with Smith-Magenis syndrome (89%) demonstrated significantly elevated maladaptive behavior scores compared with their counterparts; 12 behaviors differentiated the groups with 100% accuracy. Specifically, those with Smith-Magenis syndrome demonstrated significantly higher rates of temper tantrums (94%), disobedience (97%), attention-seeking (100%), property destruction (86%), impulsivity (86%), aggression (57%), hyperactivity (94%), distractibility (89%), toileting difficulties (80%), sleep disturbance (94%), and nail-biting behaviors (72%). Self-injurious behaviors were seen in 92% of the Smith-Magenis syndrome study group, including biting or hitting self (71–77%); nail-yanking or onychotillomania (29%), and bodily insertion or polyembolokoilamania (25%). The latter two were also associated with lower levels of delay. One or more stereotypic behaviors were demonstrated by all Smith-Magenis syndrome subjects including mouthing objects or hands in mouth (54–69%), teeth grinding (54%); "lick-and-flip" behavior (51%), self-hug, upper body spasmodic squeeze (46%), body rocking (43%), and spinning or twirling objects (40%). The most frequent stereotypies involved the mouth in some way, representing oral variants of bodily insertion. These include placing objects or fingers in the mouth (54–69%), teeth grinding (54%), and lick-and-flip behavior (51%). The high prevalence of oral insertion behavior may originate as a compensatory skill used in eating during infancy, when oral-motor dysfunction is significant and requires the use of hands/fingers to assist in propelling food back to be swallowed.

The relationship between self-abusive behaviors and decreased pain sensitivity (i.e., peripheral neuropathy) is not yet defined and warrants further study. People with Smith-Magenis syndrome in one study differed from their counterparts both in regulation of basic bodily functions (sleeping, modulating activity and affect, eating, and toileting), and in social and repetitive behaviors (Dykens and Smith, 1998). These individuals slept less, were more prone to hyperactivity, and were more emotionally labile than their counterparts. Enuresis and encopresis were singularly frequent in Smith-Magenis syndrome compared to Prader-Willi syndrome and mixed mentally retarded subjects. Socially, those with Smith-Magenis syndrome demanded more attention than their counterparts, especially in contrast to the Prader-Willi syndrome group, which was particularly high in social withdrawal. Those with Smith-Magenis syndrome also showed obsessive thinking, primarily about specific topics as opposed to food.

Sleep disturbance occurs in virtually all cases of Smith-Magenis syndrome (Greenberg et al. 1996; Smith et al., 1998b) with hypersomnolence in early infancy, changing in later childhood to fragmented and shortened sleep cycles with difficulties falling asleep, frequent and prolonged nocturnal awakenings, excessive daytime sleepiness, daytime napping, snoring, and bedwetting (see **Sleep** section below). People with Smith-Magenis syndrome who experienced snoring and labored breathing were found to exhibit more aggressive, acting-out behaviors and attention problems, consistent with published sleep studies of nonretarded children (Ali et al., 1994; Wiggs and Stores, 1996; Ball et al., 1997). The lack of longitudinal

data tracking sleep disturbance and behaviors makes it difficult to determine to what extent sleep disturbance causes or exacerbates behaviors. From the parenting standpoint, sleep deprivation experienced when dealing with their child's nighttime sleep issues may also impact parental patience and management of daytime behaviors, leading to less than optimal interventions. However, a causal role for sleep disturbance in the sleep-behavior cycle is suggested by Dykens and Smith (1998), who found an association between increased nap length and decreased aggressive and attention problems. Although age and degree of delay were correlated with behavior problems, Dykens and Smith (1998) found that sleep disturbance emerged as the strongest predictor of maladaptive behavior.

Finucane et al. (1994) described two types of self-hugging, an upper body movement and clasping the hands at chest or chin level and squeezing, often with interlocked fingers. More frequent among young children and adolescents than adults, these movements appear involuntary, with a ticlike quality. Seen in all 11 subjects with Smith-Magenis syndrome, the self-hug was observed when subjects were happy or pleased but not during temper tantrums or when subjects were unusually upset. In addition to hugging themselves, individuals with Smith-Magenis syndrome often hug others repetitively and with force. A few parents report the unfortunate demise of a family pet (gerbil, kitten) caused by such intense squeezing/hugging behaviors and excitement (Smith, 1997).

Although children with Smith-Magenis syndrome have some degree of control over their behaviors, it is important to recognize that many of the negative behaviors seen in Smith-Magenis syndrome have their origins in internally driven impulses.

The behavioral phenotype of Smith-Magenis syndrome, specifically maladaptive and self-injurious behavior and sleep disturbance, has a significant impact on family stress and support needs. A recent study by

Hodapp et al. (1998) documented high levels of parent and family problems, pessimism, and overall stress in the presence of increased numbers of family supporters. The main predictor of overall stress and parent-family problems was inversely related to the size of the family's support system. The child's degree of maladaptive behavior was the single best predictor of parental pessimism.

Evaluation

- Accurate assessment of developmental function in Smith-Magenis syndrome is often hampered by the marked speech delay and inherent bias in developmental scales, which rely on verbal skills.
- Annual multidisciplinary team evaluation is optimal, including physical, occupational, and speech therapy evaluations and pediatric assessment to assist in development of an individual educational plan.
- Periodic neurodevelopmental assessments and/or developmental pediatric consultation can be an important adjunct to the team evaluation.
- Speech/language evaluations beginning in infancy are necessary to evaluate speech and language developmental delays, optimize functional communication with the child in his/her environment, as well as provide education to parents for fostering speech and language development.
- Assessment of family support and psychosocial and emotional needs will assist in designing family interventions.

Treatment

- Early intervention should be started as soon as the diagnosis is made.
- Referral for physical, occupational, and speech therapies is important to provide support and treatment for developmental deficits.
- Educational intervention throughout the school years (at a minimum) should

include addressing individual strengths and weaknesses, taking into account the behavior disorder. This can best be done by incorporating the recommendations of a multidisciplinary developmental assessment.

- Speech/language pathology services should initially focus on facilitating swallowing and feeding problems as well as optimizing oral sensory motor development. Therapeutic goals for emphasizing increasing sensory input, fostering movement of the articulators, increasing oral motor endurance, and decreasing hypersensitivity are needed to develop the skills needed for swallowing and speech production.
- The use of sign language and total communication program as an adjunct to traditional speech/language therapy is felt to improve communication skills and also to have a positive impact on behavior (Greenberg et al., 1991). The ability to develop expressive language appears to be dependent on the early use of sign language and intervention by speech language pathologists. Functional communication with fair speech intelligibility eventually replaces the severely delayed expressive language during the school age years. Nonverbal persons with Smith-Magenis syndrome are known and frequently are older individuals who did not receive aggressive therapeutic intervention.
- Management strategies that improve nighttime sleep may have an impact on the level of maladaptive behaviors.
- Children with Smith-Magenis syndrome are very adult-oriented, with an almost insatiable need for individual attention, a key personality characteristic that has major implications both at home and in the classroom. Positive attention is clearly preferable, but negative attention may serve equally well in the quest for one-on-one adult interaction. Withholding teacher attention often prompts

negative behaviors, including verbal outburst, tantrums, aggression toward peers, and destruction of property, all of which disrupt the classroom and result in the "desired" attention. At home or in the classroom, unexpected changes in daily routine or transitions between activities as well as emotional upset can precipitate behavioral outbursts, tantrums, and aggression. Individuals with Smith-Magenis syndrome tend to respond quite positively to consistency, structure, and routine, especially with visual cues.

- Persons with Smith-Magenis syndrome have difficulties in sequential processing (i.e., counting, math tasks, multistep tasks) and short-term memory. Thus instructional strategies that recognize these inherent weaknesses while taking advantage of relative strengths in long-term memory (especially names) and visual reasoning are most effective (Dykens et al., 1997; Smith et al., 1998a).

- Inherently distractible, children with Smith-Magenis syndrome tend to function better in a smaller, calmer, and more focused classroom setting with five to seven students, a teacher, and an aide (Haas-Givler et al., 1996). In some circumstances, an individual aide in a larger classroom also works; however, with larger class sizes, competition for a teacher's attention and inherent activity level increases, risking increased behavioral problems.

- Because they are visual learners, individuals with Smith-Magenis syndrome greatly benefit from the use of pictures or visual cues/reminders to illustrate daily activities, classroom schedules, and performing self-help skills.

- Use of computer-assisted technology offers a unique educational opportunity for people with Smith-Magenis syndrome, who have a strong fascination with electronics, including VCRs, tape recorders, video games, and/or computers (Smith et al., 1998a).

- Development of a behavioral treatment plan should be initiated as soon as behavioral problems arise.

- Children with Smith-Magenis syndrome are generally eager to please and quite responsive to affection, praise, and other positive attention. In moderation, positive emotional response by the teacher or parent can strongly motivate a child to do well. Opportunities to do something they like to do, such as additional time spent on the computer, present powerful positive motivators. Time-outs have been tried, and loss of time doing a preferred activity (such as lost computer time) has been an effective strategy.

- Most patients with Smith-Magenis syndrome have been tried on a number of medications to control behavior with mixed response; adverse reactions to some medications have also been reported. Unpublished medication history data on 12 children with Smith-Magenis syndrome ages 3–16 years show a median number of five medication trials; only two children were not on medication therapy and one of these was enrolled in a strict behavior-modification program (Allen and Smith, 1997). In the multidisciplinary study conducted by Greenberg et al. (1996), the most common medications tried among 27 patients with Smith-Magenis syndrome were methylphenidate, pemoline, and thioridazine. Carbamazepine may offer some benefit to behavioral management.

- Both published (Greenberg et al., 1996; Hagerman, 1999) and unpublished data on 12 patients with Smith-Magenis syndrome showed that stimulant drugs are not particularly helpful in controlling behavior or increasing attention span (Allen and Smith, 1997). These authors found slight improvement with Adderall (1), dexedrine (1), and Ritalin (3), compared with a worsening on dexedrine (1), Ritalin (3), and marked side effects with Cylert (1). Among the antipsychotics, one child improved on stelazine; one got much worse on risperidone, and one became sedated on thoridazine. In contrast, Hagerman (1999) found marked improvement of aggression and hyperactivity in a case study of a 12-year-old female with Smith-Magenis syndrome on risperidone (1 mg bid). Greenberg et al. (1996) reported some or only transient behavior improvement for several patients with Smith-Magenis syndrome, both with and without seizures, tried on carbamazepine. Similar unpublished results (Allen and Smith, 1997) were found for eight patients with Smith-Magenis syndrome tried on anticonvulsants: three showed improvement on carbamazepine, whereas two got slightly worse; Phenobarbital showed no change (1), and valproic acid showed much improvement (1) and no change (1). Among the 12 unpublished Smith-Magenis syndrome medication histories, 3 children were tried on benzodiazepines: clonazepam showed improvement (1) or no change (1), and lorazepam showed improvement (1). Two subjects tried on tricyclic antidepressants (clomipramine or imipramine) got much worse. One subject tried on the α-2-agonist, guanfacine/Tenex, had some improvement but reported side effects. Recent use of specific serotonin reuptake inhibitors (specifically sertraline, fluoxetine) has shown considerable improvement with respect to behavioral outbursts and sleep for at least three individuals with Smith-Magenis syndrome (Smith et al., 1998a).

- Published data about the optimal intervention and behavioral strategies in Smith-Magenis syndrome are limited to anecdotal and experiential findings (Haas-Givler, 1994; Haas-Givler and

Finucane, 1995; Smith et al., 1998a). Although medication therapy may show some benefit with respect to increasing attention and/or decreasing hyperactivity, it is clear that behavioral therapies play an integral role in the behavioral management of Smith-Magenis syndrome.

- Respite care and family psychological and social support are critical to assuring the optimal environment for the affected individual.

- Referral to the national genetic support group Parents and Researchers Interested in Smith-Magenis syndrome (PRISM) as well as local, regional, or state support services is a critical need for parents and families of persons with Smith-Magenis syndrome.

Sleep

As noted above, significant symptoms of sleep disturbance are seen in virtually all persons with Smith-Magenis syndrome and have a major impact not only on the child with Smith-Magenis syndrome but on parents and other family members, many of whom also become sleep deprived themselves (Smith et al., 1998b). Greenberg et al. (1996), documented sleep abnormalities in 75% of 27 patients with Smith-Magenis syndrome, including difficulties falling asleep, frequent and prolonged nighttime awakenings, and excessive daytime sleepiness. Abnormalities of REM sleep were documented in over half of those studied with polysomnography: 12 had reduced REM sleep, 1 increased REM sleep, and 2 absent REM sleep (Greenberg et al., 1991; 1996). In contrast to the frequent nocturnal awakenings and fragmented sleep cycle characteristic of later childhood, sleep disturbance during infancy is remarkable for hypersomnolence and lethargy (Gropman et al., 1998).

A detailed study of sleep behaviors in 39 individuals with Smith-Magenis syndrome showed a significant relationship between increased age and steady decline in the total hours of sleep needed at night, earlier bedtimes, shorter nap lengths, and increased frequency of naps (Smith et al., 1998b). Total sleep cycle averaged 7.8 hours (range 3.5–10.5 hours) with mean 5:30 A.M. awakening time and mean 8:40 P.M. bedtime. Nap lengths decline sharply after age 5 years but increase in frequency from 1.2 to 1.7 after age 10 years. The most frequent problems during bedtime and nighttime periods were bedwetting (79%), bedtime rituals (74%), snoring (69%), use of sleep medications (59%), and awakening during the night either to go to the bathroom (54%) or to get a drink (54%). Parents often report that their child will not fall asleep unless one parent lies down with him or her, a bedtime habit that is difficult to end and one likely to impact the marriage as well. Early morning awakening times are the rule, even with medication treatment.

Preliminary biochemical studies (Potocki et al., 1997) document abnormally elevated urinary 6-sulfatoxymelatonin during a 24-hour sleep study in 5 of 6 affected patients studied, with aberrant melatonin profile levels skewed to daytime highs. This aberrant melatonin pattern was confirmed in two larger series of patients with Smith-Magenis syndrome: a French series of 19 subjects (deLeersnyder et al., 1999) and a U.S. series of 28 subjects (Potocki et al., 2000). Both groups independently confirmed an inversion of circadian rhythm of melatonin in virtually all subjects studied. The one American subject who failed to demonstrate this finding did not have the common SMS deletion (Potocki et al., 2000). Sleep histories similar to those published by Smith et al., (1998b) were also reported by deLeersnyder et al. (1999). The biochemical finding of complete inversion of the melatonin circadian cycle is also supported by anecdotal parental reports of general improvement of sleep patterns with the administration of over-the-counter melatonin (Smith et al., 1998b). These findings confirm the hypothesis that

an aberrant biological clock is involved in Smith-Magenis syndrome (Smith et al., 1998b). Such altered sleep patterns could be secondary to abnormalities in the production, secretion, distribution, or metabolism of melatonin (Potocki, et al., 2000).

Evaluation

- Sleep history should be elicited to document the sleep cycle to ascertain evidence of sleep apnea, snoring, and other signs of sleep abnormalities.

- Evidence of snoring or irregular nighttime breathing should precipitate a sleep study to rule out obstructive sleep apnea. This should include a sleep-deprived EEG or polysomnography.

Treatment

- Documented sleep apnea should be treated as for the general population. This may include tonsillectomy and adenoidectomy, which has been performed successfully in a few cases with possible obstruction of airway.

- The therapeutic management of the sleep disorder in Smith-Magenis syndrome remains a challenge for the physician and parents. Melatonin was shown to be effective in the treatment of chronic sleep disorder in over 90 children with a variety of diagnoses, including multiple neurological disabilities, mental retardation, Down syndrome, and other chromosome abnormalities. Not only was sleep function improved, but significant health, behavioral, and social benefits were derived from melatonin, without evidence of any side effects (Jan et al., 1994; Jan and Espezel, 1995). Although too limited to draw conclusions, early reports of therapeutic benefit from melatonin in Smith-Magenis syndrome remain encouraging (Allen and Smith, 1997; Smith et al., 1998b). A dosage of 2.5–5.0 mg (10 mg maximum) taken at bedtime has been tried without report of major adverse reactions; general improvement of sleep is reported. In the absence of formal melatonin treatment trials in Smith-Magenis syndrome, a monitored trial of 4–6 weeks on melatonin may be worth consideration in affected individuals with major sleep disturbance.

- Independently, parents have implemented similar solutions to "Smith-Magenis syndrome-proof" their child's room to minimize self-injury and maximize sleep cycle, to enhance the likelihood that the affected individual will not wake and wander in the early morning hours (Smith et al., 1998b). Strategies of removing all small objects such as toys and lamps from the bedroom and installing a door peephole for observation, an outside-locking door, and window black-out curtains have been tried with some success.

- For the most part, children with Smith-Magenis syndrome are most alert in the early morning hours, and this observation should be exploited in the educational setting. The increased frequency and duration of daytime napping with age (to make up for poor nighttime sleep) should also be recognized. Consequently, major educational activities or therapies during late afternoons are often met with increased negative behaviors and difficulties with staying on task.

Otolaryngologic

Otolaryngological findings are extremely common in Smith-Magenis syndrome, providing a physiologic explanation for the functional impairment in voice and speech previously reported. A multidisciplinary clinical study of 27 subjects with Smith-Magenis syndrome (Greenberg et al., 1996) demonstrated otolaryngological abnormalities in 94% (16/17 examined) and hearing impairment in 68% (17/25). One-third of those undergoing laryngoscopy (4/12) had laryngeal abnormalities including polyps, nodules, edema, or paralysis. These findings were confirmed by Sonies et al. (1997) in a new series of 14 affected children (9 months to 16 years). Speech impairment was exhibited in 10 of the 12 (83%) verbal children; two infants <10 months old had notably diminished vocalizations and sound production. All 14 patients demonstrated lingual findings and at least one laryngeal abnormality (polyps or nodules; plica ventricularis); structural vocal fold abnormalities without reported vocal hyperfunction were seen in all but the youngest subject. Severe oral-sensorimotor dysfunction was characterized by lingual weakness (10/14), severely limited tongue motion (11/12), lingual asymmetry (10/14), drooling (11/14), exaggerated lingual papilla (7/14), weak bilabial seal (9/14), palatal abnormalities (9/14), midline palatal pitting (6/14), and open mouth posture with an anterior tongue carriage (10/14). Velopharyngeal insufficiency was confirmed in 75%, significantly higher than observed by Greenberg et al. (1996); however, none had frank or submucous cleft palate abnormalities. Sinusitis requiring antibiotics was experienced by 10 of 14 patients; 2 required surgery. Positional vertigo was observed in 3 of 14 patients (20%). Over half reported tracheobronchial signs including recurrent pneumonia, bronchitis, aspiration, and tracheal stenosis. Other findings include significant gastroesophageal reflux (2), obstructive sleep apnea (3), subglottic stenosis (1), and hemifacial microsomia (1).

Over two-thirds of individuals with Smith-Magenis syndrome have documented hearing loss, which is conductive in 65% and sensorineural in 35% (Greenberg et al., 1996; Sonies et al., 1997). Chronic otitis media is experienced by virtually all children, beginning in early infancy and often leading to multiple ventilation tube placements. Ventilation tubes were required by 11 of 13 patients (85%), and over half had multiple sets. The increased frequency of sensorineural loss is especially interesting in light of a gene for nonsyndromic recessive deafness (*DFNB3*) that maps within the 17p.11.2 region (Friedman et al., 1995; Liang et al., 1998). *DFNB3* encodes myosin 15 (*MYO15*), an essential mechanoenzyme of the auditory system (Wang et al., 1998). The sensorineural deafness present in selected Smith-Magenis syndrome patients may result from loss of heterozygosity caused by deletion 17p11.2 and a mutation of *DFNB3* in a trans-configuration to the SMS deletion. (Liang et al., 1998). At least one patient with Smith-Magenis syndrome with high-frequency sensorineural hearing loss has been found to be hemizygous for a missense mutation in exon 29 of *MYO15* (Friedman TB, personal communication).

Evaluation

- Comprehensive otolaryngological, speech language pathology, and audiological evaluations are recommended for all newly diagnosed persons with Smith-Magenis syndrome.
- Otolaryngological evaluation is indicated to assess ear, nose, and throat problems with specific attention to ear physiology and palatal abnormalities (clefting of the palate, velopharyngeal insufficiency).
- Speech pathology evaluations are essential to evaluate oral sensorimotor skills and swallowing and possible feeding problems.
- Close otolaryngological follow-up for assessment and management of otitis media and other sinus abnormalities are recommended.
- Complete audiological evaluations should be done at regular intervals to monitor for conductive or sensorineural hearing loss.

Treatment

- Management of otolaryngological and audiological problems should begin immediately on diagnosis.

- Routine follow-up and management of all ear, nose, and throat problems in accordance with standard medical practice and professional recommendations should be conducted to optimize an affected individual's communication for developmental and educational purposes.
- Hearing amplification should be considered in the presence of documented sensorineural hearing loss.
- Otitis media is generally chronic (3–6 episodes/year) and may require prophylactic antibiotic therapies and/or ventilatory tube placement.
- Decreased immunologic function (especially IgG or IgA) is observed in over a third of cases and should be considered in the management of these infections.

Neurologic

Central nervous system abnormalities documented by neuroimaging are seen in over half of affected individuals. CT scans of 25 patients with Smith-Magenis syndrome documented ventriculomegaly in 9, enlargement of the cisterna magna in 2, and partial absence of the cerebellar vermis in one (Greenberg et al., 1998). Similar findings were seen among a group of 10 children who had undergone previous MRI: 5 had ventriculomegaly; 2 had enlarged posterior fossa; and 3 had normal scans (Gropman et al., 1998). Despite the presence of oromotor dysfunction, to date no structural abnormalities of the opercular cortex, which subserves these functions, have been reported.

The only known neuropathological study, on a patient in whom the entire 17p11.2 band was deleted, showed microcephaly and foreshortened frontal lobes with depletion of neurons frontally; a small choroid plexus hemangioma was also noted in the lateral ventricle (Smith et al., 1986).

Approximately 11–30% of people with Smith-Magenis syndrome have clinical seizures (Greenberg et al., 1991, 1996; Gropman et al., 1998). EEG abnormalities were documented in 21% of patients in the absence of a clinical history of seizures in one series (Greenberg et al., 1996). Five children (26%) had abnormal EEG in another series ($N = 19$), three of whom had no clinical history of seizures (Gropman et al., 1998). There is no single seizure type or EEG finding that is characteristic of Smith-Magenis syndrome. Recognition and treatment of seizures is important and may improve attention, behavior, and overall cognitive functioning. The prognosis depends on the type of seizure and response to anticonvulsants. Adverse side effects of medications have been reported in children with Smith-Magenis syndrome.

Clinical signs of peripheral neuropathy are reported in approximately 75% of patients with Smith-Magenis syndrome (Greenberg et al., 1996). During early infancy and childhood, signs include hypotonia (100%) with hyporeflexia (84%) and decreased sensitivity to pain (Gropman et al., 1998), although these could be caused by central abnormality. Marked flat or highly arched feet (pes planus or cavus) and unusual gait (flapping feet) are generally appreciated in childhood. In one series, distal muscle weakness was present in over half of subjects, and a previously undescribed peripheral neuropathy tremor (6–8 Hz) was evident in 21% (Gropman et al., 1998).

Peroneal motor nerve conduction velocities are generally normal. Delayed motor nerve conduction velocities due to biopsy-confirmed segmental demyelination and remyelination similar to that seen in hereditary neuropathy with liability to pressure palsy (Smith et al., 1986; Zori et al., 1993) occur rarely. *PMP22*, the gene for CMT1A, located at 17p12 (distal to the Smith-Magenis syndrome critical region), which when deleted causes hereditary neuropathy with liability to pressure palsy, is usually not deleted in Smith-Magenis syndrome (Greenberg et al., 1991 and 1996; Chevillard et al., 1993, Moncla et al., 1993). Signs of peripheral neuropathy in people with Smith-Magenis syndrome are independent of deletion of *PMP22*. It is unclear whether the peripheral neuropathy in Smith-Magenis syndrome is at all progressive.

Because of their relative insensitivity to pain, individuals with Smith-Magenis syndrome may cause injury to themselves by object insertion or persistent picking, biting or hitting during uncontrolled rages (Smith et al., 1998a). Child abuse may be suspected in these circumstances, when the child's injuries are actually self-inflicted (Smith et al., 1998a).

Evaluation

- Careful neurological evaluation should be conducted in all patients at diagnosis and annually thereafter.
- Early recognition and evaluation by physical and/or occupational therapy and implementation of services is essential.
- EEG should be obtained as a baseline in all affected individuals who have clinical seizures to guide the choice of antiepileptic agent. For those without overt seizures, EEG may be helpful to rule out subclinical events in which treatment may improve attention and/or behavior.
- Neuroimaging should be accomplished in accordance with findings such as seizures, motor asymmetry, and in some centers, language delay and/or oral motor dysfunction to rule out an anatomic basis.
- Change in behavior or attention warrants re-evaluation of both seizures and medication.
- EMG may be of benefit in individual clinical situations (Greenberg et al., 1996), especially in the setting of clinical evidence of peripheral neuropathy.

- Periodic neurodevelopmental evaluation should remain a part of the ongoing management of the individual with Smith-Magenis syndrome.

Treatment

- Seizures in individuals with Smith-Magenis syndrome typically respond to traditional antiepileptic therapies. In some cases, addition of an antiepileptic drug may have a secondary effect on behavior and/or sleep, either positive or negative. Individuals with Smith-Magenis syndrome may be particularly sensitive to the side effects of several of these agents.

- Hypotonia may be quite significant during early infancy and may impede development of gross motor skills. Therapies to improve strength and truncal tone should be included in the therapy program.

- There is no specific treatment for the peripheral neuropathy seen in Smith-Magenis syndrome. Care providers should avoid situations that may lead to pressure damage, given a possible predisposition to nerve injury. Those with larger gene deletions including *PMP22* should be managed with attention to potential pressure damage using splinting and physical therapy.

- Physical therapy and splints for foot deformities and gait instability are warranted.

Craniofacial

The facial appearance of Smith-Magenis syndrome shows considerable change with age (Smith et al., 1998a; Allanson et al., 1999) (Fig. 22.1). Although the facial features of Smith-Magenis syndrome are quite distinct in the older child (Fig. 22.1*C*), they remain quite subtle in the infant (Fig. 22.1*A*), frequently delaying diagnosis. Overall face shape is broad and square, with mild brachycephaly present in 83%. In the neonate and young infant with Smith-Magenis syndrome, the facial appearance is impressively attractive. It is characterized by a "cherubic," almost "doll-like" facial appearance, prominent "pudgy" cheeks with a flushed ("rosy") appearance, upslanting palpebral fissures with deep-set and close-set eyes, marked midfacial hypoplasia with depressed broad nasal root, and micrognathia (Smith et al., 1998a). The shape of the mouth and upper lip is quite characteristic, with a fleshy upper lip and a cupid's bow or tented appearance due to the bulky philtral pillars (Allanson et al., 1999). In infants, a "Down syndrome-like" appearance is often recognized because of the generalized hypotonia, flat midface, brachycephaly, short, broad nose, and upslanting palpebral fissures. This appearance often leads to the initial cytogenetic analysis, especially when congenital heart disease is also present (Smith et al., 1998a; Gropman et al., 1998).

The facial appearance of the older child with Smith-Magenis syndrome becomes more distinct (Fig. 22.1*B* and *C*), with a broad, square shape, marked broadening of the jaw, increasing midface hypoplasia, and relative prognathism. Brows become heavy, almost pugilistic, often extending laterally. Eyes appear deep set. The downturned mouth and characteristic cupid bow upper lip remain apparent. The "scooped" nasal bridge becomes almost "ski jump" in shape with age (Allanson, et al., 1999). In the adult, the face becomes longer but retains the square shape and prognathism. Recent anthropometric Z-score pattern profiles on 55 individuals with Smith-Magenis syndrome from 9 months to 35 years of age confirm past subjective impressions, with mandibular dimensions consistently exceeding the maxillary counterparts and craniofacial widths greater than normal (Allanson et al., 1999). Although nasal width is increased, nasal height is reduced from normal. The most striking age-related changes are increased nasal width and increased mandibular width with commensurate reduction of nasal height and midface depth.

Although velopalatal insufficiency is common in Smith-Magenis syndrome (75%), midline cleft of the palate and/or lip occurs with relatively low frequency (<10%); bifid uvula has also been seen. Prognosis is related to the degree of abnormality and its potential for surgical or medical management.

Evaluation

- Careful examination should be conducted for evidence of palatal clefts, including bifid uvula and submucous cleft palate.
- Speech and swallow evaluations are indicated in the presence of difficulties with these functions.

Treatment

- Surgical repair of lip and/or palate is indicated as for the general population.
- Parental education about special feeding techniques is needed for the child with cleft palate.

Ophthalmologic

A high frequency of eye abnormalities has been documented in Smith-Magenis syndrome, including iris anomalies, microcornea, strabismus, cataracts, and myopia. (Finucane et al., 1993b; Chen RM et al., 1996; Barnicoat et al., 1996). The frequency of ocular findings, specifically high myopia and retinal detachment, appears to be age dependent. Detached retina leading to blindness can occur (Finucane et al., 1993b; Chen RM et al., 1996). Efforts to minimize potential for retinal detachment due to trauma should be attempted. Microcornea was seen in over half of one series (Chen RM et al., 1996). The heterochromatic irides or "Brushfield-like" spots in the iris reported by several authors are actually Wolfflin-Kruckmann spots (Chen RM et al., 1996).

Other rare ocular anomalies have been reported in single patients. These include iris dysgenesis (Barnicoat et al., 1996), congenital severe right Brown's syndrome (limitation or absence of elevation in adduction of the eye) (Salati et al., 1995), and visual loss caused by bilateral macular disciform scars (Babovic-Vuksanovic et al., 1998).

Evaluation

- Annual ophthalmological evaluation with careful attention to evidence of strabismus, microcornea, iris anomalies, and refractive errors is recommended.

Treatment

- Corrective lenses for myopia have been required for several individuals with Smith-Magenis syndrome as young as 9 months. However, parents report difficulties with compliance in wearing.
- Corrective treatment for strabismus, when present, is no different than in the general population.
- The potential for detached retina related to repetitive head-banging behavior should be considered, including use of protective helmets.

Cardiovascular

The overall incidence of cardiovascular abnormalities is 27% (Greenberg et al., 1996). Anomalies include mild tricuspid or mitral valve regurgitation, ventricular septal defects, supravalvular aortic or pulmonic stenosis, and atrial septal defects.

Evaluation

- Cardiac evaluation, including echocardiogram, is recommended at the time of diagnosis.
- Follow-up should be determined by the severity of the cardiac anomaly identified.

Treatment

- Pharmacological or surgical intervention should be in accordance with customary cardiac practice for each cardiac anomaly identified.

Gastrointestinal

A history of chronic constipation is reported in 58% of cases (Smith et al., 1998b). The cause remains undefined but may stem from generalized hypotonia and/or dietary intake. Constipation may improve as diet and level of activity increase. Symptoms of encopresis are seen commonly in Smith-Magenis syndrome.

Evaluation

- Chronic constipation or alternating constipation and diarrhea warrants referral to gastroenterology and possible barium enema.
- Surgical evaluation should be performed where there is evidence of bowel obstruction.

Treatment

- Increased fluid intake, stool softeners, and dietary management are beneficial for constipation.

Genitourinary

Renal anomalies were reported in 35% of 26 patients undergoing renal ultrasound, including duplication of the collecting system (4) and one case each of unilateral renal agenesis and ectopic kidney (Greenberg et al., 1996). Nocturnal enuresis occurs in almost 80% of affected individuals (Smith et al., 1998b). Although the etiology has yet to be determined, possible causes include increased fluid intake, medications, underlying urinary tract anomalies, and/or hypotonic bladder, which have been seen in a few cases. Genital anomalies are less frequent in both sexes but include cryptorchidism, shawl or undeveloped scrotum, infantile cervix, and/or hypoplastic uterus (Smith et al., 1986; Stratton et al., 1986).

Evaluation

- It is recommended that all newly diagnosed individuals with Smith-Magenis syndrome be evaluated by baseline renal ultrasound for evidence of genitourinary anomalies.
- Routine urinalysis is appropriate at annual health maintenance exam.
- Fevers of unknown origin should precipitate an evaluation for possible urinary tract infection.

Treatment

- Suspected urinary tract infections should be treated with antibiotic therapy as in the general population.
- Surgical intervention may be necessary, in accordance with customary practice.

Musculoskeletal

A variety of hand anomalies have been described including short, broad hands (85%) and digital anomalies (66%), including cutaneous syndactyly of toes 2 and 3, clinodactyly, and/or polydactyly (Stratton et al., 1986; Smith et al., 1986; Lockwood et al., 1988; Chen et al., 1996; Yang et al., 1997). Kondo et al. (1991) noted prominent fingertip pads, fifth finger clinodactyly, and single palmar creases in all four patients described. Metacarpophalangeal pattern analysis also shows progressive shortness from metacarpal to the proximal, middle, and distal phalanges (Kondo et al., 1991; Meinecke, 1993). Short or bowed ulnae are described (12%) (Greenberg et al., 1996).

Mild to moderate scoliosis, most commonly of the midthoracic region, is seen in over two-thirds of children with Smith-Magenis syndrome age 4 years and older (Greenberg et al., 1996). Underlying vertebral anomalies are seen in a relatively low proportion of cases (Smith et al., 1986; Gropman et al., 1998).

Evaluation

- Monitoring for scoliosis should take place on an annual basis, especially during adolescence.
- Baseline spine films to rule out an underlying vertebral defect are recommended.

Treatment

- Scoliosis should be treated as for individuals in the general population. Surgical intervention is rarely required.
- Vertebral defects generally need no treatment.
- Orthopedic evaluation and use of orthotics is appropriate for positional foot deformities and/or gait disturbances.

Endocrine and Immunologic

Adrenal aplasia-hypoplasia has been described in an 11-month-old male who died unexpectedly after palatoplasty (Denny et al., 1992). The exact incidence of endocrine abnormalities in Smith-Magenis syndrome remains undefined. About one-quarter of those tested have borderline hypothyroidism. Hypercholesterolemia, specifically total cholesterol and LDL cholesterol, has been reported in two series of patients (Finucane et al., 1996; Smith et al., 1998). Precocious puberty and premature ovarian failure have been seen (personal experience).

Immunoglobulins have been mildly decreased in 23% (Greenberg et al., 1996). Diminished immunological function, specifically IgA, was also seen in one series of 20 children (personal experience).

Evaluation

- At diagnosis, routine blood chemistries, qualitative immunoglobulins, cholesterol (fasting) panel, and thyroid function should be performed.
- Baseline and adrenocorticotropic hormone-stimulated serum cortisol levels should be checked in cases of suspected hypoadrenalism.
- Specific screening of adrenal function is warranted in cases of large deletions (>half of 17p11.2 band) (Denny et al., 1992).
- Thyroid function should be evaluated at annual health maintenance visits.

- Patients with recurrent infections should have immunoglobulin electrophoresis performed.

Treatment

- Endocrine problems should be treated as in the general population.
- Treatment of hypercholesterolemia remains unstudied; dietary recommendations may be helpful, but more aggressive therapy has not yet been justified for this population.
- Immune dysfunction should be treated as in the general population.

Dermatologic

Hair and skin color are often fair, and irides are often blue. Rosy cheeks are especially evident in early childhood, possibly related to constant drooling and/or eczema. Hyperkeratotic skin over the surface of the hands, feet, and knees is noted in less than 20% of cases (Smith et al., 1986; Stratton et al., 1986; Lockwood et al., 1988). Evidence of self-injury due to hand biting on wrists, arms, and fingers is common, usually beginning at 18–24 months of age. Nail hygiene is important; hangnails often precipitate cuticle mutilation and/or nail biting and yanking.

Evaluation

- Skin assessment should be part of the routine medical examination of the individual with Smith-Magenis syndrome. Attention to areas injured in Smith-Magenis syndrome by self-injurious behaviors (wrists, arms, nails) is essential.

Treatment

- Creams can be effective in treating dry skin. Twice-daily application of over-the-counter lotions that contain either 10% urea or 5–10% lactic acid are recommended in cases of extreme dry skin.

- Long-sleeved garments can minimize injury caused by chronic self-biting and picking behavior.
- Fingered gloves and frequent manicures and pedicures for nail hygiene can minimize cuticle mutilation and nail biting, picking, and yanking.
- Recognition of stressors and events that trigger such behaviors and behavior modification may prove helpful.

RESOURCES

Parents and Researchers Interested in Smith-Magenis Syndrome (PRISMS), United States Connie Bessette, President

76 South New Boston Road
Francestown, NH 03043
Telephone 603-547-8384
Email: *cbessette@monad.net*
Internet address URL: *www.smithmagenis.org*
Contacts:
Connie Bessette, President & parent
Ann C.M. Smith, M.A., D.Sc.(hon), Chair, Professional Advisory Borad, PRISMS
Activities:
Support services: Parent-to-Parent Program; E-mail parents list; technical support; Educational materials/publications: SPECTRUM newsletter, New Parent Packet, brochures, reference materials; and National conferences (periodically)
Smith-Magenis Syndrome Foundation,
London, England
Contact:
Olga DeChassey,
P.O. Box 18802,
London, England SW7 3ZQ.
Smith-Magenis
syndromefoundation@dechassey. demon.co.uk
Smith-Magenis Syndrome — technical assistance for schools
Consultation concerning educational needs

Brenda Finucane, MS and Barbara Haas-Givler, M.Ed.
c/o Genetic Services at Elwyn, Inc.
111 Elwyn Road
Elwyn, PA 19063
Phone: 610-891-2313 FAX: 610-891-2377
Clinical research on Smith-Magenis syndrome (not exhaustive):
Baylor College of Medicine: James Lupski, MD, PhD (molecular, clinical)
National Institutes of Health: Ann C. M. Smith, MA, DSc (hon) (natural history, clinical, molecular)
University of California, Los Angeles: Elizabeth Dykens, PhD (maladaptive behaviors)
Michigan State University: Sarah Elsea, PhD (molecular cytogenetics)

DEDICATION

This chapter is dedicated to the memory of our dear friend and genetics colleague, Frank Greenberg, M.D., whose inspiration, knowledge, and contributions to our understanding of Smith-Magenis syndrome are reflected throughout this chapter.

REFERENCES

Ali NJ, Pitson D, Stradling JR (1994) Natural history of snoring and related behavior problems between the ages of 4 and 7 years. *Arch Dis Childhood* 71:74–76.

Allanson JE, Greenberg F, Smith ACM (1999) The face of Smith-Magenis syndrome: A subjective and objective study. *J Med Genet* 36:394–397.

Allen AJ and Smith ACM (1997) "Medications in Smith-Magenis syndrome: Implications for therapy." (Unpublished data on 14 Smith-Magenis syndrome patients evaluated at NIH presented at the 1997 National Conference on Smith-Magenis syndrome, Bethesda, MD.)

Babovic-Vuksanovic D, Jalal AM, Garrity JA, Robertson DM, Lindor NM (1998) Visual impairment due to macular disciform scars in a 20-year old man with Smith-Magenis syndrome: Another ophthalmologic complication. *Am J Med Genet* 80:373–376.

Ball JD, Tiernan M, Janusz J, Furr A (1997) Sleep patterns among children with attention-deficit hyperactivity disorder: A reexamination of parent perceptions. *J Pediatr Psychol* 22:389–398.

Barnicoat AJ, Moller HU, Palmer RW, Russell-Eggitt I, Winter RM (1996) An unusual presentation of Smith-Magenis syndrome with iris dysgenesis. *Clin Dysmorphol* 5:153–158.

Behjati F, Mullarkey M, Bergbaum A, Berry AC, Dochery Z (1997) Chromosome deletion 17p11.2 (Smith-Magenis syndrome) in seven new patients, four of whom had been referred for fragile-X investigation. *Clin Genet* 51:71–74.

Chen KS, Gunaratne PH, Hoheisel JD, Young IG, Miklos GLG, Greenberg F, Shaffer LG, Campbell HD, Lupski JR (1995): The human homologue of the Drosophila melanogaster flightless-I gene (FLIII) maps within the Smith-Magenis microdeletion critical region in 17p11.2. *Am J Hum Genet* 56:175–182.

Chen KS, Manian P, Koeuth T, Potocki L, Zhao Q, Chinault CA, Lee CC, Lupski JR (1997) Homologous recombination of a flanking repeat gene cluster is a mechanism for a common contiguous gene deletion syndrome. *Nat Genet* 17:154–163.

Chen KS, Potocki L, Lupski JR (1996) The Smith-Magenis syndrome (del(17)(p11.2)): Clinical review and molecular advances. *Mental Retard Dev Disabil Res Rev* 2:122–129.

Chen RM, Lupski JR, Greenberg F, Lewis RA (1996) Ophthalmic manifestations of Smith-Magenis syndrome. *Ophthalmology* 103:1084–1091.

Chevillard C, Le Paslier D, Passarge E, Ougen P, Billault A, Boyer S, Mazan S, Bachellerie JP, Vignal A, Cohen D, Fontes M (1993) Relationship between Charcot-Marie-Tooth 1A and Smith-Magenis regions: snU3 may be a candidate gene for the Smith-Magenis syndrome. *Hum Mol Genet* 2:1235–1243.

Colley AF, Leversha MA, Voullaire LE, Rogers JG (1990) Five cases demonstrating the distinctive behavioural features of chromosome deletion 17(p11.2 p11.2) (Smith-Magenis syndrome). *J Paediatr Child Hth* 26:17–21.

De Leersnyder H, Von Kleist-Retzow JC, Munnich A, Claustrat B, Lyonnet S, Vekemans M, De Bois MC (1999) Inversion of the circadian rhythm of melatonin in Smith-Magenis syndrome. *Am J Hum Genet* 65(Suppl.):A2.

Del Vecchio MA, Matika GL, Grebe TA, Butler MG, Powell CM, Smith ACM, Curry CJR, Stevenson RE, Greenberg F, Bay CA (1998) Food foraging behaviors: A phenotypic overlap between Smith-Magenis and Prader-Willi syndromes. *Am J Hum Genet* 63:557.

Denny AD, Weik LD, Lubinsky MS, Wyatt DT (1992) Lethal adrenal aplasia in an infant with Smith-Magenis syndrome, deletion 17p112. *J Dysmorph Clin Genet* 6(4):175–179.

de Rijk-van Andel JF, Catsman-Berrevoets, van Hemel JO, Hamers AJH (1991) Clinical and chromosome studies of three patients with Smith-Magenis syndrome. *Dev Med Child Neurol* 33:343–355.

Dykens E, Finucane B, Gayley C (1997) Cognitive and behavioral profiles in persons with Smith-Magenis syndrome. *J Autism Dev Disord* 27:203–211.

Dykens E, Smith ACM (1998) Distinctiveness and correlates of maladaptive behavior in children and adolescents with Smith-Magenis syndrome. *J Intellect Disabil Res* 42:481–489.

Elsea SA, Finucane B, Juyal RC, Schoener-Scott R, Hauge X, Chinault AC, Greenberg F, Patel PI (1996) Smith-Magenis syndrome due to a submicroscopic deletion in 17p11.2 allows further definition of the critical interval. *Am J Hum Genet* 59, (Suppl):A257.

Elsea SH, Fritz E, Schoener-Scott R, Meyn MS, Patel PI (1998) The gene for topoisomerase III maps within the Smith-Magenis syndrome critical region: Analysis of cell cycle distribution and radiation sensitivity. *Am J Med Genet* 75:104–108.

Elsea SH, Purandare SM, Adell RA, Juyal RC, Davis JG, Finucane B, Magenis RE, Patel PI (1997) Definition of the critical interval for Smith-Magenis syndrome. *Cytogenet Cell Genet* 79:276–281.

Elsea SA, Ramesh CJ, Jiralerspong S, Finucane BM, Pandolfo M, Greenberg F, Baldini A, Stover P, Patel PI (1995) Haploinsufficiency of cytosolic serine hydroxymethyltransferase in the Smith-Magenis syndrome. *Am J Hum Genet* 57:1342–1350.

Finucane BM, Jaeger ER, Kurtz MB, Weinstein M, Scott CI (1993b) Eye abnormalities in the Smith-Magenis contiguous gene deletion syndrome. *Am J Med Genet* 45:443–446.

Finucane, BM, Konar D, Givler BH, Kurtz MB, Scott LI (1994) The spasmodic upper-body squeeze: A characteristic behavior in Smith-Magenis syndrome. *Dev Med Child Neurol* 36:70–83.

Finucane BM, Kurtz M, Babu VR, Scott CI (1993a) Mosaicism for deletion 17p11.2 in a boy with the Smith-Magenis syndrome. *Am J Med Genet* 45:447–449.

Finucane B, Smith ACM, Elsea SH, Greenberg F, Patel PI (1996) Hypercholesterolemia in patients with del(17)(p11.2) (Smith-Magenis syndrome). *Am J Hum Genet* 59(*Suppl*):A350.

Friedman TB, Liang Y, Weber JL, Hinnant JT, Barber TD, Winata S, Arhya IN, et al. (1995) A gene for congenital recessive deafness *DFNB3* maps to the pericentromeric region of chromosome 17. *Nat Genet* 9:86–91.

Greenberg F, Guzzetta V, De Oca-Luna RM, Magenis RE, Smith ACM, Richter SF, Kondo I, Dobyns WB, Patel PI, Lupski J (1991) Molecular analysis of the Smith-Magenis syndrome: A possible contiguous-gene syndrome associated with del(17)(p11.2). *Am J Hum Genet* 49:1207–1218.

Greenberg R, Lewis RA, Potocki L, Glaze D, Parke J, Killian J, Murphy MA, Williamson D, Brown F, Dutton R, McCluggage C, Friedman E, Sulek M, Lupski JR (1996) Multidisciplinary clinical study of Smith-Magenis syndrome (deletion 17p11.2). *Am J Med Genet* 62:247–254.

Gropman A, Smith ACM, Greenberg F (1998a) Neurologic aspects of the Smith-Magenis syndrome. *Ann Neurol* 44:561.

Gropman A, Smith ACM, Allanson J, Greenberg F (1998b) Smith Magenis syndrome: Aspects of the infant phenotype. *Am J Hum Genet* 63(*Suppl*):A19.

Gropman A, Wolters P, Smith ACM (1999) Neurodevelopmental assessment and functioning in five young children with Smith-Magenis syndrome. *Am J Hum Genet* 65(*Suppl*):A141.

Haas-Givler B (1994) Educational Implications and Behavioral Concerns of SMS — From the Teacher's Perspective. *Spectrum* 1(2) 3–4 [official newsletter of PRISMS].

Haas-Givler B, Finucane B (1995) What's Teacher to Do: Classroom Strategies That Enhance Learning for Children with SMS. *Spectrum* 2(1) [official newsletter of PRISMS].

Hagerman R (1999) Smith-Magenis Syndrome. In: *Neurodevelopmental Disorders: Diagnosis and Treatment*, Hagerman R, (ed.) New York: Oxford University Press, p. 341–362.

Hodapp RM, Fidler DJ, Smith ACM (1998) Stress and coping in families of children with Smith-Magenis syndrome. *J Intellec Disabil Res* 42:331–340.

Howard-Peebles PH, Friedman JM, Harrod MJ, Brookshire GC, Lockwood JE (1985) A stable supernumerary chromosome derived from a deleted segment of 17p. *Am J Hum Genet* 37(*Suppl*):A97.

Hua X, Wu J, Goldstein JL, Brown MS, Hobbs HH (1995) Structure of the human gene encoding sterol regulatory element binding protein-1 (*SREBF1*) and localization of *SREBF1* and *SREBF2* to chromosomes 17p11.2 and 22q13. *Genomics* 25:667–673.

Jan JE, Esperzel H, Appleton RE (1994) The treatment of sleep disorders with melatonin. *Deve. Med and Child Neurol* 36:97–107.

Jan JE, Espezel H (1995) Melatonin treatment of chronic sleep disorders. *Devel Med and Child Neurol* 37:279–281.

Juyal RC, Figuera LE, Hauge X, Elsea SH, Lupski JR, Greenberg F, Baldini A, Patel PI (1996) Molecular analysis of 17p11.2 deletion in 62 Smith-Magenis syndrome patients. *Am J Hum Genet* 58:998–1007.

Juyal RC, Finucane B, Shaffer LG, Lupski JR, Greenberg F, Scott CI, Baldini A, Patel PI (1995b) Letter to the Editor: Apparent mosaicism for del(17)(p11.2) ruled out by fluorescence in situ hybridization in a Smith-Magenis syndrome patient. *Am J Med Genet* 59:406–407.

Juyal RC, Greenberg F, Mengden GA, Lupski JR, Trask BJ, van den Engh G, Lindsay EA, Christ H, Chen K-S, Baldini A, Shaffer LG, Patel PI (1995a) Smith-Magenis syndrome deletion: A case with equivocal cytogenetic findings resolved by fluorescence in situ hybridization. *Am J Med Genet* 58:286–291.

Kimura T, Arakawa Y, Inoue S, Fukushima Y, Kondo I, Koyama K, Hosoi T, Orimo A, Muramatsu M, Nakamura Y, Abe T, Inazawa J (1997) The brain finger protein gene (*ZNF179*), a member of the RING finger family, maps within the Smith-Magenis syndrome region at 17p11.2. *Am J Med Genet* 69:320–324.

Kondo I, Matsuura S, Kuwajima K, Tokashiki M, Izumikawa Y, Naritomi K, Niikawa N, Kajii T (1991) Diagnostic hand anomalies in Smith-Magenis syndrome: Four new patients with del(17)(p11.2p11.2). *Am J Med Genet* 41:225–229.

Koyama K, Fukushima Y, Inazawa J, Tomotsune D, Takahashi N, Nakamura Y (1996) The human homologue of the murine *Llglh* gene (*LLGL*) maps within the Smith-Magenis syndrome region in 17p11.2. *Cytogenet Cell Genet* 72:78–82.

Liang Y, Chen KS, Potocki L, Wang A, Fridell RA, Lupski JR, Friedman TB (1998) High frequency hearing loss in an individual with Smith-Magenis syndrome likely due to a missense mutation in *MYO15* uncovered by del(17)(p11.2p11.2). *Am J Hum Genet* 63(*Suppl*): A333.

Liang Y, Want A, Probst FJ, Arhya IN, Barber TD, Chen K-S, Deshmukh D, Dolan DF, Hinnant JT, Carter LE, Jain PK, Lalwani AK, Li XC, Lupski JR, Moeljopapiro S, Morell R, Negrini C, Wilcox ER, Winata S, Camper SA, Friedman TB (1998) Genetic mapping refines *DFNB3* to 17p11.2, suggests multiple alleles of *DFNB3*, and supports homology to the mouse model shaker-2. *Am J Hum Genet* 62:904–915.

Lockwood D, Hecht F, Dowman C, Hecht BK, Rizkallah TH, Goodwin TM, Allanson J (1988) Chromosome sub-band 17p11.2 deletion: A minute deletion syndrome. *J Med Genet* 25:732–737.

Lupski JR (1998) Genomic disorders: Structural features of the genome can lead to DNA rearrangements and human disease traits. *Trends Genet* 14:417–422.

Lupski JR, Montes de Oca-Luna R, Slaugenhaupt S, Pentao L, Guzetta V, Trask BJ, Saucedo-Cardenas O et al. (1991) DNA duplication associated with Charcot-Marie-Tooth disease type 1A. *Cell* 66:219–232.

Masuno M, Asano J, Arai M, Kuwahara T, Orii T (1992) Interstitial deletion of 17p11.2 with brain abnormalities. *Clin Genet* 41:278–280.

Meinecke P (1993) Confirmation of a particular but nonspecfic metacarpophalangeal pattern profile in patients with the Smith-Magnes syndrome due to interstitial deletion of 17p. *Am J Med Genet* 45:441–442.

Moncla A, Prias L, Arbex OF, Muscatelli F, Mattei M-G, Mattei J-F, Fontes M (1993) Physical mapping of microdeletions of the chromosome 17 short arm associated with Smith-Magenis syndrome. *Hum Genet* 90:657–660.

Patel PI, Franco B, Garcia C, Slaugenhaupt SA, Nakamura Y, Ledbetter DH, Chakravarti A, Lupski JR (1990) Genetic mapping of autosomal dominant Charcot-Marie-Tooth disease in a large French-Acadian kindred: Identification of new linked markers on chromosome 17. *Am J Hum Genet* 46:801–809.

Patel SR, Bartley JA (1984) Interstitial deletion of the short arm of chromosome 17. *Hum Genet* 67:237–238.

Potocki L, Chen K-S, Lupski JR (1999) Subunit 3 of the *COP9* signal transduction complex is conserved from plants to humans and maps within the Smith-Magenis syndrome critical region in 17p11.2. *Genomics* 57:180–182.

Potocki L, Glaze D, Tan DX, Park SS, Kashork CD, Shaffer LG, Reiter RJ, Lupski JR (2000) Circadian rhythm abnormalities of melatonin in Smith-Magenis syndrome. *J Med Genet* 37(6):428–433.

Salati R, Marini G, Degiuli A, Dalpra L (1996) Brown's syndrome associated with Smith-Magenis syndrome. *Strabismus* 4:139–143.

Schmickel RD (1986) Contiguous gene syndromes: a component of recognizable syndromes. *J Pediatr* 109:231–241.

Smith ACM 1997 personal communication at 1st SMS National Conference, Bethesda, MD.

Smith ACM, Dykens E, Greenberg F (1998a) Behavioral phenotype of Smith-Magenis syndrome (del 17p11.2). *Am J Med Genet* 81:179–185.

Smith ACM, Dykens E, Greenberg F (1998b) Sleep disturbance in Smith-Magenis syndrome (del 17p11.2). *Am J Med Genet* 81:186–191.

Smith ACM, McGavran L, Robinson J, Waldstein G, Macfarlane J, Zonona J, Reiss J, Lahr M, Allen L, Magenis E (1986) Interstitial deletion of (17)(p11.2p11.2) in nine patients. *Am J Med Genet* 24:393–414.

Smith ACM , McGavran L, Waldstein G (1982) Deletion of the 17 short arm in two patients with facial clefts. *Am J Hum Genet* 34(*Suppl*): A410.

Smith ACM, Wilkin DJ, Goker-Alpan O, Elsea SH, Patel PI, Gropman AL, Greenberg F (1998) Cholesterol abnormalities in Smith-Magenis syndrome: Haploinsufficiency of *SREBP1* in del(17)(p11.2). *Am J Hum Genet* 63(*Suppl*): A19.

Sonies BC, Solomon B, Ondrey F, McCullah L, Greenberg F, Smith ACM (1997). Oral-motor and otolaryngologic findings in 14 patients with Smith-Magenis syndrome (17p11.2): Results of an interdisciplinary study. *Am J Hum Genet* (*Suppl*)61: A5.

Stratton RF, Dobyns WB, Greenberg F, De Sana JB, Moore C, Fidone G, Runge GH, et al. (1986) Interstitial deletion of (17) (p11.2p11.2): Report of six additional patients with a new chromosome deletion syndrome. *Am J Med Genet* 24:421–432.

Sun ZS, Albrecht U, Zhuchenko O, Bailey J, Eichele G, Lee CC (1997) *RUGUI*, a putative mammalian ortholog of the Drosophila period gene. *Cell* 90:1003–1011.

Townsend-Nicholson A, Baker E, Sutherland GR, Schofield PR (1995) Localization of the adenosine A2b receptor subtype gene (*ADORA2B*) to chromosome 17p11.2-p12 by FISH and PCR screening of somatic cell hybrids. *Genomics* 25:605–607.

Trask BJ, Mefford H, van den Engh G, Massa HF, Juyal RC, Potocki L, Finucane B, Abuelo DN, Sitt Dr, Magenis E, Baldini A, Greenberg F, Lupski JR, Patel PI (1996) Quantification of flow cytometry of chromosome 17 deletions in Smith-Magenis syndrome patients. *Hum Genet* 98:710–718.

Wang A, Lian Y, Fridell RA, Probst FJ, Wilcox ER, Touchman JW, Morton CC, Morell RJ, Noben-Trauth K, Camper SA, Friedman TB (1998) Association of unconventional myosin *MYO15* mutations with human nonsyndromic deafness *DFNB3*. *Science* 280:1477–1451.

Wiggs L, Stores G (1996) Severe sleep disturbances and daytime challenging behavior in children with severe learning disabilities. *J Intellect Disabil Res* 40:518–528.

Yang SP, Bidichandani SI, Figuera LE, Juyal RC, Saxon PJ, Daldinia A, Patel PI (1997) Molecular analysis of deletion (17)(p11.2p11.2) in a family segregating a 17p paracentric inversion: Implications for carriers of paracentric inversions. *Am J Hum Genet* 60:1184–1193.

Zhao Z, Lee C-C, Jiralerspong S, Juyal RC, Lu F, Baldini A, Greenberg F, Caskey CT, Patel PI (1995) The gene for human microfibril-associated glycoprotein is commonly deleted in Smith-Magenis syndrome patients. *Hum Mol Genet* 4:589–597.

Zori RT, Lupski JR, Heju Z, Greenberg F, Killian JM, Gray BA, Driscoll DJ, Patel PI, Zackowski JL (1993) Clinical, cytogenetic, and molecular evidence for an infant with Smith-Magenis syndrome born from a mother having a mosaic 17p11.2p12 deletion. *Am J Med Genet* 47:504–511.

CHAPTER 23

SOTOS SYNDROME

TREVOR R.P. COLE

INTRODUCTION

Incidence

Sotos syndrome was first recognized as a distinct clinical syndrome in New England in 1964 (Sotos et al., 1964), although probable cases do exist in the earlier literature. One example with significant corroborating data is that of Schlesinger in 1931. Since the original report there have been several comprehensive reviews of the clinical features and literature (Jaeken et al., 1972; Wit et al., 1985; Cole and Hughes, 1994). In a survey of 40 cases of Sotos syndrome, the average age of diagnosis was 26.6 months (Cole and Hughes, 1994). However, most of the children were born in the 1970s and 1980s, and, with increasing professional knowledge, it is likely that the age at diagnosis is decreasing and the frequency of diagnosis is increasing (personal experience).

The incidence remains unknown but appears only slightly less common than one other "common" overgrowth syndrome, Beckwith-Wiedemann syndrome, for which a birth prevalence of 1 in 13,700 has been reported (Thorburn et al., 1970). The potential errors of this figure have been discussed elsewhere (Cole, 1998).

Diagnostic Criteria

There are no diagnostic tests that will confirm the diagnosis of Sotos syndrome; thus clinical diagnostic criteria need to be applied in each individual case. However, many of these are "soft" features or features common in the general population, and, therefore, "loose" interpretation will almost certainly lead to many misdiagnoses, as is evident in the literature. The four core features reported in the original paper are rapid early growth (pre- and postnatal), advanced bone age, developmental delay, and characteristic facial appearance. The first three features are relative to population normal values, and where the threshold should be drawn is obviously open to debate. Bone age may also be subject to observer error. Furthermore, these criteria are characteristic of several different overgrowth syndromes. It is also important to recognize that these features will be influenced by familial patterns, for example, parental heights that lie toward the upper limit of the normal population distribution or families that exhibit "genuine" large stature or rapid maturation. The typical growth pattern seen in Sotos syndrome is discussed in the section on growth assessment and management below.

The last feature, the characteristic facial appearance, is specific to Sotos syndrome.

Management of Genetic Syndromes, Edited by Suzanne B. Cassidy and Judith E. Allanson
ISBN 0-471-31286-X   Copyright © 2001 by Wiley-Liss, Inc.

However, this remains the most subjective of the four diagnostic criteria, despite attempts to improve the objectivity (Allanson and Cole, 1996).

The facial morphology alters during childhood and adolescence (Figs. 23.1 and 23.2), following changes similar to those seen in the general population, with lengthening of the face superimposed on the background of abnormal facial dimensions intrinsic to this disorder. This results in an evolving, yet characteristic, facial gestalt at different ages (Allanson and Cole, 1996).

The features noted in the newborn period are macrocephaly, a high bossed forehead, a high palate, and an appearance suggestive of hypertelorism because of temporal narrowing. Initially, the jaw often appears small, but within the first 1–2 years the face lengthens and the jaw becomes more prominent. The forehead remains broad and the chin remains narrow, which gives the facial outline a shape similar to an inverted pear. During this time dolichocephaly and frontal bossing become more obvious, the latter because of a striking delay in the growth of hair in the frontoparietal regions (Fig. 23.1A).

In the midchildhood period a downslant to the palpebral fissures, wear and discoloration of teeth, and a tendency to a rosy coloration to the cheeks, chin, and nasal tip, or rapid changes in facial coloring, all become more obvious. Into adulthood the face becomes longer and relatively thinner (particularly the bizygomatic diameter), but the skull still shows marked dolichocephaly and macrocephaly (Fig. 23.1B). Despite these changes and a "normalization" of the overall facial appearance, the facial gestalt can be recognized by experienced dysmorphologists and distinguished from other overgrowth or familial features, as documented in Cole and Hughes (1994).

When the above diagnostic criteria are strictly applied during childhood, all four are present in at least 75% of true cases of Sotos syndrome but in a lower percentage (<20%) of other specific and nonspecific overgrowth patterns (Wit et al., 1985; Cole and Hughes, 1994).

In 1997, Schaefer et al. examined the cranial MRI findings in 40 patients who had a characteristic facial gestalt and at least two of the other clinical criteria suggestive

(A)

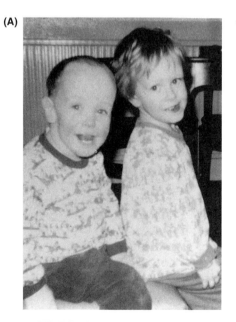

(B)

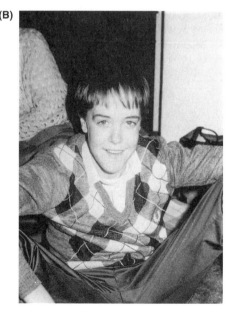

FIGURE 23.1. A. Sotos syndrome at age 18 months. B. Sotos syndrome at age 14 years.

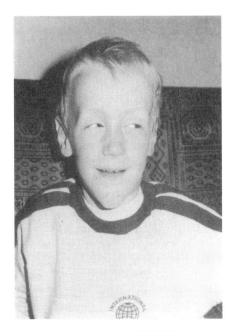 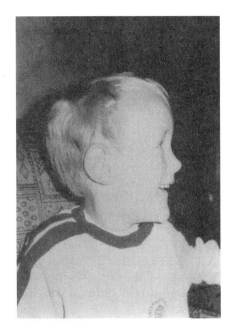

FIGURE 23.2. Sotos syndrome at age 4 years.

of Sotos syndrome listed above (Schaefer et al., 1997). The neuroradiological findings included ventricular abnormalities with a prominence of the trigone (90%), prominent occipital horns (75%), and ventriculomegaly (63%). Midline defects were also frequent, and absence or hypoplasia of the corpus callosum was found in almost all cases. It was therefore suggested that these findings could be utilized to distinguish Sotos syndrome from other mental retardation syndromes with macrocephaly. Although caution is advisable on this point, because these findings can be seen in other overgrowth patterns (personal experience), the neuroradiological findings could still be a useful adjunct to the other four diagnostic criteria.

Several other medical markers may also aid in arriving at the correct diagnosis. The more significant of these are discussed later in the text. More minor or transient features documented in early childhood include neonatal feeding difficulties, jaundice, poor nail growth (rate and quality), and tendency to increased sweating. An unexpectedly large

appetite and thirst (even allowing for size), increased sensitivity to certain sensations such as the texture of food or combing hair, but high pain threshold (the latter particularly over the trunk), are all later childhood features that have been frequently reported by parents.

Etiology, Pathogenesis, and Genetics

The etiology remains unclear. The majority of cases are sporadic, but a small number of families (<2%) appear to show autosomal dominant inheritance [4 of over 200 cases (personal experience)]. It is perhaps worth noting that the facial gestalt in those 4 families is less typical than in most sporadic cases, and this might reflect a different mutational mechanism. There are also several literature reports of vertical transmission of Sotos syndrome or affected siblings with the condition, but few are typical in their appearance and most would not meet strict diagnostic criteria. Other reports provide inadequate data to confirm the diagnosis in the extended family. In particular, tall adult stature with unspecified difficulties at school should not be considered adequate to make a diagnosis of Sotos syndrome in an adult, in light of the frequency of these findings in the general population. Furthermore, increased adult height is not necessarily characteristic of Sotos syndrome (see section on growth).

In one study, careful examination of parents and siblings of 40 probands showed no clear evidence of the condition in any of the 80 parents, 47 siblings, and 23 half-siblings (personal experience). All available parents (69) and full siblings (43) were personally examined by the author. Only 6 of 23 half-siblings were available to be examined. In addition, childhood photographs of examined and unexamined parents and siblings were studied in almost all cases. Therefore, in the absence of a definite diagnosis in a first-degree relative, the risk of recurrence is small. Parental ages have been reported as normal (Wit et al., 1985) but were subsequently reported as showing a significantly elevated paternal age in a slightly larger series (Cole and Hughes, 1994). These latter findings raise the possibility of a high frequency of de novo mutations.

The presence of overgrowth with relatively few structural abnormalities and occasional autosomal dominant families shows significant similarities to Beckwith-Wiedemann syndrome (see Chapter 4). This latter condition is caused by mutations within a cluster of imprinted genes at 11p15.5, which are either overexpressed or have "escaped" normal regulation, depending on the function of the specific gene involved (Reik and Maher, 1997). Uniparental disomy, the inheritance of both copies of a homologous pair of chromosomes from the same parent, is one mechanism resulting in excess gene expression in Beckwith-Wiedemann syndrome. Therefore, molecular studies were undertaken in 29 patients with Sotos syndrome (Smith et al., 1997). The results were negative but would only have detected nonmosaic uniparental disomy if present in greater than 10% of cases.

Diagnostic uncertainties are encountered with many case reports of different karyotypic abnormalities in children with a "Sotos-like" phenotype. One clear exception is a child with an apparently balanced translocation between 3p21 and 6p21 (Schrander-Stumpel et al., 1990) who did fulfill strict diagnostic criteria. The breakpoint at 3p21 appeared of particular interest in view of the region's association with small cell lung carcinoma, a tumor reported in a 23-year-old nonsmoker with Sotos syndrome (Cole et al., 1992). However, the breakpoint has now been reassigned to 3p22, and therefore these may be coincidental findings (Kok et al., 1999).

A paper reporting the inheritance of translocations involving 4p16.3 is of interest because duplication of 4p appears to cosegregate with overgrowth (Partington et al., 1997). However, the phenotype is rather atypical of Sotos syndrome, although it does show some similarities to a dominant overgrowth disorder reported in 1989 (Mangano et al., 1989). To date, no duplication of this region has been reported in cases of Sotos syndrome.

Differential Diagnosis

The primary feature that is likely to raise suspicion of a diagnosis of Sotos syndrome is overgrowth; therefore, the major differential diagnoses are conditions associated with excess growth. The overgrowth may involve all tissues or be tissue- or site specific. Examples of the latter include Klippel-Trenaunay-Weber syndrome, Proteus syndrome, macrocephaly syndromes, fragile X syndrome, Marfan syndrome, and Prader-Willi syndrome. These should be easily distinguishable by their own distinct clinical phenotypes and lack of generalized overgrowth.

The phenotypic overlap between Sotos syndrome and fragile X syndrome (see Chapter 10) has been the subject of several papers. However, these syndromes are usually dissimilar, and in none of the reported cases has the facial gestalt been typical. In the study of 40 typical cases of Sotos syndrome reported by Cole and Hughes (1994), all 36 children tested cytogenetically had normal karyotypes and were negative for the fragile X syndrome. Subsequently, molecular analysis of the fragile X gene was carried out in 29 of these cases and was negative in all instances (Smith et al., 1997).

Frequently, measurement of span and upper-to-lower body segment ratio reveals that much of the excess growth in Sotos syndrome is in the limbs rather than the trunk. Thus in patients with minor skeletal changes and a thin body habitus, as is common, there is some adult phenotypic overlap with Marfan syndrome (see Chapter 13). However, careful examination of other systems and childhood features confirms the distinct nature of these two conditions.

More difficult to distinguish clinically are those disorders with generalized macrosomia (Table 23.1). In a few cases there may be a reliable diagnostic test, for example, in congenital adrenal hyperplasia, ACTH receptor deficiency, pituitary or adrenal secretory tumors, and Sanfilippo syndrome. In the remaining cases there is either no diagnostic test, for example, Weaver syndrome, or it is not yet feasible to use in clinical practice, for example, Beckwith-Wiedemann and Simpson-Golabi-Beh-mel syndromes.

The overgrowth conditions of Beckwith-Wiedemann syndrome, Simpson-Golabi-Behmel syndrome, Perlman syndrome, Nevo syndrome, and MOMO syndrome have a number of hard diagnostic features, which facilitate discrimination (Table 23.2). Discussion and comparison of the clinical features of Beckwith-Wiedemann (see Chapter 4) and Simpson-Golabi-Behmel syndromes are presented in some detail elsewhere (Cohen, 1989; Cole, 1998).

The differentiation between Sotos syndrome, Weaver syndrome, Marshall-Smith

TABLE 23.1. Generalized Overgrowth Disorders

Disorders with Overgrowth as a Frequent and Major Component

Familial/sporadic constitutional gigantism
Bannayan-Riley-Ruvalcaba syndrome
Beckwith-Wiedemann syndrome
Marshall-Smith syndrome
MOMO syndrome
Nevo syndrome
Perlman syndrome
Seip-Berardinelli syndrome
Simpson-Golabi-Behmel syndrome
Sotos syndrome
Weaver syndrome

Disorders with Overgrowth as an Occasional and Minor Component

ACTH receptor deficiency
Congenital adrenal hyperplasia
Pituitary/adrenal and gonadal secretory tumors
Familial precocious maturation
Klinefelter syndrome
Sanfilippo syndrome

TABLE 23.2. Features (Excluding Overgrowth and Advanced Bone Age) in BeckwithWiedemann, Simpson-Golabi-Behmel, Perlman, MOMO, and Nevo Syndromes

Beckwith-Wiedemann Syndrome	Simpson-Golabi-Behmel Syndrome	Perlman Syndrome	Nevo Syndrome	MOMO Syndrome
Macroglossia	Macrostomia	Deep-set eyes	Dolichocephaly	Prominent forehead
Facial hemangiomas	Orofacial clefts	Wide, depressed nasal bridge	Short palpebral fissures	Large ears
	Hypertelorism			
Ear creases/pits		Gum hypertrophy	Myopia	Large nose
	Coarse facies			
Omphalocele	Large/grooved tongue	Everted lower lip	Prominent nasal bridge	Macrostomia
Abdominal wall defects	Ear creases	Sternal abnormalities	Micrognathia	Downturned corners of mouth
Visceromegaly	Polysyndactyly	Congenital heart disease	Kyphoscoliosis	Glaucoma
Abdominal tumors	Broad hands		Narrow chest	Coloboma
		Intestinal malrotation		
Hemihypertrophy	Square terminal phalanges		Contractures of large and small joints	Nystagmus
Hypoglycemia		Splenic abnormalities		Truncal obesity
	Extra ribs			
			Edema of hands and feet	Short, broad chest
Normal head circumference	Extra nipples	Pancreatic cysts		
	Segmentation defects	Congential heart disease	Tapering digits	Hypoplastic nipples
			Cryptorchidism	
	Defect of cardiac conduction	Renal cysts and dysplasia		Brachydactyly
	Abdominal wall defects	Hydronephrosis		Clubbed nails
		Nephropathy		Delayed bone age
	Visceromegaly and tumors	Wilms tumors		Cutis marmorata
		Cryptorchidism		
	Intestinal malrotation	Hypospadias		
	Renal malformations	Hypoglycemia		
	Cryptorchidism			

TABLE 23.3. Facial Dysmorphism of Sotos Syndrome, Weaver Syndrome, Marshall-Smith Syndrome, and Constitutional Large Stature

Sotos Syndrome	Weaver Syndrome	Marshall-Smith Syndrome	Constitutional Gigantism
Frontal bossing	Round forehead	Fine facial features & bones	Nonspecific features likely to be familial
High forehead	Round face (early childhood)	Thin, gaunt gestalt	
Bizygomatic narrowing	Large, dysplastic ears	Prominent eyes	
Downslanting palpebral fissures	Hypertelorism	Depressed nasal bridge	
Hypertelorism	Prominent philtrum	Anteverted nares	
Long face	Long philtrum	Micrognathia	
Long mandible	Small, distinct mandible	Choanal atresia	
Face pear-shaped outline	Dimpled/grooved mandible	Hyperextension of neck	
Facial flushing	Macrocephaly	Thick eyebrows	
High palate	<100%	Overfolded ear helix	
Slow hair growth in frontoparietal region			

syndrome, and constitutional gigantism is primarily based on subjective clinical opinion of the facial gestalt. The individual facial features are listed in Table 23.3. The most difficult differential diagnosis is between Sotos syndrome and Weaver syndrome. The facial appearance of Weaver syndrome in infancy (Fig. 23.3) includes a small chin and characteristic round face. However, during the first year of life the jaw in Sotos syndrome may also appear relatively small. A dimpled soft tissue pad on the anterior aspect of the chin in Weaver syndrome is often quite distinctive. Contractures of the large and small joints are significantly more common in Weaver syndrome. Observation of Marshall-Smith syndrome reveals that many affected children fail to thrive soon after birth, and they often die in the early childhood period. Additional features suggestive of Marshall-Smith syndrome (Fig. 23.4) include fine, gaunt facial features, "bullet"-shaped middle phalanges, and an anterior occipital spur at the base of the skull.

Consideration of the diagnosis of Sotos syndrome in patients with constitutional gigantism probably only occurs if developmental delay is also present. The concurrence of these features will often be coincidental because of the frequency of developmental delay in the population. In patients with constitutional large stature, one might predict that the absence of the typical facial gestalt and a normal bone age would exclude the

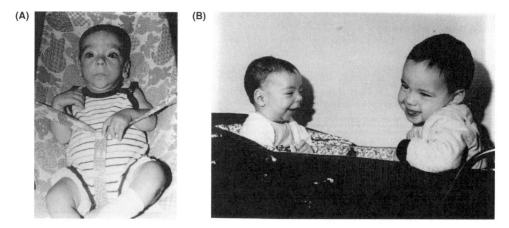

FIGURE 23.3. Weaver syndrome at ages 3 (A) and 7 (B) months.

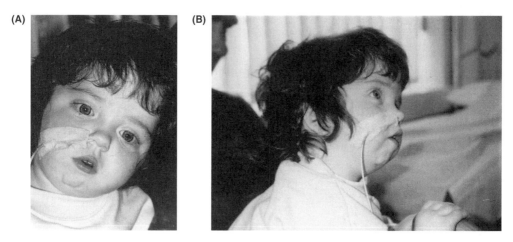

FIGURE 23.4. Marshall-Smith syndrome at age 2 years (A), 9 months (B).

diagnosis. Because neither of these features is invariably present, this is not always the case.

All cases undergoing diagnostic evaluation should have a bone age assessment. Other investigations should ideally include a karyotype and molecular fragile X analysis to exclude these anomalies. Where diagnostic doubt remains, an MRI of the brain may be beneficial. Any case demonstrating regression or early plateauing of developmental milestones requires a metabolic assessment and, in particular, exclusion of Sanfillipo syndrome.

MANIFESTATIONS AND MANAGEMENT

Growth and Feeding

Feeding difficulties are common in the neonatal period, and as many as 25% of term babies have required tube feeding (Cole and Hughes, 1994). Failure to suck and coordinate swallowing because of anatomical features, hypotonia, and immaturity may be the commonest reasons for such symptoms. Protracted feeding difficulties lasting several months have been recognized and may cause failure to thrive in the first year of life.

Most babies with Sotos syndrome will be large for gestational age at delivery. It is important to recognize that the most significantly elevated measurement is likely to be birth length (mean + 3.2 SD), followed by head circumference (mean + 1.8 SD), and weight (mean + 1.0 SD), and approximately 85% of newborn babies will have a birth weight below the 97th centile (Cole and Hughes, 1994). In the neonatal and early infant period there is also commonly a period of failure to thrive, probably secondary to feeding difficulties and medical complications, lasting as long as 3 or 4 months, which may "mask" the diagnosis (personal experience).

By 12 months of age, overgrowth is almost invariably present. Throughout childhood, height and head circumference are usually the most significantly elevated growth parameters, running parallel to but significantly above the 97th centile. Most children have relatively thin limbs and trunk, and measurement of span-to-height and upper-to-lower body segment ratios reveals that much of the excess growth is in the limbs rather than the trunk. Hands and feet are usually large, even when plotted against height age. Early height predictions are almost always excessive, and endocrine intervention in adolescence is rarely necessary (personal experience).

Final height in Sotos syndrome is influenced by parental heights (i.e., target heights). In a series of 18 British girls who had achieved their final height, this measurement had a mean value of 172.9 cm (UK population mean 163.5 cm), which was only 6.2 cm above their mean target height prediction (Agwu et al., 1999). The initial hypothesis was that the girls went through an early puberty (mean age of menarche 12.2 ± 1.8 years; UK mean 13 years) and therefore had an early cessation of growth. However, the two girls with the most delayed menarche (15.4 and 14 years) both still had heights less than the 97th centile. Therefore, it seems likely that early puberty and fusion of the epiphyses is not the complete explanation.

The situation in boys is more unpredictable, and there is a greater tendency to increased adult stature. Data are available on 9 adult males with a mean final height of 184.3 cm (UK population mean 175.5 cm). It was notable that their target height had only been 173 cm, i.e., less than the UK population mean, and that the mean excess in final height, compared to the predicted target height, was +11.3 cm with a range of +5 to +20 cm (Agwu et al., 1999). The timing of puberty in boys is also more widely distributed and less closely associated with bone age.

Evaluation

- Longitudinal monitoring of growth, bone age, and puberty may be beneficial from about 7 or 8 years of age because it can provide some clarification of the likely growth outcome.

Treatment

- There is no feasible or justifiable endocrine intervention during the first 10 years of life.
- Endocrine intervention to initiate early puberty has been prescribed in two females and one male (personal experience). There was no clear evidence of significant change in the final height outcome. If cessation of linear growth is achieved too early, the detrimental effect of changing from one of the largest to one of the smallest in a peer group, and the possible increased disproportion of height to head circumference and hand and foot lengths, must be considered.
- Experience from a large, untreated cohort would suggest that intervention is rarely necessary (personal experience).

Development and Behavior

Almost all children with Sotos syndrome present some features of development delay and cognitive impairment, but the severity is very variable and may be inconsistent across different areas within a single individual. The high frequency could be due to selection bias, because this is one of the diagnostic criteria.

All individuals exhibit some delay in achieving early milestones, and this is most noticeable for motor skills (personal experience). The degree of motor delay is a poor predictor of long-term cognitive and educational achievement. This may partly be explained by the deleterious effect of marked hypotonia and large body size, present in 100% of cases (Cole and Hughes, 1994).

Although hypotonia improves over the first few years of life, many individuals have significant coordination difficulties throughout childhood, affecting both fine and gross motor skills, the latter commonly to a greater degree (personal experience). The early excessive drooling and poor enunciation are also likely to be a result of the low tone and poor coordination.

Language delays are also usually present but display greater variability and may show some correlation with long-term educational outcome, particularly if later milestones such as use of sentences are considered. Speech delay is often exacerbated by hearing loss, but the latter is usually mild and secondary to otitis media. A small number of children have a proven sensorineural component.

The age that toilet training is achieved shows a wide range, from normal to significantly delayed.

Childhood assessment of intellectual function identifies a wide range of ability both between and within individuals with Sotos syndrome, with an IQ range between 21 and 103 with a mean of 74 (Rutter and Cole, 1991; Finegan et al., 1994). Almost half the children are in regular school, although placement will be influenced not only by IQ but also by local educational resources and the child's behavioral patterns (Rutter and

Cole, 1991; Finegan et al., 1994). Intellectual abilities may be difficult to assess reliably because of both behavior patterns and variation in skills, such as relatively good reading accuracy but more limited comprehension, which is commonly seen. Another area often significantly impaired is arithmetic skills (Rutter and Cole, 1991; Finegan et al., 1994). Although a single typical cognitive pattern is not found, more abstract or conceptual subjects caused greater difficulty than more concrete or visual processes.

Behavior is one of the key areas influencing family and personal outcome. Difficult behavior is almost universally present, although no specific or diagnostic profile is apparent and the severity is variable (Rutter and Cole, 1991; Finegan et al., 1994). From about the age of 2 years an increased tendency to tantrums and aggressive behavior, often directed against family members, has been reported anecdotally but not found at significantly increased overall rates (Finegan et al., 1994). However, the tantrums, in particular, appear to persist for a longer period than in siblings and are of greater severity, the latter feature perhaps resulting from the child's cognitive impairment, frustration, and large size.

From early childhood, poor concentration and subsequent attention deficit disorder are common, significantly affecting home and school life. The child's large size but limited intellectual and behavioral maturity often lead to very unrealistic expectations from adults and poor peer group relationships. Difficulty with social interactions results in a tendency to associate with younger children and, in later life, in a significant degree of social isolation. This latter feature is of particular concern to parents and older children and occurs even in the higher-functioning individuals with Sotos syndrome.

Other behavioral difficulties reported in the literature in general, and more specifically by Rutter and Cole (1991) and Finegan et al., (1994), are an overreliance on routines and a tendency to obsessions, for example, repetitive watching of a favorite video or pursuit of a specific pattern of play. These suggest an overlap with autistic tendencies, although a clear diagnosis of autism is very uncommon.

Although a reliance on routines is common in many children, there are other situations in which the children appear to show an impetuous nature with little thought for the consequences or for their own safety. This, taken with their more limited intellectual and motor skills, can result in significant personal dangers. Other commonly reported symptoms include poor sleep patterns and unusual degrees of anxiety and subsequent phobias. The texts of Rutter and Cole (1991) and Finegan et al., (1994) contain fuller discussions.

The data referring to adults are much more limited. Although the behaviors tend to improve, there is often some residual difficulty that might best be summarized as immaturity or naïveté (personal experience). A significant number of adults suffer from social isolation.

Evaluation

- All individuals with Sotos syndrome need a critical evaluation of their educational requirements so that an appropriate program can be structured (Finegan et al., 1994.)
- A formal behavior assessment may be necessary, and this possibility should be discussed with parents.
- Hearing should be assessed as part of routine care, and the medical team should have a low threshold for requesting further formal hearing evaluation in any child who fails routine assessments.

Treatment

- Drooling and articulation difficulties may benefit from combinations of physical therapy, occupational therapy, and speech therapy.
- Early intervention, including physical therapy and occupational therapy,

should be considered after assessment of the child's tone and coordination.

- Education programs should be based on careful assessment of cognitive function.
- At school, a classroom assistant is frequently beneficial to maintain the child's attention and effort, particularly when attention deficit disorder is present.
- Treatment of behavioral disorders has traditionally been very different in Europe and North America, with a reliance on behavioral therapy in Europe and much more frequent pharmacological intervention in the US. In Sotos syndrome, there are some successes and failures with each method. In the US, many of the children are treated with Ritalin. There are frequent anecdotal reports from the parents of improvement and numerous failures. No formal, controlled study has been done to assess the potential benefits of either approach in Sotos syndrome.
- Treatment of hearing loss is as in the general population.

Neurologic

Marked hypotonia is usually present from birth, and although this appears to improve during childhood, subtle evidence may remain even in adults. It is interesting to note that, despite this central hypotonia, reflexes are often brisk and occasional beats of clonus can be elicited when testing the knee or ankle jerks. Some difficulty with coordination is invariable, with hypotonia exacerbating this feature (Cole and Hughes, 1994). Hypotonia and incoordination appear to affect gross motor movements more than fine motor skills. Large size, hypotonia, and poor coordination make many physical activities difficult, and nonparticipation in sports events may increase social isolation in childhood. One sport many children with Sotos syndrome have excelled in is swimming. Although children with Sotos syndrome appear to have appropriate strength in the muscle groups, their families frequently describe easy fatiguability. This may reflect their immaturity, large size, and poor coordination. Special effort may be required to find appropriate-sized strollers for these large young children. These symptoms do improve with time, and there is no evidence of deterioration.

Febrile convulsions are common, present in almost 50% of cases. Almost half the individuals who have had a febrile seizure will go on to have nonfebrile seizures in later childhood and adulthood.

In 1969, Appenzeller reported a case of Sotos syndrome with apparent abnormalities of the autonomic nervous system (Appenzeller and Snyder, 1969) but these findings have not been reported subsequently. However, there is potential corroborative evidence of autonomic dysfunction from clinical observations. Parents frequently report unexplained episodes of sweating, high facial coloring or flushing, and poor control of peripheral temperature. These features have been noted to appear both concurrently and independently. To date, this is purely a clinical observation, and no associated complications, such as syncope, have been recognized.

Evaluation

- A careful neurological examination should be performed as a baseline on diagnosis and with routine physician visits.
- EEG should be performed if there is evidence of convulsions or absence spells.
- MRI may help both as a diagnostic tool and to exclude evidence of progressive hydrocephalus, but this is not necessary as a routine investigation.

Treatment

- Physical therapy and occupational therapy may be of benefit in the treatment of early hypotonia and later incoordination.

- Swimming should be encouraged.
- There is no evidence that seizures should be managed any differently in Sotos syndrome than in epilepsy due to other causes.

Immunologic

Infections appear to be very common in early childhood, particularly affecting the respiratory tract. In the newborn period, a number of individuals have been reported with pneumonias, which may be attributable to prematurity, requiring ventilation or aspiration, or low tone and poor coordination resulting in decreased pulmonary clearance of secretion with secondary infection. During early childhood, upper respiratory tract infections remain frequent. Recurrent episodes of otitis media are particularly troublesome, documented in 72% of cases; these are commonly associated with conductive hearing loss (Cole and Hughes, 1994). The most likely explanation for the frequency of infection is disruption of the normal anatomical and physiological mechanisms for drainage and clearance of secretions. To date, there has been no clear evidence of altered immunity.

Microbiologically proven urinary tract infections have been identified in up to 20% of males and females with Sotos syndrome (Cole and Hughes 1994) and appear to be caused by structural abnormalities and reflux in the majority of cases. Several authors have reported similar problems in other series or single cases.

Evaluation

- Children with recurrent upper respiratory tract infections, in particular otitis media, should be referred to an otolaryngologist for further assessment, including audiological investigations.
- In view of the potentially covert nature of urinary and middle ear infections, these should be considered in any child with Sotos syndrome who is unwell. This

is particularly relevant in view of the hypersensitivity to febrile convulsions.

- All individuals with a single proven urinary tract infection should have appropriate urological investigations in view of the high *a priori* risk of an anatomical anomaly.

Treatment

- Many children undergo surgical interventions including tonsillectomy, adenoidectomy, and insertion of ventilation tubes.
- In most instances of urinary tract infection, after detection of a structural urinary tract anomaly, prophylactic antibiotics have been necessary. In a few, surgical reimplantation of the ureters has been required (Hammadeh et al., 1995).

Ophthalmologic

The ocular manifestations of Sotos syndrome are poorly documented and frequently overlooked. In one study of 32 individuals with Sotos syndrome, 50% appeared to have some ocular disease (Maino et al., 1994). Of these, the most common disorders were refractive errors, and hyperopia, frequently greater than +2 diopters, was particularly common. Strabismus was also a relatively frequent finding, present in over 40% of cases.

Evaluation

- In view of the additional burden and correctable nature of many oculovisual abnormalities, it is important that these abnormalities are not overlooked. Assessment by an ophthalmologist or optometrist should be considered at diagnosis and at any point in time when there is evidence of visual difficulty.

Treatment

- Standard approaches to visual acuity abnormalities and strabismus have been effective.

Dental

Dental abnormalities are common in childhood. Early eruption of teeth is seen in 54% of individuals. Excessive wear and discoloration are apparent in 75% of these primary teeth. There is a relatively high frequency of gingivitis and occasional dental abscesses (personal observation). The etiology of these features is difficult to ascertain in view of the frequent administration of antibiotic and anticonvulsant syrups. However, in some individuals who have had little, if any, medication there is still evidence of the above dental features. Histologic and ultrastructural studies of the teeth do not reveal any apparent abnormalities (personal observation). Primary and secondary teeth are often malaligned secondary to the craniofacial anomalies. Anecdotal review of dental X-rays has revealed that Sotos syndrome patients have absence of secondary teeth at a frequency higher than expected (personal observation).

Evaluation

- A pediatric dentist should evaluate all children with Sotos syndrome at the point when adequate cooperation can be obtained, but no later than 3 years of age.
- Referral to an orthodontist is appropriate if dental malalignment or crowding is noted.

Treatment

- The child's reluctance to clean teeth regularly has been helped in some cases by the use of electric toothbrushes.
- Orthodontic work may be necessary but is complicated by the underlying bony abnormality and poor patient cooperation.

Cardiovascular

Overt congenital heart disease is rare but if specifically investigated may be present in up to 10% of cases (Cole et al., 1994). The most common anomaly identified is persistent patent ductus arteriosus, which requires surgical closure in approximately half the cases (personal observation). One study reported congenital heart disease in 5 of 10 patients with Sotos syndrome (Kaneko et al., 1987). However, the certainty of the diagnosis was difficult to assess in all cases. A review relying on parental recall reported that 19% of children with Sotos syndrome had congenital heart disease, with at least 8% confirmed by review of the available medical records (Lin et al., 1992). Review of all the literature identifies the most common abnormalities as simple shunts, such as atrial or ventricular septal defects and patent ductus arteriosus, or occasionally right-sided obstructive lesions. The precise proportion of individuals with mitral valve prolapse is unknown, although this has been reported anecdotally (A.E. Lin, personal communication). The author is aware of three girls who were diagnosed with an episode of cardiomyopathy, in two cases with associated pericarditis, for which the etiology remains unknown and which appears to have resolved spontaneously after supportive measures.

Evaluation

- There does not appear to be justification for routine echocardiogram in patients with Sotos syndrome, although a low threshold for investigation is appropriate.

Treatment

- Management of cardiac defects is no different from that in the general population.

Neoplasia

An association of Sotos syndrome with tumor development was documented over 30 years ago and has been a point of debate ever since. Early series may have overestimated the risk because of ascertainment bias and inclusion of nonmalignant tumors (Wit et al., 1985). Studies by Hersh et al., (1992) suggested that only 2% of patients had a tumor. This latter figure is compatible with our own experience.

The site and type of tumor in Sotos syndrome is very varied and has included embryonal tumors such as neuroblastoma, nephroblastoma, and hepatoblastoma. There are occasional reports of lymphoreticular malignancy, although in some cases the underlying diagnosis of Sotos syndrome is controversial (Corsello et al., 1996; Cole and Allanson, 1998).

Tumors occur at increased frequency in a number of the different overgrowth syndromes (Beckwith-Wiedemann syndrome, Simpson-Golabi-Behmel syndrome, Weaver syndrome, and Marshall-Smith syndrome), suggesting that these are not entirely chance occurrences and may have a common etiological mechanism. It would appear unlikely that the mechanism is loss of a tumor suppressor gene, although this cannot be excluded. An alternative explanation may be failure of adequate tissue differentiation, as would be indicated by the presence of nephroblastomatosis associated with some cases of Wilms tumor. Another alternative explanation might be hyperplasia and increased cell division at a time when full differentiation or regulation has yet to be achieved. To date, an excess of common solid tumors such as carcinoma or sarcoma in adult patients with Sotos syndrome has not been identified (personal observation).

Evaluation

- In view of the rarity, wide age range of onset, and diverse nature of the tumors in Sotos syndrome, there is not, as yet, any clear indication for or benefit from regular tumor surveillance.

Treatment

- If a tumor is identified, treatment is the same as in the general population.

Musculoskeletal

Early hypotonia, large size, and joint laxity appear to precipitate a number of orthopedic complications. Particularly problematic are foot deformities, and the reported frequency of 50%, which includes both mild and severe symptoms, could be an underestimate (Cole and Hughes, 1994). Another relatively frequent feature is kyphoscoliosis. A relatively high frequency of fractures in early childhood led to concerns about bone fragility. There is no evident excess of fractures (personal observation), which in itself is surprising, because these children are large with poor coordination. Investigations of bone density have yet to show any evidence of osteoporosis or osteopenia (M. Davie, personal communication).

Evaluation

- Careful examination of the musculoskeletal system should be performed at diagnosis and with routine medical visits.
- Foot deformities or scoliosis evident on clinical examination should be referred for orthopedic opinion.

Treatment

- Foot deformities benefit from physiotherapy and supportive orthotic intervention.
- Surgery may have to be considered for severe pes planus and valgus deformity.
- Mild scoliosis requires only observation or occasionally the use of a cast or brace, although the latter may be difficult because of patient noncompliance.
- In a small number of cases, surgical correction of scoliosis may need to be considered (Latham et al., 1994).

Gastrointestinal

A tendency to severe constipation, with or without overflow, present in over 10% of cases, exacerbates difficulties with toilet training in some children and commonly necessitates pharmacological intervention or, very rarely, surgical intervention, for example after rectal prolapse.

Evaluation

- History of bowel and bladder problems should be obtained with routine visits.

Treatment

- Symptoms are treated as in the general population.

RESOURCES

Sotos Syndrome Support Association
Three Danada Square East, #235
Wheaton, Il 60187
USA

Child Growth Foundation
2 Mayfield Avenue, Chiswick
London W4 1PW
England

Eltern-Initiative Sotos Syndrome
Steinernkreuzweg 22
D-55246 Mainz-Kosteim
Germany

REFERENCES

Agwu JC, Shaw NJ, Kirk J, Chapman S, Ravine D, Cole TRP (1999) Growth in Sotos syndrome. *Arch Dis Child* 80:339–342.

Allanson JE, Cole TRP (1996) Sotos syndrome: Evolution of the facial phenotype — subjective and objective assessment. *Am J Med Genet* 65:13–20.

Appenzeler O, Snyder RD (1969) Autonomic failure with persistent fever in cerebral gigantism. *J Neurol Neurosurg Psychiatry* 32:123–128.

Cohen MM Jr (1989) A comprehensive and critical assessment of overgrowth and overgrowth syndromes. In: *Advances in Human Genetics.* Harris H and Hirschhorn K, eds. New York: Plenum, 1989, Vol. 18; p. 181–303.

Cole TRP (1998) Growing interest in overgrowth. *Arch Dis Child* 78:200–204.

Cole T, Allanson JE (1998) Reply to "Lymphoproliferative disorders in Sotos syndrome:

Observation in two cases". *Am J Med Genet* 75:226.

Cole TRP, Hughes HE (1994) Sotos syndrome: A study of the diagnostic criteria and natural history. *J Med Genet* 31:20–32.

Cole TRP, Hughes HE, Jeffreys MJ, Williams G, Arnold M (1992) Small cell lung carcinoma in a patient with Sotos syndrome: Are genes at 3p21 involved in both conditions? *J Med Genet* 29:338–341.

Corsello G, Giffre M, Carcione A, Cuzto ML, Piccione M, Ziino O (1996) Lymphoproliferative disorders in Sotos syndrome: Observation in two cases. *Am J Med Genet* 64:588–593.

Finegan JK, Cole TRP, Kingwell E, Smith ML, Smith M, Sitarenioe G (1994) Language and behavior in children with Sotos syndrome. *J Am Acad Child Adolesc Psychiatry* 33:1307–1315.

Hammadeh MY, Dutta SN, Cornaby AJ, Morgan RJ (1995) Congenital urological anomalies in Sotos syndrome. *Br J Urol* 76:133–135.

Hersh JH, Cole TRP, Bloom AS, Bertolone SJ, Hughes HE (1992) Sotos syndrome: Is there a risk of malignancy? *J Pediatr* 120:572–574.

Jaeken J, Schueren-Lodeweyckx MVAN, Eeckels R (1972) Cerebral gigantism syndrome: A report of 4 cases and review of the literature. *Zeitsch Kinderheilkd* 112:332–346.

Kaneko H, Tsukahara M, Tachibana H, Kurashige H, Kuwano A, Kajii T (1987) Congenital heart defects in Sotos syndrome. *Am J Med Genet* 26:569–576.

Kok K, Mosselaar A, Faber H, Dijkhuisen T, Draaijers TG, van der Veen AY, Buys CHCM, Schrander-Stumpel CT (1999) Breakpoint mapping by FISH in a Sotos patient with a constitutional translocation t(3;6).

Latham JM, Marks DS, Cole T, Thompson AG (1994) Scoliosis in Sotos syndrome. *Proceedings of the 5th European Spinal Deformities Society Meeting.* 122–123(A).

Lin AE, Treat KT, Kedesdy JH (1992) Survey of behavior in Sotos syndrome. *Proc Greenwood Genet Ctr* 12:95.

Maino DM, Kofman J, Flynn MF, Lai L (1994) Ocular manifestations of Sotos syndrome. *J Am Optomet Assoc* 65:339–344.

Mangano L, Palmieri S, Dotti MT, Moschini F, Frederico A (1989) Macrosomia and mental retardation: Evidence of autosomal dominant inheritance in four generations. *Am J Med Genet* 32:67–71.

Partington MW, Fagan K, Soubjaki V, Turner G (1997) Translocation involving 4p16.3 in three families: deletion causing Pitt-Rodgers-Danks syndrome and duplication resulting in a new overgrowth syndrome. *J Med Genet* 34:719–728.

Reik W, Maher ER (1997) Imprinting in clusters: Lessons from Beckwith-Wiedemann syndrome. *Trends Genet* 13:330–334.

Rutter SC, Cole TRP (1991) Psychological characteristics of Sotos syndrome. *Dev Med Child Neurol* 33:898–902.

Schaefer GB, Bodensteiner JB, Buehler BA, Lin A, Cole TRP (1997) The neuroimaging findings in Sotos syndrome. *Am J Med Genet* 68:462–465.

Schlesinger B (1931) Gigantism (acromegalic in nature). *Proc R Soc Med* 24:1352.

Schrander-Stumpel CT, Fryns JP, Hamers GC (1990) Sotos syndrome and de novo balanced autosomal translocation (t(3;6)(p21;p21). *Clin Genet* 37:226–229.

Smith M, Fullwood P, Yu Q, Palmer S, Upadhyaya M, Cole T (1997) No evidence of uniparental disomy as a common cause of Sotos syndrome. *J Med Genet* 34:10–12.

Sotos JF, Dodge PR, Muirhead D, Crawford JD, Talbot NB (1964) Cerebral gigantism in childhood. *N Engl J Med* 271:109–116.

Thorburn MJ, Wright ES, Miller CG, Smith EHM (1970) Exomphalos-macroglossia-gigantism syndrome in Jamaican infants. *Am J Dis Child* 119:316–321.

Wit JM, Beemer FA, Barth PG, Oothuys JWE, Dijkstra PF, Van den Brande JL, Leschot NJ (1985) Cerebral gigantism (Sotos syndrome), compiled data of 22 cases. *Eur J Paediatr* 114:131–140.

CHAPTER 24

STICKLER SYNDROME

DOUGLAS J. WILKIN, RUTH M. LIBERFARB AND CLAIR A. FRANCOMANO

INTRODUCTION

Stickler syndrome, also called hereditary progressive arthro-ophthalmopathy, is a common autosomal dominant connective tissue disorder affecting primarily the ocular, orofacial, and skeletal systems (Stickler et al., 1965; Rimoin and Lachman, 1993) (Fig. 24.1). Stickler and colleagues first described the syndrome in two papers. The first paper described a new dominant syndrome consisting of progressive myopia beginning in the first decade of life and resulting in retinal detachment and blindness (Stickler et al., 1965). Affected persons also exhibited premature degenerative changes in various joints with abnormal epiphyseal development and slight joint hypermobility. In the second paper, Stickler and Pugh (1967) described changes in the vertebrae and hearing deficit as part of the syndrome, as well as the midface hypoplasia that is characteristic for the phenotype (Fig. 24.2). Opitz et al. (1972) described patients with Stickler syndrome also having features of Pierre Robin sequence. Both inter- and intrafamilial phenotypic variability is seen in this syndrome, such that affected individuals can be mildly affected, manifesting few features of the disorder, or severely affected, with manifestations of all of the features of the syndrome.

Incidence

Herrmann et al. (1975) suggested that Stickler syndrome is the most common autosomal dominant connective tissue dysplasia in the North American Midwest. Although estimates vary, it is thought that the frequency of Stickler syndrome is roughly 1:10,000. Phenotypic variability of the syndrome can make the diagnosis difficult, and the syndrome may be significantly underdiagnosed.

Diagnostic Criteria

The three major systems involved in Stickler syndrome are the ocular system, the oro-auriculo-facial system, and the musculoskeletal system. Severe myopia with onset in the first decade of life, vitreous degeneration, spontaneous retinal detachment, chorioretinal degeneration, open angle glaucoma, and presenile cataracts are ocular features of the disorder (Stickler et al., 1965; Rimoin and Lachman, 1993; Wilkin et al., 1998a). During infancy, midface hypoplasia is often evident and features of Pierre Robin sequence, including bifid uvula and submucous cleft palate, can be present and may result in severe feeding and respiratory problems (Schreiner et al., 1973). Mixed and sensorineural hearing loss in the higher frequencies is also a manifestation of the

Management of Genetic Syndromes, Edited by Suzanne B. Cassidy and Judith E. Allanson
ISBN 0-471-31286-X   Copyright © 2001 by Wiley-Liss, Inc.

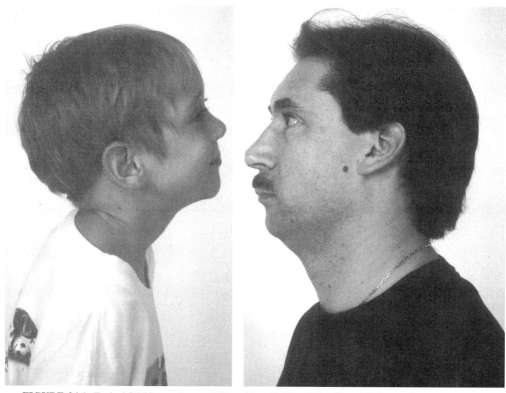

FIGURE 24.1. Typical Stickler syndrome. Affected boy (*left*) and his affected father (*right*). In addition to oro-auriculo-facial manifestations (see Fig. 24.2), affected individuals can have ocular and musculoskeletal features. Ocular features, including high myopia, are usually present in early childhood.

syndrome (Liberfarb and Goldblatt, 1986). During childhood, joint pain and stiffness may signify the onset of juvenile osteoarthritis. Early onset degenerative joint disease is a major complication in adulthood. Radiographs of the skeleton may demonstrate a mild form of spondyloepiphyseal dysplasia, even in patients without other signs of the syndrome (Stickler and Pugh, 1967; Rimoin and Lachman, 1993) (Fig. 24.3). Mitral valve prolapse has been reported in 45% of affected individuals (Liberfarb and Goldblatt, 1986). To date, no formal diagnostic criteria have been published. Babies born with a cleft palate or infants with early-onset high myopia should be evaluated for Stickler syndrome.

Characterization of the vitreoretinal phenotype in Stickler syndrome has resulted in a proposed classification of the syndrome into two subtypes, type 1 and type 2 (Snead et al., 1996a, 1996b). Vitreoretinal analysis to distinguish between the two types is best done by an ophthalomologist familiar with Stickler syndrome. However, most cases of Stickler syndrome are diagnosed without knowledge of the vitreous architecture. The clinical detail required to type the patient is not always available, nor is it necessary in order to make the diagnosis of Stickler syndrome. Snead et al. (1996a, 1996b) described the vitreous in type 1 Stickler syndrome as characterized by a vestigial gel remnant occupying the anterior vitreous cavity and extending in a thin sheet a variable distance over the pars plana and anterior retina up to, and sometimes beyond, the equator posteriorly. This finding is present at birth in these patients and remains present throughout life. According to the same authors,

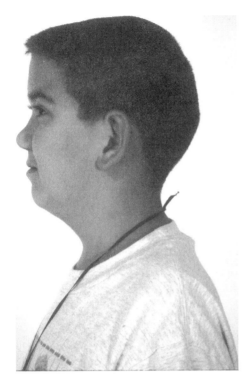

FIGURE 24.2. Midface hypoplasia in Stickler syndrome. Flat facies with depressed nasal bridge, midface or maxillary hypoplasia, and micrognathia can be characteristic of Stickler syndrome. Other oro-auriculo-facial features may include epicanthal folds, clefting of the hard or soft palate, Pierre Robin sequence, sensorineural deafness, and dental anomalies.

type 2 Stickler syndrome also has abnormal vitreous architecture, although it is distributed throughout the entire posterior segment. In type 2 Stickler syndrome there is decreased normal fibrillar gel matrix. The remaining gel matrix has gel strands of variable diameters, associated with areas of localized or complete posterior hyaloid membrane separation (Snead et al., 1996a).

The general criteria for Stickler syndrome are the same in both types. It is important to note that individuals with type 2 Stickler syndrome have much milder ocular manifestations (Snead et al., 1994); early-onset high myopia has not been reported in type 2 Stickler syndrome (Vikkulla et al., 1995).

No formal criteria have yet been published for the diagnosis of Stickler syndrome. In the

presence of cleft palate, characteristic ocular abnormalities, or high frequency sensorineural hearing loss, we have begun using a point system to aid in the diagnosis (Rose et al., 2000). A maximum of two points is awarded for each of the following systems:

Orofacial Cleft palate (2) points
          Characteristic facies (1 point)
Ocular   Characteristic vitreous
          degeneration or retinal
          detachment (2 points)
Auditory High frequency sensorineural
          hearing loss (2 points)
          Hypermobile tympanic
          membranes (1 point)
Skeletal History of femoral head failure
          (1 point)
          Radiographically demonstrated
          osteoarthritis $\leq$ age 40 (1 point)
          Scoliosis, spondylolisthesis, or
          Scheuermann-like kyphotic
          deformity (1 point)
Family History/ Molecular Data (1 point maximum)
          Independently affected 1st
          degree relative in a pattern
          consistent with autosomal
          dominant inheritance or
          presence of *COL2A1*, *COL11A1*,
          or *COL11A2* mutation
          associated with Stickler
          syndrome

The diagnosis of Stickler syndrome requires the presence of cleft palate, ocular abnormalities, or high frequency sensorineural hearing loss and a total of 5 points out of a possible 9.

Etiology, Pathogenesis, and Genetics

The observation that type II collagen is present in both cartilage and the secondary vitreous of the eye suggested that the basis of Stickler syndrome may be a defect in *COL2A1*, the gene that encodes type II collagen (Maumenee, 1979) (Table 24.1). Subsequently, Stickler syndrome was linked

TABLE 24.1. Expression of Type II Collagen and Type XI Collagen in Cartilage and the Eye

Cartilage		Eye	
Type II Collagen	Type XI Collagen	Type II Collagen	Type XI Collagen
COL2A1	COL11A1	COL2A1	COL11A1
	COL11A2		COL5A2
	COL2A1		COL2A1

Note: Type II collagen is always a homotrimer of the product of the *COL2A1* gene. In cartilage, type XI collagen is a heterotrimer of the products of the *COL11A1*, *COL11A2*, and *COL2A1* genes. However, in the eye, type XI collagen is a heterotrimer of the products of the *COL11A1*, *COL5A2*, and *COL2A1* genes. Therefore, individuals with Stickler syndrome due to a mutation in the *COL11A2* gene would not be expected to have ocular anomalies as severe as those with Stickler syndrome due to mutations in other genes.

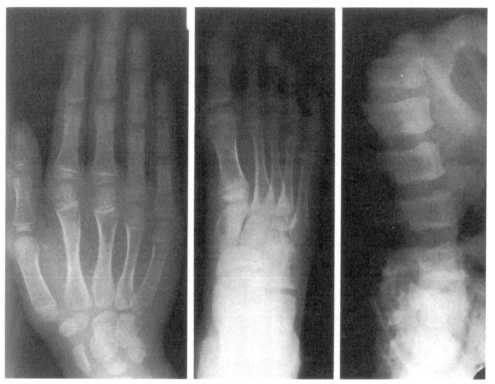

FIGURE 24.3. Radiographic findings in Stickler syndrome. Arachnodactyly, fusion of carpal centers, and a mild spondyloepiphyseal dysplasia are noticeable. Other musculoskeletal features may include hyperextensible joints, Marfanoid habitus, and arthropathy. Reprinted with permission (Jones KL, 1988).

to *COL2A1* (Francomano et al., 1987). Since then, at least 15 dominant mutations in the *COL2A1* gene have been identified in individuals or families with Stickler syndrome (Ahmad et al., 1991; Brown et al., 1995; Wilkin et al., 1998b). All of the mutations introduce a premature stop codon into the triple helical domain of the collagen

molecule, implying that the phenotype results from a quantitative defect in type II procollagen biosynthesis. Presumably, only half the normal amount of type II collagen monomers is available to be incorporated in the type II collagen fiber. Type II collagen is a homotrimer of the product of the *COL2A1* gene (Table 24.1). The collagen monomers (chains) form stable triple helices, which aggregate into the supramolecular structures of fibrillar collagen. It is hypothesized that this decreased amount of normal type II collagen results in Stickler syndrome.

Genetic heterogeneity in Stickler syndrome has been demonstrated by the exclusion of linkage to *COL2A1* in about 50% of Stickler syndrome families reported (Knowlton et al., 1989). Mutations in the genes encoding type XI collagen (*COL11A1* and *COL11A2*) have been identified in a few affected individuals (Vikkula et al., 1995, Richards et al., 1996). Clinical and molecular findings have suggested that the phenotype in Stickler syndrome families with severe ocular manifestations are the result of mutations in either *COL2A1* or *COL11A1*, while the phenotype in families with milder eye involvement results from mutations in the *COL11A2* gene (Snead et al., 1994) (Table 24.1). It appears that mutations in *COL2A1* are associated with a high risk of retinal detachment, a low likelihood of deafness and a change in facial appearance with age, while in *COL11A1* mutations commonly cause deafness and are associated with the characteristic face even in adult life (Annunen et al.). Furthermore, it has been proposed that type 1 Stickler syndrome results from mutations in *COL2A1*, while type 2 Stickler syndrome results from mutations in the other genes (Snead et al., 1994, 1996a, 1996b). Some Stickler syndrome families with severe eye manifestations are not linked to *COL2A1*, *COL11A1*, or *COL11A2*, suggesting at least a fourth gene is involved in the phenotype (Wilkin et al., 1998a).

Diagnostic Testing

DNA diagnostic testing for Stickler syndrome is complicated by the known genetic heterogeneity. The identification of a causative mutation is the only available method that is completely accurate. If linkage has not been established to one of the three known loci, or a specific mutation is not known, one cannot exclude the diagnosis. Testing is available in some clinical laboratories, as is testing through a number of research protocols. Information on testing centers is available through the GeneTests directory or by contacting the Stickler syndrome support group, Stickler Involved People (SIP; www.sticklers.org).

Differential Diagnosis

Wagner syndrome, Marshall syndrome, and the Weissenbacher-Zweymuller syndrome are often confused with Stickler syndrome. In fact, the phenotypes of each syndrome are so similar that it is often difficult to completely distinguish the disorders clinically. Some geneticists believe that these phenotypes are distinct syndromes, others believe they represent phenotypic variants of the same syndrome.

Wagner (1938) reported a family with 28 members affected by low myopia (−3.00 diopters or less), a fluid vitreous, and cortical cataracts. No extraocular features were described. This syndrome has come to be called Wagner syndrome, hyaloidoretinal degeneration of Wagner, Wagner vitreoretinal degeneration, or erosive vitreoretinopathy. Affected individuals manifest complete absence of the normal vitreal scaffolding and preretinal, equatorial, and avascular grayish-white membranes.

Retinal detachment was not noted in any of the 28 members of the original Swiss family studied by Wagner (1938). Schwartz et al. (1989) suggested that Wagner syndrome is characterized by vitreoretinal degeneration without extraocular manifestations, whereas Stickler syndrome also has extraocular manifestations in the musculoskeletal and craniofacial systems.

Fryer et al. (1990) studied a large family with Wagner syndrome. Affected individuals in this family had none of the nonocular features associated with Stickler syndrome. Recombination with the *COL2A1* locus was demonstrated, thus excluding that gene as the site of the mutation. However, the demonstration by Körkkö et al. (1993) of a *COL2A1* mutation in a family with Wagner syndrome indicates that there are at least two loci causing Wagner syndrome. Affected individuals in this family had early-onset cataracts, lattice degeneration of the retina, and retinal detachment. It has been suggested that this family may not have Wagner syndrome, but may have Stickler syndrome.

Marshall syndrome is a rare autosomal dominant skeletal dysplasia, characterized by ocular abnormalities, sensorineural hearing loss, craniofacial anomalies, and anhidrotic ectodermal dysplasia (Marshall, 1958). Affected individuals are myopic (ranging from −3 to −20 diopters) with a fluid vitreous and congenital cataracts. Retinal detachment is possible. Craniofacial characteristics are common. Micrognathia is evident in some affected individuals, as is the absence of nasal bones, producing a short nose with a very flat nasal bridge, anteverted nares, and a long philtrum.

The distinction between the Stickler and Marshall syndromes is also strongly supported by the work of Ayme and Preus (1984) who surveyed published reports on the two syndromes. A set of 18 patients with clinical description, photographs, and radiographs was used to tabulate a list of 53 features, including facial characteristics, size and habitus, and joint, limb, and hip manifestations. Analysis of these features revealed two distinct groups of patients. The authors concluded that there was no reason not to consider these two syndromes as separate disorders. The authors suggested that the facies of individuals with the two disorders differ. Patients with Marshall syndrome have a flat or retracted midface, whereas those with Stickler syndrome have a flat malar area, which is often erroneously described as a flat midface. Marshall syndrome patients have thick calvaria, abnormal frontal sinuses, and intracranial calcifications, and the eyeballs appear large, possibly because of a shallow orbit.

In affected members of a large kindred diagnosed with Marshall syndrome, Griffith et al. (1998) identified a mutation in the *COL11A1* gene. The results demonstrate that Marshall syndrome and a subset of Stickler syndrome families have mutations in the *COL11A1* gene. The distinctness of the phenotype of these two disorders may be a reflection of different kinds of mutations within this large gene.

Weissenbacher and Zweymuller (1964) described an infant with Pierre Robin sequence and chondrodysplasia. Weissenbacher-Zweymuller syndrome is characterized by neonatal micrognathia and rhizomelic chondrodysplasia with dumbbell-shaped femora and humeri, and regression of bone changes and normal growth in later years (Weissenbacher and Zweymuller, 1964; Haller et al., 1975). Radiologically there are also vertebral coronal clefts. Average growth after 2 to 3 years, "catching up" to average height, is seen.

It has been suggested that Weissenbacher-Zweymuller syndrome may be neonatal expression of Stickler syndrome (Kelly et al., 1982). Ayme and Preus (1984) did a cluster analysis of published cases and concluded that Weissenbacher-Zweymuller syndrome and Stickler syndromes are separate entities. Among the features found in Weissenbacher-Zweymuller syndrome but not in Stickler syndrome were markedly decreased body length at birth with short limbs, catch-up growth after 2 or 3 years, lack of progressive deformity, and autosomal recessive inheritance as indicated by affected siblings with phenotypically normal parents. Myopia and retinal detachment are characteristics of Stickler syndrome that are not found in Weissenbacher-Zweymuller syndrome. However, recent studies of the original patient with this syndrome document a mutation in *COL11A2* that demonstrates that Weissenbacher-Zweymuller syndrome is identical to nonocular Stickler syndrome (Pihlajamaa et al., 1998).

MANIFESTATIONS AND MANAGEMENT

Optimal management of Stickler syndrome requires an interdisciplinary team of specialists, tailored to the affected individual's specific medical needs.

Growth and Feeding

These are not an issue in Stickler syndrome except in those patients with clefts. Babies with a cleft palate have difficulty feeding. A cleft in the roof of the mouth makes it difficult for the baby to suck forcefully enough to draw milk through a nipple. It is possible to breastfeed some infants with cleft palate, though this will require extra patience. Breastfeeding is more likely to be successful in babies with less severe clefts.

Evaluation

- Babies with Stickler syndrome who have a cleft palate should be monitored for inadequate nutrition by frequent plotting of height and weight attainment, as for all babies with clefts.
- A feeding evaluation by an occupational or physical therapist may be indicated for patients with significant difficulty feeding.

Treatment

- During bottle feeding, the baby should be in a sitting position to help prevent milk from leaking into the nose through the cleft. A regular nipple for premature babies and a squeeze bottle can help a baby with cleft palate feed more easily. Occasionally, a baby may feed best with the aid of a plastic artificial palate, called an obturator, which temporarily covers a palatal cleft. Not all cleft teams favor this approach.
- Most cleft palate teams pay close attention to feeding and help parents establish good feeding practices right after

the child is born. Their recommendations usually keep problems to a minimum.

Development and Behavior

Development is not an issue in Stickler syndrome.

Ophthalmologic

Major manifestations of the ocular system in Stickler syndrome include moderate to severe myopia (at least -5 diopters), with onset in childhood, spontaneous retinal detachment, and a congenital vitreous anomaly. Minor manifestations include presenile cataract, glaucoma, and strabismus.

Early-onset high myopia must be frequently monitored, as it can lead to spontaneous retinal degeneration and detachment. Refractive errors, cataracts, and vitreoretinal abnormalities can be detected early in life in patients with Stickler syndrome (Wilson et al., 1996).

Seery et al. (1990) found cataracts of various types or aphakia in 115 of 231 eyes of patients with Stickler syndrome. The most frequent and distinctive lesions, described as wedge and fleck cataracts, accounted for 40 of the 93 cataracts observed.

Evaluation

- Frequent (at least annual) examinations by an ophthalmologist are recommended, starting in infancy, to evaluate the severity of myopia, strabismus, the vitreoretinal architecture, and the presence or absence of cataracts and glaucoma.

Treatment

- Corrective lenses should be prescribed for myopia as early as possible.
- Prophylactic laser photocoagulation of vitreoretinopathy should be considered. Leiba et al. (1996) retrospectively reviewed a large family with Stickler

syndrome (at least 42 affected members). Ten eyes were prophylactically treated with laser photocoagulation. In this family, the incidence of retinal detachment was significantly higher in nonlasered eyes than in lasered eyes.

- Surgery may be required to repair retinal detachments and remove cataracts. Lens implantation may be necessary if lenses are removed because of cataracts. Surgical procedures are the same as in the general population.
- Glaucoma should be treated as in the general population.
- Ocular prosthesis may be required if sight is lost due to retinal detachment.
- Corrective treatment for strabismus is indicated, as for the general population.

Craniofacial

Major manifestations of the oro-auriculo-facial system in Stickler syndrome include cleft palate with or without the other features of Pierre Robin sequence. Minor manifestations include midface hypoplasia, micrognathia, and sensorineural hearing loss in the higher frequencies.

A retrospective review of 90 children with Pierre Robin sequence was carried out using oximetry, apnea monitoring, and sleep studies to identify subgroups at a higher risk of developing severe airway obstruction, and response to treatment was assessed (Tomaski et al., 1995). Airway obstruction and feeding difficulties vary among patients with Pierre Robin sequence. Treatment is challenging and the appropriate management may not be readily identified, causing delay in securing the airway. Although most patients with Stickler syndrome do not suffer from debilitating airway and feeding difficulties, all babies with cleft palate or Pierre Robin sequence do have some feeding difficulties, with the severity proportional to the degree of airway obstruction (Tomaski et al., 1995). (See Chapter 19 for a more detailed

description of management of Pierre Robin sequence.)

Babies with cleft palate are especially susceptible to middle ear disease. The cleft can contribute to recurrent otitis media, which may lead to mild to moderate hearing loss. If treated properly in infancy and childhood, the hearing losses need not be permanent. If not properly managed, speech development may be affected and hearing loss may become permanent. Ear disease usually improves following cleft palate repair.

Some children with cleft palate may develop speech more slowly than other children. Their words may sound nasal and they may have difficulty producing some consonant sounds. However, after cleft palate repair, most children eventually catch up and develop normal speech, though some will require speech therapy.

Evaluation

- Otolaryngology evaluation should be done, especially to evaluate the patient for ear and palate abnormalities, including bifid uvula and submucous cleft palate. An otolaryngologist should examine all babies with cleft palate within the first 3 to 6 months of life.
- If otitis media is detected, it often can be treated with antibiotics. In some cases pressure equalizing (PE) tubes may need to be placed to drain the fluid.
- Hearing should be tested regularly in babies and children with cleft palate. Audiograms should be done at regular intervals to monitor mixed and sensorineural hearing loss.
- Speech and swallow evaluations should be accomplished for all affected patients.

Treatment

- Teaching parents feeding techniques is required when the child has a cleft palate.
- Surgery is needed to repair a cleft palate. The timing and type of surgery

will depend on a number of factors, including the preference of the individual surgeon, the general health of the baby and the nature of the cleft. Cleft palate repair is generally timed to restore the partition between the nose and mouth as early as possible, often between 12 and 18 months.

- Insertion of ventilation tubes may be necessary for persistent recurrent otitis media.
- Hearing aids may be required. Devices to help children hear in school may be beneficial when hearing loss is documented, as may preferential classroom placement.
- Speech therapy will almost always be needed in children with clefts.

Musculoskeletal

Major manifestations of the musculoskeletal system in Stickler syndrome include early-onset degenerative joint disease and radiographic evidence of a mild spondyloepiphyseal dysplasia. Minor manifestations include joint hypermobility, including hyperextensibility of the knees and elbows; joint pain or stiffness in childhood; arachnodactyly; scoliosis; and Marfanoid habitus. The joint hyperflexibility of youth usually evolves into degenerative arthritis. The musculoskeletal manifestations can be extremely variable both within and between families. Radiographic manifestations are often very mild and are infrequently reported.

Osteoarthritis, with onset as early as the third decade of life, is one of the major manifestations of Stickler syndrome. Severe osteoarthritis with an early onset has been associated with mutations in the *COL2A1* gene (Ritvaniemi et al., 1995). A specific *COL2A1* mutation (Arg519Cys) has been identified in at least five unrelated families with early-onset osteoarthritis associated with a mild spondyloepiphyseal dysplasia. The relationship between the phenotype of

affected individuals in these families and Stickler syndrome is unknown.

Radiographic evidence of a mild spondyloepiphyseal dysplasia is a significant aspect of Stickler syndrome. Spondyloepiphyseal dysplasia is characterized by typical skeletal changes. Individuals with spondyloepiphyseal dysplasia have characteristic X-ray findings, including delayed ossification of the axial skeleton with ovoid vertebral bodies. With time, the vertebral bodies appear flattened. There is delayed ossification of the femoral heads, pubic bones, and calcaneus (heel). Coxa vara (deformity of the hip joint) is common.

Evaluation

- Individuals with Stickler syndrome should have a full skeletal evaluation to determine the involvement of the skeleton in the phenotype. Orthopedic problems, spinal column instability, deformities of the legs, arthrosis of hips, and other skeletal manifestations can then be identified and appropriate treatment planned.
- Rheumatology consultation is suggested to determine onset and severity of osteoarthritis.
- Rehabilitation medicine or physical therapy consultation may be indicated to evaluate body mechanics and range of motion and strength, and to recommend strengthening exercises.
- Radiographic skeletal survey in childhood is suggested to document the presence and severity of spondyloepiphyseal dysplasia.
- If chronic pain is present, evaluation by a pain specialist may be helpful.
- Occupational therapy evaluation is recommended to determine the patient's ability to function in daily activities.

Treatment

- Pain medications should be prescribed, as needed.

- Appropriate splints may be required for strength and to stabilize lax joints, particularly during sports.
- Aids or braces may be required to assist in daily activities.
- Education of the patient and family regarding joint protection is important.
- Education of the patient regarding exercises for strengthening muscles around lax joints is recommended.
- Hydrotherapy, or other physical therapy modalities, may increase range of motion, endurance, and strength.
- An individual exercise program should be developed, such as one recommended by the rehabilitation medicine or physical therapy evaluation.

Cardiovascular

Among 57 patients with Stickler syndrome, Liberfarb and Goldblatt (1986) found that 50% of females and 43% of males had mitral valve prolapse. They suggested that Stickler syndrome should be considered in cases of dominantly inherited mitral valve prolapse with or without joint laxity and slender bones, just as it must be considered in all cases of Pierre Robin syndrome, dominantly inherited myopia with or without retinal detachment and deafness, and dominantly inherited cleft palate. Mitral valve prolapse may be associated with nonexertional chest pain or palpitations, both of which are alleviated by beta-blockade therapy.

Evaluation

- Echocardiogram should be performed in all patients.
- Cardiology consultation should be obtained if abnormalities are found.

Treatment

- Antibiotic prophylaxis for subacute bacterial endocarditis (SBE), per American Heart Association guidelines, should be recommended for all patients with mitral valve prolapse.
- Beta-blockade should be started for symptomatic patients with mitral valve prolapse.

RESOURCES

Stickler Involved People (SIP)
www.sticklers.org/sip/
Australian Stickler group
dove.mtx.net.au/~mrossnay/stickler.html
Canadian Stickler group
home.ican.net/~17976
England Stickler group
www.netcomuk.co.uk/~gfmsssg

Books and Brochures

Stickler—The Elusive Syndrome, by Wendy Hughes
This book explains, in layman terms, the condition and possible medical problems. The approach is positive and leaves the reader with hope and skills to manage Stickler syndrome. It is available from SIP.
Stickler Living Book (M. Ratchford, ed.) is a booklet written by members of SIP on living with Stickler syndrome. It is available through SIP.

Online Agencies

Greenberg Center for the Skeletal Dysplasias
http://www.med.jhu.edu/Greenberg.Center/Greenberg.htm
March of Dimes: Cleft lip and palate
http://noah.cuny.edu/pregnancy/march_of_dimes/birth_defects/cleftlip.html

REFERENCES

Ahmad NN, Ala-Kokko L, Knowlton RG, Jimenez SA, Weaver EJ, Maguire JI, Tasman W, Prockop DJ (1991) Stop codon in the procollagen II gene (*COL2A1*) in a family with the Stickler syndrome (arthro-ophthalmopathy). *Proc Natl Acad Sci (USA)*, 88: 6624–6627.

Annunen S, Korkko J, Czarny M, Warman ML, Brunner HG, Kaariainen H, Mulliken JB, Tranebjaerg L, Brooks DG, Cox GF, Cruysberg JR, Curtis MA, Davenport SL, Friedrich CA, Kaitila I, Krawczynski MR, Latos-Bielenska A, Mukai S, Olsen BR, Shinno N, Somer M, Vikkula M, Zlotogora J, Prockop DJ, Ala-Kokko L (1999) Splicing mutations of 54-bp exons in the *COL11A1* gene cause Marshall syndrome, but other mutations cause overlapping Marshall/Stickler phenotypes. *Am J Hum Genet* 65: 974–83.

Ayme S, Preus M (1984) The Marshall and Stickler syndromes: Objective rejection of lumping. *J Med Genet* 21: 34–38.

Brown DM, Vandenburgh K, Kimura AE, Weingeist TA, Sheffield VC, Stone EM (1995) Novel frameshift mutations in the procollagen 2 gene (*COL2A1*) associated with Stickler syndrome (hereditary arthro-ophthalmopathy). *Hum Mol Genet* 4: 141–142.

Francomano CA, Liberfarb RM, Hirose T, Maumenee IH, Streeten EA, Meyers DA, Pyeritz RE (1987) The Stickler syndrome: Evidence for close linkage to the structural gene for type II collagen. *Genomics* 1: 293–296.

Fryer AE, Upadhyaya M, Littler M, Bacon P, Watkins D, Tsipouras P, Harper PS (1990) Exclusion of *COL2A1* as a candidate gene in a family with Wagner-Stickler syndrome. *J Med Genet* 27: 91–93.

Griffith AJ, Sprunger LK, Sirko-Osadsa DA, Tiller GE, Meisler MH, Warman ML (1998) Marshall syndrome associated with a splicing defect at the *COL11A1* locus. *Am J Hum Genet* 62: 816–823.

Haller JO, Berdon WE, Robinow M, Slovis TL, Baker DH, Johnson GF (1975) The Weissenbacher-Zweymuller syndrome of micrognathia and rhizomelic chondrodysplasia at birth with subsequent normal growth. *Am J Roentgen Rad Ther Nucl Med* 125: 936–943.

Herrmann J, France TD, Spranger JW, Opitz JM, Wiffler C (1975) The Stickler syndrome (hereditary arthroophthalmopathy). *Birth Defects Orig Art Ser* XI: 76–103.

Jones KL (1988) *Smith's Recognizable Patterns of Human Malformation*. Philadelphia, WB Saunders, p 245.

Kelly TE, Wells HH, Tuck KB (1982) The Weissenbacher-Zweymuller syndrome: Possible neonatal expression of the Stickler syndrome. *Am J Med Genet* 11: 113–119.

Knowlton RG, Weaver EJ, Struyk AF, Knobloch WH, King RA, Norris K, Shamban A, Uitto J, Jimenez SA, Prokop DJ (1989) Genetic linkage analysis of hereditary arthro-ophthalmopathy (Stickler syndrome) and the type II procollagen gene. *Am J Hum Genet* 45: 681–688.

Körkkö J, Ritvaniemi P, Haataja L, Kääriäinen H, Kivirikko KI, Prockop DJ, Ala-Kokko L (1993) Mutation in type II procollagen (*COL2A1*) that substitutes aspartate for glycine 1-67 and that causes cataracts and retinal detachment: Evidence for molecular heterogeneity in the Wagner syndrome and Stickler syndrome. *Am J Hum Genet* 53: 55–61.

Leiba H, Oliver M, Pollack A (1996) Prophylactic laser photocoagulation in Stickler syndrome. *Eye* 10: 701–708.

Liberfarb RM, Goldblatt A (1986) Prevalence of mitral-valve prolapse in the Stickler syndrome. *Am J Med Genet* 24: 387–392.

Marshall D (1958) Ectodermal dysplasia: Report of a kindred with ocular abnormalities and hearing defect. *Am J Ophthalmol* 45: 143–156.

Maumenee IH (1979) Vitreoretinal degeneration as a sign of generalized connective tissue diseases. *Am J Ophthalmol* 88: 432–449.

Opitz JM, France T, Herrmann J, Spranger JW (1972) The Stickler syndrome. *New Engl J Med* 286: 546–547.

Pihlajamaa T, Prockop DJ, Faber J, Winterpacht A, Zabel B, Giedion A, Wiesbauer P, Spranger J, Ala-Kokko L (1998) Heterozygous glycine substitution in a *COL11A2* gene in the original patient with the Weissenbacher-Zweymuller syndrome demonstrates its identity with heterozygous OSMED (non-ocular Stickler syndrome). *Am J Med Genet* 80:115–120.

Richards AJ, Yates JR, Williams R, Payne SJ, Pope FM, Scott JD, Snead MP (1996) A family with Stickler syndrome type 2 has a mutation in the *COL11A1* gene resulting in the substitution of glycine 97 by valine in alpha 1(XI) collagen. *Hum Mol Genet* 5: 1339–1343.

Rimoin DL, Lachman RS (1993) Genetic disorders of the osseous skeleton. In: *McKusick's Heritable Disorders of Connective*

Tissue Beighton P (ed.). St Louis, Mosby, pp 557–689.

Ritvaniemi P, Körkkö J, Bonaventure J, Vikkula M, Hyland J, Paassilta P, Kaitila I, et al. (1995) Identification of *COL2A1* gene mutations in patients with chondrodysplasias and familial osteoarthritis. *Arthritis Rheum* 38: 999–1004.

Rose PS, Levy HP, Johnston JJ, Davis J, Griffith AJ, Liberfarb RM, Francomano CA. Proposed diagnostic criteria for Stickler syndrome. *Am J Hum Genet* 67 (supp): A235, 2000.

Schreiner RL, McAlister WH, Marshall RE, Shearer WT (1973) Stickler syndrome in a pedigree of Pierre Robin syndrome. *Am J Dis Child* 126: 86–90.

Schwartz RC, Watkins D, Fryer AE, Goldberg R, Marion R, Polomeno RC, Spallone A, et al. (1989) Non-allelic genetic heterogeneity in the vitreoretinal degenerations of the Stickler and Wagner types and evidence for intragenic recombination at the *COL2A1* locus. *Am J Hum Genet* 45: A218.

Seery CM, Pruett RC, Liberfarb RM, Cohen BZ (1990) Distinctive cataract in the Stickler syndrome. *Am J Ophthalmol* 110: 143–8.

Snead MP, Payne SJ, Barton DE, Yates JRW, Al-Imara L, Pope FM, Scott JD (1994) Stickler syndrome: Correlation between vitreoretinal phenotypes and linkage to *COL2A1*. *Eye* 8: 609–614.

Snead MP, Yates JRW, Pope FM, Temple IK, Scott JD (1996a) Masked confirmation of linkage between type 1 congenital vitreous anomaly and *COL2A1* in Stickler syndrome. *Graefe's Arch Clin Exp Ophthalmol* 234: 720–721.

Snead MP, Yates JRW, Williams R, Payne SJ, Pope FM, Scott JD (1996b) Stickler syndrome type 2 and linkage to the *COL11A2 gene. Ann NY Acad Sci* 785: 331–332.

Stickler GB, Belau PG, Farrell FJ, Jones JD, Pugh DG, Steinberg AG, Ward LE (1965) Hereditary progressive arthro-ophthalmopathy. *Mayo Clin Proc* 40: 433–455.

Stickler GB, Pugh DG (1967) Hereditary progressive arthro-ophthalmopathy. II. Additional observations on vertebral abnormalities, a hearing defect, and a report of a similar case. *Mayo Clin Proc* 42: 495–500.

Tomaski SM, Zalzal GH, Saal HM (1995) Airway obstruction in the Pierre Robin sequence. *Laryngoscope* 105: 111–114.

Vikkula M, Mariman ECM, Lui VCH, Zhidkova NI, Tiller GE, Goldring MB, van Beersum SEC, de Waal Malefijt MC, van den Hoogan FH, Ropers HH (1995) Autosomal dominant and recessive osteochondrodysplasias associated with the *COL11A2* locus. *Cell* 80: 431–437.

Wagner H (1938) Ein bisher unbekanntes Erbleiden des Auges (degeneratio hyaloideo-retinalis hereditaria), beobachtet im Kanton Zurich. *Klin Mbl Augenheilk* 100: 840–858.

Weissenbacher G, Zweymuller E (1964) Gleichzeitiges Vorkommen eines Syndroms von Pierre Robin und einer fetalen Chondrodysplasie. *Mschr Kinderheilk* 112: 315–317.

Wilkin DJ, Mortier GR, Johnson CL, Jones MC, De Paepe A, Shohat M, Wilden RS, Falk RE, Cohn DH. (1998a) Correlation of linkage data with clinical features in eight families with Stickler syndrome. *Am J Med Genet* 80: 121–127.

Wilkin DJ, Clark AM, Glick IE, Liberfarb R, Cohn DH, Francomano CA (1998b) Rapid identification of common sites of *COL2A1* mutations in Stickler syndrome. *Am J Hum Genet* 63: A393.

Wilson MC, McDonald-McGinn DM, Quinn GE, Markowitz GD, LaRossa D, Pacuraruk AD, Zhu X, Zackai EH. (1996) Long-term follow-up of ocular findings in children with Stickler's syndrome. *Am J Ophthalmol* 122: 727–728.

CHAPTER 25

TRISOMY 18 AND TRISOMY 13 SYNDROMES

JOHN C. CAREY

TRISOMY 18

Incidence

Trisomy 18 syndrome, also known as the Edwards syndrome, was originally described by Professor John Edwards and colleagues in a single case published in the spring of 1960. Soon after, Smith and colleagues at the University of Wisconsin described the first patients in North America and the syndromal pattern became established (Edwards et al., 1960; Smith et al., 1960). Indeed, this group was instrumental in the original descriptions of both trisomy 18 and trisomy 13. Since that time, hundreds of case reports and several series have been widely published throughout the world. Trisomy 18 represents the second most common autosomal trisomy syndrome behind trisomy 21 (Down syndrome). The pattern in trisomy 18 includes a recognizable constellation of major and minor anomalies, a predisposition to increased neonatal and infant mortality, and a significant developmental and motor disability in older children. A detailed listing of the many manifestations and their approximate frequency in the syndrome is given by Jones (1997).

On the basis of numerous studies performed in different areas of North America,

Europe, and Australia, the prevalence in live-born infants ranges from 1 in 3600 to 1 in 8500 (Root and Carey, 1994: Embleton et al., 1996). The most accurate estimate in live-births with only minimal influence by prenatal screening is from the Utah study and indicates a figure in livebirths of about 1 in 6000. Because trisomy 18 is a relatively common chromosomal cause of stillbirths, the frequency in *total* births would obviously be higher than this figure of 1 in 6000 (Root and Carey, 1994).

Birth prevalence data is altered by prenatal detection that is based on screening with maternal age or maternal serum triple marker screening and amniocentesis and followed by pregnancy termination of affected fetuses. A recent study in the United Kingdom determined the frequency of trisomy 18 at 18 weeks gestation to be 1 in 4274 and in liveborn infants to be 1 in 8333 (Embleton et al., 1996). If one assumes a birth prevalence of 1 in 6000, these figures estimate the current change in birth prevalence of trisomy 18 caused by prenatal diagnosis.

Diagnostic Criteria

The characteristic pattern of prenatal growth deficiency, craniofacial features (Fig. 25.1), distinctive hand posture of overriding fingers, nail hypoplasia, and short sternum allows for

Management of Genetic Syndromes, Edited by Suzanne B. Cassidy and Judith E. Allanson
ISBN 0-471-31286-X   Copyright © 2001 by Wiley-Liss, Inc.

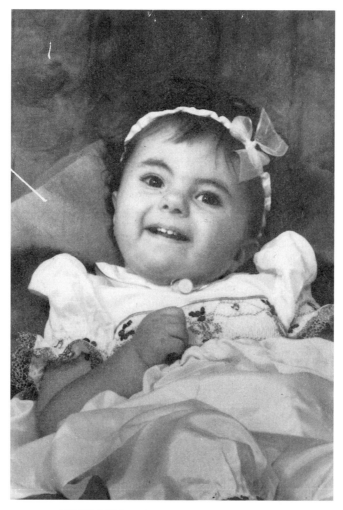

FIGURE 25.1. A 2 year old girl with trisomy 18.

clinical diagnosis in the newborn infant with trisomy 18. Marion et al. (1988) developed a bedside scoring system for the diagnosis of trisomy 18 syndrome in the newborn period that provides the clinician without specialized training in clinical genetics and dysmorphology a useful checklist to help differentiate newborns with the syndrome from other infants with multiple congenital anomalies.

The establishment of a diagnosis in trisomy 18 syndrome occurs by the performance of a standard G-banded karyotype demonstrating the extra chromosome 18 or one of the less common partial trisomy 18 findings seen in individuals with the Edwards syndrome phenotype, as discussed below.

Etiology, Pathogenesis, and Genetics

Trisomy 18 phenotype (Edwards syndrome) is usually the result of trisomy, i.e., 3 copies, of the 18th chromosome. In 4 recent large series that attempted to ascertain all cases in a region through a surveillance program, 165 of 176 neonates with the Edwards syndrome phenotype had full trisomy 18 (Carter et al., 1985; Young et al., 1986; Goldstein and

Nielsen, 1988; Embleton et al., 1996); 8 of 176, or 5%, had mosaicism, and 3 had partial trisomy 18, usually caused by an unbalanced translocation. Thus about 94% of infants labeled as having the syndrome will have full trisomy 18, whereas the remainder will have mosaicism or partial 18q trisomy.

In full trisomy 18 the extra chromosome is presumably present because of nondisjunction. A number of recent investigations have studied the mechanism of origin of the nondisjunction in trisomy 18 (Kupke and Mueller, 1989; Fisher et al., 1995; Eggermann et al., 1996; Bugge et al., 1998). The error in nondisjunction can arise as a malsegregation of chromosomes during meiosis or postzygotic mitosis, as has been demonstrated in other trisomies. From combined series, 95% of the time when determination could be made, the additional chromosome was a result of maternal nondisjunction. Of note, in the paternally derived cases the error was postzygotic in a number of situations. What was more unique, however, was the observation that about 50% of the nondisjunctional errors in oogenesis were in meiosis II. This is unlike all other human trisomies that have been investigated, which usually show a higher frequency of maternal meiosis I errors. Also, in contrast to trisomy 21, the error in maternal meiosis II showed normal recombination in the nondisjoined chromosomes. As in trisomy 21 and trisomy 13, the frequency of nondisjunctional trisomy 18 increases with advancing maternal age. However, the increased frequency of maternal meiosis II errors and the normal recombination indicate that the biology of nondisjunction in trisomy 18 is unique.

There has been much controversy regarding the critical region of chromosome 18 that results in the classical Edwards syndrome. A number of regions of the 18 long arm have been proposed to represent the important area that generates the phenotype, but no clear consensus has been reached (Wilson, 1993;

Boghosian-Sell et al., 1994). The small number of cases of partial trisomy 18, as well as the intrinsic variability of cases with full trisomy 18, makes conclusions about genotype-phenotype correlations tentative. However, the milder manifestations of patients with 18p trisomy and the Edwards syndrome-like phenotype in patients with trisomy of almost the entire long arm support a pivotal role for the 18q region, as documented by Wilson (1993). On the other hand, the fact that the two patients with trisomy of 18q.11.2 to terminus reported by Boghosian-Sell et al. (1994) do not exhibit the full classical Edwards syndrome phenotype suggests that the 18p and/or the 18q11.1 region have/has some role in generating the complete pattern. These two patients appear to have a somewhat different facial gestalt than surviving infants with trisomy 18 (personal observation), and they have better prenatal and postnatal growth than older children with full trisomy 18.

There has been a general lack of data regarding recurrence risk in both trisomy 18 and trisomy 13. Most practicing geneticists tend to use the 1–2% recurrence risk figure for nondisjunction, as calculated empirically in trisomy 21. Of note, low-grade parental mosaicism has been described on two occasions in sporadic cases of trisomy 18 (Beratis et al., 1972). In addition, a number of reported cases have demonstrated the occurrence of two different trisomies in siblings (reviewed by Baty et al., 1994a). The only empiric data on trisomies 18 and 13, which included 168 and 50 siblings, respectively, showed no chromosome abnormality (Baty et al., 1994a). However, in one family with a liveborn infant with trisomy 13, there had been a previously terminated fetus with trisomy 18 that was not part of the original study of cases of trisomy 18. If these figures are combined, they indicate a recurrence of 1 in 181 pregnancies, or a risk of 0.55%, with confidence limits of 0–1.6%. This figure obviously is close to 1% and supports the approach of the author, who quotes a recurrence risk of "1% or slightly less." The recurrence risk in partial trisomy cases would obviously depend on the presence or absence of a translocation or inversion in one of the parents. A *de novo* duplication is not associated with increased risk, whereas a familial translocation may predispose to unbalanced offspring and would have a recurrence risk larger than that of trisomy 18.

Diagnostic Testing

As mentioned above, definitive diagnosis of trisomy 18 is by detection of complete or partial trisomy of chromosome 18. This can be easily accomplished in any laboratory competent in performing chromosome analysis. Rapid diagnosis by interphase fluorescence *in situ* hybridization (FISH) in many newborns with trisomy 18 (and trisomy 13) can be helpful in making decisions regarding surgical intervention and care. Lymphocyte analysis usually takes 48 hours, but collecting bone marrow aspirate with results available in 6–8 hours may be important in some cases. More recently, buccal smears have been proposed for rapid diagnosis using DNA probes (Harris et al., 1994).

Because of the association between trisomy 18 and advanced maternal age, prenatal diagnosis of fetuses with trisomy 18 has paralleled the development of amniocentesis and chorionic villus sampling programs. In recent years, a significant body of literature has developed around the sonographic detection of patterns suggestive of trisomy 18 (and trisomy 13). Because of the common occurrence of intrauterine growth retardation in fetuses with trisomy 18 in both the second and third trimester, the diagnosis is often made during these gestational periods. In addition, polyhydramnios occurs in 30–60% of pregnancies with trisomy 18 and often leads to prenatal diagnosis. A number of characteristic prenatal signs have been described in fetuses with trisomy 18. These findings, in conjunction with intrauterine growth retardation or a major malformation

consistent with the phenotype, often bring up the diagnosis in prenatal settings after 20 weeks of gestation. Hill (1996) recently reviewed the sonographic detection of trisomy 18 comprehensively. The most publicized sonographic markers include choroid plexus cysts, large cysterna magna, and a "strawberry"–shaped calvarium.

The usefulness of choroid plexus cysts as a sign of trisomy 18 is a controversial topic in the obstetric literature, with no clear consensus on when to offer amniocentesis for karyotype when cysts are discovered, particularly when there are no other findings (Gross et al., 1995; Shields et al., 1996; Reinsch, 1997). Because some second trimester fetuses with trisomy 18 will have no other anomalies or growth findings, there is an increased risk of trisomy 18 in the presence of an isolated choroid plexus cyst (Reinsch, 1997). However, the decision about the performance of invasive prenatal diagnosis is complicated, and the author recommends reviewing the risk figures with the family in light of maternal age-specific risks and other prenatal screening. Gratton et al. (1996) presented estimates based on maternal age and multiple-marker screening in the presence of an isolated choroid plexus cyst in the clinical scenario. In the final analysis, it is the family who will make the decision based on the individual risk in the context of the procedural risk, the perceived impact of trisomy 18, and the perceived benefit of making the diagnosis in utero.

Multiple-marker screening is being used in the prenatal diagnosis of trisomy 18. Staples et al. (1991) showed that individual levels of human chorionic gonadotropin (hCG), unconjugated estriol, and α-fetoprotein (AFP) are significantly lower in pregnancies with trisomy 18 than in an unaffected pregnancy. In one recent study, the median levels of AFP, unconjugated estriol, and hCG were 0.65, 0.43, and 0.36 multiples of the unaffected population median (MoMs), respectively (Palomaki et al., 1995). With the use of a method of individual risk estimation based on these markers and maternal age, 60% of pregnancies associated with trisomy 18 can be detected.

Another controversy in the prenatal diagnosis of trisomy 18 is the utilization of FISH markers with the detection of three signals in amniocytes at interphase. The controversy centers on the utilization of this approach unaccompanied by the traditional metaphase chromosome analysis. Most clinicians feel that three FISH signals in conjunction with characteristic ultrasound abnormalities is sufficient to make the prenatal diagnosis before the availability of metaphase chromosome results. The community of cytogeneticists still expresses some discomfort in the utilization of FISH alone in making the diagnosis. The prenatal diagnosis of trisomy 18 in the mid to late second or third trimester is of significance, because it may modify management at the time of delivery (see **MANIFESTATIONS AND MANAGEMENT**).

Differential Diagnosis

The cardinal features of trisomy 18, the Edwards syndrome phenotype, include consistent findings of prenatal growth deficiency, characteristic facial appearance, overriding fingers and clenched hand, hypoplastic nails, and short sternum. Additional findings, such as short hallux and frequent malformations, help support the diagnosis. The syndromal pattern is quite discrete and, in its totality, is rarely confused with other syndromes.

The most common condition with overlapping features includes the heterogeneous group of disorders falling under the diagnosis of the fetal akinesia sequence. This condition, sometimes labeled as Pena-Shokeir syndrome type I, involves polyhydramnios, characteristic facial features, and multiple joint contractures including overriding fingers (Jones, 1997). Although this is a heterogeneous group of mostly autosomal recessive conditions, most cases do not have the structural heart defects and lack the characteristic face of trisomy 18. Of note, there

is a condition originally described in the French literature as pseudotrisomy 18 syndrome (Simpson and German, 1969). In retrospect, most children labeled with this condition probably fall into the fetal akinesia sequence category.

Because of the similarity in hand and finger positioning, some cases with the condition distal arthrogryposis type I might be confused with trisomy 18. However, infants with distal arthrogryposis type I do not have the major malformations and usually lack the prenatal growth deficiency, and they are thus easily distinguished from those with trisomy 18. Because of overlapping malformations, occasionally some infants with CHARGE association (see Chapter 5) can be confused with trisomy 18. Again, the entire pattern of findings, and the normal karyotype in CHARGE association, will distinguish the two conditions.

TRISOMY 13

Incidence

In the same issue of *The Lancet* in which the original case of trisomy 18 was published, the original case of trisomy 13 was also presented (Patau et al., 1960). Since that time there have been hundreds of case reports and a few large series. Generally, trisomy 13 syndrome presents as an obvious multiple congenital anomaly pattern, unlike trisomy 18 in which external major malformations are less notable. The combination of orofacial clefts, microphthalmia/anophthalmia, and postaxial polydactyly of the limbs allows for recognition by the clinician. However, because each of the three mentioned cardinal features have only 60–70% occurrence in the syndrome, clinical diagnosis can be challenging, especially in a child without a cleft lip or the facial features of holoprosencephaly. Trisomy 13 is usually the result of the presence of an extra 13th chromosome, leading to 47 chromosomes. The occurrence of translocations makes up a higher portion in trisomy

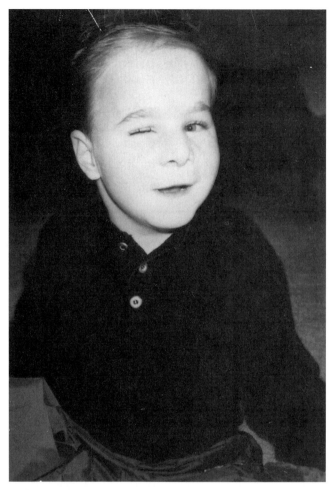

FIGURE 25.2. A $5\frac{1}{2}$ year old boy with trisomy 13. Note the distinctive facial features of the older child.

13 syndrome than in trisomy 18 syndrome. There are fewer birth prevalence studies than in trisomy 18, but estimates in early studies ranged from 1 in 5000 to 1 in 12,000 total births. Two recent studies from Denmark and the United Kingdom found birth prevalence in liveborns of approximately 1 in 20,000 to 1 in 29,000 (Goldstein and Nielsen, 1988; Wyllie et al., 1994). The concurrent influence of prenatal diagnosis and subsequent termination of affected fetuses modifies these figures. Thus, as in trisomy 18, this figure in liveborn infants is lower than the frequency of trisomy 13 at 15–16 weeks of gestation. Of note, these figures are still lower than expected from the earlier estimates of prevalence of trisomy 13 mentioned above. This is probably caused by the relatively small numbers involved in these early studies, rather than a true decreasing occurrence of trisomy 13 in recent decades. The frequency of trisomy 13 at 15–16 weeks of pregnancy in Utah (1995–1997), based on unpublished data from the Utah Congenital Malformation Registry combining livebirths, stillbirths, and terminated pregnancies, is just below 1 in 6000 (personal data). The best estimate of live births with trisomy 13 after accounting for prenatal diagnosis is approximately 1 in 10,000 to 1 in 20,000.

Diagnostic Criteria

The pattern of malformations in the most typical infants with trisomy 13 is quite characteristic and allows for clinical diagnosis by the neonatal practitioner. As mentioned, orofacial clefts, microphthalmia/anophthalmia, and postaxial polydactyly of hands and/or feet represent the cardinal signs. Trisomy 13 should always be considered in an infant with holoprosencephaly and multiple anomalies. Localized cutis aplasia of the occipital region, when present, also helps in the clinical diagnosis. In infants without cleft lip or the craniofacial features of holoprosencephaly (cyclops or cebocephaly), the facial gestalt (Fig. 25.2), especially the prominence of the nasal bridge and tip, is helpful in diagnosis. Minor anomalies such as capillary hemangiomas of the forehead, anterior cowlick, and ear malformations are also of assistance. The clinical findings are listed by Jones (1997). Of course, diagnosis must be confirmed by finding trisomy of all or most of the long arm of chromosome 13 on chromosome analysis. A number of abnormalities that are found on postmortem examination in trisomy 13 are particularly distinctive and can allow for differentiation in confusing cases (Moerman et al., 1988), including holoprosencephaly of any type and pancreatic and cystic renal dysplasia.

Etiology, Pathogenesis, and Genetics

The etiology of the trisomy 13 phenotype (Patau syndrome) is the extra chromosome 13. Many reviews cite the occurrence of translocation trisomy 13 in about 20% of cases. The above-cited population studies of Denmark and the United Kingdom indicate that about 5–10% of cases of trisomy 13 are caused by a translocation, usually a 13;14 unbalanced Robertsonian translocation. Mosaicism for trisomy 13 makes up a smaller proportion of cases in population series of Patau syndrome. A recent review of trisomy 13 mosaicism indicates the presence of only 30 well-documented cases in

the world literature (Delatycki and Gardner, 1997). As for all chromosomal mosaicism syndromes, there is little correlation between the degree of mosaicism in lymphocytes and the resultant resemblance to the classical Patau syndrome (Delatycki and Gardner, 1997).

In trisomy 13 due to nondisjunction, the origin of the extra chromosome is maternal in about 90% of cases. Most of the time the stage of nondisjunction is maternal meiosis I, unlike trisomy 18, where maternal meiosis II is as common as meiosis I (Zaragoza et al., 1994; Robinson et al., 1996). Of cases in which nondisjunction is paternal in origin, the majority are primarily postzygotic mitotic errors. In the case of trisomy 13 due to 13;13 translocations, the structural abnormalities are usually isochromosomes that originate in mitosis.

Phenotype-karyotype correlations for partial trisomies of chromosome 13 have been discussed more extensively than in most other partial trisomy syndromes (Rogers, 1984; Tharapel et al., 1986). On the basis of the summary of published cases of both proximal and distal partial trisomies, one can conclude that the orofacial clefts and scalp defects are caused by genes that are duplicated on the proximal portion of 13q. The prominent nasal bridge and polydactyly are caused by genes on the bottom half of 13q. Cases of partial 13q have a better outcome in terms of lifespan than full trisomy 13, suggesting that genes all along the chromosome are involved in the occurrence of increased neonatal mortality, as in trisomy 18. The issues surrounding the recurrence risk for trisomy 13 are similar to those of trisomy 18 and are discussed above.

Diagnostic Testing

Most of the relevant diagnostic issues in trisomy 13 are the same as those discussed above for trisomy 18. There is a recent thorough review of the prenatal ultrasound findings in trisomy 13 (Lehman et al., 1995).

About 80% of fetuses recognized in the second trimester have findings on prenatal ultrasound. Because of the high occurrence of holoprosencephaly in trisomy 13, the prenatal diagnosis of holoprosencephaly should always raise the question of trisomy 13, especially when other ultrasound abnormalities are found. The long list of sonographically detectable malformations associated with trisomy 13 has also been summarized (Hill, 1996). Unlike trisomy 18, maternal serum triple-marker screening has not shown as characteristic a pattern and will not be discussed here. Immediate diagnosis in the newborn period with bone marrow aspiration or FISH investigations is often indicated because of the need for urgent management decisions, which are discussed below. As in the case of trisomy 18, FISH probes can be used in the postmortem situation, including in stillborns, if chromosomes were not initially obtained.

Differential Diagnosis

Because the cardinal features of trisomy 13 syndrome include a number of manifestations that are seen in various other multiple congenital anomaly situations, the differential diagnosis is quite long. However, the pattern in total is distinctive and usually allows for straightforward diagnosis. The presence of postaxial polydactyly in the context of either neonatal illness or death suggests Meckel-Gruber and hydrolethalus syndromes. The characteristic renal malformations and encephalocele in Meckel-Gruber syndrome usually allow it to be distinguished from trisomy 13. Another recently described condition in the differential diagnosis is the so-called holoprosencephaly-polydactyly syndrome, also known as "pseudotrisomy 13" (reviewed by Lurie and Wulfsberg, 1993). In addition, severe Smith-Lemli-Opitz syndrome (see Chapter 21) shares important similarities. Other syndromes with holoprosencephaly and multiple anomalies also overlap with trisomy 13, but again, the chromosome finding allows for distinction.

MANIFESTATIONS AND MANAGEMENT

The approach to the management of a third-trimester fetus and newborn infant with trisomy 18 or 13 is quite complicated, and the literature is clearly controversial. The avoidance of delivery by caesarean section when a fetus is known to have trisomy 18 appears to be the trend in the U.S. and British obstetric literature (Schneider et al., 1981; Rochelson et al., 1986). However, Spinnato et al. (1995) make a strong ethical case for respecting maternal autonomy in making decisions regarding aggressive intrapartum management in conditions like trisomy 18 and related serious disorders. It is important to acknowledge that because approximately 50% of infants with trisomy 18 or 13 will live longer than a week and about 5% of infants will live past 1 year, the casually used term of "lethal abnormality" seems inappropriate and misleading. Certainly, families of children with trisomy 18 and 13 and related serious disorders assert quite eloquently their concern about the use of "lethal" in these settings (Baty et al., 1994).

The oral tradition in the pediatric literature also indicates a nonintervention approach in newborn management of trisomy 18 and 13. Bos et al. (1992) summarize these issues, arguing that early diagnosis is very important so that surgery can be withheld. The authors make a case that a patient with trisomy 18 should be viewed as having a "hopeless outlook" and "not to be subjected to invasive procedures." Arguments indicating that there is "imminent death" and profound mental retardation suggest to Bos et al. that patients with trisomy 18 should be "allowed to die." Paris et al. (1992) make the point that to support "groundless hopes or false expectations as a means for caring or protecting the parents exposes the infant to potential pain and fruitless suffering." They proceed by saying; "to be fair to the infant, the parents, and the staff, the plan for a patient afflicted with a fatal condition should be thought through before any interventions are undertaken."

There is amazingly little documentation of the precise reason for death in infancy or *in utero* for either condition. Conventionally, it is usually stated that the early mortality is due to the high occurrence of structural heart malformations. However, as will be detailed below, most of the heart lesions in both syndromes are not those that result in death in infancy. Recent investigations into the natural history of trisomy 18 and 13 have suggested that central apnea, or its presence with a combination of other health factors, is the primary pathogenesis of the increased infant mortality (Root and Carey, 1994; Wyllie et al., 1994; Embleton et al., 1996).

The most important issues and questions that emerge in the counseling and management of newborn infants with trisomy 18 or 13 are the high infant mortality and the significant developmental disability. It is not clear why, but a certain percentage of children with trisomy 18 and 13 will survive the first year of life. There are no factors in a 1-to 2-week-old infant who does not require a ventilator that predict who will survive and who will not, other than the absence of serious malformations such as hypoplastic left heart or diaphragmatic hernia (personal experience). Most children with trisomy 18 or 13 who are beyond the newborn period do not receive more aggressive or extraordinary care (Root and Carey, 1994). The older children with trisomy 18 or 13 in the literature, and in the international support group, SOFT (Support Organization for Trisomy 18, 13 and Related Disorders), are not individuals who have been maintained on home ventilators or other such extraordinary maneuvers to sustain life.

The trend in neonatal intensive care in the last two decades has placed significant weight on parental decision making, usually in the context of the "best interest for the child." This being the case, it seems prudent for the clinician to be accurate and current on the mortality risk tables and developmental outcome of older infants and children with trisomy 18 and 13. About 5% of children will be alive at 1 year of age without extraordinary measures, and all of these children will progress in developmental milestones, albeit slowly. Parents appreciate partnership in decision making. Overly simplified and value-laden terms such as "lethal," "vegetative," and "hopeless" not only are inaccurate but convey an implicit message from the outset. The recent change in approach to the neonatal care of infants with trisomy 18 and 13 is documented in the natural history section of the entry on trisomy 18 and 13 in *Smith's Recognizable Patterns of Human Malformation* (Jones, 1997). In earlier editions, recommendation was withdrawal of all treatment designed "to prolong life" once the diagnosis was made. In the newest edition the author states, "Once the diagnosis has been established, limitations of extraordinary medical means for prolongation of life should be seriously considered. Parents and individual circumstances of each infant must be taken into consideration."

There is developmental progress in children with these syndromes who survive, and initial counseling of the family should be realistic and accurate but not unnecessarily grim and bleak. Options for care and management must be explained. Families clearly appreciate an honest and straightforward approach to the challenges and decisions with the best interests of the child in mind (personal experience).

The families of infants with trisomy 18 or 13 must initially deal with the issue of low survival rate and the practical decisions in the newborn period concerning resuscitation, surgery, and life support. As time goes on, the family must then deal with the prospect of significant disability if the baby survives. Mixed and ambivalent feelings about what is best for the child are natural. The primary care practitioner has a unique opportunity and obligation to provide support on an ongoing basis. Recognition of the uncertainty of the situation and of the paradox of preparing for both the probability of death and the possibility of living is helpful in the early weeks (Carey, 1992).

In neonatal care, appropriate fluid and nutritional support are always indicated. Decisions can be made on a day-by-day, week-by-week, or month-by-month basis, and different courses can be pursued according to the status of the child and changing circumstances. Despite the reality of the life expectancy figures and the overwhelming nature of the condition, a respectful and humanistic approach that recognizes parental feelings and thoughts on each decision represents a thoughtful and caring way to proceed.

Growth and Feeding

Growth deficiency is the rule for both trisomy 18 and 13. Growth charts for older infants have been collated and published (Baty et al., 1994a). In the publication by SOFT, Barnes and Carey (1996) have formatted these growth charts to fit into the patients' regular charts. Weight and length are below the 3rd percentile, more consistently so in trisomy 18 than in trisomy 13. By the age of 1 year, the average weight in trisomy 13 is near the 5th percentile, with many cases exceeding the 5th percentile after 3 years of age. Length and height are also less affected in trisomy 13 in the third and fourth years of life than in trisomy 18. Head circumference tends to be below the 3rd percentile, on average. In trisomy 13, the head circumference is lower in the presence of holoprosencephaly in surviving children.

For surviving infants with trisomy 18 and 13, feeding difficulties remain one of the challenges of childhood. Feeding is a particularly difficult problem in neonates and infants with trisomy 18 or 13. Most infants with either condition require tube feeding from birth. In one study, 44% and 53% of children with trisomy 18 and 13, respectively, did learn bottle or breast feeding during the first few weeks or months of life

(Baty et al., 1994a). This study probably was biased toward children with prolonged survival, so overall rates may be lower. It is unusual for a child with trisomy 18 or 13 who has not established oral feeding in infancy to do so later in life; the children who are bottle fed usually establish this skill during the first few months of life (personal observation). At least three infants with trisomy 18 have been able to nurse throughout infancy (personal data). Both the sucking and swallowing stages are difficult for these infants. Many families of older infants with trisomy 18 elect to have a gastrostomy tube placed when it becomes clear that the baby will never be able to master bottle feeding. The average age of gastrostomy placement was 7 and 8 months for trisomy 13 and 18, respectively, in the only published study (Baty et al., 1994a).

Gastroesophageal reflux is a consistent finding in infants with trisomy 18 and 13 and may explain irritability and recurrent pneumonias. Aspiration during feeding or from reflux may be the cause of early death. Gastrointestinal malformations can also play a role in feeding problems after the newborn period. Pyloric stenosis has been reported in trisomy 18, and malrotation is occasionally seen in trisomy 13; these may also affect feeding. Orofacial clefts are a frequent finding in trisomy 13 and an occasional feature of trisomy 18, and their presence will complicate the feeding difficulties in both syndromes.

Thus, in the older infant, questions about monitoring, referral to a dysphagia team, and evaluation of upper airway will emerge.

Evaluation

- Length, weight, and head circumference should be measured during each health supervision visit and plotted on the published growth curves (Baty et al., 1994a)
- Referral to a dysphagia team for evaluation may be useful.

- Assessment of the presence of gastroe-sophageal reflux as a potential factor in feeding problems should occur.

- If a child with trisomy 18 or 13 is not bottle feeding by 6 months of age, consideration of gastrostomy placement is indicated.

- Even a child who appears to be able to bottle feed in the later months of life should have an evaluation of feeding to establish airway competency.

Treatment

- Evaluative and treatment decisions should be discussed with parents on a regular basis. It is appropriate to change the degree of intervention during the course of support and care.

- Training the parents in nasal or oral gastric tube feeding will be necessary in the majority of children who require tube feeding.

- Appropriate therapy for gastroesopha-geal reflux can be initiated when this is determined to be a factor. Nissan fundoplication has been successfully performed in many children who are part of the SOFT Registry.

- Gastrostomy has been successfully performed on many children recorded in the SOFT Registry (unpublished data, SOFT Registry, Barnes and Carey, 1999).

- Anesthetic risks for these or any surgical procedures for the majority of children with either condition who have structural heart malformations require consultation by cardiology.

Development and Behavior

Very little has been written about the developmental outcome of children with trisomy 18 and 13. Most review papers and chapters indicate the presence of profound mental retardation in surviving children with both trisomies. A seminal paper by Van Dyke

and Allen (1990) was the first work in the pediatric literature to discuss the challenges faced by parents of children with trisomy 18, directing primary care practitioners to approach long-term management in children with trisomy 18 as they would in any child with disabilities.

Individual case reports of older children indicate that expressive language and walking do not occur in trisomy 18 or 13. Of note, there is one report of a 4-year-old with full trisomy 18 who walked independently (Ray et al., 1986). Advancement of motor milestones was reported in detail in another case (Woldorf and Johnson, 1994). Baty et al. (1994b) published their experience with 62 older individuals with trisomy 18 and 14 with trisomy 13. Developmental records were collected on children through collaboration with SOFT. Although all these individuals were clearly functioning in the severely to profoundly developmentally handicapped range, the children did achieve some skills of childhood and continued to learn. A number of older children with trisomy 18 could use a walker, and two children with trisomy 13 were able to walk unsupported. Developmental quotients in children over 1 year of age were in the 0.2 to 0.3 range, with developmental ages in the older children with trisomy 18 averaging 6 to 7 months and those with trisomy 13 averaging 13 months. In this series many skills that are conventionally thought not to occur in trisomy 18 or 13 are seen as individual abilities in some children. These included self-feeding, sleeping independently, object permanence, and understanding cause and effect. Older infants with trisomy 18 or 13 recognize their family and smile responsively. Developmental achievements in both syndromes have been summarized using milestones from the Denver developmental screen (Baty et al., 1994b).

Evaluation

- Developmental evaluation using standard developmental screening tools, such as the Denver Developmental

Screening Test, should be performed at regular health supervision visits.

Treatment

- Referral to early intervention programs is recommended in the ongoing care of infants and children with trisomy 18 or 13.
- Programs for children with visual disabilities may be needed for those with trisomy 13 who have significant visual abnormalities.
- For children with trisomy 13 who have hearing loss as well as visual disabilities, more comprehensive programs can be utilized. Because the apparent hearing loss of trisomy 18 does not necessarily indicate functional hearing impairment, standard early intervention programs are adequate.

Neurologic

A variety of developmental abnormalities of the brain have been described in autopsy series of trisomy 18 and 13 (Moerman et al., 1988; Kinoshita et al., 1989). Cerebellar hypoplasia has been described consistently in trisomy 18 and has been noted even in prenatal ultrasound series. Other primary structural defects of the brain described in trisomy 18 include agenesis of the corpus callosum, microgyria, and hydrocephalus. Of note, about 5% of infants with trisomy 18 have meningomyelocele, which is also seen occasionally in trisomy 13.

Functional neurological findings in both conditions include hypotonia in infancy, hypertonia later in childhood, seizures, and central apnea. Seizures occur in about 25–50% of older infants with both conditions. Seizure management is usually not complicated in either syndrome, and convulsions tend to be well controlled with appropriate medications. Central apnea is reported with holoprosencephaly, but in both syndromes it usually does not have a clear anatomical basis. Recent investigations into the natural history of trisomy 18 and 13 have suggested that central apnea, or its presence with a combination of other health factors, is the primary pathogenesis of the increased infant mortality (Root and Carey, 1994; Embleton et al., 1996; Wyllie et al., 1994).

The holoprosencephaly that is commonly present in trisomy 13 deserves special mention. Holoprosencephaly of some degree is present in about 60–70% of infants with trisomy 13, either by imaging study or autopsy. This defect of early embryogenesis of the forebrain involves lack of cleavage of the frontal hemispheres, often resulting in a single holoventricle. The holoprosencephaly in trisomy 13 can be associated with the classical facial malformations that are often seen in the presence of this defect, including cyclopia, cebocephaly, or premaxillary agenesis. In one series, the majority of the infants with trisomy 13 and holoprosencephaly had the alobar variety (Moerman et al., 1988). Other primary central nervous system malformations, including cerebellar hypoplasia and agenesis of the corpus callosum, have been reported occasionally. The presence or absence of holoprosencephaly in a newborn with trisomy 13 may have prognostic significance. Although it is known that children with trisomy 13 *without* holoprosencephaly have central apnea, individuals that survive the first year of life do *not* have semilobar or alobar holoprosencephaly as commonly as in trisomy 13 in general (unpublished observations; Reynolds et al., 1991).

The central nervous system abnormalities mentioned above play a significant role in the early mortality, central apnea, and feeding difficulties of newborn and young infants with trisomy 18 and 13 syndromes. However, the precise anatomical delineation of these defects (other than holoprosencephaly) probably does not assist in management. The seizures are generally straightforward to control in both conditions but tend to be more complicated in trisomy 13, possibly related to the presence of holoprosencephaly.

Evaluation

- Neurological examination is recommended for all infants and young children with trisomy 18 and 13.
- Neuroimaging should be done if predicting prognosis is important in older infants with trisomy 13.

Treatment

- The only treatment is related to the symptomatic occurrence of seizures or muscle tone abnormalities that occur in these children. These should be treated as in the general population, usually with anticonvulsants and physical therapy, respectively.
- Referral for early intervention, which would include physical and occupational therapy, is indicated in children with trisomy 18 or 13, as mentioned above.

Cardiovascular

Congenital heart malformations are present in about 80% of children with trisomy 13 and 90% of children with trisomy 18. The observed pattern of malformations is non-random and relatively specific. Over 90% of patients with trisomy 18 in recent series have a ventricular septal defect with polyvalvular disease (Van Praagh et al., 1989; Musewe et al., 1990; Balderston et al., 1990). In one series of trisomy 18, all 15 patients had polyvalvular disease, with 6 of the 15 having involvement of all four valves (Balderston et al., 1990). The valvular dysplasia of trisomy 18 can frequently result in tetralogy of Fallot. About 10% of patients with trisomy 18 will have a more complicated cardiac malformation, especially double-outlet right ventricle, endocardial cushion defect, or left-sided obstructive lesion. Shunt lesions, i.e., atrial septal defect and ventricular septal defects, are the most common lesions in trisomy 13. Polyvalvular dysplasia is less common in this syndrome than in trisomy 18. Double-outlet right ventricle occurs in some patients with trisomy 13 as well. Of note, the polyvalvular disease of both syndromes involves a redundant or thick leaflet but most often has relatively mild hemodynamic abnormality.

One important point in this discussion is that the majority of heart lesions in both syndromes are not those that produce neonatal death. In one series, only 6% of 31 patients with trisomy 18 or 13 had a lesion that would be considered lethal in infancy (Musewe et al., 1990). However, in this series there was the occurrence of frequent cyanosis and increased right ventricular dimensions, suggesting early development of pulmonary hypertension. In another series, 8 of 25 cases of trisomy 18 in which lung histology was studied had significant hypertrophy of the media and intimal proliferation suggesting early onset of pulmonary hypertension (Van Praagh et al., 1989). These authors suggest that patients with trisomy 18 may be predisposed to develop pulmonary vascular obstructive changes earlier than other children with ventricular septal defects.

A recent series of second-trimester fetuses examined for the presence of cardiac defects found structural heart malformations in all 19 fetuses with trisomy 18, and 16 of the 19 with ventricular septal defect had polyvalvular disease (Hyett et al., 1995).

Evaluation

- Cardiac evaluation is important at the time of diagnosis in all infants with trisomy 18 or 13. This should include an echocardiogram in the newborn period, both for assistance in management decisions and so that the family and primary care doctor have the appropriate clinical data if the infant is ill for unknown reasons. Having information about the cardiac defect and its potential role in causing symptoms is important during the process of decision making regarding care.

Treatment

- Families and their physicians vary in their approach to the treatment and management of the cardiovascular malformations in children with trisomy 18 or 13. Although the majority of children have nonlethal cardiac defects, the high frequency of shunt lesions and the early development of pulmonary hypertension, in the context of central apnea, feeding difficulties, and potential aspiration, may require treatment. Decisions regarding symptomatic treatment of heart failure or placement on oxygen and monitors should be made by families and physicians jointly.

- Because the majority of infants with trisomy 18 or 13 that succumb in the newborn or early infancy period die of central apnea or related symptoms rather than their heart defect (Embleton et al., 1996), heart surgery is rarely performed. However, once an infant with a heart defect is older than 2–3 months and is thriving, the issue of early development of pulmonary hypertension emerges. Discussion of surgery as an option is now more commonplace in North America than in the past. There are only four published reports of heart surgery in children with trisomy 18 and 13 (Van Dyke and Allen, 1990; Musewe et al., 1990; Baty et al., 1994a). In addition, the SOFT Registry group has collected cases throughout North America of children with trisomy 18 or 13 who have had cardiac surgery, most since 1990. Of 12 children with trisomy 18 who had cardiac surgery with available results, 7 had open-heart surgery (mostly ventricular septal defect repair) and 5 had closed procedures (patent ductus arteriosus ligation, pulmonary banding, and Blalock-Taussig shunt). Eight of the children survived the surgery and went home; three died during the hospitalization, and the result in the remaining patient

was not recorded. Four children with trisomy 13 had cardiac surgery, two open-heart for ventricular septal defect and tetralogy of Fallot and two closed procedures. All survived and left the hospital. The age range of these patients at the time of surgery was 4 days to 22 months; the majority were between 6 and 12 months of age. In addition, a study to learn the outcome in an additional 18 cases of trisomy 18 and 3 cases of trisomy 13 who had cardiac surgery is ongoing (personal data). Although definite conclusions from these data are somewhat limited, it is evident that children with trisomy 18 or 13 can survive anesthesia, and the majority who have had surgery have left the hospital.

Ophthalmologic

A large number of ocular manifestations have been reported in both trisomy 18 and 13 syndromes. The eye manifestations in trisomy 13 are particularly consistent and well established. Over 50% of newborns with trisomy 13 syndrome have microphthalmia or anophthalmia and colobomas. Retinal dysplasia is a common autopsy finding in infants with trisomy 13. The ocular findings associated with holoprosencephaly, including cyclopia and hypotelorism, are seen. Other distinctive eye findings seen in trisomy 13 include persistent hypoplastic primary vitreous with cataract and corneal opacities. Some infants with the condition will develop a congenital or early onset glaucoma. This could be the reason for unexplained irritability or other symptoms.

Significant ocular manifestations are much less common in trisomy 18. Although short palpebral fissures are common, major intraocular pathology or structural defects are seen in less than 10% of cases (Geiser et al., 1986). Cataracts and corneal opacities are occasionally seen in infants and young children with trisomy 18 (Calderone et al., 1983). Older infants have photophobia.

Evaluation

- Ophthalmology consultation is recommended in all older infants with trisomy 13 and when signs are present in infants with trisomy 18.
- Ophthalmologic evaluation is recommended for infants over 1 year of age with either condition, because visual acuity abnormalities are common in older children.

Treatment

- Treatment of glaucoma, cataracts, or corneal clouding should be individualized. Surgery can be suggested in older infants and children depending on the risk determined by the cardiologist and/or primary care practitioner.
- Sunglasses are helpful for photophobia in older infants and children with trisomy 18.

Genitourinary

A variety of structural defects of the genital and urinary tracts have been described in patients with trisomy 18 or 13. About two-thirds of infants with trisomy 18 will have a horseshoe kidney. Cystic dysplasias of various forms are commonly present in trisomy 13. Renal failure or disease is not a common cause of chronic illness or problems in infants and children despite the high frequency of defects (personal experience).

Urinary tract infections appear to occur with increased frequency in trisomy 18 and 13, perhaps related to the structural renal defects (Baty et al., 1994a).

Evaluation

- Because of the high frequency of renal defects, a screening abdominal ultrasound is indicated in surviving patients with trisomy 18.
- Those with significant renal defects should be followed for infection and

renal insufficiency by periodic creatinine and urinalysis.

Treatment

- Management of urinary tract infection and renal obstruction are the same as in any child.

Neoplasia

It appears that older infants and children with trisomy 18 are at increased risk to develop Wilms tumor and hepatoblastoma. In a recent series of the U.S. Wilms tumor registry, the conclusion was reached that Wilms tumor occurred more than expected in surviving children with trisomy 18 (Olson et al., 1995). Six older infants with trisomy 18 who have developed this malignancy have been reported (Faucette et al., 1991; Olson et al., 1995). In addition, the author is aware of four unpublished cases through personal communications. The presence of Wilms tumor in trisomy 18 makes biologic sense, because nodular renal blastema has been described at autopsy in infants in some pathology series. The age of development of Wilms tumor is after 5 years in most cases, which suggests a different biologic basis than the typical Wilms tumor in children.

There have been 5 case reports of infants and young children with trisomy 18 who developed hepatoblastoma (Bove et al., 1996; Teraguchi et al., 1997). Because this embryonal tumor occurs together with Wilms tumor in other malformation-dysplasia syndromes (for example, Beckwith-Wiedemann syndrome, see Chapter 4), it is biologically plausible that both of these would occur with increased risk in trisomy 18.

The actual risk to develop Wilms tumor or hepatoblastoma probably is less than 1%. Prognostically, the course has been extremely variable: 3 children died of complications related to treatment (surgery, infection); 1 was treated but died from pulmonary metastasis, 4 survived, and the other 2 succumbed because of parental choice of no treatment.

Evaluation

- Because of the high frequency of intra-abdominal tumors, particularly Wilms tumor, abdominal screening is indicated in surviving infants with trisomy 18. Although there is no established timing, it is reasonable to do abdominal screening every 6 months after the age of 6 months in infants and children with trisomy 18 (personal experience). The exact time to stop screening is unknown. Because the oldest case of development of Wilms tumor in trisomy 18 is 13 years, abdominal screening for this tumor is justified into adolescence.
- Because there has been only one reported case of Wilms tumor in trisomy 13, screening for Wilms tumor and hepatoblastoma is not indicated.

Treatment

- The treatment for Wilms tumor is similar to that in the general population.

Ears and Hearing

A vast array of middle ear and temporal bone abnormalities has been described in postmortem examinations of infants with trisomy 18 and 13. In addition, moderate to severe sensorineural hearing loss has been reported in evaluated older children. Structural ear malformations, including microtia and meatal atresia, are found on occasion in both syndromes. The external auricular abnormality of trisomy 18 is particularly characteristic, and it helps in diagnosis of newborns. The ear is small and has a small lobule that is slightly unraveled and attached to the scalp (cryptotia). The helix is frequently unfolded and simple.

Evaluation

- Audiological evaluation is recommended in infants with trisomy 18 or 13 older than 6 months of age. Behavioral testing can usually be accomplished in children older than 1 year of age.

- Brain stem auditory evoked response (BAER) studies have been performed in a number of infants and older children with trisomy 18, and children with trisomy 18 appear to do better on behavioral testing than their brain stem evoked responses would indicate (Michael Page, personal communication).

Treatment

- A trial of hearing aids in older infants with trisomy 18 or 13 who have abnormal audiological evaluations is appropriate (personal experience). However, if the hearing aid does not appear to improve communication and is difficult for the child to tolerate, the decision to continue or discontinue is individualized.

Musculoskeletal

A variety of musculoskeletal abnormalities occurs in both trisomy 18 and 13 syndromes, including medically significant malformations and minor anomalies of limb and skeleton. Postaxial polydactyly, especially of the hands, is a high frequency finding in patients with trisomy 13 (60–70%). Limb reduction defects can occur occasionally in both syndromes, and radial aplasia and other preaxial limb deficiencies occur in 5–10% of children with trisomy 18. Talipes equinovarus and calcaneovalgus positional foot deformities occur in both conditions but especially in trisomy 18, where about half of all children will have such a deformity. Some children with trisomy 18 will have contractures of other joints besides the feet, which can present as "arthrogryposis." The overriding fingers, often with camptodactyly, represent a diagnostic finding in trisomy 18.

Scoliosis develops commonly in older children with trisomy 18. This usually presents at 4 or 5 years of age and appears unrelated to structural defects of the vertebrae. Scoliosis may progress between ages 5 and 10 years.

Evaluation

- X-rays of the limbs should be performed when appropriate to management.
- Scoliosis should be evaluated clinically in older children with trisomy 18 at routine health supervision visits, and spine series can be done when clinical scoliosis is present.
- Referral to orthopedics should be considered on recognition of significant musculoskeletal abnormalities.

Treatment

- Decisions regarding the placement of casts for clubfeet and/or radial aplasia should be made keeping in mind the best interest of the child.
- Because it is uncommon for a child with trisomy 18 to walk unassisted and independently, many families and primary care physicians will defer decisions of surgery for talipes equinovarus or calcaneovalgus deformities until later childhood. However, these decisions are complex, because there are children with both syndromes who walk with assistance or independently. If this skill is acquired, treatment of positional foot deformity might be of benefit.
- Decisions about surgery for scoliosis may need to be made in the older child. Three adolescent girls with trisomy 18 are known to have had scoliosis surgery with placement of rods or fusion, and all tolerated the procedure (personal data). Decisions regarding this invasive surgery should be predicated on input from the cardiologist if the child has heart disease and/or pulmonary hypertension.

Respiratory

Because over 90% of children with trisomy 18 and 80% of children with trisomy 13 have a structural heart malformation, pulmonary hypertension related to heart defects is common in infancy. There is an impression that pulmonary hypertension may develop early in infancy in trisomy 18 (Van Praagh et al., 1989). In addition, upper airway problems including laryngomalacia and undefined airway obstruction have been seen, but the precise anatomical problem is not usually documented in either syndrome.

As mentioned above, most infants with trisomy 18 and 13 who die in infancy do so because of respiratory problems. Central apnea, upper airway obstruction, early-onset pulmonary hypertension, recurrent aspiration, feeding difficulties, tube feedings, and gastroesophageal reflux all contribute to mortality and respiratory problems, and together create a symptom complex that probably accounts for most early infant deaths (Root and Carey, 1994; Embleton et al., 1996). Frequent and open discussions are particularly important in the complicated management issues that surround the respiratory difficulties.

Evaluation

- How far to proceed and what evaluations to initiate will depend on the discussions between parents and care providers.
- Pediatric pulmonology and/or a dysphagia team may be helpful in sorting out the variables of this symptom complex.
- Evaluations, if decision is made to proceed, do not differ from those in other children with similar symptoms.

Treatment

- Decisions about home monitoring and oxygen therapy can be made on an individual basis after discussions between parents and care providers.

RESOURCES

USA Support Group SOFT
Barbara Van Herreweghe, President

2982 S. Union St.
Rochester, NY 14624
(800) 716-SOFT
http://www.trisomy.org/

Chromosome 18 Registry
The Chromosome 18 Registry and
Research Society
Jannine D. Cody, Ph.D., President
6302 Fox Head
San Antonio, TX 78247
(210) 657-4968
http://chr18.uthscsa.edu/

SOFT of United Kingdom
Jenny Robbins
Tudor Lodge, Redwood, Ross-on-Wye
Herefordshire, England HR9 5UD
(01)989-67480

Christine Rose
48 Froggatts Ride, Walmsley,
Sutton Coldfield
West Midlands, England B76 2TQ
(01)21 351-3122

REFERENCES

Balderston SN, Schaffer EN, Washington RL, Sondheimer HM (1990) Congenital polyvalvular disease in trisomy 18: Echocardiographic diagnosis. *Pediatr Cardiol* 11:138–142

Barnes AM, Carey JC (1996) *Care of the Infant and Child with Trisomy 18 or 13*. Omaha, NE SOFT Distribution Center, Meyer Institute.

Baty BJ, Blackburn BL, Carey JC (1994a) Natural history of trisomy 18 and trisomy 13. I. Growth, physical assessment, medical histories, survival, and recurrence risk. *Am J Med Genet* 49:175–188.

Baty BJ, Jorde LB, Blackburn BL, Carey JC (1994b) Natural history of trisomy 18 and trisomy 13. II. Psychomotor development. *Am J Med Genet* 49:189–194.

Beratis NG, Kardon NB, Hsu LYF, Grossman D, Hirschhorn K (1972) Parental mosaicism in trisomy 18. *Pediatrics* 50:908–911.

Boghosian-Sell L, Mewar R, Harrison W, Shapiro RM, Zackai EH, Carey JC, David L, Keppen L, Hudgins L, Overhauser J (1994) Molecular mapping of the Edwards syndrome phenotype to two noncontiguous regions on chromosome 18. *Am J Hum Genet* 55:476–483.

Bos AP, Broers CJM, Hazebroek FWJ, Van Hemel JO, Tibboel D, Swaay EW, Molenaar JC (1992) Avoidance of emergency surgery in newborn infants with trisomy 18. *Lancet* 339:913–917.

Bove KE, Soukup S, Ballard ET, Rychman F (1996) Hepatoblastoma in a child with trisomy 18: Cytogenetics, liver anomalies, and literature review. *Pediat Pathol Lab Med* 16:253–262.

Bugge M, Collins A, Petersen MB, Fisher J, Brandt C, Hertz JM, Tranebjaerg L, DeLozier-Blanchet C, Nicolaides P, Brondum-Nielsen K, Morton N, Mikkelsen M (1998) Non-disjunction of chromosome 18. *Hum Mol Genet* 7: 661–669.

Calderone JP, Chess J, Borodic G, Albert DM (1983) Intraocular pathology of trisomy 18 (Edwards syndrome): Report of a case and review of the literature. *Br J Ophthalmol* 67:162–169.

Carey JC (1992) Health supervision and anticipatory guidance for children with genetic disorders (including specific recommendations for trisomy 21, trisomy 18, and neurofibromatosis I). *Pediatr Clin N Am* 39:40–43.

Carter PE, Pearn JH, Bell J, Martin N, Anderson NG (1985) Survival in trisomy 18. *Clin Genet* 27:59–61.

Delatycki M, Gardner RJM (1997) Three cases of trisomy 13 mosaicism and a review of the literature. *Clin Genet* 51:403–407.

Edwards JUH, Harnden DG, Cameron AH, Crosse VM, Wolff OH (1960) A new trisomic syndrome. *Lancet* 1:787–789.

Eggermann T, Nothem MM, Eiben B, Hofmann JD, Hinkel K, Fimmers R, Schwanitz G (1996) Trisomy of human chromosome 18: Molecular studies on parental origin and cell stage of nondisjunction. *Hum Genet* 97:218–223.

Embleton ND, Wyllie JP, Wright MJ, Burn J, and Hunter S (1996) Natural history of trisomy 18. *Arch Dis Child* 75:38–41.

Faucette KJ, Carey JC, Lemons RL, Toledano S (1991) Trisomy 18 and Wilms tumor: Is there an association? *Clin Res* 39:96A.

Fisher JM, Harvey JF, Morton NE, Jacobs PA (1995) Trisomy 18: Studies of the parent and cell division of origin and the effect of aberrant recombination on nondisjunction. *Am J Hum Genet* 56:669–675.

Geiser SC, Carey JC, Apple DJ (1986) Human chromosomal disorders and the eye. In *Goldberg's Genetic and Metabolic Eye Disease* Boston: Little, Brown.

Goldstein H, Nielsen KG (1988) Rates and survival of individuals with trisomy 18 and 13. *Clin Genet* 34:366–372.

Gross SJ, Shulman LP, Tolley EA, Emerson DS, Felker RE, Simpson JL, Elias S (1995) Isolated fetal choroid plexus cysts and trisomy 18: A review and meta-analysis. *Am J Obstet Gynecol* 172:83–87.

Gratton RJ, Hogge WA, Aston CE (1996) Choroid plexus cysts and trisomy 18: Risk modification based on maternal age and multiple-marker screening. *Am J Obstet Gynecol* 175:1493–1497.

Harris C, Wilkerson C, Clark K, Lazarski K, Meisner L (1994) Potential use of buccal smears for rapid diagnosis of autosomal trisomy or chromosomal sex in newborn infants using DNA probes. *Am J Med Genet* 53: 355–358.

Hill LM (1996) The sonographic detection of trisomies 13, 18, and 21. *Clin Obstet Gynecol* 39:831–850.

Hyett JA, Moscoso G, Nicolaides KH (1995) Cardiac defects in 1st-trimester fetuses with trisomy 18. *Fetal Diagn Ther* 10:381–386.

Jones KL (1997) *Smith's Recognizable Patterns of Human Malformation*. Philadelphia; Saunders.

Kinoshita M, Nakamura Y, Nakano R, Fukuda S (1989) Thirty-one autopsy cases of trisomy 18: Clinical features and pathological findings. *Pediatr Pathol* 9:445–457.

Kupke KG, Mueller U (1989): Parental origin of the extra chromosome in trisomy 18. *Am J Hum Genet* 45:599–605.

Lehman CD, Nyberg DA, Winter TC, Kapur RP, Resta RG, Luthy DA (1995) Trisomy 13 syndrome: Prenatal US findings in a review of 33 cases. *Radiology* 194:217–222.

Lurie IW, Wulfsberg EA (1993) "Holoprosencephaly-polydactyly" (pseudotrisomy 13) syndrome: Expansion of the phenotypic spectrum. *Am J Med Genet* 47:405–409.

Marion RW, Chitayat D, Hutcheon RG, Neidich JA, Zackai EH, Singer LP, Warman M (1988) Trisomy 18 score: A rapid, reliable diagnostic test for trisomy 18. *J Pediatr* 113:45–48.

Moerman P, Fryns JP, Van der Sten K, Kleczkowska A, Lauweryns J (1988) The pathology of trisomy 13 syndrome. *Hum Genet* 80:349–356.

Musewe NN, Alexander DJ, Teshima I, Smalhorn JF, Freedom RM (1990) Echocardiographic evaluation of the spectral cardiac anomalies associated with trisomy 18 and 13. *J Am Coll Cardiol* 15:673–677.

Olson JM, Hamilton A, Breslow NE (1995) Non-11p constitutional chromosome abnormalities in Wilms tumor patients. *Med Pediatr Oncol* 24:305–309.

Palomaki GE, Haddow JE, Knight GJ, Wald NJ, Kennard A, Canick JA, Saller DN, Blitzer MG, Dickerman LH, Fisher R (1995) Risk-based prenatal screening for trisomy 18 using alpha-fetoprotein, unconjugated oestriol and human chorionic gonadotropin. *Prenat Diagn* 15: 713–723.

Paris JJ, Weiss AH, Soifer S (1992) Ethical issues in the use of life-prolonging interventions for an infant with trisomy 18. *J Perinatol* 12:366–368.

Patau K, Smith DW, Therman E, Inhorn SL, Wagner HP (1960) Multiple congenital anomaly caused by an extra chromosome. *Lancet* 1:790–793

Ray S, Ries MD, Bowen JR (1986) Arthrokatadysis in trisomy 18. *Pediatr Orthop* 6:100–103.

Reinsch RC (1997) Choroid plexus cysts-Association with trisomy: Prospective review of 16,059 patients. *Am J Obstet Gynecol* 176:1381–1383.

Reynolds TL, Carey JC, Ward K, Kupke K (1991) Medical complications and phenotype in older children with complete trisomy 13. *Clin Res* 39:8A.

Robinson WP, Bernasconi F, Dutly F, Lefort G, Romain DR, Binkert F, Schinzel AA (1996) Molecular studies of translocations and trisomy involving chromosome 13. *Am J Med Genet* 61:158–163.

Rochelson BL, Trunca C, Monheit AG, Baker DA (1986) The use of a rapid in situ technique for third-trimester diagnosis of trisomy 18. *Am J Obstet Gynecol* 155:835–836.

Rogers JF (1984) Clinical delineation of proximal and distal partial 13q trisomy. *Clin Genet* 25:221–229.

Root S, Carey JC (1994) Survival in trisomy 18. *Am J Med Genet* 49:170–174.

Schneider AS, Mennuti MT, Zackai EH (1981) High cesarean section rate in trisomy 18 births: A potential indication for late prenatal diagnosis. *Am J Obstet Gynecol* 140:367–370.

Shields LE, Uhrich SB, Easterling TR, Cyr DR, Mack LA (1996) Isolated fetal choroid plexus cysts and karyotype analysis: Is it necessary? *J Ultrasound Med* 15:389–394.

Simpson JL, German J (1969) Developmental anomaly resembling the trisomy 18 syndrome. *Ann Genet (Paris)* 12:107–110.

Smith A, Field B, Learoyd BM (1989) Brief clinical report: Trisomy 18 at age 21 years. *Am J Med Genet* 34:338–339.

Smith DW, Patau K, Therman E, Inhorn SL (1960) A new autosomal trisomy syndrome: Multiple congenital anomalies caused by an extra chromosome. *J Pediatr* 57: 338–345.

Spinnato JA, Cook VD, Cook CR, Voss DH (1995) Aggressive intrapartum management of lethal fetal anomalies: Beyond fetal beneficence. *Obstet Gynecol* 85:89–92.

Staples AJ, Robertson EF, Ranieri E, Ryall RG, Haan EA (1991) *Am J Hum Genet* 49: 1025–1033.

Teraguchi M, Nogi S, Ikemoto Y, Ogino H, Kohdera U (1997) Multiple hepatoblastomas associated with trisomy 18 in a 3-year-old girl. *Pediatr Hematol Oncol* 14:463–467.

Tharapel SA, Lewandowski RC, Tharapel AT, Wilroy RS (1986) Phenotype-karyotype correlation in patients trisomic for various segments of chromosome 13. *J Med Genet* 23:310–315.

Van Dyke DC, Allen M (1990) Clinical management considerations in long-term survivors with trisomy 18. *Pediatrics* 85:753–759.

Van Praagh S, Truman T, Firpo A, Bano-Rodrigo A, Fried R, McManus B, Engel MA, Van Praagh R (1989) Cardiac malformations in trisomy 18: A study of 41 postmortem cases. *J Am Coll Cardiol* 13:1586–1597.

Wilson GN (1993) Karyotype/phenotype correlation: Prospects and problems illustrated by trisomy 18. In: *The Phenotypic Mapping of Down Syndrome and Other Aneuploid Conditions*, Wiley-Liss, New York: p. 157–173.

Woldorf J, Johnson K (1994) Gross motor development of a 7-year-old girl with trisomy 18. *Clin Pediatr* 33:120–122.

Wyllie JP, Wright MJ, Burn J, Hunter S (1994) Natural history of trisomy 13. *Arch Dis Child* 71:343–345.

Young ID, Cook JP, Mehta L (1986) Changing demography of trisomy 18. *Arch Dis Child* 61:1035–1936.

Zaragoza MV, Jacobs PA, James RS, Rogan P, Sherman S, Hassold T (1994) Nondisjunction of human acrocentric chromosomes: Studies of 432 trisomic fetuses and liveborns. *Hum Genet* 94:411–417.

CHAPTER 26

TUBEROUS SCLEROSIS

ROBERT F. MUELLER

INTRODUCTION

The first detailed description of the tuberous sclerosis complex is thought to have been by Bourneville, who reported tubers and sclerosis of the brain found at postmortem in individuals with mental retardation and epilepsy (Bourneville, 1880). Vogt first described the classical triad of features in tuberous sclerosis of mental retardation, epilepsy, and the misnamed facial rash of "adenoma sebaceum." He also noted the occurrence of kidney and heart tumors (1908). The hereditary nature of tuberous sclerosis was first reported by Berg (1913). It was subsequently confirmed as being inherited as an autosomal dominant disorder, often arising as a new mutation, by Gunther and Penrose (1935).

Incidence

Although early reports suggested that tuberous sclerosis is a very rare disorder, with a prevalence of approximately 1 in 100,000 individuals (Gunther and Penrose, 1935), more recent systematic ascertainment studies report age-related population prevalence figures up to 1 in 5,000 under the age of 5 years and 1 in 25,000 for individuals of all ages (Hunt, 1983; Hunt and Lindenbaum,

1984; Sampson et al., 1989; Shepherd et al., 1991; Ahlsen et al., 1994).

Life expectancy for people with tuberous sclerosis is usually normal, even in those with severe learning difficulties. Occasionally, individuals with tuberous sclerosis will die suddenly and unexpectedly because of epilepsy and/or cardiac arrhythmias or because of complications of a giant cell astrocytoma or pulmonary lymphangiomyomatosis.

Diagnostic Criteria

Tuberous sclerosis is a multisystem disorder with protean manifestations involving the central nervous system, skin, eyes, heart, kidneys, lungs, gut, bones, and teeth. Diagnostic criteria for tuberous sclerosis were first proposed and updated by Gomez (1979; 1991) and revised by a committee established by the National Tuberous Sclerosis Association (Roach et al., 1992). More recently, a panel of clinicians and geneticists at the Tuberous Sclerosis Complex Consensus Conference re-evaluated the clinical diagnostic criteria in light of new clinical and genetic information (Roach et al., 1999a; Roach et al., 1999b)(see Table 26.1).

Central nervous system involvement can manifest symptomatically as any combination

Management of Genetic Syndromes, Edited by Suzanne B. Cassidy and Judith E. Allanson
ISBN 0-471-31286-X   Copyright © 2001 by Wiley-Liss, Inc.

TABLE 26.1. **Diagnostic Criteria for Tuberous Sclerosis**

System	Primary Features	Secondary Features	Tertiary Features
Family history		Affected 1st-degree relative	
CNS	Cortical tuber		Cerebral white-matter "migration tracts" or heterotopias
	Subependymal nodule		
	Giant cell astrocytoma		Infantile spasms
Skin	Facial angiofibroma(ta)	Shagreen patch	Hypomelanotic macule
	Multiple ungual fibromata	Fibrous forehead plaque	"Confetti"-like depigmented skin lesions
Ocular	Multiple retinal astrocytomata	Other retinal hamartoma or depigmented patch	
Cardiac		Rhabdomyoma(ta)	
Renal		Angiomyolipoma(ta)	
		Cysts	
Respiratory		Pulmonary lymphangiomatosis	
Skeletal			Bone cysts
Oral/Dental			Randomly distributed enamel pits in deciduous teeth
Gastrointestinal			Hamartomatous rectal polyps

Definite tuberous sclerosis — Either 1 primary, 2 secondary, or 1 primary plus 2 tertiary features
Probable tuberous sclerosis — Either 1 secondary plus 1 tertiary, or 3 tertiary features
Suspect tuberous sclerosis — Either 1 secondary or 2 tertiary features

of epilepsy, learning difficulties/mental retardation, behavior problems, or tumors. Over three-quarters of people with tuberous sclerosis will have evidence of central nervous system structural abnormality on investigation, which can include the classical cortical tubers, subependymal glial nodules of the lateral walls of the lateral ventricles (Fig. 26.1), hamartomatous cerebral foci, dilated lateral ventricles, or subependymal giant cell astrocytoma. Occasionally, a child under 1 year of age with tuberous sclerosis will have a normal CT scan; if the diagnosis is still uncertain, it will be necessary to repeat the scan at a later age. Over three-quarters of people with tuberous sclerosis also have epilepsy of a variety of types (Hunt, 1983; Webb et al., 1991; Hunt, 1993; Ahlsen et al.,

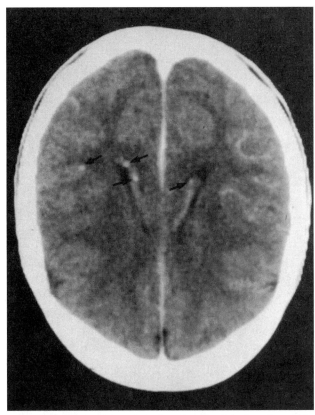

FIGURE 26.1. Subependymal glial nodules of the lateral walls of the lateral ventricles demonstrated on cranial CT.

1994). Infantile spasms are one of the most common presentations of tuberous sclerosis, and approximately one-fifth of all children presenting with this type of seizure are found to have tuberous sclerosis (Pampiglione and Pugh, 1975). In addition, about 50% of people with tuberous sclerosis will have mental retardation or learning difficulties.

There are several characteristic skin findings in tuberous sclerosis (Fig. 26.2–26.6). Depigmented or hypomelanotic patches, called ash-leaf spots because of their most common shape, can occur anywhere and are the most frequent skin manifestation (Fig. 26.2). They may be present at birth or may develop with time, and they become more apparent under a Wood lamp. Angiofibromata (previously misnamed "adenoma sebaceum") are red papules in the nasolabial

area, most frequently appearing in adulthood (Fig. 26.3). Fibrous patches occur most commonly on the forehead (Fig. 26.4), and shagreen patches, which contain a proliferation of connective tissue, most often occur on the back (Fig. 26.5). Periungual and subungual fibromas are other common skin findings, usually appearing in adulthood. They often cause ridging of the nails.

Retinal phakomata or hamartomata are found in approximately one-half of affected individuals, although they usually do not affect visual acuity.

Antenatally detected cardiac rhabdomyomas can be the presenting feature of tuberous sclerosis (Fig. 26.7). In 50–80% of instances in which a cardiac rhabdomyoma is detected antenatally, the child will be found to have tuberous sclerosis (Harding

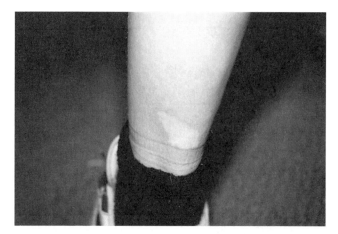

FIGURE 26.2. A depigmented or hypomelanotic "ash-leaf" patch in a person with tuberous sclerosis.

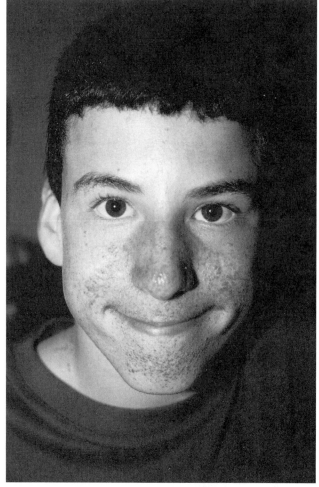

FIGURE 26.3. Symmetrical "butterfly" distribution of angiofibromata ("adenoma sebaceum") on the nasolabial folds and cheeks in a person with tuberous sclerosis.

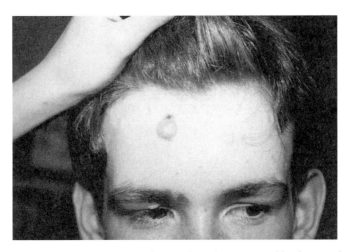

FIGURE 26.4. An enlarged forehead fibrous plaque in a person with tuberous sclerosis.

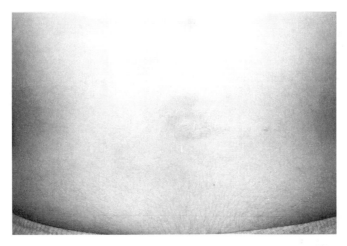

FIGURE 26.5. A shagreen patch on the lower lumbar region in a person with tuberous sclerosis.

and Pagon, 1990). Cardiac rhabdomyomas may be silent or may cause heart failure or arrhythmia. They tend to regress with age.

Unilateral or bilateral angiomyolipomata are the most common form of renal anomaly, being found in nearly two-thirds of people with tuberous sclerosis (Fig. 26.8). Cysts of the kidney are also frequent.

Cystic disease of the lung is an uncommon but well-described feature of tuberous sclerosis. Pulmonary lymphangiomyomatosis is an uncommon but serious manifestation of tuberous sclerosis, which has been reported almost exclusively in females (Polosa et al.,

1995). Cystlike areas of reduced density occur in the phalanges and calvarium in tuberous sclerosis. Gingival fibromata and dental pits are also recognized findings.

Etiology, Pathogenesis, and Genetics

Tuberous sclerosis is inherited as an autosomal dominant disorder. Between one-half and two-thirds of cases, however, arise as a new mutation (Fleury et al., 1980; Sampson et al., 1989; Ahlsen et al., 1994). Although there are reports of apparent nonpenetrance in tuberous sclerosis (Baraitser and Patton,

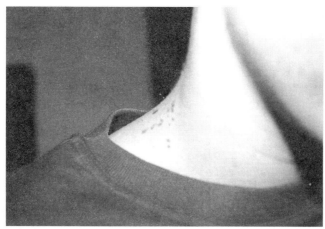

FIGURE 26.6. Soft, fleshy skin tags (molluscum fibrosum pendulum) on the side of the neck and upper shoulders in an individual with tuberous sclerosis.

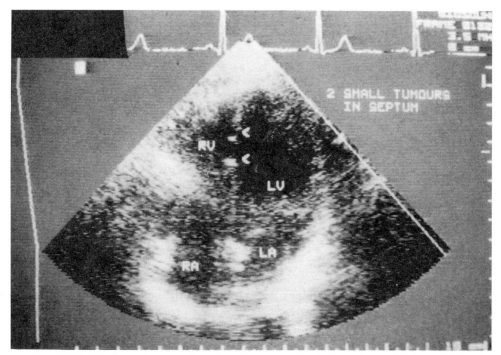

FIGURE 26.7. Still frame from a cardiac echo in a person with tuberous sclerosis showing the left and right ventricles with echodense areas in the interventricular septum (arrowed) due to presumed cardiac rhabdomyomata.

1985; Webb and Osborne, 1991), this is, in fact, uncommon.

In 1987, family studies showed linkage of tuberous sclerosis to a locus (*TSC1*) on the long arm of chromosome 9 near the ABO blood group locus at 9q34 (Fryer et al., 1987a). Detailed physical mapping and sequencing of the whole of a 900-kilobase region on the long arm of chromosome 9 led to identification of the *TSC1* gene (van

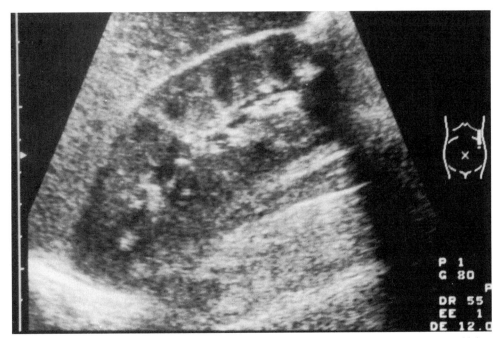

FIGURE 26.8. A still frame from a renal ultrasound in a person with tuberous sclerosis showing multiple areas of increased echogenicity due to presumed angiomyolipomata.

Slegtenhorst et al., 1997). It soon became clear, however, that a significant proportion of families with individuals affected with tuberous sclerosis in multiple generations did not show linkage to the *TSC1* locus. Although the possibility of linkage to loci on chromosomes 11 and 12 was reported, the occurrence of polycystic kidney disease in some individuals with tuberous sclerosis suggested that the region of the short arm of chromosome 16 containing the gene for adult polycystic kidney disease (*APKD1*) was a potential candidate region for a second tuberous sclerosis gene (*TSC2*), which was subsequently confirmed (Kandt et al., 1992). Individuals with both tuberous sclerosis and polycystic kidney disease were deleted for both of these physically contiguous genes.

Although studies have shown that approximately half of the multigeneration families with tuberous sclerosis are linked to each of the two loci, mutations in the *TSC2* gene account for the majority of sporadic cases, with underrepresentation of mutations in the *TSC1* gene in that group. Although there was preliminary evidence that mental retardation occurs more commonly in sporadically affected individuals with mutations in the *TSC2* gene than with mutations in the *TSC1* gene, there is no evidence at present for a consistent genotype-phenotype correlation (Jones et al., 1997; Beauchamp et al., 1998; Kwiatkowska et al., 1998; Ali et al., 1998; Au et al., 1998; van Slegtenhorst et al., 1999; Jones et al., 1999).

The two proteins encoded by the *TSC1* and *TSC2* genes have been shown to act as tumor suppressor genes, with loss of heterozygosity leading to the development of hamartomata (Sepp et al., 1996). The *TSC2* gene encodes tuberin, a putative GTPase activating protein (Xiao et al., 1997), whereas the *TSC1* gene encodes hamartin, a novel protein with no homology to tuberin or any other previously identified vertebrate protein. Although the function of their protein products is not fully understood, they colocalize within cells and interact in vivo, suggesting that they function in the same complex rather than in separate pathways (van Slegtenhorst et al., 1998; Young and Povey, 1998; Johnson et al., 1999).

Because most instances of tuberous sclerosis occur sporadically, to be able to give recurrence risk information, it is necessary to determine for each affected individual whether the tuberous sclerosis is familial or has arisen as a new mutation. This involves obtaining a detailed family history and examining the parents' skin looking for the characteristic dermatological features of tuberous sclerosis, including use of a Woods lamp (Flinter and Neville, 1986). In addition, it is necessary to arrange indirect fundoscopy, a cranial CT, and a renal scan before providing genetic counseling (Cassidy et al., 1983; Al-Gazali et al., 1989; Fryer et al., 1990).

If one of the parents has tuberous sclerosis, the recurrence risk in each future pregnancy is 50%. In providing advice to such families, this figure should be further modified by the data from unbiased prospective studies of individuals born with tuberous sclerosis. These have shown that approximately two-thirds of individuals who inherit the tuberous sclerosis gene will have epilepsy and/or mental retardation (Webb et al., 1996). If, on the other hand, the results of the family studies show that neither parent has features of tuberous sclerosis, there is still a 2% risk for subsequent children to be clinically affected. This may reflect the possibility of germline mosaicism in one of the parents (Yates et al., 1997; Rose et al., 1999; Verhoef et al., 1999), or rare instances may be the result of a second mutation arising independently in the family. Nonpenetrance in tuberous sclerosis is unusual.

Screening of apparently normal siblings of sporadically affected individuals with tuberous sclerosis is controversial. It would seem reasonable for unaffected siblings to be screened before they have a family themselves. If, on the other hand, a sibling has features that could be caused by tuberous sclerosis, such as unexplained learning difficulties or epilepsy, it would be appropriate to carry out the full range of investigations at an earlier stage. Investigation of subsequent children by noninvasive means, such as Woods lamp examination of the skin, echocardiography, and renal ultrasound, would seem reasonable for the reassurance it provides to the parents.

Diagnostic Testing

At present, diagnosis is usually based on clinical findings, using the diagnostic criteria (Table 26.1). Skin exam, ultrasound of the heart and kidneys, and cranial imaging are part of the clinical assessment. Cranial CT or MRI are among the most useful investigations in individuals with or suspected of having tuberous sclerosis, looking for cortical tubers, subependymal gliomas, dilated lateral ventricles, or hamartomatous foci (Roach et al., 1987; Braffman et al., 1992).

It was hoped that identification of the gene(s) responsible for tuberous sclerosis would help when an individual presented with features that only allowed a probable or suspect diagnosis of the disorder, for example, a child with an isolated cardiac rhabdomyoma. In addition, it was hoped that routine molecular testing would allow one to determine for certain, in a sporadically affected individual, whether the disorder was familial or had arisen as a result of a new mutation. Although the mutations identified to date cluster in specific parts of the *TSC1* and *TSC2* genes, in the majority of the families with tuberous sclerosis a unique mutation in one of these two genes is responsible for the disorder (Jones et al., 1997, Au et al., 1998; van Slegtenhorst et al., 1999; Jones et al., 1999). As a consequence, screening for mutations in the two genes responsible for tuberous sclerosis is very labor intensive and is not currently routinely available. Only a limited number of molecular laboratories are prepared to offer mutation screening in tuberous sclerosis on a clinical diagnostic service basis.

Currently, there are two instances in which molecular testing can be used diagnostically. First, if multiple individuals in different generations of a family are affected with tuberous sclerosis, linkage analysis (analysis of the pattern of segregation of alleles of closely flanking/intragenic polymorphic markers for the two tuberous sclerosis genes) can be used to determine which of the two genes is likely to be responsible for the disorder. Linkage analysis allows the possibility of presymptomatic diagnosis for people at risk in such informative families, i.e., determination, in the absence of conclusive symptoms or signs of the disorder, whether an individual at risk has inherited the tuberous sclerosis gene. Second, if a child with tuberous sclerosis is found to have polycystic kidney disease, it is likely that a deletion of the two contiguous genes (*TSC2* and *APKD1*) is responsible. Because of both locus and mutational heterogeneity, further technological developments will be required before mutation screening becomes widely available. In addition, somatic cell tissue-specific mosaicism can occur, which can further confound the interpretation of the results of molecular analyses in providing genetic counseling (Kwiatkowska et al., 1999).

Differential Diagnosis

Some features that occur as part of tuberous sclerosis can occur as occasional, isolated normal findings in the general population. For example, depigmented patches are present in up to 8 per 1000 of the general population (Alper and Holmes, 1983; Vanderhooft et al., 1996). Some features or findings could arise as a consequence of acquired causes, e.g., periungual fibromas secondary to trauma. Other features that are clearly pathological can occur as a result of another genetic disorder, for example, café au lait macules (Jozwiak et al., 1998). Café au lait macules are a hallmark feature of neurofibromatosis type 1 (see Chapter 14). Less commonly, individuals with neurofibromatosis 1

will have depigmented macules. Although some isolated findings can be hard to distinguish from other disorders, for example, retinal phakomata in tuberous sclerosis can be confused with retinoblastoma, in most instances the situation can be clarified by clinical examination and investigation, as detailed previously, looking for other features characteristic of tuberous sclerosis. The results, in conjunction with application of the diagnostic criteria for tuberous sclerosis, should help confirm or exclude the diagnosis of tuberous sclerosis.

MANIFESTATIONS AND MANAGEMENT

Growth and Feeding

Growth is generally normal in individuals with tuberous sclerosis. Children with severe mental retardation can present with feeding problems, but it is uncommon for the diagnosis of the disorder to be made at that time. Evaluation and treatment of any feeding disorder in this circumstance would not differ from that performed in the general population.

Development and Behavior

Most estimates of the frequency of mental retardation in persons with tuberous sclerosis are biased by the means of ascertainment. Estimates range from 25% to 100% (Gomez, 1979; Shepherd et al., 1991, Webb et al., 1991; Curatolo et al., 1991; Hunt, 1993; Gillberg et al., 1994). Individuals with tuberous sclerosis can have normal intelligence. The best estimate of the prevalence of mental retardation, from an unbiased series of secondarily ascertained individuals, is just under 50% (Webb et al., 1991). The severity of mental retardation reported can range from mild to severe.

Although approximately two-thirds of individuals with tuberous sclerosis who have epilepsy also have learning difficulties/mental retardation, the majority of people with tuberous sclerosis who are seizure free are of normal intelligence. Children with tuberous sclerosis who present with seizures in the first 2 years of life, particularly with infantile spasms, are more likely to have mental retardation than children who develop seizures later in childhood. There is no consistent correlation between the number of central nervous system lesions and intellectual outcome.

Many children with tuberous sclerosis who have moderate to severe cognitive impairment and epilepsy also have behavioral problems, which can include hyperactivity, autistic-like behavior, and sleep problems (Hunt and Shepherd, 1993; Gillberg et al., 1994; Bruni et al., 1995; Baker et al., 1998). In addition, individuals with tuberous sclerosis who have moderate to severe cognitive impairment have significant communication problems, which can compound any behavioral problems. Although the behavioral problems in children with tuberous sclerosis can improve with age, behavioral disturbance in a full-grown adolescent with communication difficulties can be very trying for parents. There are few published long-term follow-up studies on behavior in adults with tuberous sclerosis.

Evaluation

- Screening assessment of developmental abilities should occur at the time of diagnosis and should be repeated at least annually during childhood, because developmental delay can become evident at any age.
- In a child with tuberous sclerosis found to have developmental delay, a detailed developmental assessment is required to provide appropriately for his or her special educational needs.
- Assessing behavioral problems in a child with tuberous sclerosis with learning difficulties and epilepsy can be difficult but should include enquiry about

behavioral patterns, socialization, attention and concentration problems, and sleep pattern.

- Changes in behavior in a person with tuberous sclerosis can be a sign of underlying physical problems, especially in an individual with tuberous sclerosis who has moderate or severe mental retardation with communication difficulties. If there is a concomitant deterioration in the control of epilepsy along with behavioral changes, the possibility of a giant cell astrocytoma should be considered (Curatolo et al., 1991; Hunt and Stores, 1994).

Treatment

- Early intervention programs, including interaction with therapists, introduction to play groups, or preschool nurseries for children with special educational needs, should occur as early as possible in infancy if developmental delay is identified.
- Special educational input during the school years should be individualized and based on careful neuropsychological evaluation.
- Many of the behavioral problems in individuals with tuberous sclerosis can be dealt with by simple, straightforward measures. Referral to a multidisciplinary team specializing in behavioral management, including a clinical psychologist and psychiatrist, can be appropriate, especially in difficult cases. If the individual with tuberous sclerosis has moderate to severe cognitive impairment, identifying a team or clinic with special experience and expertise in behavioral problems for such individuals is appropriate.
- Limited reliable information is available on the use of medications for the management of behavioral problems

in individuals with tuberous sclerosis, although there is preliminary evidence that melatonin can help to treat severe sleep disorders in individuals with tuberous sclerosis (O'Callaghan et al., 1999).

Neurologic

Seizures. A variety of seizure types can occur in tuberous sclerosis, including infantile spasms and myoclonic, partial, and generalized tonic-clonic seizures. The majority of affected children who present with seizures in infancy will still have them by the age of 5 years (Hunt, 1993). Children who present with seizures in the first 2 years of life, particularly with infantile spasms, are more likely to have mental retardation than children who develop seizures later in childhood. Early recognition and treatment of seizures in children presenting with infantile spasms is felt to be associated with a better developmental outcome.

The EEG findings in people with tuberous sclerosis are not diagnostic and can show a variety of different abnormalities including hypsarrhythmia, focal spike or sharp-wave discharges, multifocal epileptiform abnormalities, and generalized spike and wave discharges.

Control of epilepsy in individuals with tuberous sclerosis is one of the most difficult aspects of management of the disorder. Although seizures in most affected individuals respond, at least to some extent, to pharmacologic treatment, a small proportion of children and adults with tuberous sclerosis have epilepsy that is refractory to anticonvulsants (Nagib et al., 1984; McLaurin and Towbin, 1985; Conzen and Oppel, 1990). Deterioration of control of epilepsy in any individual with tuberous sclerosis should be a warning sign of possible central nervous system complications.

Intracranial tumors. Over three-quarters of people with tuberous sclerosis have an abnormality in the brain, which can include the classical cortical tubers, subependymal glial nodules of the lateral walls of the lateral ventricles (Fig. 26.1), hamartomatous cerebral foci, white matter radial migration lines, or dilated lateral ventricles (Griffiths et al., 1998). These findings can be seen on investigation of an individual with tuberous sclerosis after he/she presents with epilepsy and/or mental retardation or, on occasion, as an incidental finding on routine investigation.

Individuals with tuberous sclerosis are also at risk of developing a subependymal giant cell astrocytoma, the peak age of risk being in late childhood through adolescence, although it must be kept in mind that this also occurs as a complication in adult life (Torres et al., 1998). Giant cell astrocytomas are not truly malignant, but, because they are almost always located adjacent to the foramina of Monro, they lead to raised intracranial pressure.

Evaluation

- When seizures are present, a detailed history of the age of onset, frequency, and nature should be obtained. This is important in the assessment of the appropriate anticonvulsant therapy.

- At the time of presentation with seizures, or when the control of seizures deteriorates, an EEG and cranial imaging by CT or MRI is appropriate.

- In any child with tuberous sclerosis, especially when presenting with seizures, it is vital to arrange regular neurological follow-up, both to review control of the seizures and to follow developmental progress.

- Plain skull X-rays will show areas of intracranial calcification in over one-half of people with tuberous sclerosis.

- There is no published evidence that routine periodic cranial CT or MRI is of any benefit in individuals with tuberous sclerosis.

- Classical symptoms of raised intracranial pressure caused by a giant cell astrocytoma, such as headache and vomiting, can often be difficult to evaluate in an individual with tuberous sclerosis and moderate or severe learning difficulties/mental retardation. There should be a low threshold for arranging a cranial CT or MRI to exclude the possibility of a giant cell astrocytoma. Any unexplained deterioration in the control of seizures or behavior should be taken as a possible presenting feature of this rare but serious manifestation.

Treatment

- The choice of anticonvulsants will be dependent on the nature of the seizures, along with consideration of the potential side effects and whether or not they result in control of the seizures. Although steroids have been the treatment of choice for infantile spasms in the first year of life, it has been suggested that vigabatrin is fast becoming the first-line treatment of choice (Villeneuve et al., 1998; Hancock and Osborne, 1999). Sodium valproate and carbamazepine are the drugs of choice for partial (focal) and generalized tonic-clonic seizures and can help with myoclonic seizures and drop attacks, although clonazepam or clobazepam can be used. It is important, however, to emphasize that although general recommendations about the choice of anticonsulvant therapy can be made, treatment should be tailored to the individual.

- If the epilepsy is difficult to control, a variety of different anticonvulsants are often tried individually, in sequence, or in combination. Use of multiple anticonvulsants is sometimes necessary but should be avoided if possible. If control of epilepsy proves particularly difficult, referral to a child neurologist, a neurologist with a special interest in epilepsy, or a specialist clinic for people with learning difficulties and epilepsy is appropriate.

- When seizures do not respond to standard therapies, referral to a neurology consultant is appropriate.

- Surgical removal of a giant cell astrocytoma has a significant morbidity and mortality risk. Complete surgical removal of giant cell astrocytomata is rarely possible. Recurrence of symptoms due to regrowth of the tumor is common.

- CSF shunting is often carried out to relieve the symptoms associated with raised intracranial pressure.

- Difficulty of surgical access to the tumor means that radiotherapy is a treatment option that is considered in some instances. Giant cell astrocytomata are not usually responsive to this form of treatment, and any improvement is often only temporary.

Dermatologic

The skin is often affected by tuberous sclerosis. The majority of people with tuberous sclerosis have depigmented or hypomelanotic patches, which are often oval, classically said to be "ash-leaf"in shape, and commonly located on the trunk and buttocks following the lines of the dermatomes (Fig. 26.2). They are commonly present at birth but can appear with age. Although often visible in ordinary light, they are sometimes only visible under the 360-nm-wavelength ultraviolet light of a Woods lamp. Hypomelanotic patches involving the scalp result in poliosis (patches of white hair).

Angiofibromata are present in over three-quarters of people with tuberous sclerosis but are rarely present in early childhood. They appear as pink or red papules usually occurring symmetrically in a so-called "butterfly" distribution on the naso-labial folds and cheeks (Fig. 26.3). Misnamed as "adenoma sebaceum," histologically they are hamartomatous, consisting of fibrous connective tissue and vascular elements of the skin.

The forehead fibrous plaque is a relatively recently described feature of tuberous sclerosis, occurring in approximately one-quarter of affected individuals (Fryer et al., 1987b). This appears as a raised, reddish area, sometimes present early in infancy and enlarging with age (Fig. 26.4). Histologically this is similar to an angiofibroma. Between 40% and 80% of people with tuberous sclerosis develop an area of elevated, thickened discolored skin, likened to the appearance of "untanned leather," or what is called a shagreen patch. This is usually located to one side over the lower lumbar portion of the back and, although occasionally present at birth, often develops later in life (Fig. 26.5). Histologically, it consists of a disordered or hamartomatous proliferation of collagen along with various proportions of adipose tissue, elastic tissue, smooth muscle, vascular structures, and skin appendages. Ungual fibromata are present in up to one-fifth of people with tuberous sclerosis, usually developing in adult life. They consist of flesh-colored nodules arising from the nail beds of the fingers or toes and can lead to ridging of the nail. Histologically, they are angiofibromata. Although it is uncommon in children, about one-third of adults with tuberous sclerosis develop soft, fleshy skin tags (molluscum fibrosum pendulum), most commonly located over the back of the neck and upper shoulders (Fig. 26.6).

Evaluation

- A simple inspection of the degree of facial involvement in someone with tuberous sclerosis, along with inquiry about any associated episodes of bleeding of the angiofibromata, if extensive, is appropriate.
- Facial angiofibromata are often felt to be cosmetically disfiguring, particularly in those with tuberous sclerosis and normal intelligence. Serial facial photographs can be useful to document the progression and response to treatment of the facial rash.
- Simple inspection of the nails for the presence of periungual or subungual fibromata should be carried out along with inquiry about episodes of bleeding from them.

Treatment

- Most of the cutaneous manifestations of tuberous sclerosis either do not require treatment or have no effective treatment.
- The extent of involvement that is considered appropriate for treatment is variable, depending on the age and sex of the individual with tuberous sclerosis, being more likely to be considered in females.
- Treatment for angiofibromata has been carried out by a variety of techniques in the past including diathermy and dermabrasion. More recently, argon laser treatment has been found to be quite effective. A test patch is often performed initially, because the full benefits of treatment often are not seen for 6 months. Laser treatment of the angiofibromata can take some time to complete. It is usually carried out in several stages because it is very time-consuming and is associated with blistering and swelling of the skin in the immediate period after treatment. Recurrence of the angiofibromata after diathermy and dermabrasion is not uncommon. Although experience is limited, the results of longer-term follow-up of laser treatment are promising.
- Diathermy or liquid nitrogen is commonly used for localized ungual fibromata. Occasionally, surgical removal of the nail beds is attempted if the fibromata are particularly troublesome. Ungual fibromata have a tendency to regrow, even with aggressive surgical treatment.
- Skin tags can be removed, if desired, as in the general population.

Ophthalmologic

Ocular abnormalities represent another category of important manifestations of tuberous sclerosis. Retinal phakomata, or so-called "mulberry" lesions, are relatively flat, smooth, circular or oval semitransparent areas with an indistinct boundary, located superficial to the retinal vasculature in the early stages of development. Initially, retinal phakomata are the same color as the rest of the fundus, but they often become paler as they calcify with age. Visual acuity is rarely affected unless a retinal phakoma overlies the macula. Abnormal retinal pigmentation adjacent to retinal phakomata and "punched-out" areas of depigmentation have been reported in the periphery of the fundus in people with tuberous sclerosis. At present, it is not clear how prevalent or specific the latter finding is in affected individuals.

Evaluation

- Routine direct fundoscopy will detect the more obvious retinal phakomata that can occur in people with tuberous sclerosis. Indirect fundoscopy carried out by an ophthalmologist is recommended to determine whether there is less obvious ocular involvement, such as peripheral retinal phakomata or pigmentary changes.

Treatment

- Ocular involvement in individuals with tuberous sclerosis rarely requires treatment.

Cardiovascular

Cardiac rhabdomyomata represent the primary cardiac manifestation of tuberous sclerosis. They are usually asymptomatic, often only being detected by echocardiography (Gibbs, 1985, Nuhler et al., 1994; Jozwiak et al., 1994; Nir et al., 1995) (Fig. 26.7). Occasionally, they can obstruct blood flow or lead to cardiac failure. When present in the cardiac conducting tissues, they may lead to arrhythmia. These are generally the most refractory to treatment. Cardiac rhabdomyomata in individuals with tuberous sclerosis appear to regress spontaneously in number and reduce in size with age, being seen less frequently in adults than in children (Smith et al., 1989). The spontaneous regression of cardiac rhabdomyomata means that the prognosis for cardiac involvement in tuberous sclerosis is usually very good, provided serious arrhythmias and outflow obstruction are not encountered in the newborn period. Cardiac arrhythmias are thought to be a possible cause of the rare occurrence of sudden unexplained deaths in people with tuberous sclerosis. They have been detected prenatally, leading to prenatal diagnosis of this disorder.

Evaluation

- Clinical examination should include evaluation for an irregular heart rhythm, a heart murmur, or signs of cardiac failure.
- The definitive investigation for evidence of cardiac rhabdomyomata is echocardiography. In view of the tendency of the cardiac rhabdomyomata to decrease in number and size with age in this disorder, it is appropriate to carry out echocardiography as a diagnostic investigation sooner rather than later.
- An ECG is appropriate to confirm or exclude cardiac arrhythmias.

Treatment

- The tendency for cardiac rhabdomyomata to regress in number and reduce in size in people with tuberous sclerosis means that masterly inactivity is usually the treatment of choice.
- Appropriate symptomatic medical treatment for heart failure or cardiac arrhythmias should be provided.

Genitourinary

Hamartomatous lesions of the kidney represent another common finding in tuberous sclerosis. Angiomyolipomata are usually bilateral and multiple (Stilwell et al., 1987; Bernstein, 1993; Steiner et al., 1993; Webb et al., 1994; Zimmerhackl et al., 1994; Van Baal et al., 1994). They can occur in both the cortex and the medulla, ranging in size from microscopic to large masses (Fig. 26.8). Histologically they consist of highly vascular hamartomatous growths of smooth muscle and adipose tissue. Renal angiomyolipomata are usually not associated with symptoms but can cause pain or result in intrarenal or retroperitoneal hemorrhage or hematuria, which can be life-threatening on rare occasions. Angiomyolipomata tend to increase in prevalence and severity with age and rarely will lead to hypertension or significant renal impairment (Cook et al., 1996; Ewalt et al., 1998).

Renal cystic involvement in tuberous sclerosis is less common, occurring in approximately one in six people with tuberous sclerosis (Stapleton et al., 1980). Renal cysts are a more common finding in young children, and their prevalence does not appear to increase with age (Cook et al., 1996). They can even disappear (Ewalt et al., 1998). If extensive, cystic involvement in young children can occasionally result in hypertension and renal failure presenting as classic polycystic kidney disease (Webb et al., 1993).

Either type of renal lesion can be associated with loin pain and/or hematuria. If extensive, occasionally these lesions can lead to renal impairment (Clarke et al., 1999). A small proportion of people with tuberous sclerosis can develop serious medical complications caused by cysts or angiomyolipomata. Hemorrhage from the angiomyolipomata occasionally requires emergency embolization or surgery, and it has been suggested that this risk is related to the size of the individual angiomyolipoma(ta) (Van Baal et al., 1994).

There are rare reports of renal cell carcinoma in people with tuberous sclerosis, usually occurring in later adult life.

Evaluation

- Although renal involvement can be documented by CT or MRI, it is usually best documented by ultrasound, particularly because ultrasound is relatively easier to carry out, less invasive, and more widely available.

- There is no clear evidence to support a particular protocol for periodic evaluation of the renal involvement of tuberous sclerosis. It has been suggested that if there is no initial evidence of renal involvement, renal ultrasound should be repeated approximately once every 5 years. If, however, there is no evidence of renal involvement by the age of 30, there is probably no need to continue with regular renal ultrasounds because it is unlikely that there will be significant renal involvement in later life (Cook et al., 1996).

- If there is evidence of renal involvement, it has been suggested that regular evaluation including blood pressure measurements, serum creatinine, and renal ultrasound should be carried out more frequently, perhaps every 2–3 years (Cook et al., 1996).

- Routine blood pressure determinations at annual medical evaluations are important even in the absence of known renal lesions, because hypertension can result from renal cysts or tumors.

Treatment

- Because the angiomyolipomata are usually bilateral and multiple, if intervention is necessary it is preferable to be as conservative as possible. Thus a partial nephrectomy or selective embolization is preferable to total nephrectomy. It has been suggested that the larger the angiomyolipomata, the greater the risk of hemorrhage and that elective surgery or embolization should be carried out for lesions greater than 4 cm in diameter (Van Baal et al., 1989; Van Baal et al., 1994).

- Cystic renal involvement in tuberous sclerosis rarely requires treatment. Persistent loin pain can, on occasion, warrant consideration of surgery for symptomatic relief.

Respiratory

Very rarely, people with lung involvement caused by tuberous sclerosis can present with dyspnea, hemoptysis, or a pneumothorax (Rudolph, 1981; Torres et al., 1995; Castro et al., 1995). In individuals with tuberous sclerosis, especially females, respiratory symptoms should suggest the possibility of pulmonary cystic disease or lymphangiomyomatosis. Cystic disease of the lung is an uncommon but well-described feature of tuberous sclerosis, which on X-ray is described as a "honeycomb" lung (Lie et al., 1980). Histologically, the cystic areas are bronchial or alveolar cysts consisting of a mixture of vascular, fibrous, and muscle tissue. Lymphangiomyomatosis is an uncommon but serious manifestation of tuberous sclerosis, which has been reported almost exclusively in females (Polosa et al., 1995). Histologically, the findings are similar to those seen in cystic disease of the lung but also include disordered and hamartomatous lymphatics with smooth muscle tissue involvement. Both these types of respiratory involvement usually present in the second to the fifth decade of life (Castro et al., 1995). There is preliminary evidence that the lymphangiomyomatosis could be caused by loss of heterozygosity at the *TSC2* locus (Smolarek et al., 1998).

The limited information available suggests a poor prognosis for pulmonary lymphangiomyomatosis, especially with associated chylous peritoneal or pleural effusions, even to the extent of suggesting that the only successful treatment is lung transplantation.

Evaluation

- Pulmonary lymphangiomyomatosis can be investigated by means of chest X-ray, although a CT or MRI examination is better at confirming the diagnosis and documenting the extent of involvement (Lenoir et al., 1990).

Treatment

- It has been suggested that individuals with respiratory symptoms caused by pulmonary involvement respond to treatment with progesterone and/or tamoxifen (Luna et al., 1985; Westermann et al., 1986). The evidence published is, however, anecdotal, and no systematic review or assessment of the suggested treatments has been carried out.

Miscellaneous

Persons with tuberous sclerosis rarely have symptomatic skeletal involvement. The skeletal features include cystlike areas of reduced radiological density in the metacarpals and phalanges and areas of bony sclerosis in the calvarium (Kingsley et al., 1986). Skeletal involvement is age dependent and almost always asymptomatic.

Gingival fibromata are a recognized but uncommon feature of tuberous sclerosis. Multiple enamel pits due to areas of enamel hypoplasia are also reported as a characteristic feature of tuberous sclerosis (Lygidakis and Lindenbaum, 1987; Sampson et al., 1992; Flanagan et al., 1997).

Hepatic hamartomata are present in approximately one-quarter of people with tuberous sclerosis. They can be detected incidentally during a renal ultrasound and are usually of no clinical significance (Jozwiak et al., 1992). There are rare reports of fibromatous tumors of the gastrointestinal tract in people with tuberous sclerosis. Benign, small sessile rectal polyps are reported as being a common finding in this disorder but are rarely symptomatic (Gould, 1991).

RESOURCES

Support Groups

United States/Canada

National Tuberous Sclerosis Association
8181 Professional Place, Suite 110
Landover, Maryland
20785-2226
Tel - 001-800-225-6872
Fax - 001-301-459-0394
Email - *ntsa@ntsa.org*

United Kingdom

Janet Medcalf
National Secretary
The Tuberous Sclerosis Association of
Great Britain
Little Barnsley Farm
Catshill
Bromsgrove
Worcestershire
B61 0NQ
Tel - 044-152-787-1898
Fax - 044-152-757-7390
Email - *tsassn@compuserve.com*

World Wide Web/Internet

National Tuberous Sclerosis Association
http://www.ntsa.org

Tuberous Sclerosis Association of Great Britain *http://ourworld.compuserve.com/homepages/tsassn*

Tuberous Sclerosis International
http://crystal.feo.hvu.nl/Groepar/TSI/TSI.htm

REFERENCES

Ahlsen G, Gillberg IC, Lindblom R, Gillberg C (1994) Tuberous sclerosis in Western Sweden. A population study of cases with early childhood onset. *Arch Neurol* 51:76–81.

Al-Gazali LI, Arthur RJ, Lamb JT, Hammer HM, Coker TP, Hirschmann PN, Gibbs J, Mueller RF (1989) Diagnostic and counseling difficulties using a fully comprehensive screening protocol for families at risk for tuberous sclerosis. *J Med Genet* 26:694–703.

Ali JB, Sepp T, Ward S, Green AJ, Yates JR (1998) Mutations in the *TSC1* gene account for a minority of patients with tuberous sclerosis. *J Med Genet* 35:969–972.

Alper JC, Holmes LB (1983) The incidence and significance of birth marks in a cohort of 4641 newborns. *Pediatr Dermatol* 1:58–68.

Au KS, Rodriguez JA, Finch JL, Volcik KA, Roach ES, Delgado MR, Rodriguez E Jr, Northrup H (1998) Germ-line mutational analysis of the *TSC2* gene in 90 tuberous sclerosis patients. *Am J Hum Genet* 62:286–294.

Baker P, Piven J, Sato Y (1998) Autism and tuberous sclerosis complex: Prevalence and clinical features. *J Autism Dev Disord* 28:279–285.

Baraitser M, Patton MA (1985) Reduced penetrance in tuberous sclerosis. *J Med Genet* 22:29–31.

Beauchamp RL, Banwell A, McNamara P, Jacobsen M, Higgins E, Northrup H, Short P, Sims K, Ozelius L, Ramesh V (1998) Exon scanning of the entire *TSC2* gene for germline mutations in 40 unrelated patients with tuberous sclerosis. *Hum Mutat* 12:408–416.

Berg H (1913) Vererbung der tuberösen sklerose durch zwei bzw. drei generationen. *Z Ges Neurol Psychiatr* 19:528–539.

Bernstein J (1993) Renal cystic disease in the tuberous sclerosis complex. *Paediatr Nephrol* 7:490–495.

Bourneville DM (1880) Sclérose tubéreuse des circonvolutions cérébrales: Idiote épilepsie hémiplégique. *Arch Neurol (Paris)* 1:81–91.

Braffman BH, Bilaniuk LT, Naidisch TP, Altman NR, Post MJ, Quencer RM, Zimmerman RA, Brody BA (1992) MR imaging of tuberous sclerosis: Pathogenesis of this phakomatosis, use of gadopentetate dimeglumine, and literature review. *Radiology* 183:227–238.

Bruni O, Cortesi F, Giannotti F, Curatolo P (1995) Sleep disorders in tuberous sclerosis: A polysomnographic study. *Brain Dev* 17:52–56.

Cassidy SB, Pagon RA, Pepin M, Blumhagen JD (1983) Family studies in tuberous sclerosis.

Evaluation of apparently unaffected parents. *JAMA* 249:1302–1304.

Castro M, Shepherd CW, Gomez MR, Lie JT, Ryu JH (1995) Pulmonary tuberous sclerosis. *Chest* 107:189–195.

Clarke A, Hancock E, Kingswood C, Osborne JP (1999) End-stage renal failure in adults with tuberous sclerosis complex. *Nephrol Dial Transplant* 14:988–991.

Conzen M, Oppel F (1990) Tuberous sclerosis in neurosurgery. An analysis of 18 patients. *Acta Neurochir* 106:106–109.

Cook J, Oliver K, Mueller RF, Sampson J (1996) Cross-sectional natural history of renal disease in tuberous sclerosis. *J Med Genet* 33:480–484.

Curatolo P, Cusmai R, Cortesi F, Chiron C, Jambaque I Dulac O (1991) Neuropsychiatric aspects of tuberous sclerosis. *Ann NY Acad Sci* 615:8–16.

Ewalt DH, Sheffield E, Sparagana SP, Delgado MR, Roach ES (1998) Renal lesion growth in children with tuberous sclerosis complex. *J Urol* 160:141–145.

Flanagan N, O'Connor WJ, McCartan B, Miller S, McMenamin J, Watson R (1997) Developmental enamel defects in tuberous sclerosis: A clinical genetic marker? *J Med Genet* 34:637–639.

Fleury P, de Groot WP, Delleman JW, Verbeeten B, Frankenmolen-Witkiezwicz IM (1980) Tuberous sclerosis: The incidence of sporadic cases versus familial cases. *Brain Dev* 2:107–117.

Flinter FA, Neville BG (1986) Examining the parents of children with tuberous sclerosis. *Lancet* 2:1167.

Fryer AE, Chalmers A, Connor JM, Fraser I, Povey S, Yates AD, Yates JR, Osborne JP (1987a) Evidence that the gene for tuberous sclerosis is on chromosome 9. *Lancet* 1:659–661.

Fryer AE, Osborne JP, Schutt W (1987b) Forehead fibrous plaque: A presenting skin sign in tuberous sclerosis. *Arch Dis Child* 62:292–293.

Fryer AE, Chalmers AH, Osborne JP (1990) The value of investigation for genetic counselling in tuberous sclerosis. *J Med Genet* 27:217–223.

Gibbs JL (1985) The heart and tuberous sclerosis. An echocardiographic and electrocardiographic study. *Br Heart J* 54:596–599.

Gillberg IC, Gillberg C, Ahlsen G (1994) Autistic behaviour and attention deficits in tuberous sclerosis: A population-based study. *Dev Med Child Neurol* 36:50–56.

Gomez MR ed. (1979) *Tuberous sclerosis*. New York; Raven.

Gomez MR (1991) Phenotypes of the tuberous sclerosis complex with a revision of the diagnostic criteria. *Ann NY Acad Sci* 615:1–7.

Gould SR (1991) Hamartomatous rectal polyps are common in tuberous sclerosis. *Ann NY Acad Sci* 615:71–80.

Gould SR, Stewart JB, Temple LN (1990) Rectal polyposis in tuberous sclerosis. *J Mental Defic Res* 34:465–473.

Griffiths PD, Bolton P, Verity C (1998) White matter abnormalities in tuberous sclerosis complex. *Acta Radiol* 39:482–486.

Gunther M, Penrose LS (1935) The genetics of epiloia. *J Genet* 31:413–430.

Hancock E, Osborne JP (1999) Vigabatrin in the treatment of infantile spasms in tuberous sclerosis: Literature review. *J Child Neurol* 14:71–74.

Harding CO, Pagon RA (1990) Incidence of tuberous sclerosis in patients with cardiac rhabdomyoma. *Am J Med Genet* 37:443–446.

Hunt A (1983) Tuberous sclerosis: A survey of 97 cases. I. Seizures, pertussis immunisation and handicap. *Dev Med Child Neurol* 25:346–349.

Hunt A (1993) Development, behaviour and seizures in 300 cases of tuberous sclerosis. *J Intellect Disabil Res* 37:41–51.

Hunt A, Lindenbaum RH (1984) Tuberous sclerosis: A new estimate of prevalence within the Oxford region. *J Med Genet* 21:272–277.

Hunt A, Shepherd C (1993) A prevalence study of autism in tuberous sclerosis. *J Autism Dev Disord* 23:323–339.

Hunt A, Stores G (1994) Sleep disorder and epilepsy in children with tuberous sclerosis: A questionnaire-based study. *Dev Med Child Neurol* 36:108–115.

Johnson MW, Emelin JK, Park SH, Vinters HV (1999) Co-localization of *TSC1* and *TSC2* gene products in tubers of patients with tuberous sclerosis. *Brain Pathol* 9:45–54.

Jones AC, Daniells CE, Snell RG, Tachataki M, Idziaszczyk SA, Krawczak M, Sampson JR,

Cheadle JP (1997) Molecular genetic and phenotypic analysis reveals differences between *TSC1* and *TSC2* associated familial and sporadic tuberous sclerosis. *Hum Mol Genet* 6:2155–2161.

Jones AC, Shyamsundar MM, Thomas MW, Maynard J, Idziaszczyk S, Tomkins S, Sampson JR, Cheadle JP (1999) Comprehensive mutation analysis of *TSC1* and *TSC2* and phenotypic correlations in 150 families with tuberous sclerosis. *Am J Hum Genet* 64:1305–1315.

Jozwiak S, Pedich M, Rajszys P, Michalowics R (1992) Incidence of hepatic hamartomas in tuberous sclerosis. *Arch Dis Child* 67:1363–1365.

Jozwiak S, Kawalec W, Dluzewska J, Daszkowska J, Mirkowicz-Malek M, Michalowicz R (1994) Cardiac tumours in tuberous sclerosis: Their incidence and course. *Eur J Paediatr* 153:155–157.

Jozwiak S, Schwartz RA, Janniger CK, Michalowicz R, Chmielik J (1998) Skin lesions in children with tuberous sclerosis complex: Their prevalence, natural course, and diagnostic significance. *Int J Dermatol* 37:911–917.

Kandt RS, Haines JL, Smith M, Northrup H, Gardner RJ, Short MP, Dumars K, Roach ES, Steingold S, Wall S, Blanton SH, Flodman P, Kwiatkowski DJ, Jewell A, Weber JL, Roses AD, Pericak-Vance MA (1992) Linkage of an important gene locus for tuberous sclerosis to a chromosome 16 marker for polycystic kidney disease. *Nat Genet* 2:37–41.

Kingsley DP, Kendall BE, Fitz CR (1986) Tuberous sclerosis: A clinicoradiological evaluation of 110 cases with particular reference to atypical presentation. *Neuroradiology* 28:38–46.

Kwiatkowska J, Jozwiak S, Hall F, Henske EP, Haines JL, McNamara P, Braiser J, Wigowska-Sowinska J, Kasprzyk-Obara J, Short MP, Kwiatkowski DJ (1998) Comprehensive mutational analysis of the *TSC1* gene: Observations on frequency of mutation, associated features, and non-penetrance. *Ann Hum Genet* 62:277–285.

Kwiatkowska J, Wigowska-Sowinska J, Napierala D, Slomski R, Kwiatkowska DJ (1999) Mosaicism in tuberous sclerosis as a potential failure of the molecular diagnosis. *N Engl J Med* 340:703–707.

Lenoir S, Grenier P, Brauner MW, Frija J, Remy-Jardin M, Revel D, Cordier JF (1990) Pulmonary lymphangiomatosis and tuberous sclerosis: Comparison of radiographic and thin-section CT findings. *Radiology* 175:329–334.

Lie JT, Miller RD, Williams DE (1980) Cystic disease of the lungs in tuberous sclerosis: Clinicopathologic correlation, including body plethysmographic lung function tests. *Mayo Clin Proc* 55:547–553.

Luna CM, Gene R, Jolly EC, Nahmod N, Defranchi HA, Patino G, Elsner B (1985) Pulmonary lymphangiomatosis associated with tuberous sclerosis. Treatment with tamoxifen and tetracycline-pleurodesis. *Chest* 88:473–475.

Lygidakis NA, Lindenbaum RH (1987) Pitted enamel hypoplasia in tuberous sclerosis patients and first-degree relatives. *Clin Genet* 32:216–221.

McLaurin RL, Towbin RB (1985) Tuberous sclerosis: Diagnostic and surgical considerations. *Pediatr Neurosci* 12:43–48.

Nagib MG, Haines SJ, Erickson DL, Mastin AR (1984) Tuberous sclerosis: A review for the neurosurgeon. *Neurosurgery* 14:93–98.

Nir A, Tajik AJ, Freeman WK, Seward JB, Offord KP, Edwards WD, Mair DD, Gomez MR (1995) Tuberous sclerosis and cardiac rhabdomyoma. *Am J Cardiol* 76:419–421.

Nuhler EG, Turniski-Harder V, Engelhardt W, von Bermuth G (1994) Cardiac involvement in tuberous sclerosis. *Br Heart J* 72:584–590.

O'Callaghan FJ, Clarke AA, Hancock E, Hunt A, Osborne JP (1999) Use of melatonin to treat sleep disorders in tuberous sclerosis. *Dev Med Child Neurol* 41:123–126.

Pampilgione G, Pugh E (1975) Infantile spasms and subsequent appearance of tuberous sclerosis. *Lancet* 2:1046.

Polosa R, Magnano M, Crimi N, Vancheri C, Mistretta A (1995) Pulmonary tuberous sclerosis in a woman of child-bearing age with no mental retardation. *Respir Med* 89:227–231.

Roach ES, Williams DP, Laster DW (1987) Magnetic resonance imaging in tuberous sclerosis. *Arch Neurol* 44:301–303.

Roach ES, Smith M, Huttenlocher P, Bhat M, Alcorn D, Hawley L (1992) Diagnostic criteria: Tuberous sclerosis complex. Report of the Diagnostic Criteria Committee of the National

Tuberous Sclerosis Association. *J Child Neurol* 7:221–224.

Roach ES, Gomez MR, Northup H (1999a) Tuberous sclerosis complex consensus conference: Revised clinical diagnostic criteria. *J Child Neurol* 13:624–628.

Roach ES, DiMario FJ, Kandt RS, Northup H (1999b) Tuberous sclerosis consensus conference: Recommendations for diagnostic evaluation. *J Child Neurol* 14:401–407.

Rose VM, Au K-S, Pollom G, Roach ES, Prashner HR, Northrup H (1999) Germ-line mosaicism in tuberous sclerosis: How common? *Am J Hum Genet* 64:986–992.

Rudolph RI (1981) Pulmonary manifestations of tuberous sclerosis. *Cutis* 27:82–84.

Sampson JR, Attwood D, al Mughery AS, Reid JS (1992) Pitted enamel hypoplasia in tuberous sclerosis. *Clin Genet* 42:50–52.

Sampson JR, Scahill SJ, Stephenson JB, Mann L, Connor JM (1989) Genetic aspects of tuberous sclerosis in the west of Scotland. *J Med Genet* 26:28–31.

Sepp T, Yates JR, Green AJ (1996) Loss of heterozygosity in tuberous sclerosis hamartomas. *J Med Genet* 33:962–964.

Shepherd CW, Beard CM, Gomez MR, Kurland LT, Whisnant JP (1991) Tuberous sclerosis complex in Olmsted County, Minnesota, 1950–1989. *Arch Neurol* 48:400–401.

Smith HC, Watson GH, Patel RG, Super M (1989) Cardiac rhabdomyomata in tuberous sclerosis: Their course and diagnostic value. *Arch Dis Child* 64:196–200.

Smolarek TA, Wessner LL, McCormack FX, Mylet JC, Menon AG, Henske EP (1998) Evidence that lymphangiomyomatosis is caused by *TSC2* mutations: Chromosome 16p13 loss of heterozygosity in angiomyolipomas and lymph nodes from women with lymphangiomyomatosis. *Am J Hum Genet* 62:810–815.

Stapleton FB, Johnson D, Kaplan GW, Griswold W (1980) The cystic lesion in tuberous sclerosis. *J Pediatr* 97:574–579.

Steiner MS, Goldman SM, Fishman EK, Marshall FF (1993) The natural history of renal angiomyolipoma. *J Urol* 150:1782–1786.

Stilwell TJ, Gomez MR, Kelalis PP (1987) Renal lesions in tuberous sclerosis. *J Urol* 138:477–481.

Torres OA, Roach ES, Delgado MR, Sparanga SP, Sheffield E, Swift D, Bruce D (1998) Early diagnosis of subependymal giant cell astrocytoma in patients with tuberous sclerosis. *J Child Neurol* 13:173–177.

Torres VE, Bjornsson J, King BF, Kumar R, Zincke H, Edell ES, Wilson TO, Hattery RR, Gomex MR (1995) Extrapulmonary lymphangioleiomyomatosis and lymphangiomatous cysts in tuberous sclerosis complex. *Mayo Clin Proc* 70:641–648.

Van Baal JG, Fleury P, Brummelkamp WH (1989) Tuberous sclerosis and the relation with renal angiomyolipoma. A genetic study on the clinical aspects. *Clin Genet* 35:167–173.

Van Baal JG, Smiths NJ, Keeman JN, Lindhout D, Verhoef S (1994) The evolution of renal angiomyolipomas in patients with tuberous sclerosis. *J Urol* 152:35–38.

Vanderhooft SL, Francis JS, Pagon RA, Smith LT, Sybert VP (1996) Prevalence of hypopigmented macules in a healthy population. *J Pediatr* 129:355–361.

van Slegtenhorst M, de Hoogt R, Hermans C, et al. (1997) Identification of the tuberous sclerosis gene *TSC1* on chromosome 9q34. *Science* 277:895–808.

van Slegtenhorst M, Nellsit M, Nagelkerken B, Cheadle J, Snell R, van den Ouweland A, Reuser A, Sampson J, Halley D, van der Sluijs P (1998) Interaction between hamartin and tuberin, the *TSC1* and *TSC2* gene products. *Hum Mol Genet* 7:1053–1057.

van Slegtenhorst M, Verhoef S, Tempelaars A, Bakker L, Wang Q, Wessels M, Bakker R, Nellist M, Lindhout D, Halley D, van den Ouweland A (1999) Mutational spectrum of the *TSC1* gene in a cohort of 225 tuberous sclerosis complex patients: No evidence for genotype-phenotype correlation. *J Med Genet* 36:285–289.

Verhoef S, Bakker L, Templaars AM, Hesseling-Janssen AL, Mazurczak T, Jozwiak S, Fois A, Bartalini G, Zonnenberg BA, van Essen AJ, Lindhout D, Halley DJ, van den Ouweland AM (1999) High rate of mosaicism in tuberous sclerosis complex. *Am J Hum Genet* 64:1632–1637.

Villeneuve N, Soufflet C, Plouin P, Chiron C, Dulac O (1998) Treatment of infantile spasms with vigabatrin as a first-line therapy and in monotherapy: Apropos of 70 infants. *Arch Pediatr* 5:731–738.

Vogt H (1908) Zur diagnostik der tuberösen sklerose. *Z Erforsch Behandl Jugendl Schwach-sinns* 2:1–12.

Webb DW, Fryer AE, Osborne JP (1991) On the incidence of fits and mental retardation in tuberous sclerosis. *J Med Genet* 28: 395–397.

Webb DW, Osborne JP (1991) Non-penetrance in tuberous sclerosis. *J Med Genet* 28:417–419.

Webb DW, Super M, Normand IC, Osborne JP (1993) Tuberous sclerosis and polycystic kidney disease. *Br. Med. J.* 306:1258–1259.

Webb DW, Kabala J, Osborne JP (1994) A population study of renal disease in patients with tuberous sclerosis. *Br J Urol* 74:151–154.

Webb DW, Fryer AE, Osborne JP (1996) Morbidity associated with tuberous sclerosis: A population study. *Dev Med Child Neurol* 38:146–155.

Westermann CJ, Oostveen AC, Wagenaar SS, Hilvering C, Overbeek SE, Verheijen-Breem-haar D, Corrin B (1986) Pulmonary tuberous sclerosis treated with tamoxifen and proges-terone. *Thorax* 41:892–893.

Xiao GH, Shoarinejad F, Jin F, Golemis EA, Yeoung RS (1997) The tuberous sclerosis 2 gene product, tuberin, functions as a Rab5 GTPase activating protein (GAP) in modulating endocytosis. *J Biol Chem* 272:6097–6100.

Yates JR, Van Bakel I Sepp T, Payne SJ, Webb DW, Nevin NC, Green AJ (1997) Female germline mosaicism in tuberous sclerosis con-firmed by molecular genetic analysis. *Hum Mol Genet* 6:2265–2269.

Young JM, Burley MW, Jeremiah SJ, Jeganathan D, Ekong R, Osborne JP, Povey S (1998) A mutation screen of the *TSC1* gene reveals 26 protein truncating mutations and 1 splice site mutation in a panel of 79 tuberous sclerosis patients. *Ann Hum Genet* 62:203–213.

Young J, Povey S (1998) The genetic basis of tuberous sclerosis. *Mol Med Today* 4:313–319.

Zimmerhackl LB, Rehm M, Kaufmehl K, Kurle-mann G, Brandis M (1994) Renal involvement in tuberous sclerosis complex: A retrospective survey. *Paediatr Nephrol* 8:451–457.

CHAPTER 27

TURNER SYNDROME

VIRGINIA P. SYBERT

INTRODUCTION

Incidence

Turner syndrome, also known as Ullrich-Turner syndrome or Bonnevie-Ullrich-Turner syndrome, is defined as a disorder in females in which there is absence of a normal second sex chromosome. Ullrich (1930) reported an 8-year-old girl with pterygium colli and short stature; Bonnevie (1932) discussed a mouse mutation that led to cystic hygromas; Turner (1938) described 7 females with short stature, webbing of the neck, cubitus valgus, and sexual infantilism; and Ford et al., (1959) first demonstrated 45,X as the cause. In general, absence of a normal second sex chromosome leads to a constellation of physical findings including congenital lymphedema and resultant neck webbing, short stature, and gonadal dysgenesis. These are the hallmark features of Turner syndrome. A multiplicity of other physical and cognitive alterations are also associated.

Turner syndrome is reported to occur in 1 in 2500 to 1 in 3000 liveborn females. This number is based on screening of newborn populations. 45,X (monosomy X) occurs much more often among pregnancy losses than in liveborn infants. This has led to the theory, as yet unproven, that the 45,X

conceptions that survive to live birth must be mosaic for a second cell line containing material from a second sex chromosome.

Diagnostic Criteria

The physical phenotype of individuals with Turner syndrome (Figs. 27.1–27.3) is highly variable and is often normal, with the exception of short stature. There is really only one criterion for the diagnosis of Turner syndrome: demonstration of a cytogenetic alteration in the second sex chromosome leading to deletion of part or all of the short arm of an X or a Y chromosome in a clinically significant proportion of cells.

Etiology, Pathogenesis, and Genetics

The cause of the Turner syndrome is loss of part or all of the second sex chromosome. In particular, deletion of the short arm of the second copy of the X chromosome or homologous sequences on the Y chromosome gives the phenotype of short stature and gonadal dysgenesis. These chromosomal anomalies can arise during gametogenesis or as a result of postzygotic nondisjunction. No single feature of Turner syndrome is invariably present among affected females, with perhaps the

Management of Genetic Syndromes, Edited by Suzanne B. Cassidy and Judith E. Allanson
ISBN 0-471-31286-X   Copyright © 2001 by Wiley-Liss, Inc.

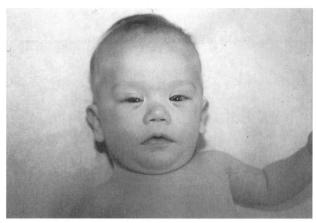

FIGURE 27.1. Three-month-old with 45,X karyotype. Note mild ptosis, epicanthal folds with flat nasal bridge and downturned mouth. Neck appears somewhat broad.

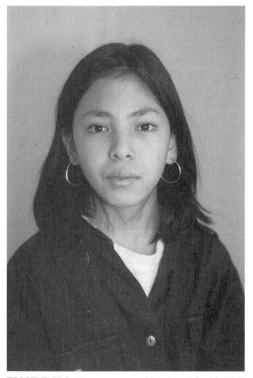

FIGURE 27.2. Fourteen-year-old Asian girl with 45,X karyotype. Appearance is essentially normal for ethnic group.

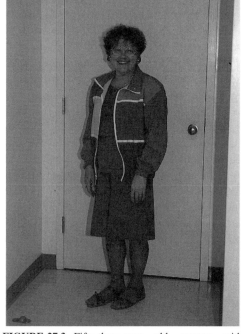

FIGURE 27.3. Fifty-three-year old woman with 45,X/46,XX/47,XXX. Appearance is normal, except for short stature.

exception of short stature in women whose chromosome complement appears to be 45,X with no evidence of a second cell line.

There has been considerable research to determine the exact chromosomal regions and the genes therein whose loss accounts for the physical stigmata of Turner syndrome and to seek the Y-linked regions that contain genes controlling stature and testicular development. It is difficult to tease out the specific effects of X chromosome deletions and rearrangements in Turner syndrome, because most patients with these alterations are also mosaic for a monosomy X cell line that may play the major role in determining physical outcome. By studying patients with pure, structural X chromosome rearrangements and no evidence of a 45,X cell line, some conclusions have been drawn. Loss of long arm material from the X chromosome, either terminal or interstitial, can result in short stature and primary or secondary ovarian failure. Loss of genes distal to Xq13 (those close to the end of the long arm of the chromosome) appears to have no effect on stature. There are interstitial long arm deletions of X that do not result in phenotypic Turner syndrome. Very distal X short arm deletions are compatible with but do not ensure normal ovarian function. Loss of this region usually confers short stature. This is believed to be caused by loss of the *SHOX* gene, located in the pseudoautosomal region of the Y and on Xp (Rao et al., 1997). *SHOX* refers to Short stature HOmeoboX-containing gene. Homozygosity for mutations in *SHOX* causes Leri-Weill dyschondrosteosis, an autosomal dominant disorder with short stature and Madelung deformity. Loss of the *SRY* gene locus, the testis-determining factor, on the short arm of the Y chromosome also leads to the phenotype of Turner syndrome, even in the absence of a 45,X cell line [for example, 46,X,del(Yp)]. In patients mosaic for a 45,X cell line, the likelihood of short stature and gonadal dysgenesis is high if the diagnosis is made postnatally, irrespective of the presence of a normal or rearranged Y or X chromosome in a second cell line.

The ring or marker X chromosome found in a subset of patients with Turner syndrome may be small or large. Its presence is sometimes associated with an atypical, more severe phenotype. It has been proposed that some of these X chromosome derivatives lack *XIST*, the region on the X chromosome that controls X inactivation. Thus, theoretically, these rings do not inactivate, causing abnormality by overexpression of X chromosome material. Some studies support this contention; others do not.

There are many karyotype alterations that can lead to the clinical entity of Turner syndrome. In the author's series of 487 patients (Sybert, 1995; unpublished data), approximately one-half of patients in whom Turner syndrome is diagnosed will have a 45,X chromosome constitution. Five to ten percent will have 46,X,i(Xq) (duplication of the long arm with loss of the short arm) as their chromosome abnormality. Most of the remaining will have mosaicism for 45,X and one or more other cell lines, some of which may contain two normal X chromosomes. For the most part, individuals mosaic for 45,X/46,XX diagnosed after birth do not have significant phenotypic differences from individuals with 45,X. Those mosaic for 45,X/46,XX or 45,X/46,XY who are diagnosed prenatally through routine amniocentesis performed for advanced maternal age and not for findings suggestive of Turner syndrome may be much more likely to exhibit no stigmata of Turner syndrome postnatally (Koeberl et al., 1995). Confusion is sometimes generated by misinterpreting the term "mosaic" as implying only mosaicism for a normal 46,XX cell line. Mosaicism for two abnormal cell lines, e.g., 45,X/46,X,i(Xq), confers the same spectrum of risk as does monosomy 45,X.

The role of genomic imprinting in Turner syndrome has been questioned. Genomic imprinting is the term used for the differential expression of genes or DNA segments depending on the parent of origin of the chromosome. There is, to date, no conclusive evidence that imprinting of specific loci on either the Y or the X chromosome leads to specific findings in patients.

There have been many attempts to establish firm karyotype-phenotype correlations in Turner syndrome. For any given individual, predictions of physical involvement based on chromosome constitution are unreliable. Women with 45,X have conceived; women with 45,X/46,XX and a preponderance of 46,XX cells may be short, infertile, and have all the associated malformations, dysmorphic features, and cognitive findings of Turner syndrome.

There are some correlations between karyotype and phenotype for chromosomally similar groups. Individuals with 45,X are more likely to have congenital lymphedema and the associated nuchal webbing; the frequencies were 67% (134/200 with 45,X) versus 11% (23/211 with other karyotypes) in the author's series (Sybert, 1995; unpublished data). Individuals with 45,X/46,XX are more likely to have spontaneous menarche compared with women with monosomy X, isochromosome X, or ring X [36% (12/33) versus 15% (30/202) in the author's series (Sybert, 1995; unpublished data)]. As a group, they are marginally taller, although the mean height is still just below the third percentile [151.0 ± 9.8 cm in 19 patients with mosaicism as compared with 146.5 ± 6.7 cm in 99 patients with 45,X in one series (Sybert, 1995; unpublished data)]. The presence of an isochromosome Xq may confer a higher risk for hypothyroidism (Sybert, 1995; unpublished data). The presence of a Y chromosome confers a risk for gonadoblastoma. Individuals with a ring or marker chromosome have an increased risk for mental retardation. Some of these patients may lack the more typical facial features of the Turner syndrome and have phenotypic features atypical for Turner syndrome, including syndactyly of fingers 3 and 4 or swirly pigment change along the lines of Blaschko.

There is little evidence to support an increased risk for offspring with Turner syndrome associated with increasing maternal age or for an increased risk within families.

Diagnostic Testing

Routine peripheral blood karyotyping, with evaluation of 20 cells, is usually sufficient to confirm the diagnosis of Turner syndrome. If the results are normal, (46,XX) and the diagnosis is suspected clinically, expansion of cell counts to 100 and examination of a second cell type, such as skin fibroblasts, are warranted to exclude mosaicism for an abnormal cell line. The buccal smear for Barr body analysis is an inadequate test for Turner syndrome.

There is some controversy regarding the extent to which a search for an occult cell line with a Y chromosome should be done in girls with a 45,X karyotype. This concern derives from two reasons: 1) the theoretical possibility that all 45,X survivors are mosaic for a normal cell line (unproven), and 2) there is a risk for gonadoblastoma in dysgenetic gonads with Y chromosome material (proven). The studies to date using FISH probes for Y sequences or H-Y antigen in such individuals have not shown compelling evidence that occult Y chromosome material in females with 45,X is a significant clinical concern. Routine screening for Y chromosome material in patients with 45,X is warranted only if there is evidence of masculinization or mosaicism for an unidentified marker or ring chromosome (Sybert, 1995; unpublished data).

Differential Diagnosis

Approximately one-fifth to one-third of girls with Turner syndrome are diagnosed at birth because of the presence of lymphedema, manifesting as puffy hands and feet. The majority of these girls will have a 45,X chromosome constitution. In the newborn period, the major disorders that lead to congenital edema of the neck and extremities are Turner syndrome and Noonan syndrome (see Chapter 15). Noonan syndrome also shares short stature in common with Turner syndrome.

The causes of short stature, the feature that leads to the diagnosis of another one-third of patients, usually between ages 5 and 10 years, are legion. Turner syndrome should be suspected and ruled out by chromosome testing in any girl with short stature, unless a clear-cut history of constitutional delay or familial short stature, coupled with an absence of any other physical stigmata of Turner syndrome, can be documented. With the exception of constitutional delay and familial short stature, no other cause of growth failure in otherwise healthy-appearing girls is more common or more likely than Turner syndrome.

The third cardinal feature that leads to the diagnosis of Turner syndrome is delay or absence of puberty, resulting from gonadal dysgenesis. The differential diagnosis includes other causes of primary ovarian failure. These are readily excluded by an abnormal karyotype. Most of the girls diagnosed with Turner syndrome in the teen years because of lack of puberty are also short. The combination of short stature and delayed or absent puberty should always lead to chromosome testing. If karyotyping is normal and mosaicism is excluded, single-gene causes for gonadal failure should be sought.

MANIFESTATIONS AND MANAGEMENT

Growth and Feeding

Prematurity is more common in pregnancies of infants with Turner syndrome, with 12% of infants delivering at gestational ages of 36 weeks or less in one study (Sybert, 1995; unpublished data)

Mean birth weight in full-term infants with Turner syndrome is between the 25th and 50th centiles for normal females (unpublished data). Curves for ponderal growth have not yet been established for Turner syndrome.

Feeding problems are common, including frequent spitting, vomiting, and difficulty in latching and in sucking. Frank gastroesophageal reflux and failure to thrive also occur. Both breast- and bottle-fed infants experience these problems. For the majority, these are mild problems. In a minority, nasogastric or gastric tube feeding has been required. How much of this is caused by anatomical differences in the oropharynx (high palate, palatal insufficiency) and how much by oral motor immaturity is not known. The one study addressing this issue evaluated 10 infants with Turner syndrome presenting to clinics for growth failure, thus selecting for infants with more severe difficulties. The authors suggested that both factors played roles, as did a component of abnormal gastroesophageal motility (Mathisen et al., 1992).

The mean birth length of full-term infants with Turner syndrome is 46 cm (18 in.), just at the fifth centile for the normal female population (Sybert, 1995; unpublished data).

Growth velocity in Turner syndrome is less than normal even in infancy, but this deceleration may go unnoticed. By 18 months, most girls are growing at or below the third centile for height. Recognition of growth failure is gradual. Many girls will not be the shortest child in kindergarten but will be the shortest by third or fourth grade, leading to diagnosis in the 5- to 10-year-old group. When the normal pubertal growth spurt does not occur, children are often brought for evaluation. It is easy to misinterpret absence of evidence of puberty and small size as constitutional delay. Unfortunately, a significant minority of those who seek diagnosis in midchildhood because of growth failure is not diagnosed until the midteens, when the continued absence of secondary sex characteristics raises suspicion (Sybert, 1995; unpublished data). All of the author's 104 patients who were diagnosed to have Turner syndrome as teenagers because of amenorrhea and short stature had evidenced growth failure much earlier in childhood. Thyroid disease can be associated with growth failure. In girls with Turner syndrome, although hypothyroidism can exacerbate growth failure, it rarely, if ever, initiates it.

In later childhood and adult life, obesity can present difficulties for individuals with Turner syndrome. This appears to be a consequence of excess caloric intake and decreased caloric expenditure. Short girls and women are less likely to engage in sports or physical activity. There does not appear to be an intrinsic metabolic abnormality resulting in inappropriate weight gain.

In 1983, a long-term study of the efficacy of recombinant human growth hormone (hGH) in Turner syndrome was undertaken in the United States. In 1997, the FDA approved the use of this medication in Turner syndrome. In most but not all centers, growth hormone treatment for Turner syndrome is a standard treatment. There is considerable literature discussing growth hormone secretion in Turner syndrome. To date, no clinically significant alteration has been consistently identified. As a rule, girls with Turner syndrome do not have insufficient or ineffective growth hormone production. For treatment, growth hormone is given in superphysiologic amounts based on the hypothesis that the skeleton in Turner syndrome may have a blunted response to endogenous hormone that can be stimulated by increased levels of hGH.

To date, 12 major studies have followed treated patients to final adult heights. Success in treatment has been based on two comparisons. The first compares the mean final height of the hGH-treated group of patients to the historical mean height of 143.2 cm derived by Lyon et al. from 4 European studies and their own patients (Lyon et al., 1985). The second approach compares the final height achieved by each subject to her projected adult height, based on her centile in the Lyon curve at age of onset of hGH treatment, or her predicted adult height using one of a number of formulas based on mid-parental height derived for that purpose. Only one published study has had a concurrent matched control group (Hochberg and Zadik, 1999). When achieved heights are compared with projected or predicted

heights, the results range from impressive to inconsequential gains, from no gain to as much as (3.8 in) 9.7 cm (Table 27.1). When final heights are compared across the board between relatively similar populations (e.g., Sybert, 1995; Plotnick et al., 1998), the differences in final height are a few centimeters. Complicating all these analyses are different treatment regimens, different ages at commencement of treatment, and different durations of therapy. Although one study suggested that all treated girls reached or exceeded their predicted adult height (Rosenfeld et al., 1998), other studies have not reported similar success (Donaldson, 1996; Bramswig, 1997; Chu et al., 1997; Donaldson, 1997). There is disagreement as to whether starting treatment before or after age 10 contributes to the positive effect of treatment, as to the effect of age of institution of concomitant estrogen, therapy, and as regards the benefit of adding oxandrolone to the regimen.

No studies have looked at the psychosocial outcomes associated with human growth hormone treatment and a real or perceived increase in height.

With or without growth hormone therapy, girls with Turner syndrome will become short adults. There is mild skeletal disproportion, usually not socially significant, but which may make alteration of clothing necessary. Most adults with Turner syndrome adjust successfully to their petite stature.

Evaluation

- It is not necessary to perform a feeding study in all newborns with Turner syndrome. However, attention should be paid to parental concerns, and complaints regarding difficulty in feeding or poor weight gain should be taken seriously.

- Referral to physical/occupational therapy for a feeding evaluation may be helpful, as are reassuring discussions with the parents and simple interventions such as nipple changes (a cleft

TABLE 27.1. Final Adult Height in Turner Syndrome After Treatment with Recombinant Human Growth Hormone ± Androgens ± Estrogens Compared with Predicted or Projected Final Heights

Reference	Country	N	FAH±SD, cm	Pre-AH±SD, cm	Pro-AH±SD, cm	Difference, cm
Rosenfeld et al., 1998	US	60	151.6±5.8		142±5.9	9.6
Retrospective controls		25	144.2±6		144.2±5.6	
Haeusler et al., 1996	Austria	20	152.9±3.5		143.7±4.0	9.2
Takano et al., 1997	Japan (0.5 IU/kg)	15	142.2±6.5		137 (historical controls)	5.2
	Japan (1.0 IU/kg)	15	144.3±3.5			7.3
Plotnick et al., 1998	US,NCGS	622	148.3±5.6		141.9±6.2	6.4
Sas et al., 1999	Holland	19	155.5±5.4	149.2±6.0		6.3±3.0
Nilsson et al., 1996	Sweden	44	152.2±5.9	146.4±5.3		5.8
Rochiccioli et al., 1995	France	117	150.1±5.6	144.9±5.2		5.1
Hochberg and Zadik 1999	Israel	25	147.3±4.9		142.6±5.2	4.7±2.9
controls		24	142.9±5.1		143.5±4.2	−0.6±7.2
Betts et al., 1999	UK (includes patients from other studies)	52	Not given	Not given		3.9 − 5.0*
Van den Broeck et al., 1995	Netherlands, UK, France, Norway, Germany	56	150.7±4.9	147.4	147.8	2.9
Massa et al., 1995	Belgium	45	152.3±5.3	149.7±5.7		2.6
Chu et al., 1997	Scotland	26	142.6		142	0.6
Taback et al., 1996	Canada	17	148		148.2	−0.2
Nonrandom controls		14	140.7		144	−3.7
Sybert	US untreated	137	147.8±8.1	146.2		1.6
	Age matched with NCGS/Genentech	15	148.9±5.3			

FAH, final adult height; Pre-AH, predicted adult height; Pro-AH, projected adult height; NCGS, National Cooperative Growth Study. *Calculated based on changes in height SDs palate nipple may be useful) and positioning after feeds.

- Growth hormone testing in girls with Turner syndrome is rarely indicated.

Treatment

- Individuals with Turner syndrome should be encouraged to maintain physical activity to avoid obesity. It should be remembered that unstable patellae might make certain forms of exercise problematic. Swimming, walking, and bicycle riding are activities that can be encouraged in childhood and maintained lifelong.

- Education regarding nutrition may be helpful. However, remember that many individuals with Turner syndrome have a naturally stocky habitus. It is gross obesity that is to be avoided.

- The decision to treat or not with growth hormone needs to be made by each family, fully informed regarding the modest gain in height that is likely to be achieved (and may not be achieved by all) contrasted with the burden of injections and monitoring. hGH appears to be safe, although long-term issues such as effect on risk for diabetes and other skeletal alterations remain unresolved. Each family will perceive the burden of short stature and the risks and benefits of treatment differently. It is appropriate to discuss this issue with an endocrinologist as well as with other physicians.

- Growth hormone treatment, if instituted, should be started at about age 4, or at the time of diagnosis during childhood thereafter.

- It is important for adults and peers to treat children with Turner syndrome as age appropriate, not height appropriate. It is easy to dismiss as cute behavior what would be unacceptable in a child of similar age who does not appear small.

Development and Behavior

This area has been extensively studied in Turner syndrome. The majority of individuals with Turner syndrome have intelligence that falls within the normal range on testing, are successful in school, and function as independent adults. Approximately 10% of affected individuals, irrespective of karyotype, will have significant delays, need special education, and require some ongoing assistance in adult life either in job placement or assisted living. The risk for mental retardation is highest in individuals with a marker chromosome (66%) or a ring (X) chromosome (30%) (Sybert, 1995; unpublished data).

Among those with normal intelligence, specific learning deficits are found in a majority, but not all. These include difficulties in processing, visual-spatial reasoning, right-left discrimination, sequencing, and speed of task completion (Money and Granoff, 1965; Lahood and Bacon, 1985; Silbert et al., 1977; Downey et al., 1991; Delooz et al., 1993; Ross et al., 1995). Performance scores on IQ testing are often significantly lower than verbal scores. These deficits translate into problems with higher mathematics and difficulties with directions, driving, and multitasking.

There have been a handful of studies using MRI or PET scans to look at the structure of the brain in individuals with Turner syndrome. No consistent alterations have been demonstrated.

In the school years, problems may surface in the later elementary grades and sometimes earlier. Behavior problems contribute, in addition, to difficulties in comprehension. As a group, girls with Turner syndrome have more difficulty with short attention span, immature behavior, hyperactivity, peer relationships, and maintaining focus. Not all girls will have these characteristics. Often the difficulties are subjectively appreciated and not evident on standard academic evaluation, creating a problem for those girls who may benefit from educational assistance and yet not qualify for it on a testing basis alone.

Adolescent girls with Turner syndrome may experience isolation from peers because their social maturation may lag behind. How much of this is due to lack of ovarian hormone effects on the brain or short stature or infantilization by others is unknown. There may be alterations in psychosocial maturation that are not hormonally mediated, because similar cognitive and social profiles can be seen despite normal ovarian function (Sybert, 1995; unpublished data). Feelings of isolation may be overwhelming, and some girls benefit from psychiatric intervention. Others appear not to be perturbed by what is perceived by their parents and other adults as progressive alienation from peers.

Most girls and women with Turner syndrome lead lives of satisfaction for themselves and their loved ones. Most are independent, productive adults. They are later to date, leave home, and marry than their age-matched cohorts (Pavlidis et al., 1995). Most are well educated. In the author's series of 202 adults, 181 have finished high school or higher, 61 have completed 4-year college programs, and 11 have graduate degrees (Sybert, 1995; unpublished data).

Surveys of adults with Turner syndrome suggest that most function successfully with reasonable levels of satisfaction in employment and social life (Pavlidis et al., 1992; Sylvén et al., 1993). As a group, they are often employed at an occupational level below that predicted by education and training. These surveys are fraught with methodological problems, not the least of which is the inherent self-selection of respondents. In adults, difficulties with coordination, fine motor control, and speed of processing can have a significant negative effect on job performance, despite normal comprehension and desire to succeed. Women with Turner syndrome often fail in jobs requiring rapid response and multitasking. This is clearly not true for all; success in highly stressful professional careers is not rare.

Adults with Turner syndrome have fewer social contacts and appear more isolated compared with women of similar age in the general population (Pavlidis et al., 1995). They do not perceive themselves to be isolated, and most report satisfaction with lifestyle. They react with appropriate depression and feelings of loss to the physical limitations conferred by their chromosome constitution but usually cope well with these feelings and appear not to be more likely to develop severe psychiatric disease than chromosomally normal individuals. Anorexia nervosa has been reported about 20 times in girls and women with 45,X and 45,X/46,XX. Estimates for the prevalence of anorexia nervosa in the general population range from 6 in 1,000,000 to 1 in 250. With such disparate estimates of occurrence, it is difficult to come to any conclusions regarding an increased risk of anorexia nervosa in Turner syndrome. Approximately 10% of individuals with Turner syndrome have psychiatric diagnoses, including major reactive depression, unipolar and bipolar disease, anorexia, bulimia, psychosis, drug and alcohol addiction, and obsessive-compulsive disorder (Sybert, 1995; unpublished data). This is probably not significantly increased from the risk in the general population.

We have seen no evidence for early onset of senility in Turner syndrome, in contrast to what has been reported for trisomy 21.

It has been suggested that females with Turner syndrome fail to read social cues appropriately. They do not recognize or they misinterpret facial expressions and body language. This is often manifested as inappropriate persistence in maintaining a conversational theme and contact (McCauley et al., 1987; Ross et al., 2000).

One important aspect of achieving independence for adolescents and adults with Turner syndrome is driving, which presents great difficulty for them. Problems with visual motor integration, impaired spatial and directional abilities, and the reality of short stature all combine to make driving difficult and frightening for the individual and her parents. With appropriate accommodation — picking the right car with a seat that can be adjusted, professional driver's education, and careful planning of routes ahead of time — vehicular independence can be achieved.

Evaluation

- The expectation is that most girls in infancy and preschool will not present with problems. Routine pediatric developmental screening is appropriate, and identified concerns should be dealt with as in any infant or toddler.
- Indications of difficulties in school, including poor performance and teacher concern, should prompt formal cognitive and educational assessment.
- Evidence of attention deficit or hyperactivity requires professional assessment.

Treatment

- Medication plays the same role in the management of girls with Turner syndrome and attention deficit/hyperactivity disorder as in children with these problems without Turner syndrome.
- As the level of schooling increases, more subtle difficulties may surface. Care should be taken to use adequate time to explain directions and to reiterate if necessary. For some girls, untimed testing is appropriate to allow them time to organize their thinking and express their knowledge.
- For many, appropriate job counseling and accommodations in the workplace may be necessary. Referral for vocational assessment and rehabilitation can be helpful for some.
- Support groups for adults are extremely valuable, as they are for parents. Teenagers tend to reject such groups, although pen pal relationships can be quite successful (Sybert, 1995; unpublished data).

Cardiovascular

Congenital heart disease is a recognized component of Turner syndrome, with estimates of prevalence ranging from 17% to 45% (Gotzsche et al., 1994; Sybert, 1998). Coarctation of the aorta and/or bicuspid aortic valve are the most common lesions, followed by other aortic valve abnormalities. Hypoplastic left heart is also associated with Turner syndrome. There are no clear phenotype-karyotype correlations.

The natural history of specific cardiac lesions appears to be no different in individuals with Turner syndrome than in individuals without Turner syndrome. Death from cardiac involvement is a significant concern in Turner syndrome. In one series of over 400 patients, 4 died in the newborn period because of hypoplastic left heart syndrome and another at age 22 years from end-stage cardiac disease related to structural malformation. Three died of aortic dissection. (Sybert, 1995; unpublished data).

Hypertension, mitral valve prolapse, and conduction defects are also features of Turner syndrome. Of these, hypertension is by far the most common. It is usually essential in nature and not associated with arteriosclerotic heart disease or renal disease. Not surprisingly, the risk for hypertension increases with age and with obesity. The risk for coronary artery disease in Turner syndrome is unclear. A handful of case reports of patients with symptomatic disease has appeared. In most, no attention was paid to family history or *a priori* risk. There have been a few reports of lipid abnormalities in small series of patients and some concern regarding the role of ovarian hormone replacement in lipid homeostasis in these patients. In the author's large series, the frequency of lipid abnormalities, myocardial infarction, and atherosclerosis was not increased over the general population (Sybert, 1995; unpublished data); however, this population was not systematically screened for triglycerides and cholesterol.

Concern regarding the occurrence of aortic dissection in Turner syndrome was raised a number of years ago by Lin and colleagues (1986). Coarctation of the aorta (unrepaired and repaired), bicuspid aortic valve, and hypertension are known risk factors for aortic dissection in the general population, and it is reasonable to attribute a significant proportion of the occurrences of aortic dissection in patients with Turner syndrome to these risk factors. There have been more than 60 reports of aortic dissection in patients with Turner syndrome to date (see Sybert, 1998 for review). In all except 5, one or more of the risk factors were present. In a self-administered survey review, 12 of 15 individuals reporting aortic dissection had recognized risk factors (Lin et al., 1998).

Evaluation

- When the diagnosis of Turner syndrome is made, an echocardiogram should be scheduled. This should include measurement of aortic root diameter. Normal parameters for aortic root diameters in this population of extremely short individuals have not been established. Physical examination alone, even by a cardiologist, is inadequate because bicuspid aortic valves may not cause a murmur in childhood.
- The need for and frequency of repeat echocardiography for assessment of aortic root diameter in those without structural cardiac abnormalities is undetermined, because it is not known whether gradual dilatation of the aortic root precedes dissection, as in Marfan syndrome. Consensus guidelines for health supervision for children with Turner syndrome recommend annual repeat echocardiography (American Academy of Pediatrics Committee on Genetics, 1995), although there are no published data to support this recommendation and considerable argument against it (Sybert, 1998; Lin et al., 1998).
- Routine physical examinations for affected individuals should always

include blood pressure check. If hypertension is found, an evaluation to exclude specific causes is appropriate, as it is in any individual.
- Monitoring lipids is reasonable but should be left to the discretion of the health care provider until a clear risk for lipid-related disease is established in Turner syndrome.

Treatment

- If a cardiac malformation is detected, referral to a cardiologist is strongly recommended.
- Recommendations for management and additional monitoring, including antibiotic prophylaxis for valve disease, repeated echocardiography, and surgery, must be individualized and are not specific to the disorder .
- Prevention of obesity is highly desirable in affected individuals. Obesity is a major factor in hypertension and diabetes in Turner syndrome. Education about diet and encouragement of exercise are important. Activities that can be maintained lifelong by an individual who is short, with problematic knees and often poor coordination, include swimming, walking, bicycling, and rowing.
- Recommendations for management of hypertension are not specific to Turner syndrome.

Endocrine

Hypothyroidism is common in Turner syndrome, occurring in about 15–30% of adults (Germain and Plotnick, 1986; Sybert, 1995). Development of clinical disease is usually preceded by the appearance of antithyroid antibodies. Acute thyroiditis is not common, although it does occur. The mean age of onset of hypothyroidism in one series was 26.7 years (Sybert, 1995). Onset in mid to late childhood occurs in 5–10% of girls with

Turner syndrome (Sybert, 1995). The occurrence of thyroid disease does not correlate with karyotype in several studies (Sybert, 1995; Radetti et al., 1995), although it has been suggested by others (Ivarsson et al., 1995) that the presence of an isochromosome Xq increases the likelihood of thyroid disease.

Gonadal dysgenesis is a cardinal feature of Turner syndrome. Ninety percent of affected individuals will require estrogen to initiate puberty and complete growth and estrogen and progesterone to maintain menses. Although the uterus may be small because of lack of estrogen, structural uterine abnormalities are rare. The vagina may be small.

Many girls with Turner syndrome will develop pubic and axillary hair changes, generally to Tanner II or III, even in the absence of functional ovaries. These changes of adrenarche should not be misinterpreted as indicative of ovarian function. Some girls with Turner syndrome have enough residual ovarian function to evidence early signs of puberty, such as breast budding or vaginal spotting, but soon thereafter they develop secondary amenorrhea. Others are able to initiate and complete puberty, and they maintain ovulatory cycles for a time. Among these women, premature ovarian failure is common. Approximately 10% of girls with 45,X will go into puberty on their own; many fewer complete it without hormone replacement. Twenty-five percent of 45,X/46,XX mosaic girls will experience spontaneous menarche; again, progressive ovarian failure may ensue (Sybert, 1995).

Spontaneous fertility does occur in Turner syndrome and is most likely in women mosaic for a normal 46,XX cell line. Women with deletions of the very distal part of the short arm of the X may also maintain fertility. Realistically, most adult women with Turner syndrome will not become pregnant with their own eggs.

To date, more than 230 pregnancies in 93 women with Turner syndrome have been reported (Sybert, 1995; Tarani et al., 1998). These are summarized in Table 27.2. The risk of spontaneous abortion is very high, but because several individuals were ascertained because of multiple pregnancy losses, the *a priori* risk in a potentially fertile patient is possibly lower. The risk for trisomy 21 is increased. Four of 128 liveborn infants had Down syndrome (3%). The risk for sex chromosome aneuploidy is clearly increased, approaching 20%. Twinning appears to be more common, with 7 sets of twins in a total of 233 pregnancies.

It is reiterated in the literature that insulin resistance and type II diabetes are increased in Turner syndrome. These assertions have been based on studies looking at response to oral and intravenous glucose loads in individuals with Turner syndrome. Among 356 subjects, ages ranging from 4.7 to 54 years, pooled from a total of 10 separate series, an average of 27% had abnormal oral glucose tolerance test results. Abnormal responses to an oral glucose load occurred in 8–15% of control groups, none of whom were matched with subjects with Turner syndrome for weight and height. In contrast, intravenous glucose tolerance testing revealed no differences between subjects ($n = 75$) and controls, even when an oral challenge had given elevated blood glucose levels. Furthermore, two studies have suggested an increased prevalence of both abnormal glucose tolerance test curves and diabetes in parents and family members of individuals with Turner syndrome (Forbes and Engel, 1963; Rimoin et al., 1970)

It has been posited that there is insulin resistance in Turner syndrome, the basis of which is not known. There is conflicting evidence regarding the salutary or deleterious effect of ovarian hormone replacement on glucose homeostasis in Turner syndrome and no information regarding long-term effects of human growth hormone. Although growth hormone treatment has an effect on carbohydrate metabolism, to date there are no data to support an increased risk for development of

TABLE 27.2. Outcome of Pregnancy in Turner Syndrome

Karyotype	Number of Women	Number of Pregnancies	SAB	SB	Liveborn Normal	Trisomy 21	X Chromosome Abnormality	Congenital Malformation
45,X	18	42	17 (40%)	2	17 (40%)	1	45,X (2) 46,X,del X (1)	Cleft palate (1)*
45,X/46,XX	34	92	45 (49%)	8‡	38 (41%)	1	45,X (1) X,XX (3) X/X,del X (1) X/X.Xp⁻ (1)	Omphalocele, tetralogy, kidney abnormalities (2 males); spina bifida (2)
Other†	41	99	30 (30%)	9	37 (37%)	2	X/XY (1) 45,X (3) X/XX (2) X/XX/XXX (4) X/X,r(X) (4) X/X,del Xp (2)	VSD (1) CHD (1)
Totals	93	233	92 (39%)	19 (8)	92 (39%)	4 (2%)	25 (11%)	7 (3%)

SAB, spontaneous abortion; SB, stillbirth; VSD, ventricular septal defect; CHD, congenital heart disease. *Father had cleft palate; †e.g., X/XXX; X/X,delXp; X/X,r(X); ‡two with anencephaly, parents were first cousins diabetes in girls and women who are taking or have received growth hormone treatment.

Among 257 adult patients from several large published series of individuals with Turner syndrome, 18 (7%) have had frank diabetes requiring treatment. In the author's adult patients, only 2% have developed diabetes (Sybert, 1995; unpublished data).

Evaluation

- In infancy and early childhood, thyroid function should be checked only if growth appears abnormal for Turner syndrome.

- As a screen, measure TSH on an alternate-year basis beginning at about 10 years of age if growth is not a concern.

- In adults, screening for thyroid function on a yearly basis, including TSH, is recommended.

- If the TSH is elevated but thyroid functions are normal, repeat the test in 3–4 months.

- Normal FSH and LH levels in the first 3–12 months of life suggest that residual ovarian function exists. However, there is no guarantee that it will remain adequate to ensure normal initiation and progression through puberty. Hence, the predictive utility of testing is not great. If FSH and LH levels are elevated at that time, one can be certain of the need for ovarian hormone replacement in the future. FSH and LH are normally suppressed in children, even in those individuals with no gonads. Thus measurement of these hormones during childhood is not useful.

- At the time of ultrasound evaluation of the kidneys, ovarian and uterine structure can also be evaluated. If normal-sized ovaries are present, endogenous ovarian function may exist.

- If there is a question regarding ovarian function in a teenager with Turner syndrome and signs of puberty, FSH, LH,

and estradiol levels can help in sorting out the need for oral replacement.

- Periodic urinalysis for glucose at routine pediatric evaluations and at adult screening visits can be followed by blood glucose level or glycosylated hemoglobin level if there are reasons for concern.

Treatment

- If TSH is persistently elevated, replacement therapy should be started. Referral to an endocrinologist may be indicated.

- Replacement guidelines are the same for individuals with Turner syndrome as for anyone with hypothyroidism.

- Ovarian hormone therapy should be initiated at about age 14 years. Starting treatment earlier may result in a decrement in final adult height. Deferring it beyond 14 years does not appear to increase final height (Sybert, 1995; unpublished data). Although 14 years of age is later than the mean age of onset of puberty in normal females, it is still within the range of normal. Psychosocial issues and patient maturity and desires also must be considered, but in general, this timing appears to work well. In girls who have received growth hormone treatment and have completed most of their growth earlier, ovarian hormone replacement can be started earlier (i.e., around age 12), if desired.

- There is no single formula for sex hormone replacement. In general, the lowest effective doses should be used. In the United States, conjugated estrogens (Premarin) or ethinyl estradiol are the estrogens most commonly used. Initial dosing with Premarin at 0.3 mg/day or ethinyl estradiol 5–10 μg/day is maintained for 3–6 months and increased to 0.625 or 1.25 mg or 20 or 50 μg, respectively, as guided by breast development. This can be in continuous daily dosing or cycled during the first year.

- After the first year of treatment, unopposed estrogen must not be given, and cycling with a progestational agent is mandatory to minimize the risk for endometrial hyperplasia and uterine adenocarcinoma. Cycling is usually on a monthly basis. A variety of schedules have been successful (e.g., estrogen days 1–21, 1–25, or 1–28; progesterone days 15–21, 15–25, or 15–28). Withdrawal bleeding occurs on those days when no medication is taken.
- Standard low-dose birth control pills are another maintenance treatment option.
- It has been suggested that transdermal estrogen may be preferable in Turner syndrome, because elevation of liver enzymes associated with oral estrogen replacement has been documented. However, the number of patients studied is small, and there is no compelling clinical evidence for an excess of liver disease in adult women with Turner syndrome.
- For adults who no longer wish to have withdrawal bleeding, a postmenopausal regimen, such as daily estrogen/low-dose progesterone combined therapy, can be used.
- The approach to the "postmenopausal" patient with Turner syndrome should be the same as for any postmenopausal female. There has not been an increased occurrence of breast cancer in Turner syndrome.
- Occasionally, an adult patient will want to stop treatment completely, and this is not contraindicated, although consideration should be given to the usual potential consequences seen in the general population, such as osteopenia.
- Dyspareunia may occur because of a small vagina or atrophic vaginal lining. It is reasonable to discuss the potential for these problems in anticipation of sexual activity and to offer options ranging from lubricants (Astroglide is excellent) to vaginal estrogen cream to dilatation. In most patients, these problems have not occurred (Sybert, 1995; Pavlidis et al., 1995).
- A matter-of-fact, honest, and straightforward approach to explaining about infertility to affected teenagers and young women, while being reassuring about sexual function, parenting abilities, and options [adoption, GIFT (gamete intrafallopian transfer), fostering, and choosing to not have children], can help families and affected individuals. It is important to acknowledge the sense of loss of the ability to have one's own biological children experienced both by parents and by the girls.
- Pregnancy, utilizing GIFT techniques with donor eggs, has been attempted in a small number of women with Turner syndrome with a success rate equal to that of the procedure in women without Turner syndrome. In two women, aortic dissection has been reported. Thus the safety of pregnancy in Turner syndrome remains uncertain. Among women with Turner syndrome who have become pregnant spontaneously, no occurrences of aortic dissection have been reported.
- Yearly pelvic examinations and Pap smears are appropriate for patients who are receiving hormone replacement.
- The best treatment for diabetes is to encourage weight control from childhood onward. The majority of patients with Turner syndrome and diabetes have adult-onset (non-insulin dependent) disease, and most of them are overweight.
- Diet, oral hypoglycemics, and insulin may all come into play in the treatment of diabetes in Turner syndrome, with treatment strategies no different from the general population

Ophthalmologic

Ocular problems were found in about half of individuals with Turner syndrome in one series of 409 patients (Sybert, 1995; unpublished data). Strabismus is fairly frequent in infants and girls with Turner syndrome, with about 18% of patients having clinically significant external ocular muscle problems. Ptosis is frequent (13%). It rarely requires surgical intervention. Hyperopia and myopia occur, but whether to a greater degree than in the general population is unclear. Cataracts and nystagmus also occur more commonly in Turner syndrome. Red-green colorblindness was found with the same frequency as in normal males (Chrousos et al., 1984; Sybert, 1995; unpublished data). Despite these findings, most individuals with Turner syndrome will have functional vision.

Evaluation

- A careful screening eye examination should be done, with a low threshold of concern for strabismus in infancy.
- Referral to an ophthalmologist is warranted if any concerns exist.

Treatment

- Management of ocular abnormalities is problem specific and not different in Turner syndrome.

Ears and Hearing

The majority of infants and children with Turner syndrome will experience recurrent otitis media. The basis for this susceptibility is thought to be a combination of small, dysfunctional eustachian tubes and palatal dysfunction. In the author's large series, 63% of patients experienced recurrent bouts of otitis media, 27% had tympanostomy tube placement, 3% had cholesteatomas, 3% had mastoidectomy, and 7.6% had chronic conductive hearing loss (Sybert, 1995; unpublished data).

In addition to these mechanical problems, sensorineural hearing loss also appears to be a feature of Turner syndrome. Its basis is not understood. In a Swedish study, 90% of 44 adult females with Turner syndrome were found to have sensorineural hearing loss by testing; in two-thirds this was clinically significant (Hultcrantz et al., 1994). Twenty-seven percent of the women wore hearing aids. The loss appeared to be progressive. In the author's series, 10% had sensorineural hearing loss, with hearing aids being required by 5% of children and 17% of adults (Sybert, 1995; unpublished data).

The frequency of ear infections decreases with age and growth of facial structures. Most teenagers and adults do not suffer recurrent otitis media.

Evaluation

- Fever, irritability, or signs of congestion in infancy and childhood should prompt evaluation for otitis media.
- Children with a history of recurrent infections should be followed carefully for conductive hearing problems. Sensorineural hearing loss in adults may be unappreciated. Adults with Turner syndrome should have audiometric exams on a regular basis, and complaints of hearing loss should be taken seriously.

Treatment

- Aggressive prophylaxis in those children with recurrent otitis media is probably appropriate.
- With early indication that recurrent otitis is likely to be a problem, referral to otolaryngology for ventilation tube placement may be considered to try to avoid long-term consequences of scarred tympanic membranes and cholesteatomas.
- Caution should be exercised with regard to adenoidectomy. The palatal dysfunction in Turner syndrome may be exacerbated by removal of adenoids. Such surgery should be undertaken only after careful evaluation of speech and palate configuration is made.
- Appropriate use of hearing aids should be encouraged. It is not uncommon for

adult individuals to fail to recognize the role a hearing deficit plays in their difficulty in comprehending instructions, negatively affecting work performance.

Craniofacial

Cleft palate, either overt or submucous, is more common in Turner syndrome, as is Pierre Robin sequence (see Chapter 19). Hypernasal speech is typical. The maxilla and mandible may be mismatched in Turner syndrome. Prognathia or micrognathia is common. Dental crowding is usual. Outcome after treatment in Turner syndrome is no different than for similar craniofacial problems in the general population.

Evaluation

- Most clinically significant problems will be self-evident. Patients should be examined for an intact uvula and palate.

Treatment

- Referral for orthodontic evaluation should be made, although orthodontic treatment may not always be required. When it is needed, it does not differ from that in the general population.
- Repair of cleft palate, when present, does not differ from repair in the general population.

Gastrointestinal

In addition to the feeding difficulties and reflux discussed earlier, gastrointestinal problems are seen with increased frequency in Turner syndrome.

Hernias, both inguinal and abdominal, occur in a minority of newborns with Turner syndrome [1% in the author's series (Sybert, 1995; unpublished data)]. Their occurrence is not associated with presence of edema or with specific karyotype.

Vascular malformations of the gastrointestinal tract have been described in more than 25 case reports. The reported vascular lesions include telangiectases, venous malformations, and hemangiomas. Sites of involvement include the esophagus, stomach, duodenum, ileum, small bowel, and large bowel. Involvement of gut mucosa or gut serosa, or both, has been reported. All of the patients came to attention for recurrent rectal bleeding. In some, more lesions appeared to develop; in others, resolution occurred, either spontaneously or associated with estrogen therapy. Ages at presentation ranged from 4 months to 57 years.

Inflammatory bowel disease in Turner syndrome, including both Crohn disease and ulcerative colitis, has been reported with a frequency similar to vascular bowel involvement. In one reported series of 135 adults with Turner, 2 had Crohn disease and 2 had ulcerative colitis syndrome (Arulanantham et al., 1980). Two others had chronic diarrhea with no specific diagnosis. A cell line containing an i(Xq) has been found in more than half of the reported cases of inflammatory bowel disease, clearly disparate from the expected 10–15% based on karyotype distribution. In another large series, of 5 patients with such chronic bowel complaints, 2 had a cell line with i(Xq) (Sybert, 1995; unpublished data). In that series there were 3 additional patients with intestinal polyposis, only one of whom had a positive family history. Recent work has suggested an increased incidence of celiac disease in Turner syndrome (Bonamico et al., 1998).

There have been isolated reports of elevated liver enzymes, of unknown cause and unassociated with liver disease, in individuals with Turner syndrome. The significance of this is not known. Gallbladder disease may be present more often than expected, not associated with diabetes or obesity (Sybert, 1995; unpublished data).

Evaluation

- Unexplained anemia or rectal bleeding should prompt evaluation for gastrointestinal vascular malformations. Many of the vascular lesions can be visualized only by direct examination by techniques external to the gut (laparoscopy or laparotomy) or internal to the gut (endoscopy) and no firm guidance for the extent of evaluation can be given. Screening for fecal occult blood is not routine.

- No presymptomatic screening for inflammatory bowel disease is indicated. The nature and scope of investigation must be individualized.

Treatment

- Surgery may be an appropriate option for resectable bleeding vascular lesions of the gut. Embolization may be effective in some situations. In numerous reports, treatment with transfusion has been adequate, and recurrent, uncontrolled bleeding episodes have not been common. Ovarian hormone therapy may play a role in management in some cases.

- Treatment for complications of inflammatory bowel disease is the same as for their occurrence in individuals without Turner syndrome. Management may be complicated, however, by ovarian hormone replacement, which can exacerbate bowel symptoms.

Renal

Structural renal malformations have long been recognized to be increased in frequency in Turner syndrome. They are found in up to 40% of affected individuals (Krawczynski et al., 1974; Sybert, 1995; unpublished data; Lippe et al., 1998). These include: renal agenesis, horseshoe kidney, malrotation, duplication of the collecting system, ureteropelvic and ureterovesicular obstruction, and aberrant renal arteries. The malformations rarely result in renal dysfunction or disease. In a minority, however, reflux, hydronephrosis, and recurrent urinary tract infections can be severe. The frequency and types of renal defects and their complications from a series of patients who have been examined by renal ultrasound or intravenous pyelogram or both (Sybert, 1995; unpublished data) are shown in Table 27.3.

Multicystic kidneys, renal stones without other renal disease, nephrotic syndrome, and benign hematuria also occur (Sybert, 1995; unpublished data). There appears to be no correlation between karyotype and presence or type of renal involvement.

TABLE 27.3. Renal Involvement in Turner Syndrome (*n* = 337)

Urinary Tract Anomaly	*n*	(%)
Horseshoe	41	(12.2)
With hydronephrosis 8; with reflux 1		
Malrotation	12	(3.5)
Duplication of part/all collecting system	35	(10.4)
With hydronephrosis 7		
Hydronephrosis without structural abnormalities	13	(3.8)
Multicystic/dysplastic kidneys	6	(1.8)
Unilateral 5; bilateral 1		
Unilateral absence of kidney	4	(1.2)
Reflux without structural abnormality	5	(1.5)
Ureteral/urethral stenosis	3	(0.8)
Recurrent urinary tract infection, normal structure	5	(1.5)
Other	13	(4.9)
TOTAL	137	(40.7)

Evaluation

- All individuals with Turner syndrome must be evaluated by renal ultrasound.
- If normal, renal ultrasound does not need to be repeated in the absence of signs of urinary infection or renal dysfunction.
- If structural renal malformations are found, repeat evaluation must be individualized and firm guidelines cannot be given.

Treatment

- Treatment is driven by and specific for the renal complication, not for Turner syndrome.

Musculoskeletal

Turner syndrome results in a skeletal dysplasia characterized by short stature, a mild epiphyseal dysplasia and typical bony alterations, including short fourth metacarpals and metatarsals. One structural skeletal alteration that can lead to dysfunction is an abnormal tibial plateau coupled with patellar changes. Frequent dislocation of the patellae and chronic knee pain are fairly common complaints (Sybert, 1995; unpublished data)

The increased carrying angle at the elbow can be more than a curiosity. Limited range of motion may interfere with some function. Although Madelung deformity is seen in individuals with Turner syndrome, it is an infrequent concern.

Osteoporosis, or a clinically significant decrease in trabecular bone mass leading to an increased risk of fractures, is claimed to be a feature of Turner syndrome. The bones appear osteopenic on radiographic evaluation, and measures of bone density by dual-photon absorptiometry are often, but not always, below age-matched controls. Ovarian hormone replacement and growth hormone treatment appear to improve these measures, although one study found no differences in regional bone mass between those patients treated with growth hormone and estrogen replacement and those treated with estrogen replacement alone, nor between these groups and an age-matched group of untreated patients with Turner syndrome (Mora et al., 1992). The number of subjects in all studies has been small, and studies are all cross-sectional. There have been very few studies to establish the "normal" range of bone mass in Turner syndrome. None has compared bone mass measurements with both height-matched and age-matched controls. None has followed a cohort of individuals over a long enough time to establish that true accelerated bone loss occurs, as opposed to an inherent lower initial endowment of bone mass without accelerated loss. Although an increased wrist fracture rate has been claimed for Turner syndrome, other studies have not found an increased rate of wrist fractures or compression fractures of the vertebrae.

To date, it has not been established whether the reduced bone mass in Turner syndrome is a specific, inherent, nonprogressive feature of a general skeletal dysplasia, or whether it is analogous to the accelerated bone loss of postmenopausal women. Few adult women have experienced unusual loss of height with aging, as would occur with vertebral compression and collapse (Sybert, 1995; unpublished data).

Evaluation

- Routine skeletal surveys in Turner syndrome are not recommended. The patient with Turner syndrome who presents with symptomatic knee problems should be referred for evaluation and management.
- Routine measurements of regional bone mass for clinical care in childhood and young adult life are probably not warranted, unless there is concern for rapid loss of height, symptoms suggestive of vertebral compression fractures, or an increased rate of other fractures.

Treatment

- Ovarian hormone replacement is important to both establish and maintain adult bone mass. With all risk factors being equal, ovarian hormone replacement should continue in these women throughout life. Switching to a postmenopausal regimen in later adult life is appropriate. However, longitudinal data to support the need for or a benefit from lifelong ovarian hormone treatment are lacking. Thus the benefits of "postmenopausal" hormone replacement should be weighed against the risks, as in the general population.

Lymphatics

Lymphedema *in utero* is a major feature of Turner syndrome. It is believed to be one of the causes of the high prenatal loss of 45,X conceptions. Its detection on ultrasound most often leads to prenatal diagnosis. Its cause is uncertain. Hypoplastic lymphatics have been demonstrated in a few patients. The residual puffiness of the hands and feet, redundant nuchal skin and webbing, and abnormal fingernail and toenail configuration are direct consequences of the lymphedema. Correlation of the presence of lymphedema with cardiac malformations has been suggested (Clark, 1984; Berdahl et al., 1995) but has not been found by others (Sybert, 1995; unpublished data).

It may take months to several years for the puffiness in the tops of the hands and feet to resolve. Rarely, lymphedema can persist, or it may recur, unilaterally or bilaterally, in the legs in late childhood, at the time of ovarian hormone replacement treatment, or later in adult life. There is usually no recognized precipitating cause, although one study demonstrated hypoplastic lymphatics of the legs in 17 of 21 patients, in those with and without clinical lymphedema (Vittay et al., 1980).

Evaluation

- Usually no evaluation is necessary.

Treatment

- Usually no treatment is required. The lymphedema slowly resolves.
- If lymphedema recurs or fails to resolve, standard treatment such as support socks, elevation, or pressure pump may be required. Persistent or recurrent lymphedema can be a difficult management problem for individuals with or without Turner syndrome.

Dermatologic

An increased number of typical melanocytic nevi has long been noted in individuals with Turner syndrome. They are often on the face. They do not appear unusual clinically or histologically. The risk of malignant melanoma arising in or associated with the presence of nevocytic nevi does not appear to be increased in Turner syndrome.

Streaky hypopigmentation or hyperpigmentation distributed along the lines of Blaschko occurs in some patients mosaic for 45,X/46,X,+mar or 45,X/46,X,+ring(X), usually associated with mental retardation and other unusual phenotypic features.

An increased risk for the development of keloids has been suggested for females with Turner syndrome. It is not clear whether this reflects an endogenous tendency for exuberant and aberrant scar formation or whether this risk is more apparent than real because the surgeries these patients typically undergo involve areas of the body known to be more likely to exhibit such scarring, such as the neck and upper chest. In the author's series in which 104 surgical procedures were done in 93 individuals, 47 of which involved the neck or chest, hypertrophic scars or keloids developed in 6 individuals (Larralde et al., 1998).

Hirsutism is not typical in Turner syndrome, although luxuriant arm and leg hair occurs in a minority (Sybert, 1995; unpublished data).

Premature fine wrinkling of facial skin, clinically similar to the wrinkling seen in heavy tobacco smokers, appears to occur commonly in women with Turner syndrome in their late thirties and early forties. It is not associated with smoking or with excessive sun exposure (personal observation).

Evaluation

- No specific evaluation is necessary.

Treatment

- Management of abnormal scarring, annoying moles, and wrinkles is not specific for Turner syndrome. Referral to a dermatologist or plastic surgeon may be advisable.

Neoplasia

There does not appear to be an intrinsic increased risk for malignancy in Turner syndrome, with the exception of the risk for gonadoblastoma in those with mosaicism for a Y chromosome. In this group, who comprise about 5% of the Turner syndrome population, the likelihood of tumor development in the presumed testicular streaks approaches 30% by age 30.

Hasle and colleagues (1996) reviewed the records of 597 women with Turner syndrome in the Danish Cytogenetic Register. Overall, there was no increase in the relative risk of malignancy compared to the general population, although there were more cases of colon cancer than expected. They also found no history of gonadoblastoma or dysgerminoma in 29 patients with a Y chromosome present, but they had no way of ascertaining whether these patients had had prophylactic gonadectomy. One patient with 45,X/46,XY had an adenocarcinoma of a gonadal streak.

Endometrial carcinoma has been reported, occurring exclusively in those women with Turner syndrome who received unopposed estrogen treatment or prolonged treatment with diethylstilbestrol, suggesting that endometrial hyperplasia was the primary risk factor, not Turner syndrome itself.

Treatment

- Prophylactic gonadectomy is indicated for all patients with Turner syndrome with a Y chromosome. The timing of surgery depends on the age and health of the patient, but there are few compelling reasons to delay surgery after diagnosis.
- Any woman receiving estrogen replacement needs to be cycled with a progestational agent to prevent endometrial hyperplasia.

Life Expectancy

Does the patient with Turner syndrome face a decrease in life expectancy? If one excludes congenital heart disease, there still appears to be some concern regarding this issue, but no firm answer. In a population survey from Edinburgh, Scotland, Price et al. (1986) found 15 deaths among their 156 patients; this they calculated to be a five-fold excess over expected. When congenital heart disease was excluded, a three-fold increase remained. In the author's series of almost 500 liveborn patients, 25 have died. Ten of these deaths were due to complications of congenital heart disease. Among the 215 adult individuals, causes of death were cardiac (5), accident (2), malignant hyperthermia (1), acute myelomonocytic leukemia (1), acute febrile syndrome (1), and old age (3).

RESOURCES

The Turner's Syndrome Society of the United States

1313 Southeast 5th Street, Suite 327
Minneapolis, MN 55414
Phone: 800-365-9944
Fax: 612-379-3619
url:http://www.turner-syndrome-us.org

The Turner Syndrome Society of Canada

814 Glencairn Ave
Toronto, Ont CA M6B 2A3

Phone: 1-800-465-6744
Fax: 416-781-7245
url:http://www.TurnerSyndrome.ca

The Turner Syndrome Society of Quebec (in French)

Phone: 1-888-9TURNER or
1-450-655-8771
url:http;//www.turnerquebec.qe.ca

The Turner Syndrome Society of UK C/o Child Growth Foundation

2 Mayfield Ave
Chiswick, London
Phone : 44(0)181-994-7625
Fax: 44(0)181-995-9075
url:http://www.tss.org.uk

Publications

Available through the Turner Syndrome Society at no cost are growth charts for Turner syndrome.

Publications also available at cost through the Turner Syndrome Society include several chapbooks:

Reiser PA, Underwood LE (1992) *Turner Syndrome: A Guide for Families.*

Rosenfeld RG (1992) *Turner Syndrome: A Guide for Physicians.*

The Society also has videotapes of its annual conferences available for a fee.

REFERENCES

American Academy of Pediatrics Committee on Genetics (1995) Health supervision for children with Turner syndrome. *Pediatrics* 96:1166–1173.

Arulanantham K, Kramer MS, Gryboski JD (1980) The association of inflammatory bowel disease and X chromosomal abnormality. *Pediatrics* 66:63–67.

Berdahl LD, Wenstrom KD, Hanson JW (1995) Web neck anomaly and its association with congenital heart disease. *Am J Med Genet* 56:304–307.

Betts PR, Butler GE, Donaldson MDC, Dunger DB, Johnston DI, Kelnar CJH, Kirk J (1999) A decade of growth hormone treatment in girls with Turner syndrome in the UK. *Arch Dis Child* 80:221–225

Boman UW, Moller A, Albertsson-Wikland K (1998) Psychosocial aspects of Turner syndrome. *J Psychosom Obstet Gynaecol* 19:1–18.

Bonamico M, Bottaro G, Pasquino AM, Caruso-Nicoletti M, Mariani P, Gemme G, Povadiso E, Ragusa MC, Spina M (1998) Celiac disease and Turner syndrome. *J Pediatr Gastroenterol Nutr* 26:496–499.

Bramswig JH (1997) Expectation bias with respect to growth hormone therapy in Turner syndrome. *Eur J Endocrinol* 137:446–447.

Chang HJ, Clark RD, Bachman H (1990) The phenotype of 45,X/46,XY mosaicism: An analysis of 92 prenatally diagnosed cases. *Am J Hum Genet* 46:156–167.

Clark EB (1984) Neck web and congenital heart defects: A pathogenic association in 45,XO Turner syndrome? *Teratology* 29:355–361

Chrousos GA, Ross JL, Chrousos G, Chu FC, Kenigsberg D, Cutler G Jr, Loriaux DL (1984) Ocular findings in Turner syndrome. *Ophthalmology* 91:926–928.

Chu CE, Connor JM (1995) Molecular biology of Turner's syndrome. *Arch Dis Child* 72:285–286.

Chu CE, Paterson WF, Kelnar CJH, Smail PJ, Greene SA, Donaldson MDC (1997) Variable effect of growth hormone on growth and final adult height in Scottish patients with Turner's syndrome Acta Paediatr 86:160–164.

Coto E, Toral JF, Menéndez MJ, Hernando I, Plasencia A, Benevides A, Lopez-Larrea C (1995) PCR-based study of the presence of Y-chromosome sequences in patients with Ullrich-Turner syndrome. *Am J Med Genet* 57:393–396.

Cutler GB Jr, Ross JL (1992) Estrogen therapy in Turner's syndrome. *Acta Paediatr Jpn* 34:195–202.

Darby PL, Garfinkel PE, Vale JM, Kirwan PJ, Brown GM (1981) Anorexia nervosa and 'Turner syndrome': Cause or coincidence? *Psychol Med* 11:141–145.

Davies MC, Gulekli B, Jacobs HS (1995) Osteoporosis in Turner's syndrome and other forms of primary amenorrhoea. *Clin Endocrinol* 43: 741–746.

Delgado JA, Trahms CM, Sybert VP (1986) Measurement of body fat in Turner syndrome. *Clin Genet* 29:291–297.

Delooz J, van den Berghe H, Swillen A, Kleczkowska A, Fryns JP (1993) Turner syndrome patients as adults: A study of their cognitive profile, psychosocial functioning and psychopathological findings. *Genet Counsel* 4:169–179.

Donaldson MDC (1996) Jury still out on growth hormone for normal short stature and Turner's syndrome. *Lancet* 348:3–4.

Donaldson MDC (1997) Growth hormone therapy in Turner syndrome — current uncertainties and future strategies. *Horm Res* 48 (Suppl 5):35–44.

Downey J, Elkin EJ, Ehrhardt AA, Meyer-Bahlburg HF, Bell JJ, Morishima A (1991) Cognitive ability and everyday functioning in women with Turner syndrome. *J Learn Disabil* 24:32–39.

Finby N, Archibald RM (1963) Skeletal abnormalities associated with gonadal dysgenesis. *Am J Roentgenol* 89:1222–1234.

Forbes AP, Engel E (1963) The high incidence of diabetes mellitus in 41 patients with gonadal dysgenesis, and their close relatives. *Metabolism* 12:428–439.

Ford CE, Jones KW, Polani PE, de Almeida JC, Briggs JH (1959) A sex-chromosome anomaly in a case of gonadal dysgenesis (Turner's syndrome). *Lancet* 1:711–712.

Garden AS, Diver MJ, Fraser WD (1996) Undiagnosed morbidity in adult women with Turner's syndrome. *Clin Endocrinol* 45: 589–593.

Gemmill RM, Pearce-Birge L, Bixenman H, Hecht BK, Allanson JE (1987) Y chromosome-specific DNA sequences in Turner syndrome mosaicism. *Am J Hum Genet* 41:157–167.

Germain EL, Plotnick LP (1986) Age-related anti-thyroid antibodies and thyroid abnormalities in Turner syndrome. *Acta Paediatr Scand* 75:750–755.

Gotzsche CO, Krag-Olsen B, Nielsen J, Sorensen KE, Kristensen BO (1994) Prevalence of cardiovascular malformations and association with karyotypes in Turner's syndrome. *Arch Dis Child* 71:433–436.

Gravholt CH, Naeraa RW, Fisker S, Christiansen JS (1997) Body composition and physical fitness are major determinants of the growth hormone-insulin-like growth factor axis aberrations in adult Turner's syndrome, with important modulations by treatment with 17β-estradiol. *J Clin Endocrinol Metab* 82:2570–2577.

Greenlee R, Hoyme H, Witte M, Crowe P, Witte C (1993) Developmental disorders of the lymphatic system. *Lymphology* 26:156–168.

Haeusler G, Frisch H (1994) Methods for evaluation of growth in Turner's syndrome: Critical approach and review of the literature. *Acta Paediatr* 83:309–314.

Haeusler G, Schmitt K, Blümel P, Plöchl E, Waldhor T, Frisch H (1996) Growth hormone in combination with anabolic steroids in patients with Turner syndrome: Effect on bone maturation and final height. *Acta Paediatr* 85: 1408–1414.

Hasle H, Olsen JH, Nielsen J, Hansen J, Friedrich U, Tommerup N (1996) Occurrence of cancer in women with Turner syndrome. *Br J Cancer* 73:1156–1159.

Held KR, Kerber S, Kaminsky E, Singh S, Goetz P, Seemanova E, Goedde HW (1992) Mosaicism in 45,X Turner syndrome: Does survival in early pregnancy depend on the presence of two sex chromosomes? *Hum Genet* 88:288–294.

Hochberg Z, Zadik Z (1999) Final height in young women with Turner syndrome after GH therapy: An open controlled study. *Eur J Endocrinol* 141:218–224.

Holl RW, Kunze D, Etzrodt H, Teller W, Heinze E (1994) Turner syndrome: Final height, glucose tolerance, bone density and psychosocial status in 25 adult patients. *Eur J Pediatr* 153:11–16.

Huisman J, Slijper FME, Sinnema G, Akkerhuis GW, Brugman-Boezeman A, Feenstra J, den Hartog L, Heuvel F (1993) Psychosocial effects of two years of human growth hormone treatment in Turner syndrome. *Horm Res* 39 (Suppl 2):56–59.

Hultcrantz M, Sylvén L, Borg E (1994) Ear and hearing problems in 44 middle-aged women with Turner's syndrome. *Hear Res* 76: 127–132.

Ivarsson SA, Carlsson A, Bredberg A, Alm J, Aronsson S, Gustafsson J, Hagens L, Hager A, Kristom B, Marcus C, Moell C, Nilsson KO, Tuvemo T, Westphal O, Albertsson-Wildand K, Aman J (1999) Prevalence of coeliac disease in Turner syndrome. *Acta Paediatr* 88:933–936

Ivarsson SA, Ericsson UB, Nilsson KO, Gustafsson J, Hagenas L, Hager A, Moell C, Tuvemo T, Westphal O, Albertsson-Wildand K (1995) Thyroid autoantibodies, Turner's syndrome and growth hormone therapy. *Acta Paediatr* 84:63–65

James RS, Coppin B, Dalton P, Dennis NR, Mitchell C, Sharp AJ, Skuse DH, Thomas NS, Jacobs PA (1998) A study of females with deletions of the short arm of the X chromosome. *Hum Genet* 102:507–516.

Jospe N, Orlowski CC, Furlanetto RW (1995) Comparison of transdermal and oral estrogen therapy in girls with Turner's syndrome. *J Pediatr Endocrinol Metab* 8:111–116.

Keats TE, Burns TW (1964) The radiographic manifestations of gonadal dysgenesis. *Radiol Clin North Am* 2:297–313.

Koeberl DD, McGillivray B, Sybert VP (1995) Prenatal diagnosis of 45,X/46,XX mosaicism and 45,X: Implications for postnatal outcome. *Am J Hum Genet* 57:661–666.

Krawczynski M, Maciejewski J, Grzybkowska B, Bartkowiak K (1974) Les anomalies de la vascularisation du système urogénital dans le syndrome de Turner. *Pédiatrie* 29:413–422.

Kushnick T, Irons TG, Wiley JE, Gettig EA, Rao KW, Bowyer S (1987) 45X/46X,r(X) with syndactyly and severe mental retardation. *Am J Med Genet* 28:567–574.

Lahood BJ, Bacon GE (1985) Cognitive abilities of adolescent Turner's syndrome patients. *J Adolesc Health Care* 6:358–364.

Larralde M, Gardner SS, Torrado M, Fernhoff PM, Santos Munoz AE, Spraker MK, Sybert VP (1998) Lymphedema as a postulated cause of cutis verticis gyrata in Turner syndrome. *Pediatr Dermatol* 15:18–22.

Lin AE, Lippe BM, Geffner ME, Gomes A, Lois JF, Barton CW, Rosenthal A, Friedman WF (1986) Aortic dilation, dissection, and rupture in patients with Turner syndrome. *J Pediatr* 102:47–50.

Lin AE, Lippe B, Rosenfeld RG (1998) Further delineation of aortic dilation, dissection, and rupture in patients with Turner syndrome. *Pediatrics* 102(1). URL:http://www.pediatrics.org/cgi/content/full/102/1/e12

Lippe B, Geffner ME, Dietrich RB, Boechat MI, Kangarloo H (1988) Renal malformations in patients with Turner syndrome: Imaging in 141 patients. *Pediatrics* 82:852–856.

Lyon AJ, Preece MA, Grant DB (1985) Growth curve for girls with Turner syndrome. *Arch Dis Child* 60:932–935.

Massa G, Otten BJ, de Muinck Keizer-Schrama SM, Delemarre-van de Waal HA, Jansen M, Vulsma T, Oostdijk W, Waelkens JJ, Wit JM (1995) Treatment with two growth hormone regimens in girls with Turner syndrome: Final height results. Dutch Hormone Working Group. *Horm Res* 43:144–146.

Mathisen B, Reilly S, Skuse D (1992) Oral-motor dysfunction and feeding disorders of infants with Turner syndrome. *Dev Med Child Neurol* 34:141–149.

McCauley E, Ito J, Kay T (1986) Psychosocial functioning in girls with Turner's syndrome and short stature: Social skills, behavior problems, and self-concept. *J Am Acad Child Psychiatry* 25:105–112.

McCauley E, Kay T, Ito J, Treder R (1987) The Turner syndrome: Cognitive defects, affective discrimination, and behavioral problems. *Child Dev* 58:464–473.

McCauley E, Ross JL, Kushner H, Cutler G Jr (1995) Self-esteem and behavior in girls with Turner syndrome. *J Dev Behav Pediatr* 16:82–88.

Migeon BR, Luo S, Jani M, Jeppesen P (1994) The severe phenotype of females with tiny ring X chromosomes is associated with inability of these chromosomes to undergo X inactivation. *Am J Hum Genet* 55:497–504.

Money J, Granoff D (1965) IQ and the somatic stigmata of Turner's syndrome. *Am J Ment Def* 70:69–77.

Mora S, Weber G, Guarneri MP, Nizzoli G, Pasolini D, Chiumello G (1992) Effect of estrogen replacement therapy on bone mineral content in girls with Turner syndrome. *Obstet Gynecol* 79:747–751.

Muhs A, Lieberz K (1993) Anorexia nervosa and Turner's syndrome. *Psychopathology* 26:29–40.

Netley C, Rovet J (1982) A typical hemispheric lateralization in Turner syndrome subjects. *Cortex* 18:377–384.

Nilsson KO, Albertsson-Wikland K, Alm J, Aronson, S, Gustafsson J, Hagenas L, Hagar A, Ivarsson SA, Karlberg J, Kinstrom B, Marais C, Moell C, Ritzen M, Tuvemo T, Wattsg ard C, Westgren U, Westphal O, Aman J (1996) Improved final height in girls with Turner's syndrome treated with growth hormone and oxandrolone. *J Clin Endocrinol Metab* 81:635–640.

Ogata T, Matsuo N (1995) Turner syndrome and female sex chromosome aberrations: Deduction of the principal factors involved in the development of clinical features. *Hum Genet* 95:607–629.

Orten JL (1990) Coming up short: The physical, cognitive, and social effects of Turner's syndrome. *Health Soc Work* 15:100–106.

Page DC (1987) Hypothesis: A Y-chromosomal gene causes gonadoblastoma in dysgenetic gonads. *Development* 101, *Suppl*:151–155.

Pavlidis K, McCauley E, Sybert VP (1995) Psychosocial and sexual functioning in women with Turner syndrome. *Clin Genet* 47:85–89.

Plotnick L, Attie KM, Blethen SL, Sy JP (1998) Growth hormone treatment of girls with Turner syndrome: The National Cooperative Growth Study Experience. *Pediatrics* 102:479–481.

Press F, Shapiro HM, Cowell CA, Oliver GD (1995) Outcome of ovum donation in Turner's syndrome patients. *Fertil Steril* 64:995–998.

Price WH, Clayton JF, Collyer S, De Mey R, Wilson J (1986) Mortality ratios, life expectancy, and causes of death in patients with Turner's syndrome. *J Epidemiol Community Health* 40:97–102.

Radetti G, Mazzanti L, Paganini C, Bernasconi S, Russo G, Rigon F, Caccian E (1995) Frequency, clinical and laboratory features of thyroiditis in girls with Turner's syndrome. The Italian Study Group for Turner's Syndrome. *Acta Paediatr* 84:909–912

Ranke MB (1995) Growth hormone therapy in Turner syndrome. *Horm Res* 44 (*Suppl*) 3:35–41.

Rao E, Weiss B, Fukami M, Rump A, Niesler B, Merk A, Muroya K, Binder G, Kirsch S, Winklemann M, Nordsick G, Helnrich U, Breuning MH, Ranke MB, Rosenthal A, Ogata T,

Rappold GA (1997) Pseudoautosomal deletions encompassing a novel homeobox gene cause growth failure in idiopathic short stature and Turner syndrome. *Nat Genet* 16:54–63.

Rimoin DL, Harder E, Whitehead B, Packman S, Peake GT, Sly WS (1970) Abnormal glucose tolerance in patients with gonadal dysgenesis and their parents. (Abstract) *Clin Res* 18:395.

Rochiccioli P, Battin J, Bertrand AM, Bost M, Cabrol S, leBouc Y, Chaussain, JL, Chatelain P, Colle M, Czernichow P (1995) Final height in Turner syndrome patients treated with growth hormone. *Horm Res* 44:172–176.

Rosenfeld RG, Tesch L-G, Rodriguez-Rigau LJ, et al. (1994) Recommendations for diagnosis, treatment, and management of individuals with Turner syndrome. *The Endocrinologist* 4:351–358.

Rosenfeld RG, Attie KM, Frane J, Brasel JA, Burstein S, Cara JF, Chernausek S, Gotlink W, Kuntze J, Lippe BM, Mahoney CP, Moore NV, Saenger P, Johanson AJ (1998) Growth hormone therapy of Turner's syndrome: Beneficial effect on adult height. *J Pediatr* 132:319–324.

Ross JL, Stefanatos G, Roeltgen D, Kushner H, Cutler GB Jr (1995) Ullrich-Turner syndrome: Neurodevelopmental changes from childhood through adolescence. *Am J Med Genet* 58:74–82.

Ross J, Zinn A, McCauley E (2000). Neurodevelopmental and psychosocial aspects of Turner syndrome. *Ment Retard Devel Disabil Res Rev* 6:135–141.

Rovet J, Ireland L (1994) Behavioral phenotype in children with Turner syndrome. *J Pediatr Psychol* 19:779–790.

Rubin K (1998) Turner syndrome and osteoporosis: Mechanisms and prognosis. *Pediatrics* 102:481–485.

Saenger P (1997) Turner's syndrome. *Curr Ther Endocrinol Metab* 6:239–243.

Sas TCJ, de Muinck Keizer-Schrama SMPF, Stijnen T, van Teunenbroek A, Hokken-Koelega ACS, Waelkens JJJ, Massa GG (1999) Final height in girls with Turner's syndrome treated with once or twice daily growth hormone injections. *Arch Dis Child* 80:36–41.

Shaw NJ, Rehan VK, Husain S, Marshall T, Smith CS (1997) Bone mineral density in Turner's syndrome — a longitudinal study. *Clin Endocrinol* 47:367–370.

Silbert A, Wolff PH, Lilienthal J (1977) Spatial and temporal processing in patients with Turner's syndrome. *Behav Genet* 7:11–21.

Silverman BL, Friedlander JR (1997) Is growth hormone good for the heart? *J Pediatr* 131: S70–S74.

Skuse DH, James RS, Bishop DVM, Coppin B, Dalton P, Aamodt-Leeper G, Bacarese-Hamilton M, Creswell C, McGurk R, Jacobs PA (1997) Evidence from Turner's syndrome of an imprinted X-linked locus affecting cognitive function. *Nature* 387:705–708.

Sybert VP (1995) The adult patient with Turner syndrome. In: *Turner Syndrome in a Life Span Perspective: Research and Clinical Aspects*, Albertsson-Wikland K and Ranke MB, eds. New York; Elsevier, 205–218.

Sybert VP (1998) Cardiovascular malformations and complications in Turner syndrome. *Pediatrics* 101(1). URL:http://www.pediatrics.org/cgi/content/full/101/1/e11

Sylvén L, Magnusson C, Hagenfeldt K, von Schoultz B (1993) Life with Turner's syndrome — a psychosocial report from 22 middle-aged women. *Acta Endocrinol* 129:188–194.

Sylvén L, Hagenfeldt K, Ringertz H (1995) Bone mineral density in middle-aged women with Turner's syndrome. *Eur J Endocrinol* 132: 47–52.

Taback SP, Collu R, Deal CL, Guydatt HJ, Salisbury S, Dean HJ, Van Vliet G (1996) Does growth-hormone supplementation affect adult height in Turner's syndrome? *Lancet* 348: 25–27.

Takano K, Shizume K, Hibi I (1989) Turner's syndrome: Treatment of 203 patients with recombinant human growth hormone for one year. A multicentre study. *Acta Endocrinol* 120:559–568.

Takano K, Ogawa M, Tanaka T, Tachibana K, Fujita K, Hizuka N (1997) Clinical trials of GH treatment in patients with Turner's syndrome in Japan — a consideration of final height. The Committee for the Treatment of Turner's Syndrome. *Eur J Endocrinol* 137:138–145.

Tarani L, Lampariello S, Raguso G, Colloridi F, Pucarelli I, Pasquino AM, Bruni LA (1998) Pregnancy in patients with Turner's syndrome: Six new cases and review of the literature. *Gynecol Endocrinol* 12:83–87.

Turner HH (1938) A syndrome of infantilism, congenital webbed neck, and cubitus valgus. *Endocrinology* 23:566–574.

Ullrich O (1949) Turner's syndrome and status Bonnevie-Ullrich. A synthesis of animal phenogenetics and clinical observations on a typical complex of developmental anomalies. *Am J Hum Genet* 1:179–202.

Van den Broeck J, Massa GG, Attanasio A, Matranga A, Chaussain JL, Price DA, Aarskog D, Wit JM (1995) Final height after long-term growth hormone treatment in Turner syndrome. *J Pediatr* 127:729–735.

Vittay P, Bösze P, Gaál M, László J (1980) Lymph vessel defects in patients with ovarian dysgenesis. *Clin Genet* 18:387–391.

Wolff DJ, Brown CJ, Schwartz S, Duncan AMV, Surti U, Willard HF (1994) Small marker X chromosomes lack the X inactivation center: implications for karyotype/phenotype correlations. *Am J Hum Genet* 55:87–95.

Yorifuji T, Muroi J, Kawai M, Tanaka K, Kiwaki K, Endo F, Matsuda I, Nagasaka H, Furosho K (1998) Uniparental and functional X disomy in Turner syndrome patients with unexplained mental retardation and X derived marker chromosomes. *J Med Genet* 35:539–544.

Zinn AR (1997) Growing interest in Turner syndrome. *Nat Genet* 16:3–4.

Zinn AR, Tonk VS, Chen Z, Fleiter WL, Gardner HA, Guerra R, Kushner H, Schwartz S, Sybert VP, Van Dyke DL, Ross JL (1998) Evidence for a Turner syndrome locus or loci at Xp11.2-p22.1. *Am J Hum Genet* 63:1757–1766.

CHAPTER 28

VATER ASSOCIATION

BRYAN D. HALL

INTRODUCTION

Incidence

VATER association is an acronym for a sporadic constellation of findings that occur together more often than by chance alone (Quan and Smith, 1973). The major anomalies associated with this constellation are listed in Table 28.1. VATER association is a relatively common, nonrandom multiple-malformation condition (Fig. 28.1) with an incidence of 1.6 in 10,000 (Khoury et al., 1983). No specific recurring etiology has been established. The term VACTERL association (Nora and Nora, 1975) is sometimes used in place of VATER because two additional features (cardiac = C, limb/radial = L) are more specifically identified in the

acronym. Table 28.1 illustrates which anomaly each letter represents in the two acronyms.

Diagnostic Criteria

The VATER/VACTERL association represents a core group of 7 anomalies (see Table 28.1 and Fig. 28.1). Very few patients have all 7 features, the average number of features per patient being three to four (Botto et al., 1997). Unfortunately, no minimum criteria have been agreed on regarding which of these features or what combination of these constitutes a secure diagnosis. It seems prudent to require at least 1 anomaly in each of the 3 geographic regions of involvement (limb, thorax, and pelvis/lower abdomen) for a secure diagnosis and at least 2 anomalies

TABLE 28.1. Core Features of VATER/VACTERL Association

VATER Association	VACTERL Association
V = vertebral defects	V = vertebral defects
A = anal atresia	A = anal atresia
	C = cardiac anomalies*
T = tracheoesophageal fistula	T = tracheoesophageal fistula
E = esophageal atresia	E = esophageal atresia
R = renal/radial defects	R = renal
	L = limb (radial)

*Quan and Smith noted cardiac anomalies but did not include them in the acronym.

Management of Genetic Syndromes, Edited by Suzanne B. Cassidy and Judith E. Allanson
ISBN 0-471-31286-X   Copyright © 2001 by Wiley-Liss, Inc.

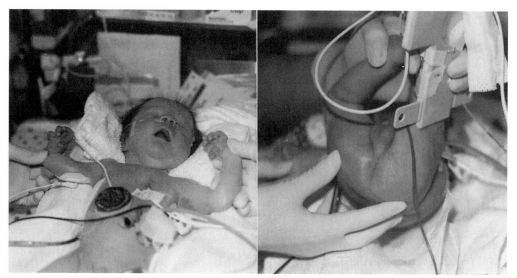

FIGURE 28.1. Newborn with VATER/VACTERL association showing bilateral radial/thumb hypoplasia and imperforate anus.

in each of 2 geographic areas to qualify as probable VATER/VACTERL association.

Etiology, Pathogenesis, and Genetics

No consistent or recurring etiology has been established for the VATER/VACTERL association (Khoury et al., 1983). Most cases of the VATER/VACTERL association occur as sporadic events in their families (Rittler et al., 1997) with a low recurrence risk. It is generally felt to be a heterogeneous disorder with the various yet-to-be established etiologies working through a common embryological pathway (Botto et al., 1997).

Other anomalies and abnormalities do occur in the VATER/VACTERL association. Some are common, like single umbilical artery (70%), and others less common, like cleft lip, polydactyly (preaxial), small intestinal atresia, auricular aberrations, and genital/urogenital defect (Botto et al., 1997). Rare instances of caudal regression and lower extremity defects have also been reported (Temtamy and Miller, 1974). Intrauterine growth retardation of unexplained etiology is occasionally present.

Diagnostic Testing

The VATER/VACTERL association has no specific inclusive tests for confirmation of the diagnosis. Consideration of the possibility of the VATER/VACTERL association is usually raised when a neonate presents with imperforate anus, tracheoesophageal fistula/esophageal atresia, and/or radial/thumb hypoplasia, because these features are externally obvious and/or symptomatic within a short time after birth. Once the possibility of VATER/VACTERL association exists, certain diagnostic tests for identification of cryptic anomalies should be automatically performed. These tests include renal scan, echocardiogram, and full X-rays of the spine. This empiric approach not only is useful in further supporting or ruling out the diagnosis of VATER/VACTERL association but potentially can identify additional anomalous organ systems that will allow for earlier therapeutic intervention.

VATER/VACTERL represents a classic example of a diagnosis of exclusion. There is no facial gestalt to aid pattern recognition, and its core features are commonly found in other situations and syndromes.

These problems mandate the need to exclude all other similar clinical entities and to have obtained a normal chromosome analysis. It remains important to exclude teratogenic exposure during early gestation and to obtain a careful family history for similar anomalies.

Differential Diagnosis

The differential diagnosis list when considering the VATER/VACTERL association is long (Khoury et al., 1983) because so many of its accompanying anomalies can be found as components of other syndromes. Certainly, any syndrome associated with radial defects and anal atresia (e.g., Fanconi anemia, trisomy 18, Townes-Brock syndrome) should be ruled out. Vertebral, limb, and cardiac anomalies can all be seen in the embryopathy of infants of diabetic mothers (Weaver et al., 1986). Holt-Oram (hand-heart) syndrome should also be considered in patients who have primarily cardiac and radial abnormalities. This is autosomal dominant with highly variable expressivity, so that a careful family history is needed and the parents of the affected patient should be examined and hand radiographs and cardiac evaluations considered.

Recently, hydrocephalus has been reported in some patients with VATER/VACTERL features resulting in a new acronym, VACTERL-H (Lomas et al., 1998). Familial occurrences in some of these cases have suggested autosomal recessive and/or X-linked recessive inheritance. These familial instances in the presence of a rarely observed anomaly (hydrocephalus) suggest that these patients are unlikely to represent true VATER/VACTERL association. This assumption is important because true VATER/VACTERL association is rarely genetic and carries a generally good prognosis for intelligence. Additionally, a few patients with Fanconi anemia have been reported with hydrocephalus and anal defects (e.g., stenosis, atresia). Given the high incidence of radial and renal anomalies in Fanconi anemia (Porteous et al., 1992), such patients could be misdiagnosed as having VATER/VACTERL association. Chromosome breakage studies should be done on all patients who have hydrocephalus in association with VATER/VACTERL features.

The presence of esophageal atresia and tracheoesophageal fistula in syndromes such as trisomy 18 (see Chapter 25) and Fanconi anemia, and occasionally CHARGE association (see Chapter 5), can also be confusing. It is not usually necessary to rush too quickly into making the diagnosis of VATER/VACTERL association. It can be a tentative diagnosis until all test results are back and you have had the opportunity to follow the child's progress over time. This is the burden and blessing of an exclusion diagnosis.

MANIFESTATIONS AND MANAGEMENT

The VATER/VACTERL association is very complex from the clinical management standpoint. All seven of its core features may necessitate surgical intervention.

Table 28.2 lists the physician specialists most commonly required to adequately deal with individuals affected with VATER/VACTERL association. Up to 13 different physician specialists could be required for any 1 child. This impressive number of potential specialists dealing with the child's surgical and medical problems can be expanded further by including important support personnel such as a physical therapist, developmentalist (infant stimulation), nutritionist, psychologist/behaviorist, and social worker. The need for long-term follow-up by most of the specialists is labor intensive for the child and family, but it is exceedingly important. Hopefully, one physician, ideally the child's primary care doctor, can maintain a timely and efficient balance between the child's needs and the specialists' requirements. The primary care physician is

TABLE 28.2. Specialists Required and Areas of Involvement in VATER/VACTERL Association

Medical Specialist	Major Areas of Involvement
Neonatologist	Neonatal care, coordinating other specialists
Geneticist	Diagnosis, counseling, long-term follow-up
Pediatric surgeon	Surgery (anal, tracheoesophageal fistula, esophageal atresia), long-term follow-up
Orthopedist	Surgery/medical therapy (spine/limbs), long-term follow-up
Nephrologist	Diagnosis, medical therapy (urinary tract), long-term follow-up
Urologist	Surgery (genitalia, urinary tract), long-term follow-up
Cardiac surgeon	Surgery (heart), possible long-term follow-up
Gastroenterologist	Diagnosis/medical therapy (reflux, obstruction, diarrhea, gastrostomy problems), long-term follow-up
Pulmonologist	Diagnosis/medical therapy (pneumonia, aspiration), long-term follow-up
Gynecologist	Diagnosis/surgery (genital/reproductive tract), long-term follow-up
Physical therapist	Diagnosis/medical therapy, long-term follow-up
Developmentalist	Physical/intellectual stimulation, long-term follow-up
Nutritionist	Adequate nutrition, long-term follow-up
Psychologist/behaviorist	Body image/personality therapy, long-term follow-up
Social worker	Assistance to child/family with system/bureaucracy, long-term follow-up
Primary care physician	Underpinning all of the above, long-term follow-up

the most critical factor in assuring the best outcome for these children. Follow-up with the geneticist may be of help in this difficult situation as problems may be noticed that require referral back to the specialist or indicate additional testing. In addition, the geneticist may be able to answer difficult questions the primary doctor is not comfortable in answering.

The multiple individual anomalies in patients with VATER/VACTERL association clearly require a concerted and extended effort to minimize or ameliorate the adverse effects, both singly and in combination. There remains a whole person who still has problems, which may need intervention.

The long-term prognosis for children with the VATER/VACTERL association is variable. Each surgical anomaly seems, prognostically, independent of the other. If each surgical defect can be satisfactorily repaired and/or medically treated, the prognosis is excellent. If some defects cannot be totally repaired or persist with sequelae, then the prognosis is the sum total of the residual problems with critical organs (e.g., heart, kidneys) having a greater negative impact.

Growth and Feeding

Congenital heart failure, renal dysfunction, or gastrointestinal disorder can cause poor growth. An endocrinologist may need to be consulted if the poor growth cannot be explained by ongoing medical problems.

Evaluation

- Adequacy of caloric intake should be assessed.
- The child should be evaluated for occult cardiac, renal, or gastrointestinal problems through standard imaging and functional studies.
- An endocrinology consultation should be obtained if another source of growth compromise cannot be found.

Treatment

- If a source of growth failure is identified, it should be treated by standard means.
- Temporary measures such as increasing caloric concentration per ounce of formula may help.
- Gastrostomy tube feedings may be indicated if the child is too sick to feed

adequately or when increased metabolic output exceeds caloric intake.

Development and Behavior

Early psychomotor delay, poor body image, and behavioral problems can occur and need attention. A poor body image is often noted in those children with limb deficiencies, short stature, complicated anal atresia with persisting intestinal problems, recurrent esophageal complications, chronic cardiac symptomatology, and external genital abnormalities. Developmental progress may be compromised by problems such as congestive heart failure, renal dysfunction, or gastrointestinal difficulties.

A loving, supportive family can help the child overcome many of these potential problems, but medical personnel working with the child should be no less supportive.

Evaluation

- Formal periodic developmental evaluation should be carried out if development is delayed.
- If seizures, abnormal cranial size, or neurological signs (e.g., hypo-/hypertonia) are recognized, a neurological consultation should be obtained.

Treatment

- Physical therapy and infant stimulation are particularly important because of the frequent and prolonged hospitalizations.
- Treatment of cardiac, renal, gastrointestinal, or nutritional problems is critical in promoting developmental progress.
- Occasionally, a referral to a psychologist or behavioral pediatrician may abort a worsening body image or ongoing behavioral problem. Intervention by these specialists before the child has started to develop a body image is of critical importance

Musculoskeletal

Vertebral anomalies are generally not extensive and most often occur in upper to mid thoracic and lumbar regions, with sacral and lower cervical defects being less common. Hemivertebrae are most common, but dyssegmented and fused vertebral bodies can also be found. Bifid, hypoplastic, or absent ribs are not uncommon accompaniments of thoracic vertebral anomalies. The presence of tracheoesophageal fistula/esophageal atresia and imperforate anus dramatically increases the likelihood of thoracic and lumbar vertebral defects, respectively.

Scoliosis is sometimes present, with its nidus closely related to the location of the abnormal vertebrae. The scoliosis is usually mild but occasionally can be of modest to severe degree, requiring immediate orthopedic attention. Figure 28.2 shows a young teenage girl with the VATER/VACTERL association who had vertebral defects without congenital scoliosis but was not followed closely and developed moderately severe scoliosis that went unrecognized by her and her family.

Limb anomalies are restricted to the upper limbs in the VATER/VACTERL association, and they are usually preaxial, involving underdevelopment or agenesis of the thumbs and radial bones (Botto et al., 1997). These preaxial defects are usually bilateral but often asymmetric in degree. They run the gamut of mild to severe. Occasionally, only the thenar muscle mass is reduced in size, with or without a slightly reduced thumb circumference and hypoplastic flexion creases. These subtle features are often missed, resulting in a valuable and critical feature of the VATER/VACTERL association diagnosis not being recognized and a secure diagnosis not being made.

Evaluation

- Regular orthopedic follow-up is very important whether or not scoliosis is present.

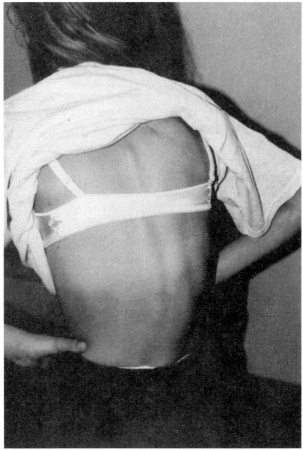

FIGURE 28.2. Teenage girl with VATER/VACTERL association who developed unrecognized scoliosis secondary to lumbar hemivertebrae.

- It is uncommon for the spinal cord to be injured by the vertebral defects, but any neurological sign, including bladder incontinence, encopresis, or paresis, should prompt further evaluation (e.g., CT or MRI spinal scan, myelogram).

- If limb abnormalities are noted, X-rays of the abnormal limb segment should be done by the physician coordinating the child's care and, if anomalies are confirmed, orthopedic assessment should be arranged.

Treatment

- Bracing and/or surgery are the two therapeutic modalities utilized to treat scoliosis, using standard methods.

- Orthopedic or plastic hand surgeons will be necessary to correct the preaxial defects from both a cosmetic and a functional standpoint.

- If the radius is significantly hypoplastic, the hand angulates sharply toward the radial side of the wrist in what is termed a radial clubbed hand. This will need to be straightened, and the procedure is a difficult surgery with mixed results.

- The thumb, if functional and of reasonable size, should be left alone, but hypoplastic thumbs are often removed and the second finger reoriented to function as an opposable thumb.

- Staged surgeries for more severe preaxial defects with postsurgical casting mandate long-term involvement and follow-up by the treating surgeon.

Gastrointestinal

Tracheoesophageal fistula and esophageal atresia are discussed together here, although only 80% of patients with esophageal atresia have tracheoesophageal fistula. Fifty to sixty percent of patients with VATER/VACTERL association have either tracheoesophageal fistula or esophageal atresia (Botto et al., 1997). Esophageal atresia manifests shortly after birth with copious oral secretions with or without respiratory problems.

The majority of children with tracheoesophageal fistula and esophageal atresia survive if their other associated anomalies are amenable to therapy. It is noteworthy that almost 37% of patients with tracheoesophageal fistula and esophageal atresia have cardiac defects, so evaluation of the heart is critical in this situation.

Anal atresia (imperforate anus) is a severe problem that requires immediate attention in the newborn period. The presence of anal atresia also is associated with an increased incidence of external anomalies of the genitalia, internal anomalies of the urinary and reproductive tracts, and vertebral defects of the lumbar and sacral spine (Sofatzis et al., 1983).

Evaluation

- Failure to be able to pass a nasogastric tube into the stomach is a strong indication of esophageal atresia. Radiopaque tubes can be seen rolled up in the blind esophageal pouch when passage into the stomach is attempted. Lack of air in the stomach indicates that there is no fistula between the lower esophagus and trachea (types A and B). A large gap between both atretic ends of the proximal and distal esophagus complicates later reanastomosis. Type C and D tracheoesophageal fistula/esophageal atresia (type C represents 80% of the cases)

have a longer lower esophageal segment with attachment to the trachea, making reanastomosis much easier but increasing the risk of retrograde chemical irritation of the respiratory tract.

- Long-term follow-up by the pediatric surgeon and gastroenterologist after tracheoesophageal repair is usually a necessity. If recurrent pneumonias persist, a pediatric pulmonologist is required to evaluate the functional integrity and anatomical status of the tracheobronchial tree.

- No clinical evidence of an anal opening is usually obvious, but sometimes the anus must be digitally probed or contrast utilized to evaluate patency.

- The urinary and reproductive tracts should be evaluated in any patient with anal atresia whether the atresia is isolated, part of a specific syndrome, or a component of the VATER/VACTERL association.

- Renal ultrasound and voiding cystourethrogram will adequately evaluate the urinary tract. Direct vaginal exam and pelvic ultrasound may be necessary in females.

- Frequently, contrast may be put into the rectum or vagina to detect fistulous connections and better clarify the anomalous anatomy.

Treatment

These anomalies are always treated surgically.

- In type A and B esophageal atresia it is usually necessary to keep the proximal esophagus dry via constant suction for 2-3 months or to exteriorize the proximal esophageal pouch via a cervical esophagostomy. A feeding gastrostomy is placed in anticipation of future direct or colon graft anastomosis. This, like all the surgeries, includes tying off the tracheoesophageal fistula/esophageal atresia (Cozzi and Wilkinson, 1967).

- Short- and long-term complications of repaired tracheoesophageal fistula/esophageal atresia include fistula formation, leakage at the anastomosis site, pneumonia, swallowing difficulties, esophageal stricture requiring repeated dilatations, and poor growth (Okada et al., 1997).

- The tracheoesophageal fistula is surgically tied off or separated with each end tied off.

- For anal anomalies, immediate surgery (anoplasty) is performed only if there is a membranous atresia or a very low atresia (Touloukian and Pickett, 1969).

- Most anal atresias are higher (above the puborectalis portion of the levator ani muscle) and require a temporary diverting colostomy. These higher atresias are also associated with an increased incidence of fistulas connecting the rectum with the urinary tract (e.g., bladder, urethra), and reproductive tract (e.g., vagina). This makes the surgery more complicated.

- Those patients with a diverting colostomy (Fig. 28.3) will have an abdominoperineal pull-through operation later when they are older and larger (12–20 pounds).

- Long-term problems of both types of surgery can be fecal impaction, megacolon, soiling, persistent fistula, and anal stenosis requiring dilatation.

Cardiovascular

Cardiac anomalies are the most common defects found in the VATER/VACTERL association, with a frequency of approximately 80% (Khoury et al., 1983). The cardiac anomalies can be of any type and any severity; consequently, they may be very obvious in the neonatal period or may be cryptic. Death and poor health remain major complications in those children with complex or untreatable congenital heart defects. Frequently, growth retardation may be ascribed to the heart problems when other medical problems are responsible. Nevertheless, some children show marked catch-up growth after delayed cardiac surgery is performed.

Evaluation

- All patients who are suspected to have VATER/VACTERL association should have an immediate cardiology consult.

- An echocardiogram should be done regardless of auscultatory or electrocardiogram results. Surgical and/or medical

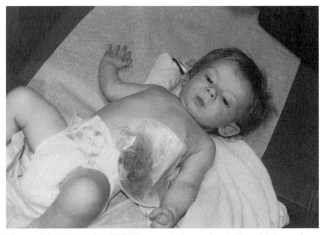

FIGURE 28.3. Infant with VATER/VACTERL association who had a high anal atresia requiring a temporary diverting colostomy. Note mild right radial and thumb underdevelopment.

therapy will be determined on the basis of these studies.

- Long-term cardiology follow-up is particularly important if a cardiac anomaly is present.

Treatment

- Treatment of the congenital heart defects and other cardiac problems does not differ from that in children with similar problems in the general population.

Respiratory

In addition to the previously mentioned respiratory complications related to tracheoesophageal atresia, laryngeal stenosis (Corsello et al., 1992) and tracheal atresia (Milstein et al., 1985) have also been reported in the VATER/VACTERL association. These latter problems generally present with moderate to severe respiratory obstruction and, in the case of tracheal atresia, ultimately lead to death. Laryngeal stenosis, depending on its degree, may go undiagnosed for months. Tachypnea, laryngotracheomalacia, and sternal, intercostal and costal retractions are common resulting symptoms.

Evaluation

- A chest X-ray should be obtained to evaluate for atelectasis and/or infiltrate and to assess obvious anatomical abnormalities.
- Blood gases should be obtained if the child appears sick.
- Swallowing studies (sometimes with contrast) and/or visualization of the larynx should be carried out, if indicated.
- Laryngoscopy is needed if symptoms persist or worsen (pre- or post-surgically).

Treatment

- Surgical correction of tracheoesophageal fistula should be accomplished, using standard techniques.

- Treatment of any pneumonia with antibiotics is appropriate.
- If recurrent aspiration occurs, steroid therapy may be required.
- Reflux precautions should be used after surgery.

Genitourinary

Renal anomalies are very common (80%) (Botto et al., 1997) in the VATER/VACTERL association. There is a high frequency of renal anomalies if anal atresia, genital defects, or lower spine defects are present. All types of renal defects have been noted including renal agenesis/dysplasia, obstructive hydronephrosis, cystic kidney(s), and ectopic kidney. The lower urinary tract may be abnormal because of fistulas between the rectum and bladder or urethra. Genital defects such as hypospadias, bifid scrotum, and labial hypoplasia are more often associated with anal atresia but both have an increased association with renal defects.

Evaluation

- The entire urinary tract should be evaluated by ultrasound in all patients with VATER/VACTERL.
- The renal system should be followed closely, generally by ultrasound, if abnormalities are discovered.
- A urologist and/or a gynecologist may be of great benefit if the child has external genital abnormalities that can be improved or corrected.

Treatment

- Urinary tract anomalies are treated the same as in nonsyndromic patients.
- Reproductive tract anomalies may require surgical reconstruction once the anomalous anatomy is accurately ascertained.
- Fistulous tracts need to be closed, but sometimes they are left open until other surgery is accomplished.

RESOURCES

TEF / VATER International Support Network
c/o Greg and Terri Burke
15301 Grey Fox Road
Upper Marlboro, MD 20772
Voice/Fax: 301.952.6837

VATER Connection Web Site
(Nancy McCarley and Angie Schreiber)
http://www.vaterconection.org/main.htm

REFERENCES

Botto LD, Khoury MJ, Mastroiacovo P, Castilla EE, Moore CA, Skjaerven R, Mutchinick OM, Borman B, Cocchi G, Czeizel AE, Goujard J, Irgens LM, Lancaster PAL, Martinez-Frias ML, Merlob P, Ruusinen A, Stoll C, Sumiyoshi Y (1997) The spectrum of congenital anomalies of the VATER association: An international study. *Am J Med Genet* 71:8–15.

Brown AB, Roddam AW, Spitz L, Ward SJ (1999) Oesophageal atresia, related malformations, and medical problems: A family study. *Am J Med Genet* 85:31–37.

Corsello G, Maresi E, Corrao AM, Dimita U, Cascio ML, Cammarata M, Giuffre L (1992) VATER/VACTERL association: Clinical variability and expanding phenotype including laryngeal stenosis. *Am J Med Genet* 44: 813–815.

Cozzi F, Wilkinson AW (1967) Esophageal atresia. *Lancet* 2:1222–1225.

Khoury M, Cordero JF, Greenberg F, James LM, Erickson JD (1983) A population study of the VACTERL association: Evidence for its etiologic heterogeneity. *Pediatrics* 71:815–820.

Lomas FE, Dahlstrom JE, Ford JH (1998) VACTERL with hydrocephalus: Family with X-linked VACTERL-H. *Am J Med Genet* 76:74–78.

Lurie IW, Ferencz C (1997) VACTERL-hydrocephaly, DK-phocomelia, and cerebro-cardio-radio-rectal community. *Am J Med Genet* 70:144–149.

Milstein JM, Lau M, Bickers RG (1985) Tracheal agenesis in infants with VATER association. *Am J Dis Child* 139:77–80.

Nora AH, Nora JJ (1975) A syndrome of multiple congenital anomalies associated with teratogenic exposure. *Arch Environ Health* 30: 17–21.

Okada A, Usui N, Inove M, Kawahara H, Kubota A, Imura K, Kamata S (1997) Esophageal atresia in Osaka. Review of 39 years experience. *J Pediatr Surg* 32:1570–1574.

Porteous ME, Cross I, Burn J (1992) VACTERL with hydrocephalus: One end of the Fanconi anemia spectrum of anomalies. *Am J Med Genet* 43:1032–1034.

Rittler M, Paz JE, Castilla EE (1997) VACTERL: An epidemiologic analysis of risk factors. *Am J Med Genet* 73:162–169.

Quan L, Smith DW (1973) The VATER association. *J Pediatr* 82:104–107.

Sofatzis JA, Alexacos L, Skouteli HN, Tiniakos G, Padiatellis C (1983) Malformed female genitalia in newborns with the VATER association. *Acta Paediatr Scand* 72:923–924.

Temtamy SA, Miller JD (1974) Extending the scope of the VATER association: Definition of the VATER syndrome. *J Pediatr* 85:345–349.

Touloukian RJ, Pickett LK (1969) Management of the newborn with imperforate anus. *Clin Pediatr* 8:389–397.

Weaver DD, Mapstone CL, Yu P (1986) The VATER association. Analysis of 46 patients. *Am J Dis Child* 140:225–229.

CHAPTER 29

VELO-CARDIO-FACIAL SYNDROME

ROBERT J. SHPRINTZEN

INTRODUCTION

Incidence

Velo-cardio-facial syndrome is a pleiotropic and highly variable disorder affecting the face, palate, and heart, among other tissues, that is caused by a microdeletion of chromosome 22q11.2.

There have been no studies to confirm the birth incidence of velo-cardio-facial syndrome, but estimates of population prevalence have been made. In part, there is a problem in calculating prevalence because the condition goes under multiple names, including velo-cardio-facial syndrome, Shprintzen syndrome, DiGeorge syndrome (or more properly, DiGeorge sequence), CATCH 22, deletion 22q11 syndrome, Cayler syndrome, Sedlačková syndrome, and conotruncal anomalies-face syndrome. Some clinicians are under the mistaken impression that these are actually separate disorders caused by the same genetic deletion, but, as is discussed below, these all represent the same disorder, which has a highly variable expression. Many clinicians have accepted a population prevalence statistic of 1 in 4000, which is based on the diagnosis of DiGeorge sequence. However, the large majority of patients with velo-cardio-facial syndrome do not have

DiGeorge sequence and the 1 in 4000 statistic is likely an underestimate of the prevalence of the entire spectrum. Perhaps the best ascertainment of patients with velo-cardio-facial syndrome has been recorded in a prospective study from a large craniofacial center (Shprintzen et al., 1985b). An analysis of 1000 consecutive cases at the center showed that 5% of all patients with clefting of the lip and/or palate had velo-cardio-facial syndrome and that 8.1% of the patients in the series who had cleft palate without cleft lip (including submucous cleft palate) had velo-cardio-facial syndrome. A subsequent study from Australia (Lipson et al., 1991) confirmed these prevalence data, as have larger studies of the population of children with clefts (personal experience). The prevalence of cleft palate (without cleft lip) in the general population, including submucous cleft, is also variable depending on the method of ascertainment. In a complete ascertainment of children from a general pediatric practice (Shprintzen et al., 1985a), the frequency of submucous cleft palate was found to be approximately 0.75% (1 in 150, or 6.7 in 1000). Overt cleft palate has a frequency of approximately 1 in 1000. Therefore, the frequency of cleft palate (overt and submucous inclusive) in the general population is conservatively 7.7 in 1000, or

Management of Genetic Syndromes, Edited by Suzanne B. Cassidy and Judith E. Allanson
ISBN 0-471-31286-X   Copyright © 2001 by Wiley-Liss, Inc.

1 in 130. Because velo-cardio-facial syndrome constitutes approximately 8.1% of the cleft palate sample, an estimated population prevalence would be 1 in 1600 living individuals, or more conservatively, 1 in 2000. The birth incidence is clearly higher because some babies with velo-cardio-facial syndrome die at birth or shortly thereafter because of severe heart anomalies (frequency unknown), and other secondary malformation sequences incompatible with life have also been reported in velo-cardio-facial syndrome including Potter sequence (Devriendt et al., 1997) and holoprosencephaly (Wraith et al., 1985). The frequency of these associations is unknown, but they are probably uncommon. However, the minimal expected birth incidence would be 1 in 2000, which would make velo-cardio-facial syndrome one of the most common genetic disorders in humans.

Diagnostic Criteria

Over 180 clinical features (Table 29.1), both physical and developmental/behavioral, have been reported in velo-cardio-facial syndrome (Shprintzen et al., 1997). None of the findings occurs with 100% frequency, indicating that there are no pathognomonic or obligatory features. However, there are some cardinal features that should raise a strong index of suspicion. In infancy, the association of cleft palate with conotruncal heart anomalies is a strong indication for suspecting velo-cardio-facial syndrome because this is the most common syndrome associated with both cleft palate and conotruncal heart anomalies. Velo-cardio-facial syndrome is the second most common syndrome associated with Robin sequence (Stickler syndrome being the most common), and therefore a diagnosis of Robin sequence should immediately raise an index of suspicion. If any of the following anomalies occur together with the palate and heart malformations, then the diagnosis is even more likely: asymmetric crying facies, laryngeal web,

TABLE 29.1. Clinical Features of Velo-cardio-facial Syndrome

Craniofacial/Oral Findings

1. Overt, submucous, or occult submucous cleft palate
2. Retrognathia (retruded lower jaw)
3. Platybasia (flat skull base)
4. Asymmetric crying facies in infancy
5. Structurally asymmetric face
6. Functionally asymmetric face
7. Vertical maxillary excess (long face)
8. Straight facial profile
9. Congenitally missing teeth
10. Small teeth
11. Enamel hypoplasia (primary dentition)
12. Hypotonic, flaccid facies
13. Downturned oral commissures
14. Cleft lip (uncommon)
15. Microcephaly
16. Small posterior cranial fossa

Eye Findings

17. Tortuous retinal vessels
18. Suborbital congestion ("allergic shiners")
19. Strabismus
20. Narrow palpebral fissures
21. Posterior embryotoxon
22. Small optic disk
23. Prominent corneal nerves
24. Cataract
25. Iris nodules
26. Iris coloboma (uncommon)
27. Retinal coloboma (uncommon)
28. Small eyes
29. Mild orbital hypertelorism
30. Mild orbital dystopia
31. Puffy eyelids

Ear/Hearing Findings

32. Overfolded helix
33. Attached lobules
34. Protuberant, cup-shaped ears
35. Small ears
36. Mildly asymmetric ears
37. Frequent otitis media
38. Mild conductive hearing loss
39. Sensorineural hearing loss

TABLE 29.1. (*continued*)

40. Ear tags or pits (uncommon)
41. Narrow external ear canals

Nasal Findings

42. Prominent nasal bridge
43. Bulbous nasal tip
44. Mildly separated nasal domes (appearing bifid)
45. Pinched alar base, narrow nostrils
46. Narrow nasal passages

Cardiac Findings

47. Ventricular septal defect
48. Atrial septal defect
49. Pulmonic atresia or stenosis
50. Tetralogy of Fallot
51. Right-sided aorta
52. Truncus arteriosus
53. Patent ductus arteriosus
54. Interrupted aorta
55. Coarctation of the aorta
56. Aortic valve anomalies
57. Aberrant subclavian arteries
58. Vascular ring
59. Anomalous origin of carotid artery
60. Transposition of the great vessels
61. Tricuspid atresia

Vascular Anomalies

62. Medially displaced internal carotid arteries
63. Tortuous, kinked, absent, or accessory internal carotids
64. Jugular vein anomalies
65. Absence of vertebral artery (unilateral)
66. Low bifurcation of common carotid
67. Tortuous or kinked vertebral arteries
68. Raynaud's phenomenon
69. Small veins
70. Circle of Willis anomalies

Neurological and Brain Findings

71. Periventricular cysts (mostly at anterior horns)
72. Small cerebellar vermis
73. Cerebellar hypoplasia/dysgenesis

TABLE 29.1. (*continued*)

74. White matter unidentified bright objects (UBOs)
75. Generalized hypotonia
76. Cerebellar ataxia
77. Seizures
78. Strokes
79. Spina bifida/meningomyelocele
80. Mild developmental delay
81. Enlarged sylvian fissure

Pharyngeal/Laryngeal/Airway Findings

82. Upper airway obstruction in infancy
83. Absent or small adenoids
84. Laryngeal web (anterior)
85. Large pharyngeal airway
86. Laryngomalacia
87. Arytenoid hyperplasia
88. Pharyngeal hypotonia
89. Asymmetric pharyngeal movement
90. Thin pharyngeal muscle
91. Unilateral vocal cord paresis

Abdominal/Kidney/Gut Findings

92. Hypoplastic/aplastic/cystic kidneys
93. Hirschsprung megacolon (2 cases)
94. Inguinal hernias
95. Umbilical hernias
96. Malrotation of bowel
97. Hepatoblastoma (single case)
98. Diaphragmatic hernia
99. Anal anomalies (displaced, imperforate)

Limb Findings

100. Small hands and feet
101. Tapered digits
102. Short nails
103. Rough, red, scaly skin on hands and feet
104. Morphea
105. Contractures
106. Triphalangeal thumbs
107. Polydactyly (both preaxial and postaxial)
108. Soft tissue syndactyly

Problems in Infancy

109. Feeding difficulty, failure to thrive
110. Nasal vomiting

(*continued overleaf*)

TABLE 29.1. (*continued*)

111. Gastroesophageal reflux
112. Nasal regurgitation
113. Irritability
114. Chronic constipation (usually not Hirschsprung megacolon)

Speech/Language Findings

115. Severe hypernasality
116. Severe articulation impairment
117. Language impairment (usually mild delay)
118. Velopharyngeal insufficiency (usually severe)
119. Dyspraxia
120. High-pitched voice
121. Hoarseness

Cognitive/Learning Findings

122. Learning disabilities (math concept, reading comprehension)
123. Concrete thinking, difficulty with abstraction
124. Drop in IQ scores in school years (test artifact)
125. Borderline normal intellect
126. Occasional mild mental retardation
127. Attention deficit/hyperactivity disorder

Miscellaneous anomalies

128. Spontaneous oxygen desaturation without apnea
129. Thrombocytopenia
130. Bernard-Soulier disease
131. Juvenile rheumatoid arthritis

Psychiatric/Psychological Findings

132. Bipolar affective disorder
133. Manic depressive illness and psychosis
134. Rapid or ultrarapid cycling of mood disorder
135. Mood disorder
136. Depression
137. Hypomania
138. Schizoaffective disorder
139. Impulsiveness
140. Flat affect

TABLE 29.1. (*continued*)

141. Dysthymia, cyclothymia
142. Schizophrenia
143. Social immaturity
144. Obsessive-compulsive disorder
145. Generalized anxiety disorder
146. Phobias

Immunologic Findings

147. Frequent upper respiratory infections
148. Frequent lower airway disease (pneumonia, bronchitis)
149. Reduced T cell populations
150. Reduced thymic hormone
151. Reactive airway disease

Genitourinary Findings

152. Hypospadias
153. Cryptorchidism
154. Genito-Urinary reflux

Endocrine Findings

155. Hypocalcemia
156. Hypoparathyroidism
157. Pseudohypoparathyroidism
158. Hypothyroidism
159. Mild growth deficiency, relative small stature
160. Absent/hypoplastic thymus
161. Hypoplastic pituitary gland

Skeletal/Muscle/Orthopedic/Spine Findings

162. Scoliosis
163. Hemivertebrae
164. Spina bifida occulta
165. Butterfly vertebrae
166. Fused vertebrae (mostly cervical)
167. Tethered spinal cord
168. Syrinx
169. Osteopenia
170. Sprengel's anomaly, scapular deformation
171. Talipes equinovarus
172. Small skeletal muscles
173. Joint dislocations
174. Chronic leg pains
175. Flat foot arches
176. Hyperextensible/lax joints

TABLE 29.1. (*continued*)

177. Extra ribs
178. Rib fusion

Skin/Integument Findings

179. Abundant scalp hair
180. Thin-appearing skin (venous patterns
     easily visible)

Secondary Sequences/Associations

181. Robin sequence
182. DiGeorge sequence
183. Potter sequence
184. CHARGE association
185. Holoprosencephaly (single case)

nasal regurgitation, hypocalcemia, or over-folded helices of the ears. The presence of clubfoot, laryngomalacia and/or obstructive apnea, retrognathia, tapered digits, inguinal hernia, umbilical hernia, hypospadias, hypotonia, or failure to thrive should also increase suspicion, although not to the same extent because they also occur commonly in association with many other syndromes. The heart anomalies that occur more commonly in association with velo-cardio-facial syndrome than in other syndromes are aortic arch anomalies (right-sided, double, or interrupted aortic arch type B), ventricular septal defect (typically malalignment type), pulmonary atresia or stenosis, tetralogy of Fallot, and truncus arteriosus. Abnormal major vessels, such as tracheal ring or aberrant right or left subclavian arteries, are also strong indicators of the diagnosis, especially if they occur in the absence of structural heart anomalies.

A variety of other anomalies occur with increased frequency in velo-cardio-facial syndrome, including short stature, hooded eyelids, suborbital congestion (Fig. 29.1), tapered digits, minor ear anomalies (Fig. 29.2), scoliosis, Sprengel deformity, flat feet with tight heel cords, leg pains, cryptorchidism, and anal anomalies.

In older patients with velo-cardio-facial syndrome, the presentation becomes more obvious because many of the most common anomalies in the syndrome are developmental, behavioral, and psychiatric (personal experience). This includes developmental and social delay, hypernasal speech, anxiety, and psychiatric problems. The most frequent of such findings (in descending order of frequency) are mild developmental delay, learning disabilities, social immaturity, hypernasal speech, impulsivity, heightened anxiety or phobias, and in adult life, psychiatric illness.

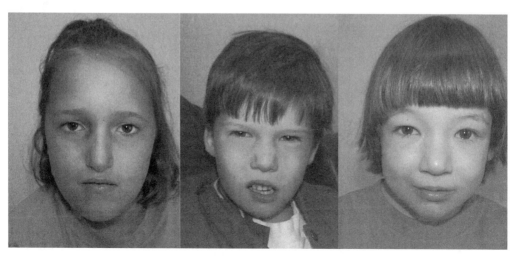

FIGURE 29.1. Variable facial phenotype in velo-cardio-facial syndrome.

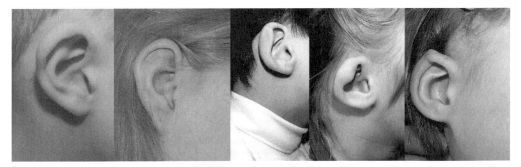

FIGURE 29.2. Variations in ear morphology in velo-cardio-facial syndrome.

Therefore, the presence of any of these behavioral manifestations in association with hypernasal speech, cleft palate, or congenital heart disease should alert clinicians to the possible diagnosis of velo-cardio-facial syndrome. Immune disorders are often encountered in infancy and persist into late childhood, leading to chronic upper and/or lower respiratory infections.

The diagnoses of DiGeorge sequence, conotruncal anomaly face syndrome, and Cayler cardiofacial syndrome have also been associated with 22q11.2 deletions. The deletions of chromosome 22 are the same for all of these disorders. The cardinal features of DiGeorge syndrome are absent thymus, hypocalcemia, immune deficiency, characteristic facial appearance, and heart anomalies. Although many cases of DiGeorge sequence are associated with deletion 22q11.2, other cases are caused by different genetic alterations. Characteristic facies and conotruncal anomalies are also associated with 22q11.2 deletions and have been called conotruncal anomaly-face syndrome. Asymmetric crying facies and heart anomalies (Cayler syndrome) can also be seen as the primary or only features of 22q11.2 deletion.

Etiology, Pathogenesis, and Genetics

In the first report describing the syndrome (Shprintzen et al., 1978), an autosomal dominant mode of inheritance was suspected based on mother-to-daughter transmission. In 1981, four mother-to-daughter transmissions were reported (Shprintzen et al., 1981). An autosomal dominant mode of inheritance was confirmed in 1985 when the first male-to-male transmission was described (Williams et al., 1985). In 1992, the first report of a microdeletion of chromosome 22 at the q11.2 band was reported (Scambler et al., 1992), followed by several other reports confirming this deletion (Driscoll et al., 1992b; Kelly et al., 1993). Subsequent studies have defined the critical region and the typical deletion. In approximately 15% of cases, a visible deletion can be detected on high-resolution karyotype. The typical deletion that occurs in the large majority of patients encompasses approximately three million base pairs, with smaller deletions of several hundred thousand base pairs also being found. Therefore, the typical deletion is large enough to contain nearly a hundred genes. To date, the size of the deletion has not been correlated with the expression of the syndrome (Morrow et al., 1995). Although a number of candidate genes have been proposed, none has been confirmed at this time (Funke et al., 1997; Sirotkin et al., 1996, 1997). It is still not known whether the syndrome is a contiguous gene syndrome or whether the majority of the phenotypic features are caused by a single gene. In several large studies of cases ascertained from multiple sources (Driscoll et al., 1993; Morrow et al., 1995), approximately 80% of patients in whom the clinical diagnosis was made were confirmed to be deleted. It is possible that the non-deleted cases represent point mutations that can not be detected by fluorescence in situ hybridization (FISH) or PCR-based microsatellite studies or that mutations elsewhere in the genome can cause the syndrome. However, it is likely that in most nondeleted cases the clinical diagnosis is incorrect and that the true number of nondeleted cases of velo-cardio-facial syndrome is very small, well under 5% (personal experience).

The pathogenesis of the syndrome has been related to a number of possible mechanisms. The earliest reports suggested a developmental abnormality of the third and fourth pharyngeal pouches (Driscoll et al., 1992a). Neural crest migration anomalies have also been suggested (Lammer and Opitz, 1986), although these are hypothetical positions at the current time. The neural crest hypothesis is based on what is known about the migration of neural crest cells to the third and fourth branchial pouches and the subsequent formation of the heart's conotruncus, the thymus gland, and the parathyroid glands. However, other anomalies in velo-cardio-facial syndrome are related to the first and second branchial arches (the ears, palate, and face). Additionally, there are many anomalies associated with velo-cardio-facial syndrome that have nothing to do with neural crest migration, including the vascular malformations and thrombocytopenia. At this point in time, there is no direct evidence that the primary mechanism in the pathogenesis of velo-cardio-facial syndrome is specific to the neural crest. More recently, it was suggested that many of the anomalies associated with velo-cardio-facial syndrome are actually the result of secondary developmental sequences, perhaps related to an early developmental anomaly of the embryonic vasculature (Shprintzen et al., 1997) because of the large variety of vascular anomalies associated with the syndrome and because many aspects of the phenotype can be explained by vascular insufficiency or disruption. A recent report (Morita et al., 1999) described a gene in the deleted region that is directly related to the formation of the endothelial lining of blood vessels affecting vascular permeability, consistent with the hypothesis presented by Shprintzen et al. (1998). Animal studies are currently under way to determine potential gene effects and the mechanism of syndrome development (Puech et al., 1997).

Diagnostic Testing

Genetic laboratory tests for velo-cardio-facial syndrome include cytogenetics, fluorescence in situ hybridisation (FISH), and molecular (microsatellite) analysis. Because chromosome analysis alone reveals only about 15% of the deletions associated with the syndrome, the easiest diagnostic procedure is FISH, which is available in most commercial or hospital labs. A number of probes have been available for FISH studies. Initially, the probe N25 from Oncor was used for the majority of FISH studies, but this probe was removed from the market in 1999 and since that time, the primary probe available has been the TUPLE probe. The FISH studies are typically done in conjunction with a karyotype, preferably high resolution, because of the possibility that the deletion may be related to a chromosome rearrangement such as an unbalanced translocation or because the constellation of anomalies could be related to a different chromosome anomaly. Molecular genetic techniques are currently used as an investigational tool in research laboratories, primarily to define the boundaries of the smallest deletion that causes the syndrome as well as for haplotyping (to determine the parental chromosome of origin) and determining the presence or absence of specific markers and genes in the deleted region. At this time, FISH remains the best clinically available laboratory test.

Because some cases of velo-cardio-facial syndrome are familial, and because the disorder is highly variable, the issue of whether or not to test the parents arises. This is particularly important if the parents or other family members are of reproductive age, because the information could be extremely valuable for genetic counseling purposes. If there is an unbalanced translocation in the child, karyotyping must be done on the parents to identify the source of the balanced translocation. If the proband has the deletion of 22q11.2 and an otherwise normal karyotype, parental FISH studies are recommended, particularly if either parent or another close relative shows any signs or symptoms of the disorder (including psychiatric problems) or if a complete family history reveals any of these common findings. Because of the subtlety of some of the clinical findings in this disorder, the physician inexperienced in the phenotype and manifestations of the condition may not identify an affected parent. Therefore, it is appropriate to refer the family for evaluation by an experienced clinical geneticist. It is important to be certain as to whether or not one of the parents is affected, given the 50% risk of transmission for an individual who has the deletion, before reviewing reproductive options and providing genetic counseling.

A few patients in whom the phenotype is convincing do not have a detectable deletion. It is possible that these individuals have velo-cardio-facial syndrome due to another genetic cause or a mutation in a single gene within 22q11.2. However, it is still most likely that cases that are clinically diagnosed as velo-cardio-facial syndrome but are FISH negative represent misdiagnosis or a possible phenocopy of velo-cardio-facial syndrome with a different etiology. In such cases, which constitute well under 5% of all patients, it is suggested that the patient be referred to a clinical geneticist or other specialist familiar with the disorder, who can in turn contact one of the molecular genetics laboratories studying velo-cardio-facial syndrome in detail, if indicated.

Differential Diagnosis

Because the phenotypic manifestations of velo-cardio-facial syndrome are so expansive, there are a number of syndromes that have multiple features in common. This is especially true of the association of congenital heart disease, cleft palate, developmental delay, and behavioral anomalies. Niikawa-Kuroki syndrome (often called Kabuki syndrome or Kabuki make-up syndrome) shares many clinical features with velo-cardio-facial syndrome, including heart anomalies, cleft palate, and hypotonia, but the facial appearance is quite different and the ears in Niikawa-Kuroki syndrome are typically large, unlike the small ears in velo-cardio-facial syndrome. Fetal alcohol syndrome (see Chapter 9) also has significant overlap with velo-cardio-facial syndrome, including relatively small stature, heart anomalies, DiGeorge sequence, chronic respiratory illness, cleft palate, Robin sequence, developmental delay, and behavioral disorders. There is some facial resemblance between Langer-Giedion syndrome and velo-cardio-facial syndrome, as well as developmental delay and eye anomalies. Bzranchio-oto-renal syndrome (BOR, or Melnick-Fraser syndrome) has ear anomalies, facial asymmetry, hearing loss, and kidney anomalies in common with velo-cardio-facial syndrome. Opitz syndrome (formerly labeled G syndrome and BBB syndrome) has cleft palate, hypertelorism, and laryngeal and feeding anomalies along with developmental delay, but the facial phenotype is quite different. Although some reports have suggested that a form of Opitz syndrome that is not X-linked is also caused by a deletion at 22q11 (Fryburg et al., 1996; McDonald-McGinn et al., 1996), the cases reported appear to fall within the clinical spectrum of velo-cardio-facial syndrome (personal opinion based on photographs and case reports). There is also some overlap between velo-cardio-facial syndrome and Oculo-auriculo-vertebral dysplasia (see Chapter 16), including cleft palate, facial asymmetry, and ear tags or pits (low-frequency features of velo-cardio-facial syndrome). Several patients with velo-cardio-facial syndrome have had mild webbing of the neck with low-set ears. In association with heart anomalies, cleft palate, developmental delay, and relative short stature, there is phenotypic overlap with both Noonan (see Chapter 15) and Turner (see Chapter 27) syndromes, although, once again, the facial gestalt should discriminate between these alternatives, and chromosome analysis will distinguish Turner syndrome. There are a number of rare syndromes associated with Robin sequence and a number of single-family syndromes that also have phenotypic overlap with velo-cardio-facial syndrome. Testing for deletion 22q11.2 by FISH will differentiate velo-cardio-facial syndrome from these disorders.

Because DiGeorge sequence is etiologically nonspecific and related to a number of genetic, chromosomal, and teratogenic causes, DiGeorge is not a final diagnosis but rather a launching point for evaluation and investigation. DiGeorge sequence is known to be caused by alcohol teratogenesis, deletions of the short arm of chromosome 10, and deletions of the long arm of chromosome 4, among others. However, the largest number of cases of DiGeorge sequence is caused by 22q11.2 deletions. Less than 15% of patients with velo-cardio-facial syndrome meet the diagnostic criteria for DiGeorge sequence (personal experience), but conversely, all patients with DiGeorge sequence who have 22q11.2 deletions meet the criteria for velo-cardio-facial syndrome.

CHARGE association is also an etiologically nonspecific disorder based on the symptomatic acronym *c*oloboma (of the eye), *h*eart anomalies, *a*tresia choanae, *r*etarded growth and development, *g*enital anomalies, and *e*ar anomalies or deafness (see Chapter 5). All of the anomalies consistent with CHARGE association occur with varying frequency in velo-cardio-facial syndrome.

The broadness of the velo-cardio-facial syndrome phenotype also has resulted in some confusion over diagnostic labels attached to the disorder. Some clinicians believe that velo-cardio-facial syndrome, DiGeorge sequence, Cayler syndrome, and conotruncal anomalies-face syndrome are separate disorders. All cases of velo-cardio-facial syndrome, DiGeorge sequence, Cayler syndrome, and conotruncal anomalies-face syndrome that are deleted at 22q11.2 represent the same disorder. Because velo-cardio-facial syndrome has so expansive a phenotype with no obligatory findings, the difference in names for the disorder has resulted from ascertainment bias, historical connotations, and a degree of scientific rivalry. Wulfsberg et al., (1996) have discussed the confusion associated with the "naming" dilemma related to velo-cardio-facial syndrome, DiGeorge sequence, and other disorders.

MANIFESTATIONS AND MANAGEMENT

Growth and Feeding

Early feeding and airway problems in some cases are related to major cardiovascular malformations and concomitant hypotonia. Vascular ring, a right-sided aorta that may impinge on the trachea or esophagus, and other major vessel anomalies can all result in constriction of the esophagus and/or trachea. It is possible to have major vascular anomalies in the absence of structural heart anomalies. Feeding disorders also occur independently of heart anomalies associated with velo-cardio-facial syndrome. One of the earliest manifestations of feeding abnormalities in velo-cardio-facial syndrome is nasal regurgitation of milk. Many clinicians become concerned that nasal regurgitation is a possible indicator of an increased risk of aspiration. This notion may be further reinforced by the presence of early pneumonia because of the immune disorder associated with velo-cardio-facial syndrome. Aspiration in velo-cardio-facial syndrome is not common, and nasal regurgitation does not increase the risk. Nasal regurgitation in velo-cardio-facial syndrome is related to hypotonia, a hypoplastic soft palate, and an extremely large nasopharynx. Pharyngeal hypotonia, one of the most common findings in velo-cardio-facial syndrome, is also likely to lead to nasal regurgitation of fluids if vomiting occurs. Vomiting is a frequent finding in velo-cardio-facial syndrome and is related to a number of factors.

- Hypotonia is present in the majority of the digestive tract, including the esophagus. Therefore, peristalsis of the esophagus on swallowing may be disordered, including a slow response time once swallowing has been initiated.

- The stomach may empty slowly because of chronic constipation. The chronic constipation in velo-cardio-facial syndrome is also related to a generalized hypotonia of the digestive tract so that emptying of the small and large bowel is less efficient than normal.

- Babies with velo-cardio-facial syndrome swallow a large amount of air during feeding because of uncoordinated breathing and swallowing. Therefore, air becomes trapped in the stomach and when expelled orally may cause substantial vomiting. This is not truly gastroesophageal reflux but, actually, emesis. Although gastroesophageal reflux can occur in velo-cardio-facial syndrome, vomiting is far more common.

Robin sequence is actually the most common secondary sequence associated with velo-cardio-facial syndrome. An analysis of 100 consecutive cases of Robin sequence showed that 11% had velo-cardio-facial syndrome (Shprintzen and Singer, 1992), and 17% of velo-cardio-facial syndrome cases initially present with the Robin sequence (Shprintzen and Singer, 1992). The feeding and growth problems seen in Robin sequence

(see Chapter 19) would be relevant to patients with velo-cardio-facial syndrome who have this anomaly.

Evaluation

- The feeding disorder associated with velo-cardio-facial syndrome is often labeled as "reflux" even though the problem is one of frank emesis. However, because the appearance of any degree of nasal discharge of fluids or food is incorrectly labeled as "reflux" by many clinicians, pH probe studies are often ordered. The pH probe study will always be strongly positive in patients with emesis because the gastric contents will be discharged through the esophagus into the oropharynx and hypopharynx. Therefore, pH probes have little diagnostic value in infants or children with velo-cardio-facial syndrome when there are obvious signs of emesis.

- Clinicians also often request a barium swallow, or, in older children who have progressed to pureed or solid foods, a modified barium swallow. Although a barium swallow may have value in some children with velo-cardio-facial syndrome, interpretation must take into account the other manifestations of the syndrome, including chronic constipation, hypotonia, and structural vascular anomalies (such as vascular ring or aortic arch anomalies that might impinge on the esophagus).

- The more appropriate study in many cases is fiber optic endoscopic evaluation of swallowing (FEES). FEES allows direct observation of the pharynx, palate, posterior tongue, and larynx of babies during swallowing. In infants, FEES can be performed either by oral endoscopy using a specialized nipple adaptor for endoscopes or through the nose (Fig. 29.3). Endoscopic studies can rule out aspiration and actually provide a better view of the

(A)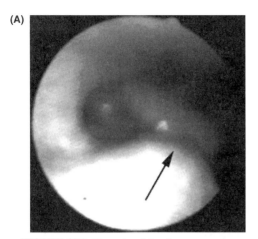

(B)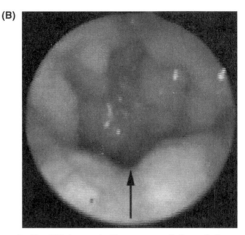

FIGURE 29.3. Normal palate shown nasopharyngoscopically (A) demonstrating convex bulge of the midline muscle mass (arrow) compared to an occult submucous cleft palate (B) showing midline notch (arrow).

glottis during swallowing than radiographic procedures. FEES has special value in velo-cardio-facial syndrome because of the high frequency of laryngeal anomalies that require endoscopic assessment for confirmation.

- Vascular anomalies in velo-cardio-facial syndrome, especially of the neck and brain, are best assessed by magnetic resonance angiography (MRA) (Mitnick et al., 1996). This technique does not involve radiation and provides excellent views of major blood vessels that can be viewed in three dimensions by many magnetic resonance machines. It is not necessary to use contrast in MRA studies, further reducing the risk of the procedure. However, in most patients with velo-cardio-facial syndrome, it is necessary to perform these studies under anesthesia to have the patient still for an extended period of time.

- In some cases, magnetic resonance cannot be used because of previous heart surgery that may have left metal clips or wires in the patient's chest. In these cases, CT angiography is typically recommended, although standard angiography can be performed. CT angiography also requires anesthesia, contrast

is necessary to define the arteries and veins, and the radiation exposure is fairly high, but the images are essentially as good as in magnetic resonance studies and can also be manipulated in three dimensions.

Treatment

- Unfortunately, because of persistent vomiting and concerns over aspiration, many children with velo-cardio-facial syndrome are treated with gastrostomy or long-term gavage feeding. This is rarely necessary. Once the source of the vomiting is isolated, treatment can be implemented along with oral feeding techniques, which would overcome the problem of hypotonia.

- It is recommended that children with velo-cardio-facial syndrome be fed with a soft nipple such as the one used for premature babies, with a large crosscut that allows the formula to flow with minimal tongue pressure. The infant should be held upright and burped frequently (at least every 3–4 minutes). Feeding should be confined to 20–30 minutes beginning with a 3-hour schedule. If a full feeding tends to induce vomiting, then more frequent, short, small feedings may be used. This approach may need to be modified if the child is medically fragile as a result of heart anomalies.

- Constipation should be treated aggressively so that a bowel movement is assured every day. This may mean using mineral oil or other dietary supplements, or even a suppository if a bowel movement has not occurred each day.

- Feeding of the child with Robin sequence is more complex and is discussed in Chapter 19.

Development and Behavior

Educational problems occur in nearly all patients with velo-cardio-facial syndrome. Mental retardation is found in a small percentage of patients with velo-cardio-facial syndrome, although diminished IQ test scores for the family are more common than true intellectual deficiency. After early developmental delay and language impairment, children with velo-cardio-facial syndrome tend to show some "catch-up" in cognitive skills at approximately 4 years of age. At this age, concrete learning skills in children with velo-cardio-facial syndrome typically are similar to those of most children of similar age, and IQ scores are usually within normal limits (Golding-Kushner et al., 1985). However, as more abstract learning develops in older normal children, people with velo-cardio-facial syndrome maintain strong concrete skills but have poor abstract reasoning and problem-solving skills. School-age children with velo-cardio-facial syndrome have IQ scores that are as much as 20 points lower than obtained previously (Golding-Kushner et al., 1985). They have specific learning disabilities in math and reading comprehension. There is typically a marked disparity between verbal IQ scores (often within the normal range) and performance IQ scores (often far below verbal scores). Although full-scale scores may place children with velo-cardio-facial

syndrome in the borderline or mildly retarded range, cognitive abilities are not as deficient as the IQ scores would suggest.

A common concern among the parents of affected individuals is the communication disorder that is found in over 90% of patients with velo-cardio-facial syndrome. Language is typically delayed and impaired, although the delay is usually mild. Achievement of speech milestones is typically several months later than normal, although in some cases more severe delay has been noted. After the onset of the first word, the use of phrases and sentences is often delayed until 3 or 4 years of age, at which time there is usually a rapid acceleration of language development, both receptive and expressive. The onset of expressive language is largely affected by the severe hypernasality found in over 70% of cases. In addition, children with velo-cardio-facial syndrome take an alternative approach to articulation development, substituting glottal stop consonants for nearly all speech sounds (Golding-Kushner et al., 1985). This abnormal pattern of compensation renders their speech unintelligible and often leads to a misdiagnosis of apraxia in many affected individuals.

Psychiatric problems are common in patients with velo-cardio-facial syndrome, particularly in adulthood. Both bipolar disorder and schizophrenia have been reported in velo-cardio-facial syndrome, and approximately 20% of affected individuals have been estimated to develop psychosis as adults (Papolos et al., 1996; Shprintzen et al., 1992; Murphy et al., 1999). Attention deficit disorder with or without hyperactivity is also common. The onset of abnormal behavior patterns has been documented in young children with the syndrome (Papolos et al., 1996). Papolos et al. (1996) reported that the psychiatric illness in velo-cardio-facial syndrome involves a spectrum of bipolar disorders and that the early presentation of attention deficit/hyperactivity disorder, obsessive-compulsive disorder, dysthymia, and cyclothymia represent prodromal manifestations of bipolar illness. Lachman et al., (1996) found that one of the genes in the deleted region of 22q11.2, *COMT* (catechol-*O*-methyltransferase), had a polymorphism involving two alleles. *COMT* encodes for catecholamines, enzymes responsible for breaking down dopamine in the brain. One version of the *COMT* polymorphism encodes for low enzymatic activity, resulting in higher levels of dopamine in the brain. In deleted patients with the low-activity *COMT* allele, only half of the gene complement for *COMT* is present, and that single copy is a low-activity allele. These authors found that patients who were hemizygous for the low-activity allele had severe rapid-cycling bipolar disorder. The other polymorphism results in high enzymatic activity and is not associated with as severe a psychiatric phenotype as the low-activity allele.

Evaluation

- Careful developmental, neuropsychological, and educational testing is indicated for all children with velo-cardio-facial syndrome.
- Children and adults should be monitored for behavioral or psychiatric problems.
- Nasopharyngoscopy and multiview videofluoroscopy are the best approaches to evaluating the cause of hypernasality.
- A detailed psychiatric assessment using standardized tests and detailed history and interview are essential for reaching a DSM diagnosis. Because the onset of psychiatric illness is evident even in young children, it is suggested that evaluations be performed by qualified child psychiatrists.

Treatment

- Because the learning problems are related to deficiencies in abstract reasoning, children with velo-cardio-facial

syndrome are best taught using concrete examples and dividing complex problems into simple components. Learning is also effective using drill and repetition.
- Children with velo-cardio-facial syndrome have a strong affinity for computers and learn well using them (personal experience).
- They also learn very well using music, especially as young children (personal experience).
- Resolution of hypernasality is almost always a surgical problem that is complicated by abnormal location and course of the internal carotid arteries (Mitnick et al., 1996; Shprintzen, 1998). Pharyngeal flap surgery could potentially sever the internal carotids.
- It has therefore been recommended that all pharyngeal surgery be preceded by MRA or CT angiography to alert the surgeon to the potential risks for aberrant internal carotid arteries (Mitnick et al., 1996; Shprintzen, 1998).
- In some instances, clinicians may choose to use sign language as an early approach to communication, but this approach is rarely necessary (personal experience) and proper speech therapy techniques can be used to improve articulation.
- The treatment of the psychiatric problems is often confusing and difficult because the early manifestations of the psychiatric disorder may include attention deficit disorder, with or without hyperactivity, obsessive-compulsive disorder, dysthymia, and cyclothymia. The standard treatments for these conditions may actually prompt adverse reactions in children with velo-cardio-facial syndrome.
- The common association of attention deficit disorder and attention deficit/hyperactivity disorder in velo-cardio-facial syndrome presents a treatment dilemma

because the standard treatment for attention deficit disorder or attention deficit/hyperactivity disorder is the administration of stimulants such as methylphenidate or dexedrine, both of which increase the secretion of dopamine in the brain. Therefore, the use of stimulants in patients with velo-cardio-facial syndrome may enhance the psychiatric symptoms in patients with the low-activity *COMT* allele.

Craniofacial

The craniofacial anomalies associated with velo-cardio-facial syndrome are among the most common manifestations of the disorder. The smallest percentage of clefts are overt clefts of the palate, constituting approximately 18% of all palate anomalies in velo-cardio-facial syndrome. Nearly half of the palate anomalies in velo-cardio-facial syndrome (44%) are submucous clefts of the palate, typically indicated by bifid uvula. The remaining 38% of the palate anomalies represent a disorder known as occult submucous cleft palate (Shprintzen, 1982). Occult submucous cleft palate refers to muscle abnormalities of the soft palate that can not be detected by oral examination. In other words, there are no signs of bifid uvula or muscle anomalies that can be seen on oral examination, but abnormal landmarks can be detected on nasopharyngoscopic examination of the soft palate, including absence of major muscle groups and notches in the palatal tissues (Fig. 29.3). Many clinicians do not have the facilities for routine nasopharyngoscopy and therefore may not diagnose the presence of an occult submucous cleft in many cases. Therefore, in many instances, hypernasal speech is reported in the absence of "cleft palate." In midsagittal radiographic views of the head and neck, the palate in patients with velo-cardio-facial syndrome is often extremely short and thin, indicating a severe tissue deficiency.

Although individuals with velo-cardio-facial syndrome have a characteristic facial appearance, it rarely stands out as being very abnormal. Increased vertical length of the face is probably the most common manifestation, even at an early age. The increase in facial length is related to vertical maxillary excess resulting in an increased height of the lower third of the face (Arvystas and Shprintzen, 1984). Vertical maxillary excess is a common finding in individuals with generalized hypotonia, and may represent a secondary manifestation of a lax envelope of facial musculature.

Retrognathia is found in approximately one-third of individuals with velo-cardio-facial syndrome. Retrognathia refers to retrusion of the lower jaw rather than small size of the jaw. Individuals with velo-cardio-facial syndrome have been found to have an abnormally obtuse cranial base angle (Arvystas and Shprintzen, 1984) that rotates the glenoid fossa and the temporomandibular joint posteriorly. Individuals with velo-cardio-facial syndrome have mandibles of generally normal size and shape, but because the mandible sits in a posteriorly positioned glenoid fossa, it is retruded in relation to the maxilla. Mandibular retrusion in velo-cardio-facial syndrome is responsible for the high frequency of Robin sequence (see Chapter 19).

Another key finding of facial morphology, hooded upper eyelids (often referred to as vertically short palpebral fissures), is also caused by this same rotational defect of the cranial base. Because the posterior skull base is rotated back, the forehead (frontal bone) tends to be positioned more forward than normal (Arvystas and Shprintzen, 1984), creating some redundancy of tissue of the upper eyelids (hooding). Mild hypertelorism is also a common finding in velo-cardio-facial syndrome, but it is rarely severe and typically does not require treatment. An upslant to the palpebral fissures is common.

Evaluation

- Assessment of facial landmarks should be done in all patients.

- Cephalometric radiographs can be used to measure the skull base angle for possible platybasia. Platybasia may be a sign that the posterior cranial fossa is small, a possible precursor to identification of Arnold-Chiari anomaly. Flatness of the skull base may also explain the presence of retrognathia and velopharyngeal insufficiency.

- In the absence of an overt cleft of the palate, careful peroral examination of the palate should be performed for bifid or hypoplastic uvula, indicative of a submucous cleft palate.

- All patients should have a speech evaluation by a speech pathologist familiar with speech disorders associated with velo-cardio-facial syndrome and/or cleft palate. Such individuals are often affiliated with a cleft palate or craniofacial team.

- Nasopharyngoscopy should be performed to detect palatal anomalies and dysfunction of the velopharyngeal mechanism during speech, if available.

- Multiview videofluoroscopy should be performed to assess deficient length and thickness of the palate, as well as dysfunction during speech.

Treatment

- Speech therapy is rarely useful in treating hypernasality in children with velo-cardio-facial syndrome, although speech therapy is very important for the correction of other speech and language impairments.

- Palate repair or reconstruction is rarely ever successful at eliminating speech problems in children with velo-cardio-facial syndrome. Secondary operations are frequently necessary to eliminate hypernasality. Pharyngeal flap surgery is most typically recommended if the surgeon is capable of creating a very wide pharyngeal flap, necessary in patients with velo-cardio-facial syndrome because of pharyngeal hypotonia and severe tissue deficiency of the palate.

- Prosthetic management of velopharyngeal insufficiency is not typically recommended in children with velo-cardio-facial syndrome because of poor compliance and lack of a permanent result.

- Orthodontic treatment is often recommended for children with velo-cardio-facial syndrome, typically in the late mixed-dentition stage, although in some cases, earlier intervention may be necessary if retrognathia is severe. Onset of orthodontic treatment may vary from 7 to 12 years.

- In cases with severe discrepancies of the facial skeleton, orthognathic surgery may be indicated to improve malocclusion and facial balance.

Respiratory

The airway problems associated with velo-cardio-facial syndrome can also be intricate and complicated. Both upper and lower airway obstruction may occur, sometimes together. Upper airway obstruction may be caused by hypotonia and/or retrognathia, either or both of which may result in glossoptosis. Lower airway obstruction in velo-cardio-facial typically involves vascular rings, abnormal major vessel placement, or laryngeal webs. Laryngomalacia is typically supraglottic with hypertrophic arytenoids being sucked into the glottis. This type of laryngomalacia does cause brief oxygen desaturation

Evaluation

- Nasopharyngoscopy can identify glossoptosis, pharyngeal vascular anomalies, laryngeal web, and laryngomalacia.

- Oxygen desaturation episodes associated with laryngomalacia are brief and typically resolve by themselves within a few months so that treatment is not necessary.

- Magnetic resonance angiography (MRA) can delineate aberrant major neck arteries.
- The source of lower airway obstruction may be determined radiographically or by bronchoscopy. The mechanism of upper airway obstruction is best visualized endoscopically because the problem is typically a functional one that must be seen in motion.

Treatment

- Lower airway obstruction in velo-cardio-facial syndrome is typically addressed surgically by removal of the vascular ring or laryngeal web.
- Laryngomalacia resolves with time and without treatment.
- Glossoptosis and hypotonia of the upper airway also typically resolve with time, but in some cases, especially those resulting in Robin sequence, glossopexy may be necessary in the newborn period to tether the tongue forward (see Chapter 19). Tracheotomy in velo-cardio-facial syndrome is rarely necessary.

Cardiovascular

The heart malformations in velo-cardio-facial syndrome are of the components derived from the conotruncus. The single most common anomaly among children with velo-cardio-facial syndrome is ventricular septal defect, typically of the malalignment type. However, because ventricular septal defects are so common in the general population (actually one of the most common anomalies in humans) and in children with other syndromes, the percentage of individuals with this defect who have velo-cardio-facial syndrome is probably relatively small. Velo-cardio-facial syndrome is a much more common diagnosis among children with aortic arch anomalies associated with heart malformations, especially interrupted aortic arch

type B and coarctation of the aorta. Detection of interrupted aortic arch type B should prompt FISH testing for deletion 22q unless another obvious syndrome is diagnosed, such as Down syndrome. Velo-cardio-facial syndrome is also common among children born with tetralogy of Fallot, pulmonary atresia or stenosis, and aberrant major vessels, such as aberrant subclavian arteries. Other heart malformations present in velo-cardio-facial syndrome include truncus arteriosus, bicuspid aortic valve, atrial septal defects, transposition of the great vessels, and anomalous origin of the carotid artery (see Table 29.1 for a complete listing of heart anomalies).

Anomalies of the internal carotids and other major neck arteries are among the most frequent clinical findings in velo-cardio-facial syndrome (Fig. 29.4). The internal carotids are ectopic and directly beneath the pharyngeal mucosa in approximately 20–30% of patients with velo-cardio-facial syndrome.

Evaluation

- All patients suspected of having velo-cardio-facial syndrome should have a cardiology assessment, even if there are no obvious manifestations of heart anomalies. This should include echocardiography to delineate the cardiovascular anatomy.
- MRA can delineate aberrant major neck arteries.

Treatment

- Heart anomalies are treated surgically following the normal protocols for such malformations. In many cases, the heart anomalies require emergent repair (as in interrupted aortic arch) and may be accomplished before the diagnosis of velo-cardio-facial syndrome is established by FISH.
- Vascular anomalies typically do not require repair unless they compromise cardiovascular perfusion. Vascular rings

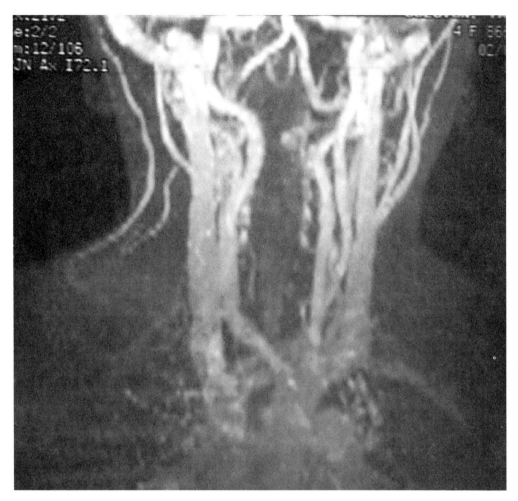

FIGURE 29.4. Severe medial deviation of the internal carotid arteries.

are one exception, because they may interfere with respiration or feeding.

Neuromuscular

In some cases, seizures are an early manifestation of velo-cardio-facial syndrome. Seizures in velo-cardio-facial syndrome are a complex problem because there are multiple possible causes that may be qualitatively difficult to distinguish. Seizures may be related to hypocalcemia, stroke, cerebellar or cerebral cortical atrophy, and transient or chronic ischemia (Shprintzen et al., 1997). Febrile seizures are also common. Seizures often

come in clusters for several months at a time and then may disappear for several years.

Chronic leg pains are a common feature of velo-cardio-facial syndrome and are often related to a combination of hypotonia and flattened arches that cause the feet to pronate and stretch the muscles. Severe muscle cramps may result, especially at night, often causing frequent waking and discomfort. Children will often ask to be picked up and carried after walking only short distances. Tight heel cords are common. However, two conditions with clinical overlap with muscle cramping may also cause lower limb problems. Tethered spinal cord has been observed in some cases, which may result in lower limb weakness. Talipes equinovarus has been found in about 5–10% of newborns with velo-cardio-facial syndrome, which may indicate that minor anomalies of the lower limb skeleton could contribute to gait and stance abnormalities.

Evaluation

- Serum calcium level should be obtained during seizure episodes.
- Brain imaging techniques, particularly MRI, can identify stroke and cortical atrophy.
- MRI of the spine is indicated to evaluate for possible tethered cord or syrinx or possible meningocele.
- EEG is typically not indicated as a routine assessment. Seizures may prompt EEG assessment, but they are most often normal.

Treatment

- Seizure management is highly dependent on identification of the source of the problem. In the minority of patients with velo-cardio-facial syndrome, hypocalcemia may be prompting seizures and calcium supplementation is recommended.
- Most seizures in velo-cardio-facial syndrome are not hypocalcemic and are best managed with appropriate anticonvulsants, such as valproic acid. Many anticonvulsant medications may have an added benefit in velo-cardio-facial syndrome because they have mood stabilizing effects. These include drugs such as valproic acid, gabapentin, carbamazepine, and lamotrigine.
- Strokes may result in seizures or neurologic sequelae. They should be managed as in the general population or, if seizures result, as stated above. It likely that such strokes are related to the vascular anomalies associated with the syndrome.

- Massage and locally applied heat are effective for acute episodes of leg pain. The use of soft shoe inserts to lift the arch is also recommended for this problem.
- Tethered cord, tight heel cords, and talipes equinovarus should be treated as for the general population. Surgery may be indicated if there is loss of motor function, weakness, or marked sensory change.

Immunologic

Immune disorders are common in the syndrome, usually presenting as chronic upper or lower respiratory illness that occurs most frequently in early childhood (ages birth to 4 years) and then subsides in frequency (Cunningham et al., 1997). Chronic middle ear disease occurs in approximately 75% of affected individuals, with subsequent conductive hearing loss. Sensorineural hearing loss, often unilateral and mild to moderate, is found in 15% of cases. The chronic infections and illnesses may occur in the absence of any detectable immune deficiency on laboratory testing, although reduced T lymphocyte counts have been observed in many, but not the majority, of these cases. Mild thrombocytopenia is also common beginning in the teen years.

Evaluation

- Standard laboratory analysis of immune function is indicated in those patients with velo-cardio-facial syndrome who have a history of chronic upper and lower respiratory infections. Although an actual immune deficiency (i.e., reduced T cells) may not be found in many cases, the history of illness should be carefully considered in determining an appropriate treatment plan. Specific laboratory tests should include complete blood count and differential, lymphocyte subsets, total immunoglobulins, mixed lymphocyte culture, and lymphocyte proliferation assay.

- In children over the age of 2 years for whom Pneumovax has been recommended, pre- and postantibody titers are recommended. Pre- and postantibody titers for other vaccines such as varicella and influenza should also be checked.

Treatment

- The presence of persistent infections in infancy and childhood often leads primary care physicians to prescribe potent broad-spectrum antibiotics for extended periods of time or even as prophylaxis. This is rarely indicated in velo-cardio-facial syndrome and may often lead to the development of opportunistic infections, including the establishment of upper and lower airway pathogens that may resist treatment once established. It is therefore recommended that each infection be treated as an acute episode with the standard course of antibiotic therapy.

- In some cases of severe immune deficiency, careful consideration must be given to the use of live virus vaccines. Modification of immunization schedules and protocols may be considered in cases with documented immune deficiency.

- In the most severe cases, some clinicians have recommended the use of gamma globulins to reduce the frequency and severity of infections. There are no published data or documented responses to this type of treatment in a controlled study of children with velo-cardio-facial syndrome.

Endocrine

Hypoparathyroidism occurs less frequently than hypothyroidism, and neither are common findings. Hypocalcemia occurs in approximately 25% of patients with velo-cardio-facial syndrome. Hypocalcemia is typically intermittent and may not be evident until the second or third decade of life.

Evaluation

- Serum calcium levels should be checked if there is a history of seizures, tremors, or other clinical manifestations consistent with hypocalcemia.

- Serum calcium should also be checked in all infants for whom the diagnosis of velo-cardio-facial syndrome or DiGeorge sequence has been established. Annual assessment of serum calcium during well-child examinations is recommended for all identified patients. Patients who have been identified as having hypocalemia and have been treated should have follow-up studies performed with frequency because of the transient nature of the problem.

- Hypothyroidism should be ruled out in children who become sluggish or who display other manifestations consistent with abnormal thyroid function. Decreased vitality and fatigue may be manifestations of the psychiatric illness associated with velo-cardio-facial syndrome, but hypothyroidism is a common enough feature of the syndrome to warrant assessment.

Treatment

- Identification of hypocalcemia should lead to treatment as in the general population.

- Hypothyroidism should also be treated when identified, as in the general population.

Genitourinary

A very wide range of other anomalies can be found in velo-cardio-facial syndrome (Table 29.1), most of which are relatively uncommon. These should be kept in mind when evaluating for unexpected findings in individual patients. Anomalies of the kidney are relatively common.

Evaluation

- Renal ultrasound should be used to identify the presence or absence of kidney aplasia or hypoplasia. Although unilateral hypoplasia/aplasia of the kidneys is typically asymptomatic, early identification is important for sound preventive care.

Treatment

- Kidney anomalies should be treated as in the general population.

Ophthalmologic

Visual impairment is common and can include strabismus, anomalies of the retinal vessels, small optic disk, ocular colobomas, prominent corneal nerves, and posterior embryotoxon. In velo-cardio-facial syndrome, the majority of eye anomalies do not impair vision.

Evaluation

- To assure that there are no visual impairments, baseline ophthalmologic assessment should be done, including full dilation.

Treatment

- Strabismus is sufficiently common in the syndrome to warrant assessment and treatment with spectacles or surgery.
- Other eye manifestations should be treated as in the general population.

RESOURCES

Velo-Cardio-Facial Syndrome Educational Foundation, Inc.
www.vcfsef.org
c/o Robert Shprintzen, Ph.D.
Jacobsen Hall, 714
SUNY Health Science Center at Syracuse
750 East Adams St.
Syracuse, NY 13210
Phone: (315) 464-6590

Fax: (315) 464-5321
E-mail: *vcfsef@email.upstate.edu*
The 22q11 Group (U.K.)
E-mail: *22q11@melcom.cix.co.uk*
The VCF Foundation of Australia
E-mail: *vcfsta@pnc.com.au*

REFERENCES

Arvystas M, Shprintzen FJ (1984) Craniofacial morphology in the velo-cardio-facial syndrome. *J Craniofacial Genet Devel Biol* 4:39–45.

Cunningham CK, Weiner LB, Shprintzen RJ (1997) Respiratory infections in children with velo-cardio-facial syndrome *Am J Hum Genet* 61:528, 95A.

Devriendt K, Moerman P, Van Schoubroeck D, Vandenberghe K, Fryns JP (1997) Chromosome 22q11 deletion presenting as the Potter sequence. *J Med Genet* 34:423–425.

Driscoll DA, Budarf ML, Emanuel BS (1992a) A genetic etiology for DiGeorge syndrome: Consistent deletions and microdeletions of 22q11. *Am J Hum Genet* 50:924–933.

Driscoll DA, Salvin J, Sellinger B, Budarf ML, McDonald-McGinn DM, Zackai EH, Emanuel BS (1993) Prevalence of 22q11 microdeletions in DiGeorge and velocardiofacial syndromes: Implications for genetic counseling and prenatal diagnosis. *J Med Genet* 30:813–817.

Driscoll DA, Spinner NB, Budarf ML, McDonald-McGinn DM, Zackai EH, Goldberg RB, Shprintzen RJ, Saal HM, Zonana J, Jones MC, Mascarello JT, Emanuel BS (1992b) Deletions and microdeletions of 22q11.2 in velo-cardio-facial syndrome. *Am J Med Genet* 44:261–268.

Fryburg JS, Lin KY, Golden WL (1996) Chromosome 22q11.2 deletion in a boy with Opitz (G/BBB) syndrome. *Am J Med Genet* 62:274–275.

Funke B, Saint-Jore B, Puech A, Sirotkin H, Edelmann L, Carlson C, Raft S, Pandita RK, Kucherlapati R, Skoultchi A, Morrow BE (1997) Characterization and mutation analysis of goosecoid-like (*GSCL*), a homeodomain-containing gene that maps to the critical region for velo-cardio-facial syndrome/DGS on 22q11. *Genomics* 46:364–372.

Golding-Kushner K, Weller G, Shprintzen RJ (1985) Velo-cardio-facial syndrome: Language and psychological profiles. *J Craniofac Genet Dev Biol* 5:259–266.

Kelly D, Goldberg R, Wilson D, Lindsay E, Carey A, Goodship J, Burn J, Cross I, Shprintzen RJ, Scambler PJ (1993) Velo-cardio-facial syndrome associated with haplo-insufficiency of genes at chromosome 22q11. *Am J Med Genet* 45:308–312.

Lachman HM, Morrow B, Shprintzen RJ, Veit S, Parsia SS, Faedda G, Goldberg R, Kucherlapati R, Papolos DF (1996) Association of codon 108/158 catechol-o-methyl transferase gene polymorphism with the psychiatric manifestations of velo-cardio-facial syndrome. *Am J Med Genet* 67:468–472.

Lammer EJ, Opitz JM (1986) The DiGeorge anomaly as a developmental field defect. *Am J Med Genet*. 2, Suppl:113–127.

Lipson AH, Yuille D, Angel M, Thompson PG, Vanderwoord JG, Beckenham EJ (1991) Velo-cardio-facial syndrome: An important syndrome for the dysmorphologist to recognize. *J Med Genet* 28:596–604.

McDonald-McGinn DM, Emanuel BS, Zackai EH (1996) Autosomal dominant "Opitz" GBBB syndrome due to a 22q11.2 deletion. *Am J Med Genet* 64:525–526.

Mitnick RJ, Bello JA, Golding-Kushner KJ, Argamaso RV, Shprintzen RJ (1996) The use of magnetic resonance angiography prior to pharyngeal flap surgery in patients with velo-cardio-facial syndrome. *Plast Reconstr Surg* 97:908–919.

Morita K, Sasaki H, Furuse M, Tsukita S (1999) Endothelial claudin. Claudin-5/tmvcf constitutes tight junction strands in endothelial cells. *J Cell Biol* 147:185–194.

Morrow B, Goldberg R, Carlson C, Gupta RD, Sirotkin H, Collins J, Dunham I, O'Donnell HO, Scambler P, Shprintzen RJ, Kucherlapati R (1995) Molecular definition of the 22q11 deletions in velo-cardio-facial syndrome. *Am J Hum Genet* 56:1391–1403.

Murphy KC, Jones LA, Owen MJ (1999) High rates of schizophrenia in adults with Velo-cardio-facial syndrome. *Arch Gen Psychiatry* 56:940–945.

Papolos DF, Faedda GL, Veit S, Goldberg R, Morrow B, Kucherlapati R, Shprintzen RJ (1996) Bipolar spectrum disorders in patients diagnosed with velo-cardio-facial syndrome: Does a hemizygous deletion of chromosome 22q11 result in bipolar affective disorder? *Am J Psychiatry* 153:1541–1547.

Puech A, Saint-Jore B, Funke B, Gilbert DJ, Sirotkin H, Copeland NG, Jenkins NA, Kucherlapati R, Morrow B, Skoultchi AI (1997) Comparative mapping of the human 22q11 chromosomal region and the orthologous region in mice reveals complex changes in gene organization. *Proc Natl Acad Sci USA* 94:14608–14613.

Scambler PJ, Kelly D, Lindsay E, Williamson R, Goldberg R, Shprintzen RJ, Wilson D, Goodship J, Cross I, Burn J (1992) Velo-cardio-facial syndrome associated with chromosome 22 deletions encompassing the DiGeorge locus. *Lancet* 339:1138–1139.

Shprintzen RJ (1982) Palatal and pharyngeal anomalies in craniofacial syndromes. *Birth Defects* 18(1):53–78.

Shprintzen RJ (1998). Discussion: Limited value of preoperative cervical vascular imaging in patients with velocardiofacial syndrome. *Plast Reconstr Surg* 101:1196–1199.

Shprintzen RJ, Goldberg R, Golding-Kushner KJ, Marion R (1992) Later-onset psychosis in the velo-cardio-facial syndrome. *Am J Med Genet* 42:141–142.

Shprintzen RJ, Goldberg RB, Lewin ML, Sidoti EJ, Berkman MD, Argamaso RV, Young D (1978) A new syndrome involving cleft palate, cardiac anomalies, typical facies, and learning disabilities: Velo-cardio-facial syndrome. *Cleft Palate J* 15:56–62.

Shprintzen RJ, Goldberg R, Young D, Wolford L (1981) The velo-cardio-facial syndrome: A clinical and genetic analysis. *Pediatrics* 67:167–172.

Shprintzen RJ, Morrow B, Kucherlapati R (1997) Vascular anomalies may explain many of the features of velo-cardio-facial syndrome (Abstract) *Am J Hum Genet* 61:34A.

Shprintzen RJ, Schwartz R, Daniller A, Hoch L (1985a) The morphologic significance of bifid uvula. *Pediatrics*, 75, 553–561.

Shprintzen RJ, Siegel-Sadewitz VL, Amato J, Goldberg RB (1985b) Anomalies associated with cleft lip, cleft palate, or both. *Am J Med Genet* 20:585–596.

Shprintzen RJ, Singer L (1992) Upper airway obstruction and the Robin sequence. *Int Anesthesiol Clin* 30:109–114.

Sirotkin H, Morrow B, DasGupta R, Goldberg R, Patanjali SR, Shi G, Cannizzaro L, Shprintzen R, Weissman SM, Kucherlapati R (1996) Isolation of a new clathrin heavy chain gene with muscle-specific expression from the region commonly deleted in velo-cardio-facial syndrome. *Hum Mol Genet* 5:617–624.

Sirotkin H, O'Donnell H, DasGupta R, Halford S, St. Jore B, Puech A, Parimoo S, Morrow B, Skoultchi A, Weissman SM, Scambler P, Kucherlapati R (1997) Identification of a new human catenin gene family member (*ARVCF*) from the region deleted in velo-cardio-facial syndrome. *Genomics* 41:75–83.

Williams MA, Shprintzen RJ, Goldberg RB (1985) Male-to-male transmission of the velo-cardio-facial syndrome: A case report and review of 60 cases. *J Craniofac Genet Dev Biol* 5:175–180.

Wraith JE, Super M, Watson GH, Phillips M (1985) Velo-cardio-facial syndrome presenting as holoprosencephaly. *Clin Genet* 27:408–410.

Wulfsberg EA, Leana-Cox J, Neri G (1996) What's in a name? Chromosome 22q abnormalities and the DiGeorge, velocardiofacial, and conotruncal anomalies face syndromes. *Am J Med Genet* 65:317–319.

CHAPTER 30

WILLIAMS SYNDROME

COLLEEN A. MORRIS

INTRODUCTION

Incidence

Williams Syndrome has been variably termed Williams-Beuren syndrome, idiopathic hypercalcemia, and supravalvar aortic stenosis syndrome. Although Williams (Williams et al., 1961) and Beuren (Beuren et al., 1962), both cardiologists, are commonly credited with the first detailed descriptions of the syndrome, there are earlier reports in the literature of idiopathic hypercalcemia (see Fanconi et al., 1952). Garcia et al., (1964) first documented the occurrence of both supravalvar aortic stenosis and idiopathic hypercalcemia, and since then, there have been several reviews detailing the Williams syndrome phenotype (Beuren, 1972; Jones and Smith, 1975; Burn, 1986; Morris et al., 1988). In 1993, Ewart et al. discovered a microdeletion of chromosome 7q11.23 encompassing the elastin gene that is detectable by fluorescent *in situ* hybridization (FISH) in 99% of individuals with the clinical phenotype of Williams syndrome (Ewart et al., 1993; Lowery et al., 1995; Mari et al., 1995; Nickerson et al., 1995). The true incidence of Williams syndrome is unknown, although estimated at between 1 in 10,000 and 1 in 20,000. Before the avail-

ability of a diagnostic test, the average age of diagnosis was 6.4 years (median 4 years).

Diagnostic Criteria

The diagnosis of Williams syndrome is based on recognition of the characteristic pattern of dysmorphic facial features, developmental delay, short stature relative to the family background, connective tissue abnormality (including cardiovascular disease), unique cognitive profile, and typical personality. Diagnostic scoring systems are available (Preus 1984; American Academy of Pediatrics, 2000) that may help the clinician determine whether diagnostic FISH testing is warranted. The facial characteristics of Williams syndrome are distinctive. Infants and young children typically have a broad forehead, bitemporal narrowing, low nasal root, periorbital fullness, stellate/lacy iris pattern, strabismus, bulbous nasal tip, malar flattening, long philtrum, full lips, wide mouth, full cheeks, dental malocclusion with small widely-spaced teeth, small jaw, and prominent earlobes (Fig. 30.1). Older children and adults usually have a more gaunt appearance of the face with a prominent supraorbital ridge, narrow nasal root of normal height, full nasal tip, malar flattening, wide mouth

Management of Genetic Syndromes, Edited by Suzanne B. Cassidy and Judith E. Allanson
ISBN 0-471-31286-X Copyright © 2001 by Wiley-Liss, Inc.

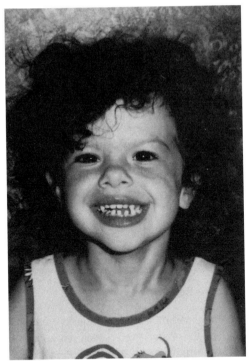

FIGURE 30.1. A 3-year old girl with Williams syndrome. Note the periorbital fullness, bulbous nasal tip, long philtrum, wide mouth, full lips, full cheeks, and small widely spaced teeth.

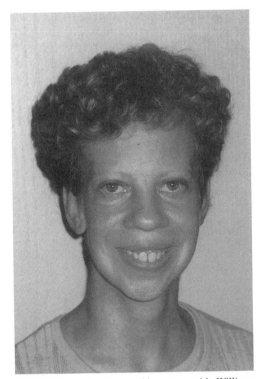

FIGURE 30.2. A 30-year old woman with Williams syndrome. Note the prominent supraorbital ridge, narrow nasal root, wide mouth with full lips, small jaw, and long neck.

with full lips, small jaw, dental malocclusion, and a long neck (Fig. 30.2). The connective tissue abnormalities include a hoarse/deep voice, hernias, bladder/bowel diverticulae, soft/loose skin, joint laxity or limitation, and cardiovascular disease (an elastin arteriopathy most commonly manifested as supravalvar aortic stenosis). Despite the historical association of the syndrome with hypercalcemia, its documented incidence is only 15%. Most children have developmental delay, but scores on full-scale IQ tests range widely, from severe mental retardation to low average; most have mild mental retardation. The unique cognitive profile of Williams syndrome consists of strengths in language and auditory memory accompanied by weakness in visuospatial construction (e.g., building an object from diagram). The Williams syndrome personality is typified by overfriendliness, attention problems, and anxiety.

Etiology, Pathogenesis and Genetics

Williams syndrome usually occurs sporadically; however, there is a 50% risk of transmitting the deletion to offspring, and familial cases, including male-to-male transmission, have been reported (Morris et al., 1993; Sadler et al., 1993). This disorder is caused by a submicroscopic deletion of chromosome 7q11.23. The deletion arises by unequal crossing over in a chromosome region predisposed to such meiotic error by the presence of a large number of repetitive DNA sequences (Dutly and Schinzel, 1996). The origin of the deletion may be maternal or paternal, without any parent-of-origin effect on the phenotype. (Wu et al., 1998). The commonly deleted region spans approximately 1.5 megabases, and 14 genes have thus far been mapped within this region. Many of the manifestations of Williams syndrome are caused by deletion of the elastin gene. The connective tissue abnormalities are the result of abnormal elastin protein production, and, interestingly, mutations within the elastin (*ELN*) gene also cause the autosomal dominant disorder, supravalvar aortic stenosis (Li et al, 1997). This condition is associated with elastin arteriopathy, hoarse voice, and hernias, but lacks other aspects of the Williams syndrome phenotype, such as mental retardation. There is no difference in the histologic appearance of diseased arteries in familial supravalvar aortic stenosis versus Williams syndrome (O'Connor, 1985).

Insight into the pathogenesis of the arterial disease has come from the study of mice hemizygous for *ELN*, which have a 47% decrease in *ELN* mRNA (Li et al., 1998). Lamellar units (an elastic fiber lamella alternating with a ring of smooth muscle around the arterial lumen) were observed to be increased in number in the experimental mice during fetal development. In humans hemizygous for *ELN*, there is a 2.5-fold increase in lamellar units, resulting in a thickened arterial media that leads to obstructive vascular disease.

Lim kinase 1 (*LIMK1*), a gene contiguous to *ELN*, is the second gene implicated in the Williams syndrome phenotype (Frangiskakis et al., 1996). Although most families with supravalvar aortic stenosis have a mutation in *ELN*, a few rare families have deletions within the Williams syndrome region that are much smaller than the deletions observed in Williams syndrome. Genotype-phenotype analysis of four families with such small deletions has shown that the Williams syndrome cognitive profile is associated with *LIMK1* deletion. These families have normal intelligence but have impaired visuospatial constructive cognition. Because *LIMK1* is expressed in the brain, it may thus be important in the development of neural pathways responsible for visual motor integration. The role of other deleted genes in the Williams syndrome phenotype is unknown;

further study of individuals and families with partial phenotypes may elucidate the pathogenetic mechanisms of other Williams syndrome features.

Diagnostic Testing

FISH testing will demonstrate *ELN* deletion in 99% of individuals with Williams syndrome. The only caveat is that some rare supravalvar aortic stenosis families will also have *ELN* deletion but do not have mental retardation, growth deficiency, and the unique personality seen in Williams syndrome, allowing a clinical distinction. Prenatal diagnosis by FISH is also available.

Differential Diagnosis

Williams syndrome should be distinguished from other syndromes that feature short stature, congenital heart disease, and developmental delay. In one study of 65 patients with a previous diagnosis of Williams syndrome but negative FISH testing, other syndromes were diagnosed in 15% of the cases (Morris et al., 1998). Overlapping clinical features in this group of 65 children were developmental delay (92%), attention deficit disorder (50%), short stature (30%), and congenital heart disease (25%). The correct diagnoses included isolated supravalvar aortic stenosis associated with *ELN* mutation, velo-cardio-facial syndrome associated with microdeletion of chromosome 22, Noonan syndrome, FG syndrome, Kabuki syndrome, fetal alcohol syndrome, and the fragile X syndrome confirmed by DNA studies. The clinical diagnosis of Williams syndrome must be confirmed by FISH testing for 7q11.23 microdeletion to avoid misdiagnosis, especially in young children. A negative FISH study should prompt a search for other diagnoses.

The differential diagnosis of Williams syndrome should include Noonan syndrome (see Chapter 15), which is characterized by short stature, broad or webbed neck, chest deformity, congenital heart disease (most commonly pulmonary stenosis), and dysmorphic facial features. In infancy, the nose of Williams syndrome and Noonan syndrome is similar, but the philtrum is usually deeply grooved in Noonan syndrome with defined peaks of the upper vermilion border, whereas the philtrum in Williams syndrome may appear thick, with loss of the cupid's bow of the upper lip. In infancy, Noonan syndrome and Williams syndrome may also share peripheral pulmonic stenoses and hernias, contributing to diagnostic confusion. The facial gestalt, pattern of other cardiovascular lesions, and the FISH test will distinguish the two. Smith-Magenis syndrome, a condition associated with a microdeletion of 17p, is also associated with short stature, congenital heart disease, hoarse voice, hearing loss, iris dysplasia, scoliosis, behavior problems, and dysmorphic facial features (see Chapter 22). The dysmorphic facies of Smith-Magenis syndrome are distinguishable from Williams syndrome by the presence of a broad square face with heavy brows, deep-set eyes, broad short nose, and thickened philtrum. Smith-Magenis syndrome has a very different cognitive profile with significant weakness in expressive language, and FISH for the Smith-Magenis syndrome 17p deletion will confirm that diagnosis. Another microdeletion syndrome that is in the differential diagnosis is the more common condition, velo-cardio-facial syndrome (see Chapter 29). Velo-cardio-facial syndrome is associated with relative short stature, cleft palate, congenital heart disease (most commonly conotruncal defects), learning disability, hearing loss, velopharyngeal insufficiency, and dysmorphic facial features. The facial features of velo-cardio-facial syndrome include a long narrow face, high nasal root, long nose with bulbous tip and small nares, supraorbital fullness, and small mandible. The facial gestalt is quite different from Williams syndrome, especially after age 2 years, and the pattern of congenital heart disease also distinguishes the

conditions. FISH for deletion 22q will confirm the diagnosis in the majority of patients with velo-cardio-facial syndrome.

Other genetic syndromes in the differential diagnosis of Williams syndrome include Kabuki syndrome, FG syndrome, Coffin-Lowry syndrome, and fragile X syndrome. Kabuki syndrome has developmental delay, short stature, congenital heart disease (most commonly coarctation of the aorta), and dysmorphic facial features. Although Kabuki syndrome shares midfacial flattening, micrognathia, and prominent earlobes with Williams syndrome, the appearance of the eyes is quite different, with long palpebral fissures and everted lateral one-third of the lower lid in Kabuki syndrome. FG syndrome, an X-linked mental retardation syndrome, shares hypotonia, constipation, overfriendliness, and attention deficit disorder with Williams syndrome but may be distinguished by the facial features that include high forehead and hypertelorism. Coffin-Lowry syndrome, an X-linked mental retardation syndrome, has dysmorphic facies that include full lips and connective tissue problems including scoliosis but does not have other Williams syndrome features such as cardiovascular disease. Fragile X syndrome (see Chapter 10) has developmental delay and hypotonia but typically has more severe mental retardation (in males) than Williams syndrome and features a shy personality when compared to Williams syndrome. DNA testing for fragile X syndrome will make that diagnosis.

One teratogenic syndrome in the differential diagnosis is fetal alcohol syndrome, characterized by short stature, developmental delay, congenital heart disease (most commonly septal defects), attention deficit disorder, and dysmorphic facial features (short palpebral fissures, midfacial flattening, thin upper lip, long, smooth philtrum, and small jaw) (see Chapter 9). Although young children with fetal alcohol syndrome often demonstrate overfriendliness and attention deficit/hyperactivity disorder, fetal alcohol syndrome may be distinguished from Williams syndrome by the different appearance of the lower face and the different pattern of heart defect.

MANIFESTATIONS AND MANAGEMENT

Growth and Feeding

Short stature relative to the family background is common in Williams syndrome, and the rate of linear growth is 75% of normal (Jones and Smith, 1975). Studies of growth employing both longitudinal and cross-sectional data have shown that the mean final height is below the 3rd centile (Morris et al., 1988, Pankau et al., 1992). The growth pattern in Williams syndrome is characterized by prenatal growth deficiency in 25–70%, and poor linear growth and weight gain in the first 2–4 years of life. Statural growth then improves in childhood, although 70% remain below the 3rd centile for midparental height. Bone age studies are normal, and head circumference is typically commensurate with height. Puberty commonly occurs early in Williams syndrome and is associated with a briefer growth spurt than normal (Pankau et al., 1992). Growth curves for Williams syndrome are available (Morris et al., 1988; Saul et al., 1998; Pankau et al., 1992).

The poor weight gain and linear growth of the young child with Williams syndrome is likely due to the severe difficulties with feeding. It is important to note that fall-off in growth should prompt investigation, because both hypothyroidism and growth hormone deficiency have been reported, although the incidence of these complications is unknown. Diabetes mellitus has been reported in 15% of adults.

Failure to thrive (80%), feeding problems (70%), and prolonged colic (70%) are commonly observed in infants with Williams syndrome (Morris et al., 1988), and gastrointestinal complications in this age group include gastroesophageal reflux, constipation, and rectal prolapse. In the young child,

sensory aversion to textures adversely affects the transition to solid foods. Abnormal posture of jaw and neck (secondary to hypotonia and ligamentous laxity) provokes gagging, and dental malocclusion and persistent tongue thrust compromise efficient chewing and swallowing.

The feeding problems do improve with medical treatment of the gastroesophageal reflux and the hypercalcemia, combined with oral/motor and feeding therapy. The hypercalcemia and hypercalciuria often improve over time, but may recur.

Evaluation

- Growth measurements should be plotted on Williams syndrome growth charts, and any deviation downward across centiles should be investigated, including thyroid function testing, followed by growth hormone testing, if indicated.
- Oral motor function and feeding should be assessed in infants.
- A complete nutritional and feeding assessment should be conducted in the infant with failure to thrive.
- Initial laboratory evaluation should include thyroid function tests, serum calcium, and a random spot urine for calcium- to-creatinine ratio.
- Infants with Williams syndrome who demonstrate failure to thrive deserve consultation with a nutritionist to assess dietary calcium intake, including taking into account the calcium content of the local water supply, which may be significant in some areas.

Treatment

- Small, frequent feedings of high caloric density are recommended for infants.
- Feeding and oral motor therapy should be instituted.
- Pureed foods will often be required for a longer period of time in the child with Williams syndrome, because there are increased problems with gagging.

Development and Behavior

Delayed development is present in most children with Williams syndrome, including delays in early speech and motor milestones. There is a wide range of intellectual ability, with full-scale IQs ranging from severe mental retardation to low average intelligence. Most individuals have mild mental retardation. Full-scale IQ scores are misleading, however, because individuals with Williams syndrome have a unique cognitive profile. They usually have higher scores on verbal subtests, contrasted with low scores on visuospatial construction subtests. The Williams syndrome cognitive profile is characterized by relative strengths in auditory rote memory and language and extreme weakness in visuospatial constructive cognition (Frangiskakis et al., 1996, Mervis et al., 1999). Despite mild mental retardation, 48% score in the normal range on vocabulary tests and 65% score in the normal range on digit recall tests (Mervis et al., 1999). At least 95% of individuals with Williams syndrome have difficulty with visual motor integration.

Fine motor tasks adversely affected by this disability include handwriting, buttoning, drawing, and pattern construction (e.g., duplicating a pattern of blocks). Scores on subtests that measure visuospatial construction are typically lower than one would expect for the overall level of cognitive ability. Gross motor skills are affected by abnormality of depth perception, leading to difficulty in negotiating uneven surfaces and stairs. Because visual-motor skills are processed by the occipitoparietal visual pathway (dorsal stream), it is possible that a gene in the Williams syndrome region is involved in the development of this specific central neural pathway. In contrast, visual recognition skills, processed by the occipitotemporal pathway (ventral stream) are relatively good (Atkinson, 1997).

Individuals with Williams syndrome typically have higher achievement in reading than in other academic areas; the mean reading level is grade 5, with a wide range from grade 1 to college observed. Mathematics poses a greater problem; most master simple addition and some learn to use a calculator. Handwriting is difficult at all ages. Visual motor skills, including drawing ability, do improve over time with therapy and practice. Adults with Williams syndrome typically live with their parents or in group homes and work in sheltered environments (Davies et al. 1997). However, with recent improvements in vocational training with job coaches and assistance with daily living skills, more adults with Williams syndrome are achieving more independence within the community.

The behavioral phenotype is characterized by attention deficit disorder, overfriendliness (especially toward adults), and generalized anxiety. Attention deficit disorder, with or without hyperactivity, is present in 73% (Greer et al. 1997), and overfriendliness to strangers is observed in 97% (Sarimski 1997). Compared with other children with mental retardation, Einfeld et al., (1997) found an increased prevalence of behavioral problems including anxiety, attention problems, and preoccupations. Although adaptive behavior is commensurate with overall intellectual ability in children with Williams syndrome, there is a characteristic pattern of strength in interpersonal skills with weakness in daily living skills (Morris and Mervis, 1999).

Evaluation

- As part of the comprehensive history, the clinician should ascertain and record developmental milestones and school performance and determine whether symptoms of attention problems and/or anxiety are present.

- A multidisciplinary approach including speech, physical, and occupational therapy is recommended to assess the developmental disabilities and to plan appropriate interventions.

- Psychological and educational assessment is important in the older child and especially in the adolescent. The School Age Differential Ability Scales (Elliott, 1990) have the advantage of clearly showing the cognitive strengths and weaknesses. The Kaufman Brief Intelligence Test (Kaufman and Kaufman 1990), which does not include a visuospatial construction component, is useful in indicating the potential intellectual ability (Morris and Mervis, 1999).

- In the evaluation of behavior problems, adaptive behavior scales and attention deficit disorder scales are often used. Results from these tests are helpful in planning behavioral or medical interventions.
- Adults require vocational testing.
- Referral to a psychiatrist experienced in treatment of individuals with mental retardation may be helpful in the evaluation of attention problems or anxiety.

Treatment

- The abnormality of visual-motor integration requires intensive occupational therapy that includes sensory integration techniques.
- Children should be taught to use their verbal and auditory strengths to remember and process spatial information.
- Handwriting should be separated from other cognitive tasks, so as not to impede academic progress in other areas.
- Speech therapy can assist with the pragmatics of language and staying on topic.
- Attention deficit disorder may be treated with methylphenidate (Power et al., 1997).
- Anxiety often requires medical treatment, and, in addition to psychotropic medication, adolescents and adults respond particularly well to a program of regular counseling (personal observation).

Neurologic

Hypotonia is a common finding (80%), and peripheral hypertonia (50%) with increased deep tendon reflexes (especially in the lower extremities) is observed in children and adults. Neuroimaging studies have shown reduced cerebral volume but preservation of cerebellar size compared to controls (Jernigan et al., 1993) and rare cases of Chiari I malformation (Kaplan et al., 1989; Wang et al., 1992). Cerebrovascular accidents associated with multiple intracranial arterial stenoses have also been reported (Ardinger et al., 1994; Wollack et al., 1996).

Evaluation

- The baseline physical examination should include a complete and careful neurologic examination including assessment of muscle tone and strength and documentation of neurologic abnormalities.
- Symptoms of headache, dysphagia, dizziness, or weakness should prompt the clinician to obtain magnetic resonance imaging of the cranium to evaluate for Chiari I malformation.
- Symptoms of stroke will require standard investigation with Magnetic Resonance Angiography (MRA) or conventional angiography.

Treatment

- Treatment of neurologic problems does not differ from that in the general population.

Endocrine

Idiopathic hypercalcemia of infancy has been documented in 15% of individuals with Williams syndrome and, when present, most commonly occurs in the first 18 months of life. However, many affected infants have historical symptoms that could have been related to hypercalcemia (e.g., vomiting, anorexia, constipation, and irritability), but unfortunately serum calcium determinations were not performed. It is important to note that the disturbance of calcium metabolism is not limited to infancy. Adults with symptomatic hypercalcemia have been reported (Morris et al., 1990), and hypercalciuria occurs in 30% of individuals with Williams syndrome. Despite numerous studies of calcium metabolism, the etiology of these abnormalities remains unknown (Kruse et al., 1992). It should be noted that hypercalcemia, although more common in infants, may occur at any age.

Evaluation

- Serum calcium (either ionized or total) should be measured 2–3 hours after feeding, and repeat measurements should be performed at the same time of day.
- If the individual is normocalcemic, blood calcium should be checked every 2–4 years throughout life.
- A random spot urine for calcium-to-creatinine ratio should be checked at the time of diagnosis and every 2 years thereafter if it is normal. Hypercalciuria on a random spot urine is diagnosed if the calcium-to-creatinine ratio is greater than 0.86 in infants less than age 7 months, 0.6 from 7 to 18 months, 0.42 from 19 months to 6 years, and 0.22 from 6 years to adult (Sargent et al., 1993).
- If hypercalciuria is found on a random sample, then a repeat spot urine should be checked for the calcium-to-creatinine ratio on a morning and evening sample, and, ideally, a 24-hour urine for calcium-to-creatinine ratio should be obtained.
- If there is persistent hypercalciuria, serum calcium measurements should be repeated and a renal ultrasound obtained to evaluate for nephrocalcinosis.
- Referral to a nephrologist for management should be considered when hypercalcemia does not respond to dietary restriction, when nephrocalcinosis is present, or when hypercalciuria is persistent.

Treatment

- In infants with hypercalcemia or hypercalciuria, if dietary calcium is greater than the recommended daily allowance, it should be decreased appropriately.
- If hypercalcemia or hypercalciuria persists with a normal calcium intake, then dietary calcium should be reduced in conjunction with a nutritionist. Low-calcium formulas are available, and vitamin D supplements are not recommended. While the patient is on a low-calcium diet, careful monitoring of serum calcium levels is important, because iatrogenic rickets has been reported in children with Williams syndrome (Martin et al., 1984). Thus it is important to counsel parents not to eliminate calcium-containing foods from the diet without close medical supervision.
- In infants with borderline high serum calcium values who also have hypercalcemic symptoms and failure to thrive, careful reduction of the calcium intake may result in symptomatic improvement; again, serum calcium levels must be carefully monitored (personal experience).
- It is important to note that manipulation of dietary calcium alone will not solve the feeding problems in Williams syndrome. Feeding therapy and treatment of gastroesophageal reflux must be offered at the same time for significant clinical improvement to occur.
- Dietary restriction of calcium, while under careful medical and nutritional observation, is sufficient in most cases, but refractory cases of hypercalcemia may be treated with oral steroids.

Cardiovascular

The cardiovascular effect of the *ELN* deletion is the most significant cause of morbidity and mortality in Williams syndrome. The elastin arteriopathy is generalized, and thus any artery may be narrowed. The most commonly detected abnormality is supravalvar aortic stenosis, with a prevalence of 75% in most reported series (Morris et al., 1988). However, the detection of supravalvar aortic stenosis depends on the sensitivity of the examination method; two-dimensional echocardiography with Doppler flow analysis is preferred (Ensing et al., 1989). Peripheral pulmonic stenosis is more often observed in infants (50%), because it typically improves over time (Wren et al., 1990). However, in angiography series, peripheral pulmonic stenosis is found in 75% (Kececioglu et al., 1993). In contrast to the pulmonary circulation, arterial stenoses in the systemic circulation may worsen over time (Ino, 1988); thus lifelong monitoring of the cardiovascular system is important. The overall prevalence of any cardiovascular abnormality is 80%, including the less frequently reported lesions such as discrete supravalvar pulmonic stenosis (25%), renal artery stenosis (40%), ventricular septal defect (10%), and other peripheral arterial stenoses (20%). Coronary artery stenosis has been documented in some cases of sudden death in Williams syndrome (Bird et al., 1996), and renal artery stenosis has been associated with hypertension (Deal et al., 1992). Cerebrovascular accident associated with arteriopathy of the neurovasculature has rarely been reported (Ardinger et al., 1994; Wollack et al., 1996). In adults, aortic insufficiency (20%) and mitral valve prolapse (15%) may occur (Kececioglu et al., 1993).

Supravalvar aortic stenosis typically presents with a systolic murmur heard best in the aortic area, radiating to the carotids, and often accompanied by a thrill in the suprasternal notch. Because of the Coanda effect, the blood pressure in the right arm is often higher than that measured in the left (French and Guntheroth, 1970). Supravalvar aortic stenosis occurs most commonly as an hourglass stenosis above the aortic valve but may also occur as a more diffuse long segment aortic hypoplasia. It should be noted that the term "hypoplasia" traditionally refers to the size of the lumen and thus may be misleading, because the aortic wall is actually thickened. The aortic stenosis causes increased resistance to blood flow, resulting in elevated left heart pressures and cardiac hypertrophy. In severe cases, cardiac failure and death will result if the lesion is untreated. There is a high degree of variability among affected individuals, with supravalvar aortic pressure gradients ranging from 0 to 110 mmHg. Thirty percent of individuals will ultimately require surgical correction (Kececioglu et al., 1993).

Hypertension is commonly observed (50%) in Williams syndrome, and the risk for its development increases with age. In a study of 95 patients aged 2–43 years, Kececioglu and colleagues (1993) found that both systolic and diastolic blood pressures were elevated in 47%, systolic elevated in 25%, and diastolic elevated in 9%.

Evaluation

- A baseline cardiology evaluation by a cardiologist is recommended at the time of diagnosis and should include measurement of the blood pressure in all four limbs and two-dimensional echocardiography with Doppler flow studies.

- If no cardiac anomaly is detected in the young child at initial evaluation, then yearly clinical cardiology evaluations should be performed until age 5 years.

- In older children and adults without previous evidence of significant cardiovascular disease, periodic monitoring by a cardiologist is warranted for potential late-onset complications.

- On a yearly basis, the physician should check and record blood pressure measurements from both arms, auscultatory findings of murmurs and bruits, and peripheral pulse assessments.

- Cardiovascular status should be reviewed before any surgery, and inpatient surgical settings are preferred over outpatient facilities.
- In children with Williams syndrome, pediatric anesthesia consultation should be considered for all surgical procedures.

Treatment

- The need for patch aortoplasty will be determined by the severity of the stenosis and the pressure gradient.
- Transcatheter balloon dilatation is used to treat some arterial stenoses, especially in the pulmonary arteries.
- Surgical treatment of supravalvar aortic stenosis has a perioperative mortality of 3–7% (Kececioglu et al., 1993; van Son et al., 1994). In one series, survival was 92% at 10 years and 88% at 20 years (van Son et al., 1994). In a series of cardiology patients, the actuarial curve was stable at 90% from ages 10 to 40 years (Kececioglu et al., 1993). Sudden death has been reported in Williams syndrome (Bird et al., 1996), most often secondary to coronary artery stenosis unrelated to the severity of supravalvar aortic stenosis. At particularly high risk are those individuals with severe bilateral outflow tract obstruction and biventricular hypertrophy, who have decreased myocardial perfusion during periods of hemodynamic stress. This condition poses a risk of myocardial compromise during induction of anesthesia.
- Hypertension is usually treated medically, unless renal arterioplasty is indicated. Beta-blockers are usually successful in the treatment of hypertension.

Gastrointestinal

Infants with Williams syndrome require treatment for feeding problems, gastroesophageal reflux, and constipation, as detailed in the **Growth and Feeding** section. In older children and adults, chronic constipation continues to be a problem in 40%, and diverticulosis is common (Morris et al., 1990). Chronic abdominal pain may be debilitating for adolescents or adults with a myriad of etiologies including hiatal hernia, gastroesophageal reflux, peptic ulcer disease, cholelithiasis, diverticulitis, ischemic bowel disease, constipation, and somatization of anxiety.

The pathogenesis of many of the gastrointestinal complaints and complications such as diverticulosis and rectal prolapse is probably an abnormality of elastic fibers. Hypercalcemia may also contribute to the symptomatology by causing anorexia, abdominal pain, and constipation. (See **Endocrine** section for evaluation and management of hypercalcemia.)

Constipation is a lifelong problem requiring ongoing management. Gastroesophageal reflux may occur at any age and, if untreated, will lead to dysphagia, esophagitis, and esophageal stricture.

Evaluation

- Evaluation should include oral motor, nutritional, and gastrointestinal assessment in infancy.
- Calcium levels should be monitored in serum and urine.
- Radiographic analysis of the upper and lower gastrointestinal tract may be warranted, especially if abdominal pain is noted. Radiographic evaluation, pH studies, or gastroenterology referral is appropriate if symptoms suggest gastroesophageal reflux
- If other causes have been eliminated, angiography may be needed to determine whether mesenteric arterial stenosis is present as the etiology of the pain.

Treatment

- Treatment of abdominal pain will depend on its cause.

- The dietary regimen will be dictated by the results of investigations for gastroesophageal reflux and hypercalcemia.
- Gastroesophageal reflux may be treated with positioning, small-volume feedings, and antireflux medication. If gastroesophageal reflux does not respond to medical treatment, fundoplication will be required.
- Constipation should be aggressively managed at all ages.
- Rectal prolapse may require surgical treatment, as in the general population.
- Individuals with diverticulosis are at increased risk for diverticulitis.

Ophthalmologic

Ophthalmologic abnormalities and deficits in visual-motor integration adversely affect function in individuals with Williams syndrome (Morris et al., 1988). Strabismus, usually esotropia, typically affects 50% of infants. However, reduced stereoacuity has been documented in children who do not have measurable strabismus, suggesting that abnormalities of binocular vision are even more prevalent and have a central nervous system origin (Sadler et al., 1996). The outcome of strabismus surgery in the Williams syndrome population is similar to that in the general population with infantile esotropia (Kapp et al., 1995).

The most common refractive error is mild to moderate hyperopia, present in 50%. Tortuosity of retinal vessels is reported in 20%. Hypoplasia and coarse architecture of the iris stroma (70%) result in a lacy/stellate iris pattern clinically visible in blue irides and visible on slit lamp examination in dark irides (Winter et al., 1996).

Evaluation

- Every individual with Williams syndrome should have a complete ophthalmologic evaluation at the time of diagnosis.

Treatment

- Aggressive treatment of strabismus is warranted to prevent amblyopia and may include corrective lenses, patching, or, in 30% of cases, medial rectus muscle recession.
- Hyperopia requires corrective lenses.

Ears and Hearing

Chronic otitis media is reported in 50% of individuals with Williams syndrome and is treated surgically in 25% (Morris et al., 1988; Klein et al., 1990). It is likely that hypotonia combined with elastin-mediated connective tissue abnormalities of the pharynx and eustachian tube are causal. Hypersensitivity to sound occurs in 85–95% and is not related either to a history of chronic otitis media or to attention deficit disorder (Van Borsel et al., 1997). Responses to sound, especially to loud or sudden noises, range from crying and/or covering ears with hands in children to complaints by adults of distress and a "nervous feeling." With aging, individuals with Williams syndrome have improved noise tolerance. The etiology of the hypersensitivity is unknown, although possibilities include a conduction disturbance resulting from an abnormality of connective tissue, an abnormality of central nervous system processing of auditory input, or failure of central nervous system habituation to auditory stimuli.

The voice of the individual with Williams syndrome is typically low-pitched, deep, or hoarse. Because elastin is an important component of the lamina propria of the vocal folds (Hammond et al., 1998), the presumption is that the voice quality is likely related to the elastin abnormality.

Evaluation

- Audiological evaluation is recommended in children with Williams syndrome.

Treatment

- As in the general pediatric population, chronic otitis media tends to improve with age, but aggressive treatment with antibiotics and tympanotomy tubes may be helpful (25%).

- The family should be counseled to avoid situations with loud noises when possible and to use earplugs when necessary.
- Older children and adults benefit from warnings before noise occurs, explanations regarding the origin of the sound, and having some control over the sound (such as turning on a noisy appliance).

Dermatologic

In addition to elastin arteriopathy, other connective tissues are affected in Williams syndrome. The skin is typically soft and loose in both infants and adults. The skin is not hyperextensible, however, and wound healing is normal. Similar to cutis laxa, adults with Williams syndrome may appear older than their age. Hernias are common, ranging from 5% for umbilical hernias to 40% for inguinal hernias. An extra sacral crease is often seen in infants with Williams syndrome. Because of the connective tissue abnormality, hernias may occur at any age, and occasional recurrences are noted.

Evaluation

- Physical examination for hernia should be performed.

Treatment

- Surgical repair of inguinal hernia may be necessary, as in the general population.

Genitourinary

The incidence of renal anomalies is increased in Williams syndrome, and detection of an abnormality is dependent on the type of investigation. In series of renal ultrasound studies, the incidence of structural renal anomalies (small, asymmetric, dystrophic, duplicated or absent kidney) is 20% (Ingelfinger and Newburger, 1991; Pober

et al., 1993; Pankau et al., 1996). Nephrocalcinosis is found in less than 5%. When renal angiography is performed, several studies have found a 50% incidence of renal artery stenosis. Bladder diverticulae are common; 60% in children (Babbitt et al., 1979) and 75% in adults (Morris et al., 1988). They are best demonstrated by voiding cystourethrogram.

Urinary frequency is nearly universal in children with Williams syndrome and may be the result of decreased bladder capacity, impulsivity, hypercalciuria resulting in increased urine production, or a combination of these factors. Enuresis is reported in 50% of children, and recurrent urinary tract infections are seen in 30% of adults. The risk for recurrent urinary tract infections and bladder diverticulae increases with age.

Evaluation

- Because the prevalence of renal structural anomalies is high, a baseline renal ultrasound is recommended at the time of diagnosis.
- Other investigations will depend on signs and symptoms.
- Performance of renal artery angiography should be considered at the time of cardiac catheterization or as part of the investigation of the significantly hypertensive patient.
- A voiding cystourethrogram may be indicated in cases of chronic urinary tract infections, persistence of enuresis beyond age 10 years, or chronic problems with micturition.
- Tests of renal function and urinalysis should be periodically checked (every 2 years).
- Structural abnormalities require referral to an urologist.

Treatment

- In patients with persistent hypercalciuria or nephrocalcinosis, referral to a nephrologist is recommended for ongoing management (see also **Endocrine** section).

- Urinary tract infections respond to standard treatment modalities.

Musculoskeletal

Hyperextensible joints are commonly observed (90%) in infants and young children with Williams syndrome, and they contribute to joint instability and delayed walking. As a result, abnormal compensatory postures to achieve stability may be noted. Many patients complain of leg pain, especially at night after a day of high physical activity. Gradually, tightening of the Achilles tendons and hamstrings occurs, resulting in a stiff and awkward gait by adolescence. Radioulnar synostosis (10%) results in limitation of supination of the forearm and does not improve with either therapy or surgery. Joint contractures, especially of the lower extremities, have been reported in 50% of children with Williams syndrome (Morris et al., 1988, Kaplan et al., 1989) and in 90% of adults (Morris et al., 1990). Scoliosis (20%), kyphosis (20%), and lordosis (40%) are common complications. The majority of the musculoskeletal abnormalities are presumably secondary to abnormal connective tissue, the result of the *ELN* deletion.

Evaluation

- A range of motion study should be performed on a yearly basis.
- Screening for spine abnormalities should be done annually.
- Orthopedic referral is required for evaluation and treatment of scoliosis.

Treatment

- A program of physical therapy to promote normal posture and normal range of motion is recommended. With physical therapy and a program of regular exercise, function, mobility, and posture improve.

- If pes planus is present, a medial wedge or insole may be of benefit, and high-top shoes may provide ankle stability in young children.
- Nocturnal leg pains may be ameliorated with physical therapy, anti-inflammatory agents, and use of elastic bandages at the knees and ankles during periods of high physical activity
- Regular low-impact exercise is important.
- The expertise of a physical therapist is helpful both in evaluation and in designing appropriate therapeutic programs.
- Exercise programs that include calming/relaxation techniques, such as yoga, have the added benefit of addressing the anxiety that is part of the Williams syndrome phenotype (personal observation).

Dental

Dental abnormalities reported in Williams syndrome include malformed teeth (10% in primary dentition and 40% in permanent dentition), missing teeth, usually incisors (10%), localized areas of enamel hypoplasia (15%), small teeth (95%), and increased space between the teeth (50%) (Hertzberg et al., 1994). Malocclusion (85%) is the most significant clinical complication, with deep bite, open bite, anterior crossbite, and posterior crossbite all being reported. The occlusal abnormalities are likely the combined result of several factors, including hypotonia, tongue thrust, and connective tissue abnormality. Orthodontic treatment has been successful in improving occlusion.

Evaluation

- In addition to early dental evaluation, orthodontic referral at age 8 years is recommended.

Treatment

- In addition to routine dental care, orthodontic treatment has improved dental relationships, the mechanics of chewing, and the appearance in many individuals with Williams syndrome.

- Oral motor and speech therapy are of value in improving chewing and swallowing.
- Because there is a propensity to enamel hypoplasia, fluoride sealants may be helpful.

RESOURCES

National Organizations

Williams Syndrome Association
P.O. Box 297
Clawson, MI 48017-0297
Phone: (248) 541-3630
Fax: (248) 541-3631
E-mail-*WSAoffice@aol.com*
World Wide Web:
http://www.williams-syndrome.org

Other Internet Resources

Williams Syndrome Foundation
World Wide Web: http://www.wsf.org

ACKNOWLEDGMENTS

The author's research is supported by Grant NS-35102 from the National Institute of Neurological Disorders and Stroke. I am thankful to the Williams Syndrome Association and its Medical Advisory Board, the Williams Syndrome Foundation, and the individuals with Williams syndrome and their families who have given generously of their time in support of research. I am grateful for the expert collaboration of researchers Dr. Carolyn Mervis, Dr. Mark Keating, and Dr. A. Dean Stock, for the assistance of research associate Stephanie Nelson and Steven LoMastro, and for critical review of the manuscript by Dr. Jack Lazerson.

REFERENCES

American Academy of Pediatrics Committee on Genetics (2000) Healthcare supervision for children with Williams syndrome. *Pediatrics.* In press.

Ardinger RH, Goertz KK, Mattioli LF (1994) Cerebrovascular stenosis with cerebral infarction in a child with Williams syndrome. *Am J Med Genet* 51:200–202.

Atkinson J, King J, Braddick O, Nokes L, Anker S, Braddick F (1997) A specific deficit of dorsal function in Williams' syndrome. *Neurol Rep* 8:1919–1922.

Babbitt DP, Dobbs J, Boedecker RA (1979) Multiple bladder diverticula in Williams "elfin-facies" syndrome. *Pediatr Radiol* 8:29–31.

Beuren AJ (1972) Supravalvular aortic stenosis: A complex syndrome with and without mental retardation. *Birth Defects* 8:45–56.

Beuren AJ, Apitz J, Harmjanz D (1962) Supravalvular aortic stenosis in association with mental retardation and a certain facial appearance. *Circulation* 27:1235–1240.

Bird LM, Billman GF, Lacro RV, Spicer RL, Jariwala LK, Hoyme HE, Zamora-Salinas R, Morris CA, Viskochil D, Frikke MJ, Jones MC (1996) Sudden death in Williams syndrome: Report of ten cases. *J Pediatr* 129:926–931.

Burn J (1986) Williams syndrome. *J Med Genet* 23:389–395.

Davies M, Howlin P, Udwin O (1997) Independence and adaptive behavior in adults with Williams syndrome. *Am J Med Genet* 70:188–195.

Deal JE, Snell MF, Marratt TM, Dillon MJ (1992) Renovascular disease in childhood. *J Pediatr* 131:378–384.

Dutly F, Schinzel A (1996) Unequal interchromosomal rearrangements may result in elastin gene deletions causing the Williams-Beuren syndrome. *Hum Mol Genet* 5: 1893–1898.

Einfeld SL, Tonge BJ, Florio T (1997) Behavioral and emotional disturbance in individuals with Williams syndrome. *Am J Ment Retard* 102:45–53.

Elliott CD (1990) *Differential Ability Scales.* San Diego, CA: Harcourt, Brace, Jovanovich.

Ensing GJ, Schmidt MA, Hagler DJ, Michels VV, Carter GA, Feldt RH (1989) Spectrum of findings in a family with nonsyndromic autosomal dominant supravalvular aortic stenosis: A Doppler echocardiographic study. *J Am Coll Cardiol* 13:413–419.

Ewart AK, Morris CA, Atkinson D, Jin W, Sternes K, Spallone P, Stock AD, Leppert M, Keating MT (1993) Hemizygosity at the elastin locus in a developmental disorder, Williams Syndrome. *Nat Genet* 5:11–16.

Fanconi G, Giradet P, Schlesinger B, Butler N, Blade JS (1952) Chronische Hypercalcaemie kombiniert mit Osteosklerose, Hyperazotaemie, Minderwuchs, und kongenitalen Missbildungen. *Helv Paediatr Acta* 7:314–334.

Frangiskakis JM, Ewart AK, Morris CA, Mervis CB, Bertrand J, Robinson BF, Klein BP, Ensing GJ, Everett LA, Green ED, Pröschel C, Gutow NJ, Noble M, Atkinson DL, Oldelberg SJ, Keating MT (1996) LIM-kinase 1 hemizygosity implicated in impaired visuospatial constructive cognition. *Cell* 86:59–69.

French JW, Guntheroth WG (1970) An explanation of asymmetric upper extremity blood pressures in supravalvular aortic stenosis. *Circulation* 42:31–36.

Garcia RE, Friedman WF, Kaback MM, Rowe RD (1964) Idiopathic hypercalcemia and supravalvular aortic stenosis. *N Engl J Med* 271:117–120.

Greer MK, Brown FR, Pai GS, Choudry SH, Klein AJ (1997) Cognitive, adaptive, and behavioral characteristics of Williams syndrome. *Am J Med Genet* 4:521–525.

Hammond TH, Gray SD, Butler J, Zhou R, Hammond E (1998) Age- and gender-related elastin distribution changes in human vocal folds. *Otolaryngol Head Neck Surg* 119:314–322.

Hertzberg J, Nakisbendi L, Neddleman HL, Pober B (1994) Williams syndrome—oral presentation of 45 cases. *Pediatr Dent* 16:262–267.

Ingelfinger JR, Newburger JW (1991) Spectrum of renal anomalies in patients with Williams syndrome. *J Pediatr* 119:771–773.

Ino T, Nishimoto K, Iwahara M, Akimoto K, Boku H, Daneko K, Tokita A, Yabuta K, Tanaka J (1988) Progressive vascular lesions in Williams-Beuren syndrome. *Pediatr Cardiol* 9:55–58.

Jernigan TL, Bellugi U, Sowell E, Doherty S, Hesselink JR (1993) Cerebral morphological distinctions between Williams and Down syndromes. *Arch Neurol* 50:186–191.

Jones KL, Smith DW (1975) The Williams elfin facies syndrome. *J Pediatr* 86:718–723.

Kaplan P, Kirschner M, Watters G, Costa T (1989) Contractures in patients with Williams syndrome. *Pediatrics* 84:895–899.

Kapp ME, von Noorden GK, Jenkins R (1995) Strabismus in the Williams syndrome. *Am J Ophthalmol* 119:355–360.

Kaufman AS, Kaufman JL (1990) *Kaufman Brief Intelligence Test*. Circle Pines, MN: American Guidance Services.

Kececioglu D, Kotthoff S, Vogt J (1993) Williams-Beuren syndrome: A 30-year follow-up of natural and postoperative course. *Eur Heart J* 14:1458–1464.

Klein AJ, Armstrong BL, Greer MK, Brown FR (1990) Hyperacusis and otitis media in individuals with Williams syndrome. *J Speech Hear Disord* 55:339–344.

Kruse K, Pankau R, Gosch A, Wohlfahrt K (1992) Calcium metabolism in Williams-Beuren syndrome. *J Pediatr* 121:902–907.

Li DY, Faury G, Taylor DG, Dais EC, Boyle WA, Mecham RP, Stenzel P, Boak B, Keating MT (1998) Novel arterial pathology in mice and humans hemizygous for elastin. *J Clin Invest* 102:1783–1787.

Li DY, Toland AE, Boak BB, Atkinson D, Ensing GJ, Morris CA, Keating MT (1997) Elastin point mutations cause an obstructive vascular disease, supravalvular aortic stenosis. *Hum Mol Genet* 6:1021–1028.

Lowery MC, Morris CA, Ewart A, Brothman L, Zhu XL, Leonard CO, Carey JC, Keating MT, Brothman AR (1995) Strong correlations of elastin deletions, detected by FISH, with Williams syndrome: Evaluation of 235 patients. *Am J Hum Genet* 57:49–53.

Mari A, Amati F, Mingarelli R, Giannotti A, Sebastio G, Colloridi V, Novelli G, Dallapiccola B (1995) Analysis of the elastin gene in 60 patients with clinical diagnosis of Williams syndrome. *Hum Genet* 96:444–448.

Martin NDT, Snodgrass GJAI, Cohen RD (1984) Idiopathic infantile hypercalcemia: A continuing enigma. *Arch Dis Child* 59:605–613.

Mervis CB, Morris CA, Bertrand J, Robinson BF (1999) Williams syndrome: Findings from an integrated program of research. In *Neurodevelopmental Disorders*; H. Tager-Flusberg, ed. Cambridge, MA: MIT Press.

Morris CA, Dilts C, Dempsey SA, Leonard CO, Blackburn B (1988) The natural history of Williams syndrome: Physical characteristics. *J Pediatr* 113:318–326.

Morris CA, Leonard CO, Dilts C, Demsey SA (1990) Adults with Williams syndrome. *Am J Med Genet Suppl* 6:102–107.

Morris CA, Lu X, Greenberg F (1998) Syndromes identified in patients with a previous diagnosis of Williams syndrome who do not have elastin deletion. *Proc. Greenwood Genet Cent* 17:116.

Morris CA, Mervis CB (1999) Williams syndrome. In *Handbook of Neurodevelopmental and Genetic Disorders in Children*, Goldstein S and Reynolds C, eds. New York: Guilford.

Morris CA, Thomas IT, Greenberg F (1993) Williams syndrome: Autosomal dominant inheritance. *Am J Med Genet* 47:478–481.

Nickerson E, Greenberg F, Keating MT, McCaskill C, Shaffer LG (1995) Deletions of the elastin gene at 7q11.23 occur in ~90% of patients with Williams syndrome. *Am J Hum Genet* 56:1156–1161.

O'Connor W, Davis J, Geissler R, Cottrill C, Noonan J, Todd E (1985) Supravalvular aortic stenosis: Clinical and pathologic observations in six patients. *Arch Pathol Lab Med* 109:179–185.

Pankau R, Partsch C-J, Gosch A, Oppermann HC, Wessel A (1992) Statural growth in Williams-Beuren syndrome. *Eur J Pediatr* 151:751–755.

Pankau R, Partsch C-J, Winter M, Gosch A, Wessel A (1996) Incidence and spectrum of renal abnormalities in Williams-Beuren syndrome. *Am J Med Genet* 63:301–304.

Pober BR, Lacro RV, Rice C, Mandell V, Teele RL (1993) Renal findings in 40 individuals with Williams syndrome. *Am J Med Genet* 46:271–274.

Power TJ, Blum NJ, Jones SM, Kaplan PE (1997) Response to methylphenidate in two children with Williams syndrome. *J Autism Dev Dis* 27:79–87.

Preus M (1984) The Williams syndrome: Objective definition and diagnosis. *Clin Genet* 25:422–428.

Sadler S, Olitsky SE, Reynolds JD (1996) Reduced stereoacuity in Williams syndrome. *Am J Med Genet* 66:287–288.

Sadler LS, Robinson LK, Verdaasdonk KR, Gingell R (1993) The Williams syndrome: Evidence for possible autosomal dominant inheritance. *Am J Med Genet* 47:468–470.

Sargent JD, Stukel TA, Kresel J, Klein RZ (1993) Normal values for random urinary calcium to creatinine ratios in infancy. *J Pediatr* 123:393–397.

Sarimski K (1997) Behavioral phenotypes and family stress in three mental retardation syndromes. *Eur Child Adolesc Psychiatry* 6:26–31.

Saul RA, Stevenson RE, Rogers RC, Skinner SA, Prouty LA, Flannery DB (1998) Growth references from conception to adulthood. *Proc Greenwood Genet Cent Suppl* 1:204–209.

Van Borsel J, Curfs LMG, Fryns JP (1997) Hyperacusis in Williams syndrome: A sample survey study. *Genet Couns* 8:121–126.

van Son JAM, Edwards WD, Danielson GK (1994) Pathology of coronary arteries, myocardium, and great arteries in supravalvular aortic stenosis. *J Thoracic Cardiovasc Surg* 108:21–28.

Wang PP, Hesselink JR, Jernigan TL, Doherty S, Bellugi U (1992) Specific neurobehavioral profile of Williams syndrome is associated with neocerebellar hemispheric preservation. *Neurology* 42:1999–2002.

Williams JCP, Barratt-Boyes BG, Lowe JB (1961) Supravalvular aortic stenosis. *Circulation* 24:1311–1318.

Winter M, Pankau R, Amm M, Gosch A, Wessel A (1996) The spectrum of ocular features in the Williams-Beuren syndrome. *Clin Genet* 49:28–31.

Wollack JB, Kaifer M, LaMonte MP, Rothman M (1996) Stroke in Williams syndrome. *Stroke* 27:143–146.

Wren C, Oslizlok P, Bull C (1990) Natural history of supravalvular aortic stenosis and pulmonary artery stenosis. *J Am Coll Cardiol* 15:1625–1630.

Wu Y-Q, Sutton V, Nickerson E, Lupski JR, Potocki L, Korenberg JR, Greenberg F, Tassabehji M, Shaffer LG (1998) Delineation of the common critical region in Williams syndrome and clinical correlation of growth, heart defects, ethnicity, and parental origin. *Am J Med Genet* 78:82–89.

INDEX